Basic Chemistry for Life Science Professionals

Introduction to Organic Compounds and Drug Molecules

Basic Chemistry for Life Science Students and Professionals

Introduction to Organic Compounds and Drug Molecules

By

Solomon Habtemariam

University of Greenwich, UK;
Pharmacognosy Research & Herbal Analysis Services UK
Email: s.habtemariam@herbalanalysis.co.uk

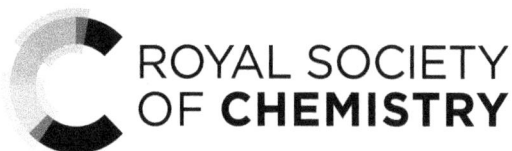

ROYAL SOCIETY
OF **CHEMISTRY**

Print ISBN: 978-1-83916-787-4
PDF ISBN: 978-1-83767-108-3
EPUB ISBN: 978-1-83916-808-6

A catalogue record for this book is available from the British Library

The Royal Society of Chemistry is a charity, registered in England and Wales, Number 207890, and a company incorporated in England by Royal Charter (Registered No. RC000524), registered office: Burlington House, Piccadilly, London W1J 0BA, UK, Telephone: +44 (0) 20 7437 8656.

Visit our website at books.rsc.org

Preface

This highly informative textbook is based on the author's decades of teaching experience at university, primarily modules/courses on basic chemistry for life sciences and pharmacology topics. University students and professionals in life science areas may include biology-related fields as well as health-allied subjects, including medical, nursing, dental, biomedical, pharmacological, and nutrition sciences. We also have students/professionals studying at the chemistry–biology interface, including subjects such as pharmaceutical sciences, pharmacy-associated disciplines, and forensic sciences. Often with a 'not so strong' chemistry background, such students and professionals usually rely on secondary-school chemistry textbooks for general knowledge on basic organic chemistry topics. These resources are, however, limited in scope, particularly as learning materials for university-level education. On the other hand, specialist subject textbooks in this field (organic chemistry, medicinal chemistry, *etc.*) are designed for higher-level chemistry studies, which are either too complex or are above the level required for life science students and professionals. This book is therefore designed to address this scenario – to provide readers in life science fields with sufficient basic chemistry knowledge on organic compounds with added focus on drug molecules.

The book is divided into four sections. The first part (Section I) addresses basic chemistry on the 'WHAT' of organic compounds and drug molecules. Starting from covalent bonding, the various classes of organic compounds and functional groups are presented along with some basic reactions. The interaction between atoms to form

Basic Chemistry for Life Science Students and Professionals: Introduction to Organic Compounds and Drug Molecules
By Solomon Habtemariam
© Solomon Habtemariam 2023
Published by the Royal Society of Chemistry, www.rsc.org

molecules and intermolecular interactions that give organic compounds their unique physical and chemical properties are discussed. Further structural diversity based on isomerism and significance in biology are discussed primarily by addressing the issue of efficacy and safety/toxicity of drugs. In Section II, organic biological molecules from low molecular weight monomers to macromolecules (proteins, carbohydrates, lipids, and nucleic acids) and their relevance to fundamental biological processes, and those compounds serving as drugs, are discussed. Section III addresses common units of measurements and physicochemical properties (including common reaction types) of organic compounds and drug molecules. Touching on the processes of pharmacodynamics and pharmacokinetics, the chemical basis of drug–target interactions is addressed in Section IV. The bulk of this section is dedicated to presenting the structural diversity and sources of drug molecules based on inspiration from natural products. The various classes of drugs from natural sources, how they are obtained through semi-synthesis and total synthesis, and also approaches of recombinant DNA technology in drug discovery are highlighted. All chapters are structured with specific learning outcomes, box summaries of key facts, a chapter summary, and exemplary problems and solutions.

Solomon Habtemariam

Acknowledgements

An academic author faces the challenges of not only preparing a manuscript in their specialist field, but also making their published work accessible to the intended audience at a reasonable price. In the latter case, I am delighted to associate myself (as a fellow member) with the Royal Society of Chemistry, a not-for-profit publisher, which made this textbook available at the indicated price tag. I extensively used scientific databases such as PubChem, ChemSpider, PubMed, and ScienceDirect to source chemical/pharmacological information on the organic compounds and drugs discussed in this text. Some images of plants and animals were sourced from Wikipedia, to which I am very grateful. I thank my students for being my inspiration to write this book, and my iconic friends in the field of organic/medicinal chemistry, Professor Giovanni Lentini (University of Bari) and Professor John Nicholson (Queen Mary University of London), for their encouragement. Although the idea of writing this book was conceived long ago, it was realised during the COVID-19 lockdown in 2021. I am grateful to my family for allowing me to have the time to work on the project.

Basic Chemistry for Life Science Students and Professionals: Introduction to Organic Compounds and Drug Molecules
By Solomon Habtemariam
© Solomon Habtemariam 2023
Published by the Royal Society of Chemistry, www.rsc.org

Author Biography

Dr Solomon Habtemariam received his BSc degree in Biology (minor – Chemistry) from the University of Addis Ababa, Ethiopia, and his master's degree (combined studies) in Pharmacology and Phytochemistry from the University of Strathclyde, Glasgow, UK. He stayed on at Strathclyde, carrying out drug discovery research, and obtained his PhD in Pharmaceutical Science. After several years in teaching and post-doctoral research at the Strathclyde Institute for Drug Research and University of Strathclyde, he joined the School of Science, University of Greenwich, in September 1998, since when he has been a leader of taught programmes and research on bioassays and natural products-based drug development. The various research projects that he has undertaken include the identification of novel compounds of mainly natural origin but also synthetic sources with potential, antimicrobial, anticancer, anti-inflammatory, antidiabetic, and anti-obesity properties, among others. As a Director of Herbal Analysis Services UK, which he established to serve as a global collaboration forum for research, Dr Habtemariam has published more than 250 scientific publications and filed over three families of patents. He is the author of a book entitled *The African and Arabian Moringa Species: Chemistry Bioactivity and Therapeutic Applications*. His most comprehensive self-authored books also include *Medicinal Foods as Potential Therapies for Type-2 Diabetes and Associated Diseases: The Chemical and Pharmacological Basis of Their Action*. Details of his research activities

Basic Chemistry for Life Science Students and Professionals: Introduction to Organic Compounds and Drug Molecules
By Solomon Habtemariam
© Solomon Habtemariam 2023
Published by the Royal Society of Chemistry, www.rsc.org

and publications are available *via* the website http://www.herbalanalysis.co.uk. With a distinguished pharmacological and analytical/medicinal chemistry background, Dr Habtemariam has decades of experience in teaching life science students (pharmaceutical, biological, forensic, biomedical, *etc.*) various topics including basic organic chemistry, instrumental/analytical methods, and pharmacology.

Contents

Basic Chemistry for Life Science Students and Professionals: Introduction to Organic Compounds and Drug Molecules
By Solomon Habtemariam
© Solomon Habtemariam 2023
Published by the Royal Society of Chemistry, www.rsc.org

2   Polarity of Bonds, Electronegativity, and Intermolecular Forces   33

3   Types of Organic Compounds, Nomenclature, and Basic Reactions: Alkanes and Cycloalkanes   51

4   Types of Organic Compounds, Nomenclature, and Basic Reactions: Alkenes, Cycloalkenes, and Other Unsaturated Hydrocarbons   65

5 Types of Organic Compounds, Nomenclature, and Basic Reactions: Functional Groups 92

6 Isomerism in Organic Compounds and Drug Molecules: Chemistry and Significance in Biology   149

SECTION II: ORGANIC MACROMOLECULES IN CELLULAR STRUCTURES, METABOLISM, AND AS DRUGS   195

7 Organic Macromolecules in Cellular Structures, Metabolism, and as Drugs: From Amino Acids to Proteins   197

8 Organic Macromolecules in Cellular Structures, Metabolism, and as Drugs: From Monosaccharides to Complex Carbohydrates 225

9 Organic Macromolecules in Cellular Structures, Metabolism, and as Drugs: From Fatty Acids to Complex Lipids and Fats 254

10 Organic Macromolecules in Cellular Structures, Metabolism, and as Drugs: From Nucleotides to Nucleic Acids 283

SECTION III: PHYSICOCHEMICAL PROPERTIES OF ORGANIC COMPOUNDS AND DRUG MOLECULES 315

11 Physicochemical Properties of Organic Compounds and Drug Molecules 317

SECTION IV: DRUG–TARGET INTERACTIONS AND COMMON SOURCES OF DRUGS AND THEIR STRUCTURAL CLASSES: INSPIRATION FROM NATURE, SYNTHESIS AND RECOMBINANT TECHNOLOGY 367

SECTION I
Basic Chemistry of Organic Compounds and Drug Molecules

1 Introduction to Organic Compounds and Covalent Bonding

Periodic Table of the Elements

Atomic number → 6 C
Average mass → 12.011

Group 1	Group 2	Group 3	Group 4	Group 5	Group 6	Group 7	Group 8	Group 9	Group 10	Group 11	Group 12	Group 13	Group 14	Group 15	Group 16	Group 17	Group 18
1 H 1.008																	2 He 4.003
3 Li 6.94	4 Be 9.012											5 B 10.81	6 C 12.011	7 N 14.007	8 O 15.999	9 F 18.998	10 Ne 20.180
11 Na 22.990	12 Mg 24.305											13 Al 26.982	14 Si 28.085	15 P 30.974	16 S 32.06	17 Cl 35.45	18 Ar 39.948
19 K 39.098	20 Ca 40.078	21 Sc 44.956	22 Ti 47.867	23 V 50.942	24 Cr 51.996	25 Mn 54.938	26 Fe 55.845	27 Co 58.933	28 Ni 58.693	29 Cu 63.546	30 Zn 65.38	31 Ga 69.723	32 Ge 72.630	33 As 74.922	34 Se 78.971	35 Br 79.904	36 Kr 83.798
37 Rb 85.468	38 Sr 87.62	39 Y 88.906	40 Zr 91.224	41 Nb 92.906	42 Mo 95.95	43 Tc [98]	44 Ru 101.07	45 Rh 102.906	46 Pd 106.42	47 Ag 107.868	48 Cd 112.414	49 In 114.818	50 Sn 118.710	51 Sb 121.760	52 Te 127.60	53 I 126.904	54 Xe 131.293
55 Cs 132.905	56 Ba 137.327	*	72 Hf 138.905	73 Ta 180.948	74 W 183.84	75 Re 186.207	76 Os 190.23	77 Ir 192.217	78 Pt 195.084	79 Au 196.967	80 Hg 200.592	81 Tl 204.38	82 Pb 207.2	83 Bi 208.980	84 Po [209]	85 At [210]	86 Rn [222]
87 Fr [223]	88 Ra [226]	**	104 Rf [267]	105 Db [268]	106 Sg [269]	107 Bh [270]	108 Hs [269]	109 Mt [278]	110 Ds [281]	111 Rg [280]	112 Cn [285]	113 Nh [286]	114 Fl [289]	115 Mc [289]	116 Lv [293]	117 Ts [294]	118 Og [294]

*	57 La 138.905	58 Ce 140.116	59 Pr 140.908	60 Nd 144.242	61 Pm [145]	62 Sm 150.36	63 Eu 151.964	64 Gd 157.25	65 Tb 158.925	66 Dy 162.500	67 Ho 164.930	68 Er 167.259	69 Tm 168.934	70 Yb 173.045	71 Lu 174.967	Lanthanides
**	89 Ac [227]	90 Th 232.038	91 Pa 231.036	92 U 238.029	93 Np [237]	94 Pu [244]	95 Am [243]	96 Cm [247]	97 Bk [247]	98 Cf [251]	99 Es [252]	100 Fm [257]	101 Md [258]	102 No [259]	103 Lr [262]	Actinides

Basic Chemistry for Life Science Students and Professionals: Introduction to Organic Compounds and Drug Molecules
By Solomon Habtemariam
© Solomon Habtemariam 2023
Published by the Royal Society of Chemistry, www.rsc.org

Learning Objectives

After completing this chapter, you are expected to be able to:

- Define organic compounds.
- Understand the difference between atoms, elements, and compounds.
- Explain how valence electrons are identified for a given atom.
- Be able to give examples of homonuclear and heteronuclear covalent bonding.
- Explain the difference between sp^3, sp^2, and sp hybridisations in carbon chemistry.
- Explain how single, double, and triple covalent bonds in a molecule are formed.

1.1 Organic Compounds *versus* Inorganic Compounds

One way of classifying chemistry as a subject is based on the nature of the compounds to be studied: 'organic compounds' for organic chemistry and 'inorganic compounds' for inorganic chemistry. We might then first ask, what makes a chemical compound organic? In life science subjects, we study the processes of life where macromolecules as chemical compounds include DNA or RNA carrying genetic information; structural proteins in muscles and the skeletal system or functional proteins as enzymes and receptors; fats and lipids including membrane structures; or carbohydrates as energy stores in the form of starch and glycogen. These macromolecules also have monomers such as amino acids for proteins, nucleotides for nucleic acids, fatty acids for fats, and simple sugars for polysaccharides (carbohydrate macromolecules). There are also thousands of chemicals involved in metabolic reactions for building (anabolism) macromolecules or for breaking them down (catabolism) such as those in the energy generation process. Such life processes are linked to what we call organic compounds, some of which are listed in Table 1.1.

One common feature of all organic compounds is that they are made from carbon. A carbon atom also bonds with other carbon atoms (the C–C bond) and/or in many cases a carbon atom is also bonded to a hydrogen atom (the C–H bond). The oxides and sulfides of carbon (carbon dioxide, carbon monoxide, carbonic acid, and carbonyl sulfide) without these C–C or C–H bonds are considered inorganic (Table 1.1). Another important feature of organic compounds is

Table 1.1 Common examples of organic and inorganic compounds.

Organic compounds	Inorganic compounds
Acetic acid, acetone, adenosine, alanine, amphetamine, arginine	Ammonia, ammonium bicarbonate, ammonium hydroxide, ammonium nitrate, ammonium sulfate, aluminium sulfide, aluminium sulfate, aluminium chloride, aluminium fluoride, aluminium hydroxide, aluminium nitrate, aluminium sulfate
Benzene, butane, butene	Boron oxide, barium bromide, barium hydroxide, borax, boron trichloride, boron oxide
Caffeine, cellulose, chloramphenicol, citric acid, cyclohexanone	Calcium chloride, calcium hydroxide, calcium sulfate, cadmium oxide, caesium carbonate, carbon dioxide, carbon monoxide, carbonic acid, carbonyl sulfide, chromic acid, cobalt(II) chloride, copper(II) sulfate, cyanogen, cyanogen thiocyanate
DNA, DDT, diethyl ether, digitonin, dioxin, dopamine	Disulfur dichloride
Ethanol, ephedrine, epinephrine, ethyl acetate, ethylene	Europium(II) sulfate, europium(III) bromide
Fatty acids, folic acid, fructose, formic acid	Francium hydroxide, francium iodide, francium oxide
Glucose, galactose, gibberellic acid, glutamine, glycerol, guanine, guanosine	Germanium oxide, germanium(II) iodide, gold(III) chloride, gold(III) oxide
Histamine, hexane, homocysteine, heptane	Hydrogen peroxide, hydrogen cyanide (HCN), hydrogen chloride, hydrogen fluoride
Ibuprofen, indole, inositol, isoleucine	Iodic acid, indium(I) oxide, iron(II) bromide, iron(III) phosphate, iron(II) sulfate
Jasmone	
Kanamycin	
Lactic acid, lactose, leucine, linoleic acid, lysergic acid diethylamide (LSD), lysine	Lead nitrate, lead(II) chloride, lithium oxide, lithium sulfate
Maltose, melatonin, menthol, methanol, morpholine	Magnesium phosphate, magnesium fluoride, magnesium hydroxide, manganese(II) oxide, mercury(II) chloride, molybdenum(IV) fluoride
Nicotine, neomycin, naphthalene, nitroglycerine, noradrenaline, norepinephrine	Nitrous oxide, nitrogen dioxide, nitrogen monoxide, neodymium(III) chloride, neptunium(III) fluoride, nickel(II) oxide, niobium(V) fluoride
Oleic acid, octane, ornithine	Osmium trioxide
Propane, palmitic acid, pentane, phenol, phenol red, phenylalanine, polystyrene, procaine, progesterone, proline, purine, pyruvic acid	Potassium hydroxide, potassium carbonate, palladium(II) chloride, plutonium(III) bromide, polonium dioxide, praseodymium(III) sulfate, promethium(III) oxide
Quinine, quinone	
Retinol (vitamin A), ribose, riboflavin (vitamin B$_2$)	Radium bromide, rhenium(VII) oxide, rhodium(III) iodide, ruthenium hexafluoride
Sucrose, salicylic acid, serine, sorbic acid, spermidine, stearic acid, sulfanilamide	Sodium chloride, sodium hydroxide, silicon dioxide, sodium nitrate, samarium(III) iodide, scandium(III) nitrate, selenic acid, selenium tetrachloride, strontium oxide, sulfur dioxide, sulfuric acid

(continued)

Table 1.1 (continued)

Organic compounds	Inorganic compounds
Thyroxine, tannin, thalidomide, thymidine, thymine, thymol, thyroxine, trypan blue, tryptophan, tyrosine	Tantalum pentafluoride, thallium(I) bromide, thionyl chloride, tin(II) bromide, titanium(II) sulfide, titanium(III) phosphide, tungsten(VI) chloride, tungsten boride
Uracil, uric acid, uridine, urea	Uranium sulfate, uranium hexafluoride, uranium tetrafluoride
Vitamins (A, B, B_1, B_2, B_3, B_4, B_5, B_6, B_{12}, C, D, E, F, H, K, M, P, S), vanillin, valium	Vanadium(II) chloride, vanadium(IV) oxide, vanadium tetrachloride
Warfarin	Water
Xylene, xylose, xanthan gum	Xenon difluoride, xenic acid
Yohimbine	
Zingiberene	Zinc phosphate, zinc oxide, zinc carbonate, zirconium hydroxide

the C–C and/or C–H bonding that we call *covalent bonding*. Many biological molecules such as proteins, sugars, and nucleic acids are soluble in water, but other organic compounds are less soluble in water and rather dissolve in organic solvents.

What Makes a Molecule an Organic Compound? – Key Facts

- It is a chemical compound made with covalent bonding.
- This covalent bonding contains at least one carbon atom, and a C–C bond is a common feature.
- Simple oxides of carbon are not considered organic as there tends to be C–H bonding in many organic compounds.
- Organic chemistry deals with the chemical structures, physical and chemical properties, and reactions of *organic compounds*.

Many mineral salts such as metallic chlorides, sulfates, hydroxides, nitrates, phosphates, *etc.* are highly polar water-soluble chemical compounds. These compounds are considered inorganic – they lack carbon and mostly involve *ionic bonding*. The list of inorganic compounds (see Table 1.1) is large, however, and includes many water-insoluble chemical compounds, and covalent bonding may also be involved in bringing elements together to form chemical compounds. Hence the main difference between organic and inorganic compounds is the C–C and C–H covalent bonding that we are addressing in this chapter. Before we go into the details of covalent bonding, however, we need to revise the distinction between elements and molecules, although our focus will remain on the chemistry of carbon.

In biological molecules, many inorganic ions may also be incorporated. For example, we have proteins that we call metalloproteins because they contain one or more metal ions tightly bound to their amino acid side chains. Many enzymes also incorporate metal ions while other proteins such as haemoglobin and myoglobin incorporate iron ions. Chlorophyll is an example of an organic compound that incorporates a magnesium ion.

1.2   Atoms, Elements, and Compounds

An element is a substance that contains one type of atom. The Periodic Table of the elements shown at the beginning of this chapter lists over 100 elements. These elements are the building blocks for all substances that we encounter. An atom is the smallest amount or particle of an element. The physical and chemical behaviour of an element at the smallest unit is therefore represented by its atoms.

Two or more atoms join together chemically to form a chemical compound. The smallest unit of this chemical combination product is a *molecule*. This bonding could be between two atoms of the same element to form diatomic molecules such as hydrogen (H_2), oxygen (O_2), nitrogen (N_2), chlorine (Cl_2), bromine (Br_2), or iodine (I_2). Alternatively, a molecule is made when two or more different atoms are involved in chemical bonding, such as hydrogen and oxygen to form water (H_2O) or carbon and hydrogen to form methane (CH_4). In organic compounds, the molecules may be made from combinations of more than two elements. As atoms are the smallest units of elements, molecules represent the smallest units in chemical compounds. The physical and chemical properties of a given organic compound are therefore represented at the smallest possible unit as a molecule.

The Periodic Table shows the elements grouped vertically in columns called groups and horizontally in rows called periods. These groupings provide valuable information about the elements in terms of their reactivity. The Periodic Table also shows metals, non-metals, and semimetals. It further gives information on atomic and subatomic structures. All atoms are composed of a nucleus, which contains protons and neutrons, and electrons circulating around the nucleus. The mass number of an atom is the sum of the protons and neutrons, which is represented by a superscript number, along with the proton number (subscript) for each atom. This *atomic notation for carbon,*

$^{12}_{6}\text{C}$, shows that its proton number is 6 and the sum of neutrons and protons or mass number is 12. Thus, carbon also has six neutrons. For oxygen, with a mass number of 16 and a proton number of 8, its atomic notation is represented as $^{16}_{8}\text{O}$, also indicating the presence of eight neutrons in its nucleus.

Hydrogen Isotopes – Key Facts

- Isotopes differ from each other by having a different number of neutrons.
- For hydrogen, the most abundant isotope is protium – with no neutrons and one proton.
- Deuterium is a hydrogen isotope with one proton and one neutron.
- Tritium is a hydrogen isotope with one proton and two neutrons.
- All hydrogen isotopes have one electron and one proton.

The proton number is also called the *atomic number* and is a fixed number for a particular element. On the other hand, atoms of an element may have different numbers of neutrons and are called *isotopes*. Some elements such as hydrogen exist mainly as one isotope; nearly all (natural abundance ~99.98%) hydrogen atoms exist with a mass number of 1 ($^{1}_{1}\text{H}$) but traces of mass number 2 ($^{2}_{1}\text{H}$) and 3 ($^{3}_{1}\text{H}$) also exist. For carbon atoms, there are far more isotopes but the predominant one is $^{12}_{6}\text{C}$ and others such as $^{13}_{6}\text{C}$ and $^{14}_{6}\text{C}$ are useful in experimental studies. Because of the presence of isotopes, the mass number of an element is presented as the average calculated based on their natural abundance. For example, for carbon, although usually presented as $^{12}_{6}\text{C}$, the actual mass may be given as 12.0101 and hydrogen as 1.00794. Some isotopes are called *radioisotopes* because their nuclei are unstable and they release excess energy through spontaneous radiation such as alpha, beta, and gamma rays. In doing so, the element is transformed into a more stable form. For carbon atoms, $^{14}_{6}\text{C}$ is a radioisotope that occurs naturally and remains for thousands of years without breaking down. Its half-life is said to be ~5730 years and hence it has uses in geological survey studies. Radioisotopes can also be produced in reactors and their main use is to generate energy, for example in the form of electricity. Radioisotopes are also used extensively in medicine for both diagnosis and therapy.

Carbon Isotopes – Key Facts

- Carbon has two stable isotopes (^{12}C and ^{13}C) and one unstable or radioactive isotope (^{14}C).
- The natural abundances of ^{12}C and ^{13}C are ~98.89% and ~1.11%, respectively.
- Radiocarbon dating is a method for determining the age of an organic material using the radioactive properties of ^{14}C. It is used extensively in archaeological studies.
- ^{13}C studies are applied in the structural elucidation of organic compounds using nuclear magnetic resonance (NMR) spectroscopy.

1.3   Valence Electrons

We adopt here a simple model of electronic configuration that allows us to understand easily the bonding interactions between atoms, as quantum mechanics is beyond the scope of this book. Molecular bonding, be it formed through ionic or covalent interactions, is a function of electrons and the useful information about the number of electrons for a given element comes from the proton number shown in the Periodic Table. Protons in the nucleus are positively charged and the negatively charged electrons circle around the nucleus. Looking into the three-dimensional structure of the nucleus, we should assume that the electrons occupy different shells or energy levels, with the energy level (n) dictating the maximum number of electrons possible in the shell as $2n^2$. The first energy level therefore has a capacity of 2, the second shell 8, the third shell 18, and the fourth shell 32 electrons. At this stage, we assume that there are large energy differences between these levels – the energy increases as we move from the first to the second level and so on. We will learn later that there are also subshells or orbitals that electrons occupy within these energy levels.

Let us consider group 14 elements of the Periodic Table: carbon, silicon, and germanium. Their atomic numbers (the same as the electron number) and their electron configurations are given in Table 1.2. For carbon, with a total of 6 electrons, the first energy level (shell) is occupied with the maximum possible 2 electrons, and the remainder go into the second energy level, which has a capacity of 8. For silicon, with 14 electrons, both the first and second shells are filled with the maximum possible number of electrons allowed (2 and 8, respectively), and the remaining 4 go into the third shell. Germanium, with

32 electrons, has the third shell filled with the maximum possible 18 electrons and the remaining 4 are in the fourth shell. Since all these elements have four electrons in their outermost shells, they were previously called group IV (now group 14) elements. On this basis, we can now see that group 1 elements have one electron in their outer shell, group 2 elements have two, and so on.

You may notice from Table 1.2 that the electronic arrangement of potassium is 2.8.8.1, not 2.8.9. This is defined by what we call the *octet rule*, referring to the tendency of atoms to prefer to have eight electrons in the outermost shell. Hence, if the third shell is not filled with 18 electrons, the tendency is to fill it with eight electrons and move the remaining electrons to the next shell. Another good example is calcium (Table 1.2).

Valence Shell and the Octet Rule – Key Facts

- The electrons in the outermost shell of the electronic configuration are valence electrons.
- The octet rule refers to the tendency of atoms to prefer to have eight electrons in the outermost shell.
- In chemical bonding, an atom tends to make a bond with another atom so as to have eight electrons in its valence shell.
- The metallic and non-metallic characteristics of elements are based on this tendency.
- Elements with fewer than four outer-shell electrons show a tendency to lose electrons, whereas those with more than four show a tendency to gain electrons.
- Group 1 and group 17 elements are the two extremes with metallic and non-metallic characteristics, respectively.
- Carbon has four electrons in its valence shell and is right in the middle between metals and non-metals. It is involved in covalent bonding.

The electrons in the outermost shell, the number of which governs the group name, are called *valence electrons*. Hence the number of valence electrons of a particular element is its group number in the Periodic Table. The reactivity of the element towards other elements is dependent on these valence electrons. As mentioned above, the octet rule states that the preferred number of electrons in the outer shell is eight. Group 18 elements already meet this requirement, and the elements are inert or unreactive. Hence neon (Ne) and argon (Ar) are also known as inert gases. The same applies to helium (He), where

Table 1.2 Electron configurations of some selected elements.[a]

| Atomic number | Element (symbol) | Energy level (n) (Maximum occupancy as $2n^2$) | | | | Group[b] |
		$n=1$ (2)	$n=2$ (8)	$n=3$ (18)	$n=4$ (32)	
1	Hydrogen (H)	**1**				1
3	Lithium (Li)	2	**1**			
11	Sodium (Na)	2	8	**1**		
19	Potassium (K)	2	8	8	**1**	
4	Beryllium (Be)	2	**2**			2
12	Magnesium (Mg)	2	8	**2**		
20	Calcium (Ca)	2	8	8	**2**	
6	Carbon (C)	2	**4**			14
14	Silicon (Si)	2	8	**4**		
32	Germanium (Ge)	2	8	18	**4**	
7	Nitrogen (N)	2	**5**			15
15	Phosphorus (P)	2	8	**5**		
8	Oxygen (O)	2	**6**			16
16	Sulfur (S)	2	8	**6**		
34	Selenium (Se)	2	8	18	**6**	
9	Fluorine (F)	2	**7**			17
17	Chlorine (Cl)	2	8	**7**		
35	Bromine (Br)	2	8	18	**7**	
10	Neon (Ne)	2	**8**			18
18	Argon (Ar)	2	8	**8**		

[a]The outer-shell electrons are called *valence electrons* and are shown in bold.
[b]Group number in the Periodic Table.

the two electrons fully occupying the first shell make it unreactive. On this basis, we can now see the tendency of elements to either lose or gain electrons to fulfil this rule. Group 17 elements with seven valence electrons need only one more electron to fill them up and prefer to gain one rather than lose seven. On the other hand, group 1 elements with one valence electron tend to lose this electron. Hence group 1 elements have good metallic characteristics with a tendency to lose an electron, and group 17 elements (also called the halogen series) have good non-metallic characteristics with a tendency to gain an electron. How this works out in the formation of chemical bonds is discussed in the following sections. We can represent valence electrons as dots around the atomic symbol (see the following sections and Figure 1.1).

Having the valence electrons and the various groups of the Periodic Table explained, we can also make some generalisations about the periods – the horizontal rows in the Periodic Table. You might ask what is common for period 1 elements (H and He), what is common for all period 2 elements (Li, Be, B, C, N, O, F, and Ne), and so on. If we consider group 1 elements (first column of the Periodic

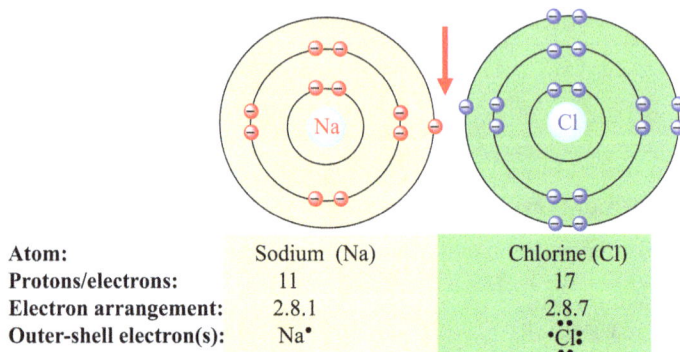

Atom:	Sodium (Na)	Chlorine (Cl)
Protons/electrons:	11	17
Electron arrangement:	2.8.1	2.8.7
Outer-shell electron(s):	Na•	•Cl:

Figure 1.1 Electron dot representation of sodium and chlorine atoms. As an exercise, you can show the electron dot representation of the elements listed in Table 1.2.

Table), moving down from hydrogen (H) to francium (Fr), the atomic size increases. In electronic configuration, period 1 elements have one shell whereas period 2 elements have two shells. As the numbers of electrons and shells increase, the tendency for electrons to be lost (instead of gained) or the metallic character increases. Note that a larger atomic size (greater atomic radius) means an increased distance from the nucleus (positively charged protons) that hold electrons, *i.e.* a greater tendency to lose an electron or an increased metallic character. Hence the metallic character increases as we move from right to left horizontally and from top to bottom vertically in the Periodic Table.

1.4   Ionic Bonding

Before we move to covalent bonding, let us investigate ionic bonding, which occurs through the interaction between metal (*e.g.* sodium, Na) and non-metal (*e.g.* chlorine, Cl) atoms to make a salt (*e.g.* sodium chloride, NaCl). Sodium with 11 electrons has a 2.8.1 electronic arrangement whereas chlorine with 17 electrons has a 2.8.7 electronic arrangement. Since the third shell has a capacity of 8 electrons, sodium with 1 electron (as a group 1 element of the Periodic Table) favours losing the single electron in the outer shell rather than trying to gain 7 electrons, whereas chlorine as a group 17 element favours gaining 1 electron instead of losing 7 (Figure 1.1).

The electron(s) in the outer shell, which is the furthest from the positively charged nucleus, may be either lost or gained to establish stability. This results in Na losing an electron and Cl gaining an electron as follows:

$Na - e^- \rightarrow Na^+$ (sodium loses an electron and is positively charged)
$Cl + e^- \rightarrow Cl^-$ (chlorine gains an electron and is negatively charged)

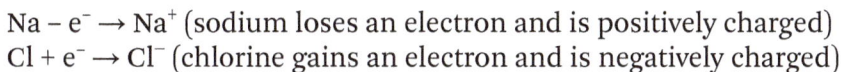

The resulting ions and attractions of oppositely charged particles to make ionic bonds is shown in Figure 1.2.

The strong attraction between these two oppositely charged particles forms the ionic bond. Chemical compounds or molecules formed through ionic interactions make a uniform solid lattice or crystal structure with a high melting point. The solid lattice structure, however, crumbles when water is added to salts as the water molecules surround the two ionic species such as Na^+ and Cl^-, *i.e.* salts dissolve in water. In later sections of this book, we will address how to make organic compounds water soluble by changing them into a salt form – meaning changing them into charged species and making ionic bonds. This has implications for how drug molecules are administered orally in aqueous solutions, how they are made, how they are absorbed from the gut, and how they interact with biological targets.

Ionic Bonding – Key Facts

- A bond is formed when an atom (such as a metal) transfers electrons to another atom (such as a non-metal).
- An ionic bond is formed by electrostatic attraction between oppositely charged ions.
- Ionic compounds undergo dissociation in water to form ions – NaCl dissociates to form Na^+ and Cl^-.

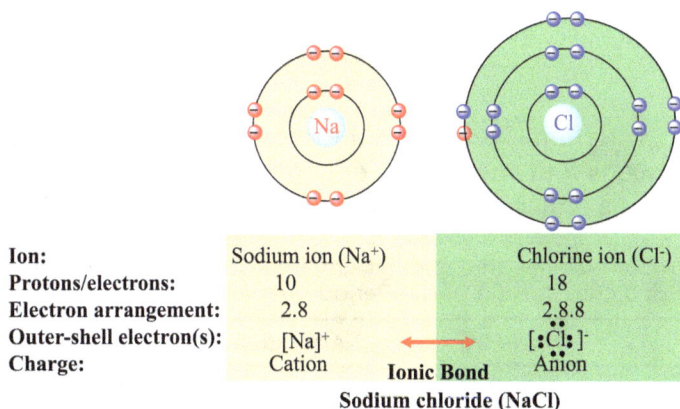

Ion:	Sodium ion (Na^+)	Chlorine ion (Cl^-)
Protons/electrons:	10	18
Electron arrangement:	2.8	2.8.8
Outer-shell electron(s):	$[Na]^+$	$[:\overset{..}{\underset{..}{Cl}}:]^-$
Charge:	Cation	Anion

Ionic Bond

Sodium chloride (NaCl)

Figure 1.2 Ionic bonding between sodium and chlorine to form sodium chloride salt. The electronic configuration of each atom in the molecule following the ionic bonding is shown.

1.5   Covalent Bonding

In ionic bonding, we have seen how atoms gain stability through bonding by either losing or gaining an electron or electrons from their outer shells. Ionic bonding works perfectly with a combination of atoms highly deficient in electrons in their outer shells (metals) and an electron excess (non-metals), particularly group 17 elements. In other elements, this 'give and take' may not be appropriate to achieve stability and they rather form bonds by sharing some electrons. This is what we call *covalent bonding*, and it is a common feature of bonding between non-metallic elements.

As in ionic bonding, the electrons involved in covalent bonding are in the outer shells of the atoms. The goal is still to gain a stable form of a molecule with complete electron sets in the outer shell. Thus, in the simplest example of covalent bonding, we expect a pair of electrons shared between two atoms to make a bond. The number of bonds involved depends on the number of electrons available for the sharing process in the outer shell. Let us consider the first elements from group 14 to group 17 of the Periodic Table as shown in Table 1.3.

Valence Electrons *versus* Valency – Key Facts

- Valency means the combining capacity of any element to make a bond.
- Valency indicates how many electrons are needed to be gained or lost in making a stable atom – a full electron shell.
- Seven valence electrons mean that the element has a valency of 1.

Carbon, with four electrons in the outer shell, which has a capacity of eight, needs four more electrons to achieve a stable atom in the formation of a molecule through bonding with other elements. This

Table 1.3   Examples of electronic arrangements for selected atoms in the indicated group of the Periodic Table.

Group	Element[a]	Arrangement	Valency/bond
Group 14	Carbon	2.4	4
Group 15	Nitrogen	2.5	3
Group 16	Oxygen	2.6	2
Group 17	Fluorine	2.7	1

[a]The first element in the indicated group of the Periodic Table is listed.

means that it must share two pairs of electrons – its valency is four and it can make four bonds. Oxygen (group 16 element) always has a valency of two as it needs two electrons to fill its shell, whereas group 17 elements, as shown in Table 1.3 for fluorine, have a valency of one.

Covalent Bonding – Key Facts

- A shared pair of electrons make a covalent bond.
- The number of electrons in the outer shell governs the number of bonds that an element can make in a covalent bond.
- Atoms form molecules through covalent bonding.

1.5.1 Types of Molecules Formed Through Covalent Bonding

1.5.1.1 Homonuclear Diatomic Molecules

Perhaps the simplest form of covalent bonding to visualise is that between the same atoms to form diatomic molecules. Elements that form covalent bonds through this process are shown in Table 1.4. Since two atoms of the same element are involved in the bonding process, a *homonuclear molecule* is the terminology used to describe a diatomic molecule. In single bond formation, one pair of electrons is shared as shown for hydrogen (H_2) and the group 17 diatomic elements fluorine (F_2), chlorine (Cl_2), bromine (Br_2), and iodine (I_2). For the group 16 element oxygen, two pairs of electrons contribute to the diatomic molecular bonding with two or double bonds. Nitrogen (N_2), as a group 15 element, needs three pairs of electrons in the sharing process to make a three- or triple-bonded molecule (see Figure 1.3).

1.5.1.2 Heteronuclear Covalent Bonding

Using the diatomic model of atoms forming a molecule through covalent bonding, let us consider hydrogen (H) and chlorine (Cl) atoms forming hydrogen chloride (HCl). As shown in Figure 1.4, hydrogen is a group 1 element with just one electron in its shell whereas chlorine, as explained in the previous section, has seven electrons in its outer shell. Both elements need one electron to complete their shell and hence make a diatomic *heteronuclear molecule*, hydrogen chloride.

Table 1.4 Diatomic elements.

Element	Ball-and-stick model[a]	Space-filling model[a]
Hydrogen (H_2)		
Nitrogen (N_2)		
Oxygen (O_2)		
Fluorine (F_2)		
Chlorine (Cl_2)		

Table 1.4 (continued)

Element	Ball-and-stick model[a]	Space-filling model[a]
Bromine (Br_2)		
Iodine (I_2)		

[a]The three-dimensional molecular structures can be represented visually using the ball-and-stick model (spheres and rods) or space-filling model (spheres without rods). The ball-and-stick model shows how the atoms are connected to each other, with the relative bond lengths and bond angles (see the following sections) illustrated. We will also learn how the relative atomic size (radius) can be presented using the space-filling model.

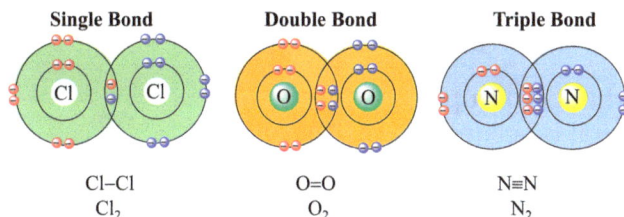

Figure 1.3 Electronic arrangement in diatomic molecules to make single, double, and triple bonds.

1.5.2 Understanding Covalent Bonding Through Atomic Orbitals

We have already explained that the electronic arrangement for atoms is based on energy levels or shells with the maximum capacity of electrons in the shell being $2n^2$. We also have subshells or orbitals that electrons occupy within these energy levels. These are what we call the s, p, d, and f orbitals. The maximum numbers of electrons in these subshells are as follows:

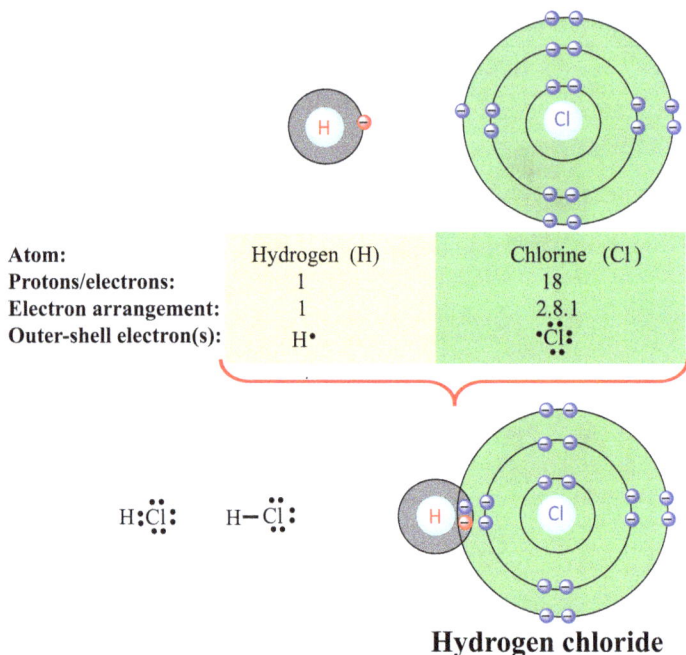

Atom:	Hydrogen (H)	Chlorine (Cl)
Protons/electrons:	1	18
Electron arrangement:	1	2.8.1
Outer-shell electron(s):	H•	•C̈l⋮

$$H{:}\ddot{\underset{\cdot\cdot}{Cl}}{:} \qquad H-\ddot{\underset{\cdot\cdot}{Cl}}{:}$$

Hydrogen chloride

Figure 1.4   Formation of a heteronuclear diatomic molecule, hydrogen chloride. The covalent bond formation between the atoms shown by a line at bottom left represents a pair of electrons shared between the two atoms (*i.e.* a single bond in a molecule represents sharing of a pair of electrons).

- an s orbital is occupied by 2 electrons
- a p orbital is occupied by 6 electrons
- a d orbital is occupied by 10 electrons
- an f orbital is occupied by 14 electrons.

In a simplistic presentation, the first four energy levels or shells for the indicated maximum capacity can be presented as shown in Table 1.5.

We can indicate the number of electrons occupying the orbitals as follows:

- $1s^2$ means 2 electrons occupying the s orbital in the first shell.
- $2s^2$ means 2 electrons occupying the s orbital in the second shell.
- $3p^1$ means 1 electron occupying the p orbital in the third shell.
- For neon (Ne) with 8 electrons (2 in the first shell and 6 in the second shell), $1s^2 2s^2 2p^6$.
- For sodium (Na) with 11 electrons (2 in the first shell, 8 in the second shell, and 1 in the third shell), $1s^2 2s^2 2p^6 3s^1$.
- For fluorine (F) with 9 electrons (2 in the first shell and 7 in the second shell), $1s^2 2s^2 2p^5$.

Table 1.5 Energy levels, shells, and subshells and their maximum capacities (number of electrons).

Energy level (shell)	Subshell (orbital)[a]	Total number of electrons
1 (first shell)	1s	2
2 (second shell)	2s, 2p	$2 + 6 = 8$
3 (third shell)	3s, 3p, 3d	$2 + 6 + 10 = 18$
4 (fourth shell)	4s, 4p, 4d, 4f	$2 + 6 + 10 + 14 = 32$

[a]The number before the subshell/orbital indicates the shell to which it belongs.

For covalent bonding involving carbon atoms, or organic compounds, we focus only on the s and p orbitals. The s orbital is spherical and has a maximum capacity for a pair of electrons, whereas p orbitals have a dumbbell shape with a capacity for a pair of electrons. For the three p orbitals of the second shell (2p subshells), we have x, y, and z orientations, as shown in Figure 1.5. These $2p_x$, $2p_y$, and $2p_z$ subshells hold a maximum of six electrons (3×2 electrons for each subshell). The s orbitals in the various electronic shells are denoted 1s, 2s, 3s, 4s, ... , *etc.*, whereas p orbitals are denoted 2p, 3p, 4p, 5p, ... , *etc.*

Let us consider the electronic configuration of chlorine, which has 17 electrons. As already highlighted in the preceding section (see Figure 1.4), the electrons are arranged as a 2.8.7 order of shells. This can be written as $1s^2 2s^2 2p^6 3s^2 3p^5$. The three p orbitals in the second shell are full (six electrons) whereas only two p orbitals in the third shell are full, leaving one p orbital with an unpaired electron. This can be presented as shown in Figure 1.6.

Although not relevant to carbon, we also have other orbitals such as d and f and their maximum electron occupancy for each shell is shown in Figure 1.7. Given that the energy levels of these orbitals are different, for elements with a large number of protons (or electrons) the order of arrangement is as shown in Figure 1.7 in the direction of the arrows. The orbitals of lowest energy fill first and follow the order shown by the arrows.

1.5.3 Covalent Bonding *via* Overlapping of Orbitals

In the previous example of covalent bonding using a homonuclear diatomic molecule, we considered hydrogen with one electron in the 1s orbital. A hydrogen molecule (H_2) is therefore made when two 1s orbitals overlap with each other to allow the sharing of the electrons as shown in Figure 1.8.

The single covalent bond formed by sharing of the electron pair in the overlapped s orbitals is a *sigma (σ) bond*. In the previous example,

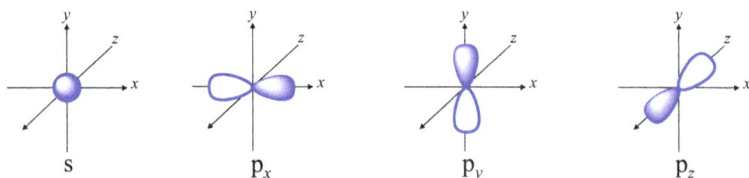

Figure 1.5   Schematic representation of the s and p orbitals. Note the p orbital's alignment along the perpendicular axis.

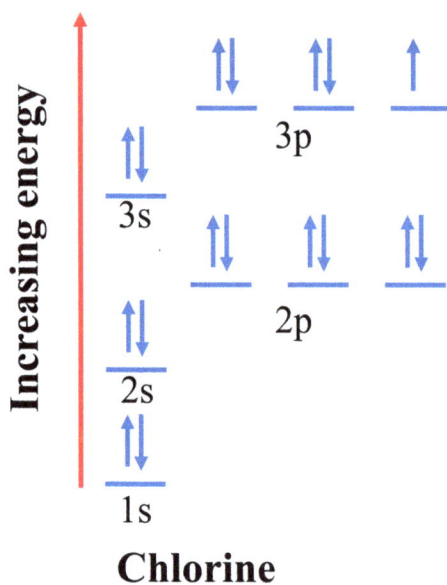

Chlorine

Figure 1.6   Electronic configuration of chlorine. Note the unpaired electron in one of the 3p orbitals.

	s	p	d	f
Highest energy	$7s^2$	$7p^6$	$7d^{10}$	
	$6s^2$	$6p^6$	$6d^{10}$	
	$5s^2$	$5p^6$	$5d^{10}$	$5f^{14}$
	$4s^2$	$4p^6$	$4d^{10}$	$4f^{14}$
	$3s^2$	$3p^6$	$3d^{10}$	
	$2s^2$	$2p^6$		
Lowest energy	$1s^2$			

Figure 1.7   Electronic configuration. The order of energy levels in the direction of the arrows is as follows: 1s 2s 2p 3s 3p 4s 3d 4p 5s 4d 5p 6s 4f 5d 6p 7s 5f 6d 7p ...

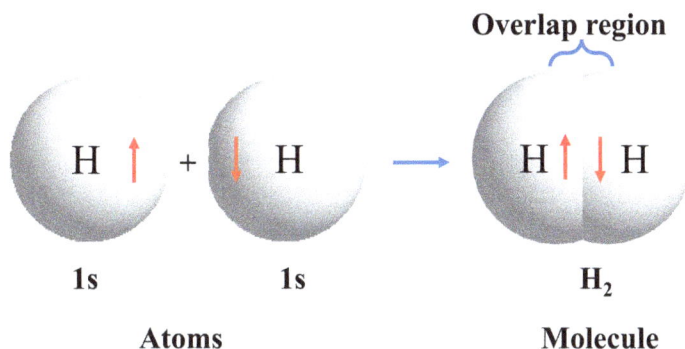

Figure 1.8   Overlapping of 1s orbitals to make a hydrogen molecule.

we also mentioned that two chlorine atoms form the diatomic chlorine molecule. As shown in Figure 1.6, the electron configuration of chlorine shows one unpaired electron in one of the 3p orbitals. This means that the sigma bonding in diatomic chlorine molecules is formed by the overlapping of two p orbitals. Sigma bonding also occurs between two different atoms, as we have seen for hydrogen and chlorine combining to form hydrogen chloride. In this case, the s orbital of the hydrogen atom overlaps the 3p orbitals of chlorine to form a sigma bond (Figure 1.9).

1.5.4   Covalent Bonding Involving Carbon

Carbon has six electrons with an arrangement of its electrons in the two shells as 2.4, *i.e.* it has a valency of four and can make bonds by sharing them with another carbon atom or other elements. Through covalent bonding, it can form single, double, or triple bonds, which can be explained better by looking into hybrid orbitals or orbital hybridisation. Let us first consider sp^3 hybridisation that allows carbon to undergo four sigma (or single) bonding.

Ground-state carbon has a $1s^2 2s^2 2p^2$ configuration whereas the excited state has a promotion of one electron from 2s to a higher energy p orbital, leading to a configuration of $1s^2 2s^1 2p^3$. In sp^3 hybridisation, a lower energy orbital of four sp^3-hybridised orbitals can be achieved, *i.e.* 2s and 2p orbitals can combine to give hybrid orbitals that we call sp^3 (Figure 1.10), *i.e.* s + ppp = sp^3.

Note that in sp^3 hybridisation, there is no unhybridised p orbital, *i.e.* we have four sp^3 orbitals that take a *tetrahedral* geometry about the carbon nuclei. One unique feature of sp^3-hybridised orbitals in carbon is the bond angle of the orbitals from each other of 109.5°, *i.e.*

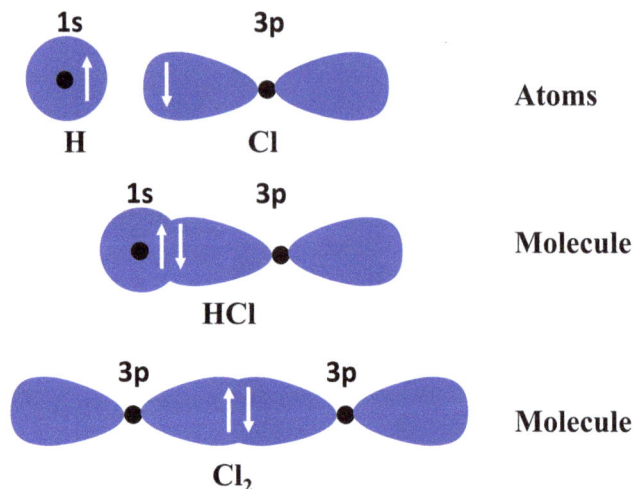

Figure 1.9   Sigma bond formation by chlorine through the overlapping of p orbitals.

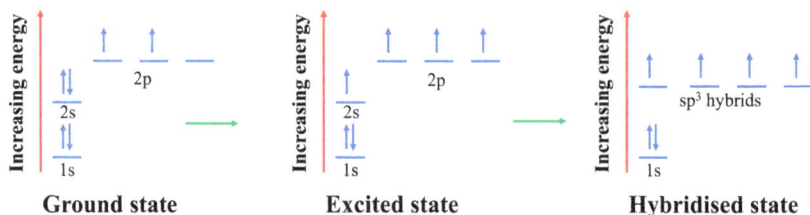

Figure 1.10   Energy levels of electronic orbitals in carbon and sp^3 hybridisation. Note that the four sp^3 orbitals occupy the same energy level higher than the 2s but lower than the 2p orbitals. Each sp^3 hybrid orbital has the capacity for two electrons. Promotion of electrons from the s to p orbitals can occur because of the small energy gap between these two orbitals. Since the energy level of the sp^3 orbital is lower than that of the p orbital, sp^3 orbital formation is favoured: the energy loss in forming sp^3 is higher than the energy input for promotion of electrons.

a tetrahedral geometry arrangement with a bond angle of 109.5° is a characteristic feature of sp^3 hybridisation in carbon (Figure 1.11).

The head-to-head overlapping of these sp^3-hybridised atomic orbitals with other orbitals from another atom forms sigma bonding. Let us consider carbon bonding with hydrogen atoms in an sp^3 fashion to make methane (CH_4). Figure 1.12 shows this bonding, and more examples of this in carbon chemistry are discussed in the following chapters.

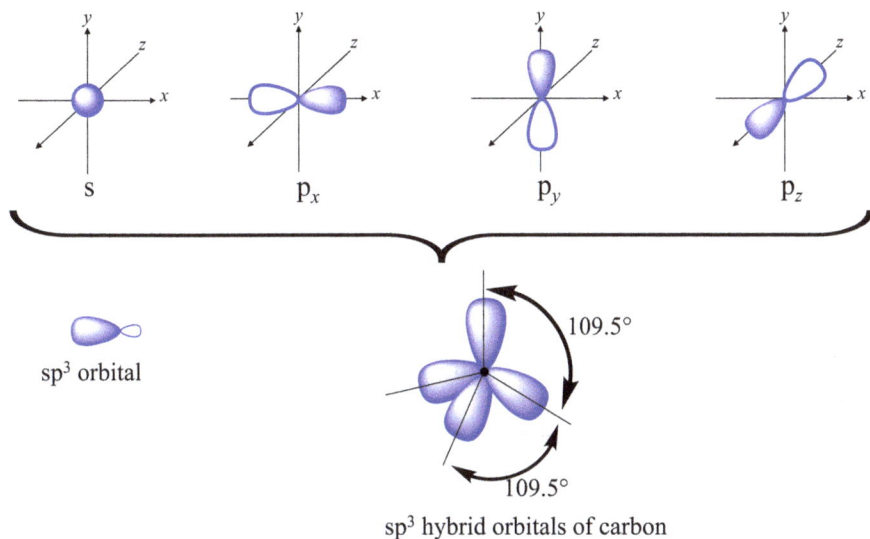

sp³ orbital

109.5°

109.5°

sp³ hybrid orbitals of carbon

Figure 1.11 sp³ hybridisation in carbon.

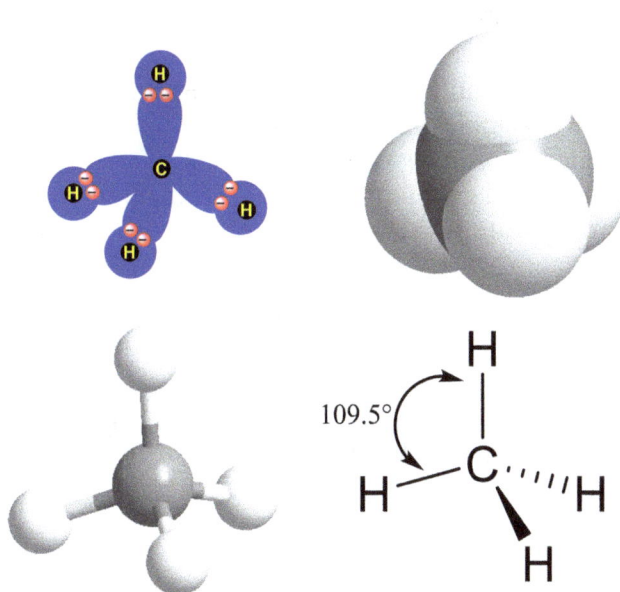

109.5°

Figure 1.12 Sigma bond formation between carbon and hydrogen to form methane.

The principle behind sp² hybridisation is depicted in Figure 1.13. In this case, a 2s orbital and two 2p orbitals are involved to form sp² hybridisation. This leaves one p orbital unchanged that appears perpendicular to the plane of the three sp² orbitals (Figure 1.14). The sp² orbitals on the plane are separated from each other by 120°.

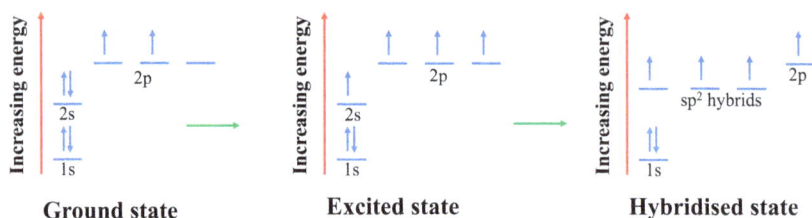

Figure 1.13   Electron arrangement of carbon in sp^2 hybridisation.

In sp^2 hybridisation, the unhybridised p orbitals of the two carbons in ethene form pi (π) bonds, *i.e.* the p atomic orbitals overlap side-to-side to share an electron pair in the space just above and below the σ bond between the two carbons. This is what we call *sideways overlapping*. Hence, in the sp^2-hybridised carbon system, we have three sigma bonding, which is similar to sp^3-hybridised orbitals and one π bond. This is exemplified by ethene (C_2H_6) in Figures 1.14 and 1.15.

Hybridised Orbitals in Carbon – Key Facts

sp^3 hybridisation:
  - Mixing of one s and three p atomic orbitals.
  - Has 25% s orbital characteristics.
  - The angle between sp^3 orbitals is 109.5°.
  - Has tetrahedral geometry of orbital arrangement.
  - All p orbitals are hybridised.

sp^2 hybridisation:
  - Mixing of one s and two p atomic orbitals.
  - Has 33% s orbital characteristics.
  - Angle between sp^2 orbitals is 120°.
  - Has trigonal planar geometry of orbital arrangement.
  - There is one unhybridised p orbital.

sp hybridisation:
  - Mixing of one s and one p atomic orbital.
  - Has 50% s orbital characteristics.
  - Angle between sp orbitals is 180°.
  - Has linear geometry of orbital arrangement.
  - There are two unhybridised p orbitals.

In sp orbitals, a 2s orbital and only one of the 2p orbitals of carbon hybridise (Figure 1.16). This forms two hybrid orbitals, leaving two p orbitals untouched. The two p orbitals lie at a right-angle to each

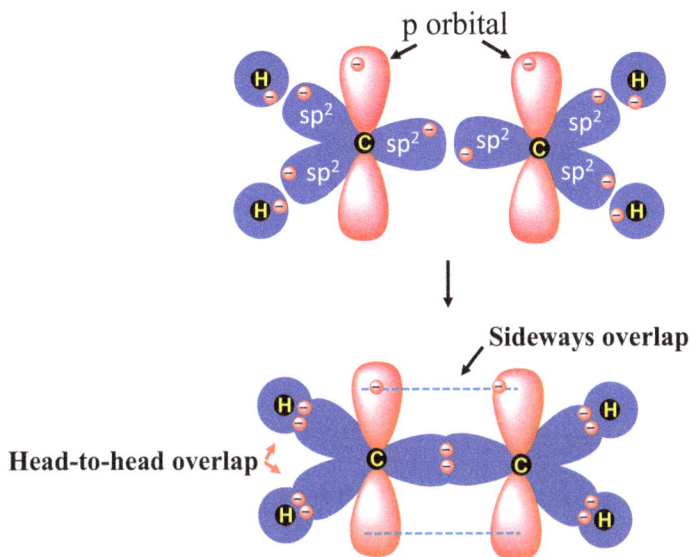

Figure 1.14 sp^2 hybridisation and covalent bond formation in ethene.

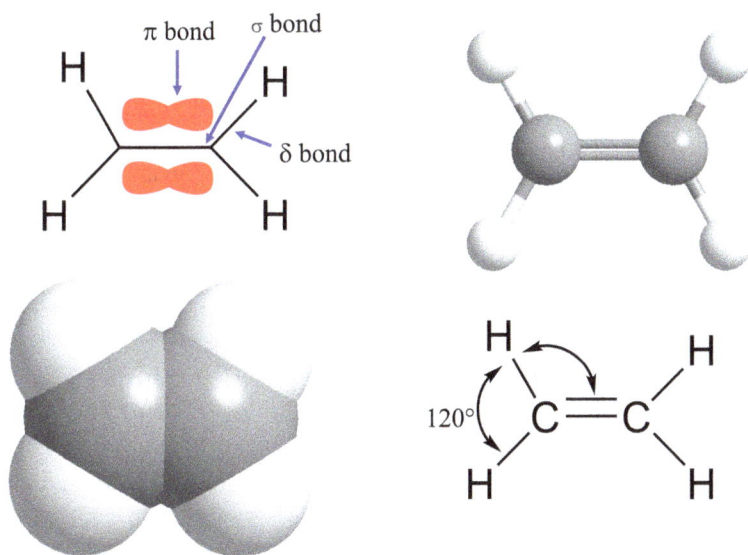

Figure 1.15 Schematic presentation of π and σ bonds in ethene. Ethene has three sp^2-hybridised orbitals of each carbon, which are involved in σ bond formation through head-to-head overlapping of orbitals, while sideways overlapping of the unhybridised p orbitals forms π bonds. Note that all double bonds in carbon chemistry that we will be referring to in this book are composed of a σ and a π bond.

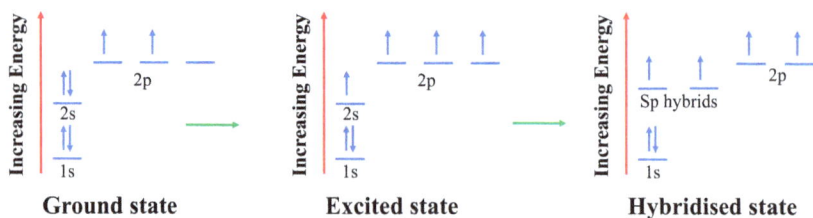

Figure 1.16 Electron arrangement of carbon in sp hybridisation.

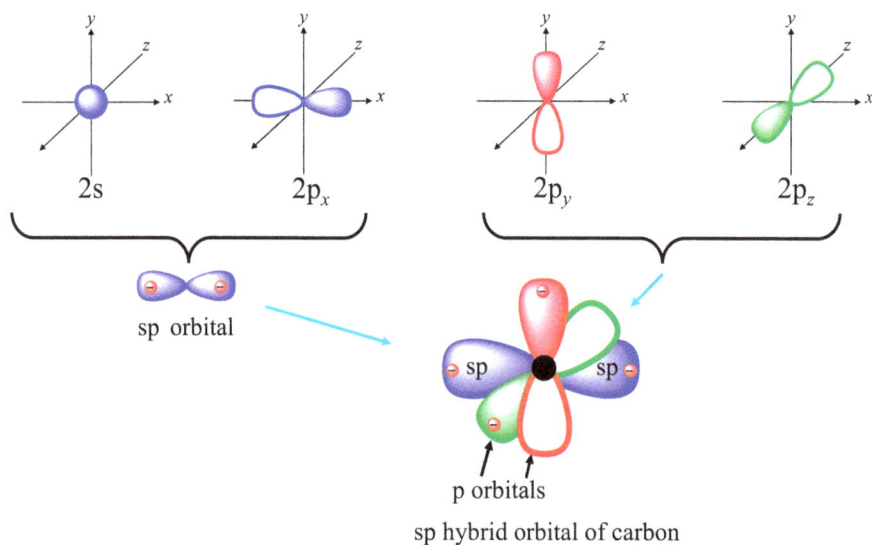

sp hybrid orbital of carbon

Figure 1.17 Schematic representation of sp hybridisation.

other whereas the sp orbitals are separated from each other by 180° (Figure 1.17).

Let us consider ethyne (acetylene) as a classic example of sp hybridisation in carbon. Through head-to-head overlap of the sp orbitals from each carbon, a σ bond is formed, whereas each carbon also makes a σ bond with a hydrogen atom (Figure 1.18). The unhybridised two sets of p orbitals form two π bonds between the carbons. As a result, a triple bond between the carbons is formed. The characteristic feature of sp-hybridised carbon is the 180° bond angle of the H–C≡C axis (Figure 1.18).

A good summary of orbital hybridisation in carbon is shown in Table 1.6. We have now seen examples of carbon bonding with hydrogen or another carbon atom through these three forms of orbital hybridisation. Carbon also makes bonds with various other elements and the

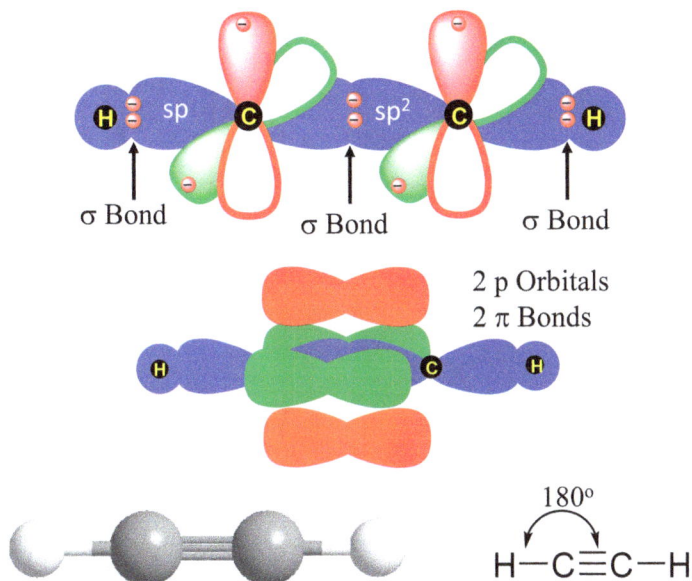

Figure 1.18 sp hybridisation in carbon with ethyne as an example. Note that two sideways overlaps make two π bonds: one above and below the sigma bond (red) in the same manner as sp² hybridisation (ethene as an example), and one in front and behind the molecule (green).

Table 1.6 Summary of hybridisation in a carbon atom.

No. of orbitals	Hybrid type	Bonding	Geometry	Bond angle/°
4	sp³		Tetrahedral	109.5
3	sp²		Trigonal planar	120
2	sp	—C≡	Linear	180

rule of hybridisation still applies in its covalent bonding with non-metal atoms such as nitrogen, sulfur, and oxygen. We will address more of this topic in the following chapters.

In C–C bonding, the various combinations of hybrid orbitals are as summarised in Figure 1.19. A molecule may possess only C–C single bonds that are formed by head-to-head overlapping of sp³–sp³ orbitals to make σ bonding. A C=C double bond has a sigma bond through overlapping of sp²–sp² orbitals and a C≡C triple bond has a sigma

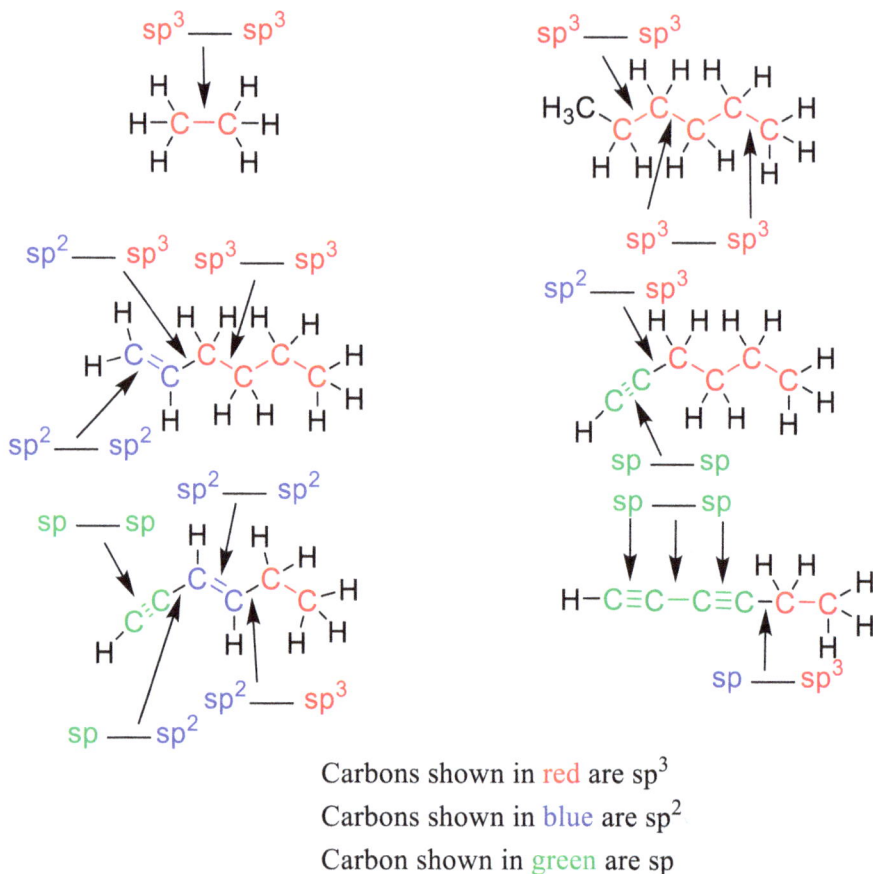

Carbons shown in red are sp^3

Carbons shown in blue are sp^2

Carbon shown in green are sp

Figure 1.19   Molecules showing the various kinds of atomic hybridisation in carbon.

bond component through overlapping of sp–sp orbitals. Molecules that possess a C=C (sp^2–sp^2) bond may also have sp^2–sp^3 σ bonding (Figure 1.19). The same applies for a CC triple (sp–sp) bond, which could undergo σ bonding with either an sp^2 or an sp^3 carbon (Figure 1.19). Complex organic compounds and their systematic classifications are addressed in the following chapters.

1.6   Summary

In this book, the emphasis is to scrutinise the basic chemistry of organic compounds and drug molecules. One common feature of all organic compounds is that they contain carbon, which forms bonds with other elements through covalent bonding. In this chapter we have answered the following questions:

- What are organic compounds and in what way do they differ from inorganic compounds?
- What are the distinguishing features of atoms, elements, and compounds?
- What are isotopes?
- What are valence electrons and what is the valency of an element?
- What are shells and subshells/orbitals and what are their maximum capacities for electrons?
- What are groups and periods in the Periodic Table?
- How is an ionic bond formed?
- How is a covalent bond formed?
- What are homonuclear and heteronuclear diatomic molecules?
- What are the distinguishing features of sp^3, sp^2, and sp hybridisations?

1.7 Problems

1. If the number of neutrons in an element is 7 and the number of electrons is 6, what is the atomic mass?
2. The atomic mass of hydrogen is 1.00794 not 1. Explain.
3. How many neutrons are in a carbon-14 (^{14}C) isotope?
4. If the natural abundances of ^{12}C and ^{13}C are 98.9 and 1.1%, respectively, what is the fractional abundance of the two forms and their fractional sum?
5. Atoms have no overall electrical charge – why?
6. What is the valency of an element with the electronic configuration 2.8.6?

Questions 7–11 are based on Figure 1.20.

7. Indicate the hybridisation state for the six carbons shown in structure 1. What would be the bond angle at each carbon?
8. What is the hybridisation of each carbon atom in benzene (structure 2)?
9. What is the hybridisation state of each carbon in structure 3? What would be the bonding geometry?
10. How many π bonds are in the molecule shown as structure 2 or benzene?
11. How many sigma bonds are present in structure 4?

Structure 1

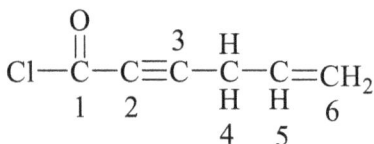

Structure 2

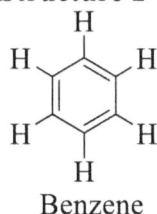

Benzene

Structure 3

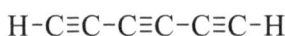

Structure 4

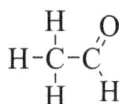

Figure 1.20 Questions 7–11 are based on this figure.

12. When potassium loses an electron to become a potassium ion (K^+), its electronic configuration becomes the same as that of which inert gas?
13. When a covalent bond is formed between two atoms, what happens to their valence electrons.
14. The number of bonds that an element can form is called what?
15. Complete Table 1.7.
16. What is the difference between a σ bond and a π bond in carbon?

1.8 Solutions to Problems

1. The number of neutrons is given as 7 and the number of electrons given as 6:

   - number of electrons = number of protons = 6;
   - atomic mass = number of neutrons + number of protons = 6 + 7 = 13.

2. Hydrogen has three isotopes: protium (^1_1H), deuterium (^2_1H), and tritium (^3_1H). The predominant isotope is protium and calculation of their natural abundances gives the average mass unit as 1.00794, *i.e.* the sum of the atomic masses of its naturally occurring isotopes, with each one multiplied by their respective abundance.

Table 1.7   Question 15 is based on this table.

Question	Ionic bond (*e.g.* NaCl, KI)	Covalent bond (methane, caffeine, *etc.*)
In what way is the bond formed by valence electrons?		
Bond is between elements of what?		
Position of elements in the Periodic Table?		
Solubility in water?		
Melting temperature?		

3. Carbon has six protons and therefore has six neutrons in ^{12}C, seven in ^{13}C, and eight in ^{14}C.
4. An abundance of 98.9% for ^{12}C means a fractional abundance of $0.989 \times 12 = 11.868$:

    - a 1.1% abundance of the ^{13}C means a fractional abundance of $0.011 \times 13 = 0.143$;
    - $11.868 + 0.143 = 12.011$. Note that this is an exemplary calculation and does not take into account the other isotopes of carbon.

5. There must be a balance between the positively charged protons and the negatively charged electrons. Hence atoms must have equal numbers of protons and electrons.
6. A valency of two needs two electrons to be gained to make up a stable eight electrons in the shell.
7. For structure 1 (Figure 1.20):

    - carbon 1 sp^2; a carbon double bond, whether it is a bond with carbon or oxygen, is still sp^2; bond angle 120°;
    - carbon 2 sp; bond angle 180°;
    - carbon 3 sp; bond angle 180°;
    - carbon 4 sp^3; bond angle 109.5°;
    - carbon 5 sp^2; bond angle 120°;
    - carbon 6 sp^2; bond angle 120°.

8. All carbons in benzene are sp^2 hybridised.
9. All carbons in the molecule are sp hybridised. The molecule is therefore linear as all the bonds have a 180° bond angle.
10. Structure 2 (benzene): three double bonds mean three pi bonds.
11. Six sigma bonds. Note that a double bond has one sigma bond and one pi bond.
12. Potassium has 19 electrons and losing one leaves 18 electrons, which is of the same configuration as argon (Ar).

Table 1.8 Answer for question 15.

Question	Ionic bond (*e.g.* NaCl, KI)	Covalent bond (methane, caffeine, *etc.*)
In what way is the bond formed by valence electrons?	Transfer of electrons	Sharing of electrons
Bond is between elements of what?	Metals and non-metals	Non-metals
Position of elements in the Periodic Table?	Opposite sides	Close together
Solubility in water?	Soluble	Some do, some don't; methane is not soluble in water whereas caffeine is
Melting temperature?	Strong bond means high melting temperature	Relatively low melting temperature

13. A covalent bond is formed by sharing some of the valence electrons. The valency of the element tells us how many electrons are involved in the sharing process.
14. Valency.
15. The answers are given in Table 1.8.
16. A sigma bond is formed by end-to-end overlapping of two hybridised s or p orbitals. A π bond is formed by sideways overlapping of p orbitals.

2 Polarity of Bonds, Electronegativity, and Intermolecular Forces

Learning Objectives

After completing this chapter, you are expected to be able to:

- Distinguish polar from non-polar bonds.
- Identify factors that influence molecular dipoles.
- Define the characteristic features of intermolecular forces.
- Be able to predict the physical features of organic compounds such as solubility and boiling point.

2.1 Electronegativity and Polarity of Bonds

2.1.1 Non-polar Bonds

Chapter 1 described covalent bonding in homonuclear and hetero-nuclear diatomic molecules. Returning to the homonuclear diatomic molecules such as hydrogen (H_2), oxygen (O_2), and nitrogen (N_2), they represent covalent bonding with the sharing of one, two, and three pairs of electrons, respectively. They also form single, double, and triple bonds, respectively (Figure 2.1). In these examples, the two atoms in the molecule share the electrons almost equally. This

Basic Chemistry for Life Science Students and Professionals: Introduction to Organic Compounds and Drug Molecules
By Solomon Habtemariam
© Solomon Habtemariam 2023
Published by the Royal Society of Chemistry, www.rsc.org

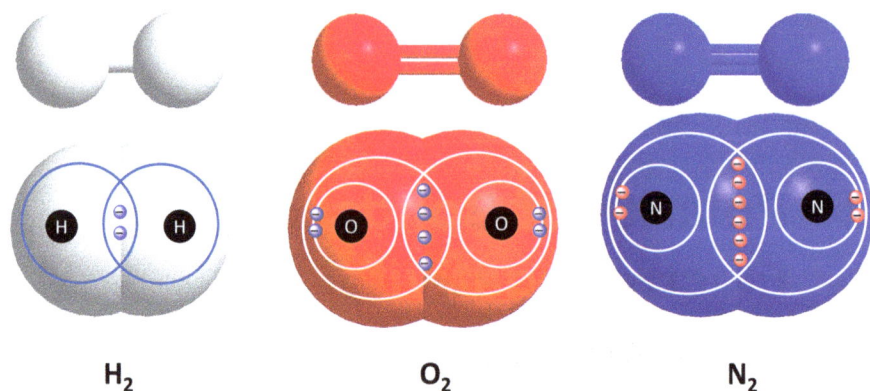

H₂   **O₂**   **N₂**

Figure 2.1 Non-polar bonding between atoms to make homonuclear diatomic molecules. Three examples representing a single bond (H_2), double bond (O_2), and triple bond (N_2) are shown. The bonds formed are truly covalent, which is based on almost equal sharing of electrons between the two atoms in the molecule. The bond is not polarised and is called non-polar.

also means that the two atoms on either side of the covalent bond do not show a significant charge difference. Since the bond that joined the two atoms to hold them together is not polarised, it is called a *non-polar bond*.

2.1.2   Overview of the Electronegativity of Elements

Before we investigate polar bonds in organic molecules, it is useful to revisit the Periodic Table of the elements and understand the relative electronegativity of the common atoms that one encounters in organic chemistry. Depending on the electronic configuration or valence electrons in the outer shell of the atom, each element may have a general tendency to either lose or gain electrons during reaction to achieve stability. Metals in group 1 or the extreme left of the Periodic Table have a tendency to lose electrons as there is only one electron in the outer shell. On the other hand, group 17 elements of the halogen series on the far right of the Periodic Table with just one electron required to fill the outer shell have a tendency to gain instead of lose an electron. This relative tendency to gain or lose electrons is a measure of *electronegativity* and is generally defined as the tendency to attract a bonding pair of electrons. As shown in Figure 2.2, the electronegativity of the elements increases as we move from the left to the right side of the Periodic Table. The

Electronegativity

Group 1	Group 2	Group 3	Group 4	Group 5	Group 6	Group 7	Group 8	Group 9	Group 10	Group 11	Group 12	Group 13	Group 14	Group 15	Group 16	Group 17	Group 18
1 H 1.008																	2 He 4.003
3 Li 6.94	4 Be 9.012											5 B 10.81	6 C 12.011	7 N 14.007	8 O 15.999	9 F 18.998	10 Ne 20.180
11 Na 22.990	12 Mg 24.305											13 Al 26.982	14 Si 28.085	15 P 30.974	16 S 32.06	17 Cl 35.45	18 Ar 39.948
19 K 39.098	20 Ca 40.078	21 Sc 44.956	22 Ti 47.867	23 V 50.942	24 Cr 51.996	25 Mn 54.938	26 Fe 55.845	27 Co 58.933	28 Ni 58.693	29 Cu 63.546	30 Zn 65.38	31 Ga 69.723	32 Ge 72.630	33 As 74.922	34 Se 78.971	35 Br 79.904	36 Kr 83.798
37 Rb 85.468	38 Sr 87.62	39 Y 88.906	40 Zr 91.224	41 Nb 92.906	42 Mo 95.95	43 Tc [98]	44 Ru 101.07	45 Rh 102.906	46 Pd 106.42	47 Ag 107.868	48 Cd 112.414	49 In 114.818	50 Sn 118.710	51 Sb 121.760	52 Te 127.60	53 I 126.904	54 Xe 131.293
55 Cs 132.905	56 Ba 137.327	★	72 Hf 138.905	73 Ta 180.948	74 W 183.84	75 Re 186.207	76 Os 190.23	77 Ir 192.217	78 Pt 195.084	79 Au 196.967	80 Hg 200.592	81 Tl 204.38	82 Pb 207.2	83 Bi 208.980	84 Po [209]	85 At [210]	86 Rn [222]
87 Fr [223]	88 Ra [226]	★★	104 Rf [267]	105 Db [268]	106 Sg [269]	107 Bh [270]	108 Hs [269]	109 Mt [278]	110 Ds [281]	111 Rg 280]	112 Cn [285]	113 Nh [286]	114 Fl [289]	115 Mc [289]	116 Lv [293]	117 Ts [294]	118 Og [294]

★	57 La 138.905	58 Ce 140.116	59 Pr 140.908	60 Nd 144.242	61 Pm [145]	62 Sm 150.36	63 Eu 151.964	64 Gd 157.25	65 Tb 158.925	66 Dy 162.500	67 Ho 164.930	68 Er 167.259	69 Tm 168.934	70 Yb 173.045	71 Lu 174.967	Lanthanides
★★	89 Ac [227]	90 Th 232.038	91 Pa 231.036	92 U 238.029	93 Np [237]	94 Pu [244]	95 Am [243]	96 Cm [247]	97 Bk [247]	98 Cf [251]	99 Es [252]	100 Fm [257]	101 Md [258]	102 No [259]	103 Lr [262]	Actinides

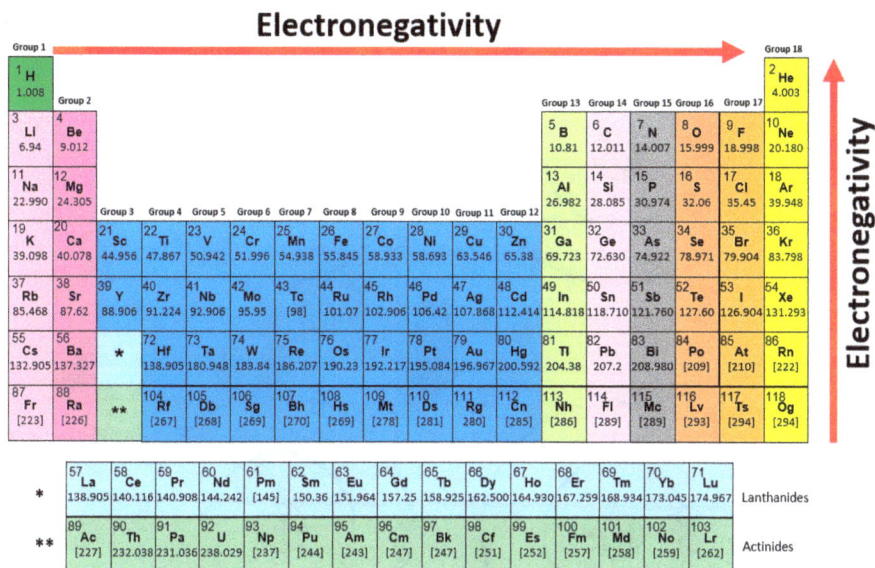

Figure 2.2   The Periodic Table of the elements – electronegativity. The trend of electronegativity increases in the direction of the arrows as shown.

electronegativity also increases as we move up the Periodic Table from the bottom to the top:

- For period 2 elements, electronegativity increases from lithium (Li) on the left to fluorine (F) on the right.
- For group 17 elements, electronegativity decreases in the order F > Cl > Br > I.

2.1.3   Extreme Electronegativity Difference – Ionic Bonding

In Chapter 1, we used sodium chloride (NaCl) salt as an example of ionic bonding between metallic and non-metallic elements. In the Periodic Table example (Figure 2.2), lithium is a group 1 element with a 2.1 electronic arrangement in its shells, whereas fluorine is a group 17 element with a 2.7 electronic arrangement, *i.e.* fluorine has just a one-electron deficiency to fill the maximum capacity in its second shell and hence its electronegativity is far higher than that of lithium. These two elements are on the opposite sides of electronegativity in the Periodic Table: highly electropositive lithium and highly electronegative fluorine. As shown in Figure 2.3, ionic

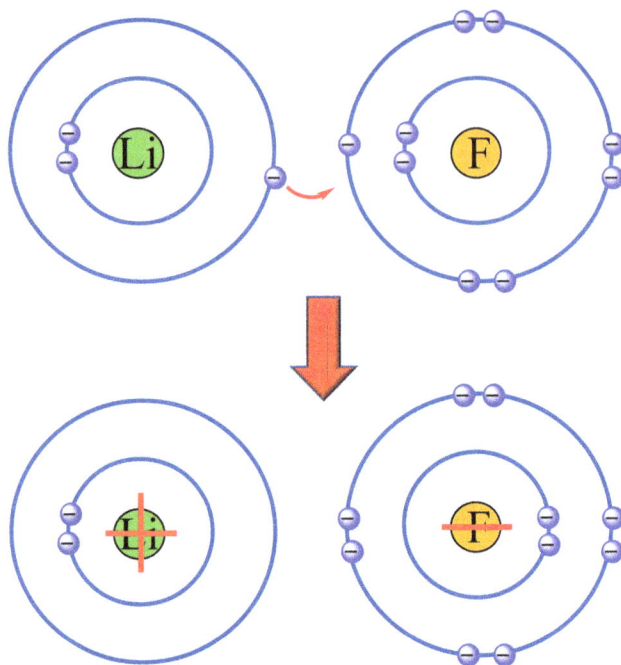

Figure 2.3 Ionic bonding between lithium and fluorine. Lithium loses an electron to become positively charged whereas fluorine accepts an electron to become negatively charged. The bonding with complete transfer of electrons is called *ionic bonding*.

bonding between these two elements occurs *via* a *complete electron transfer* from lithium to fluorine. This results in both elements being charged: the electron loser (lithium) positively, and the electron acceptor (fluorine) negatively. *Thus, ionic bonds are formed through complete transfer of electrons from an electropositive element to a highly electronegative element.*

2.1.4   Polar Covalent Bonds

Let us now consider polar bonds between elements other than carbon. Figure 2.4 shows three examples: hydrogen fluoride (HF), water (H_2O), and ammonia (NH_3). These three molecules are examples of covalent bonding with hydrogen bonded with either nitrogen, oxygen, or fluorine. However, hydrogen is far lower on the electronegativity scale than the other three elements (F, O, and N) (Figure 2.2). Note that the electronegativity difference between hydrogen and these elements (F, O, and N) is not large enough for ionic bonding through complete

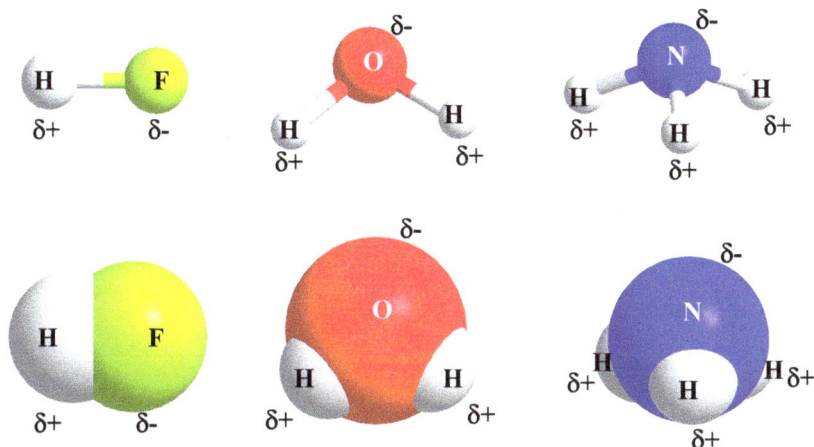

Figure 2.4   Examples of polarised bonds. Partial charge distribution with slightly positive (δ+) and slightly negative (δ−) regions in the molecule are shown for HF, H_2O, and NH_3. Fluorine, oxygen, and nitrogen are more electronegative than hydrogen and hence hold the electrons more tightly on their side than hydrogen.

electron transfer but will create unequal sharing of electrons in covalent bonding, *i.e.* the bonds exhibit a tendency for more of the electrons to be attracted to one end (F, O, or N) than the other (H) atom. We call this a *polarised bond* and designate the molecule as slightly more negative (δ−) at one end (F, O, or N) and slightly more positive (δ+) at the hydrogen end (Figure 2.4). As explained in the following sections, this kind of partial charge distribution (not as complete as an ionic bond) will be the basis for governing the physical and chemical properties of these molecules.

By using electronegativity differences, we have explained the formation of polar covalent bonds in HF, H_2O, and NH_3. In other words, a polarised bond has a *dipole*: a positive and a negative pole. As shown in Figure 2.5, the dipole can be illustrated by the plus sign on the hydrogen end of the bond towards the electronegative end.

Having explained the dipole nature of polar covalent bonds, we can apply the same principle to organic compounds. The electronegativity difference between carbon and hydrogen (Figure 2.6) is similar and the bond formed between them (*e.g.* methane, CH_4) does not show polarisation, *i.e.* a covalent bond between carbon and hydrogen is non-polar. On the other hand, the electronegativity differences between carbon and oxygen, carbon and nitrogen, and carbon and the group 17 halogen series elements (F, Cl, Br, and I) are large enough to

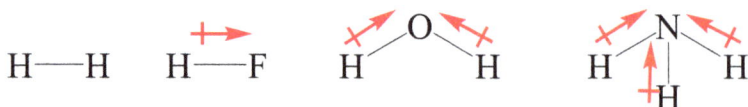

Figure 2.5 Representation of a dipole in hydrogen fluoride, water, and ammonia. Equal sharing of electrons such as in a diatomic hydrogen molecule, which has non-polar bonding, does not give a dipole. The electronegativity difference in covalent bond formation leads to a small charge difference or dipole. The base or plus (+) end of the arrows is where the partial positive charge ($\delta+$) is located.

Electronegativity: F > O > N > Cl > Br > C > H

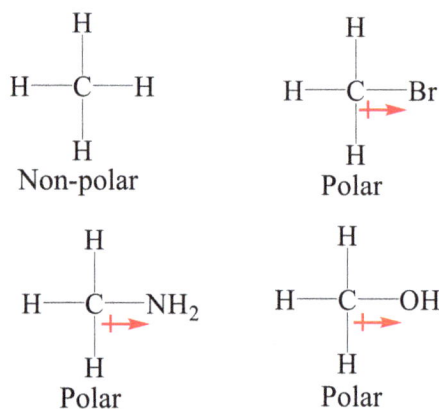

Figure 2.6 Dipole bond representation for carbon bonded with electronegative elements such as oxygen, nitrogen, and bromine.

give a polarised bond. This means that carbon is slightly more positively charged than these elements and hence a dipole bond is created (Figure 2.6).

There are, however, exceptions where a molecule has polarised bonds and yet it does not show a dipole. Let us consider carbon dioxide (CO_2). As shown in Figure 2.7, the molecular geometry of CO_2 is linear and the two polar bonds due to the electronegative oxygens attract electrons to the oxygen side but with the same magnitude in the opposite direction, *i.e.* two sets of dipole moments or vectors in the opposite direction give a net zero molecular dipole. As a result, CO_2 is non-polar. In a similar fashion, carbon tetrachloride (CCl_4, Figure 2.7) has no overall dipole (it has a molecular dipole of zero).

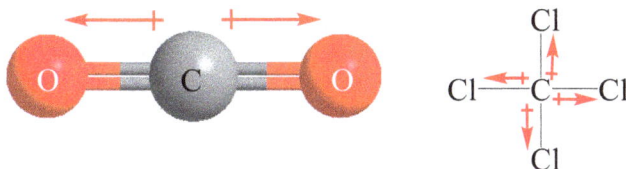

Figure 2.7 The presence of polar bonds may not be sufficient to make the molecule a dipole. Carbon dioxide (CO_2) and carbon tetrachloride (CCl_4) are used as examples to show that polarised bonds with the same magnitude in the opposite direction could lead to an overall net molecular dipole of zero, *i.e.* CO_2 and CCl_4 are non-polar.

Molecular Dipole – Key Facts

- Called the dipole moment of the molecule.
- Is a measure of overall polarity of the molecule.
- Depends on the magnitude of the individual polar bonds.
- Depends on the direction of the individual polar bonds.
- Depends on dipole moments of the individual polar bonds.

2.1.5 Electronegativity of Hybridised Orbitals in Carbon

In Chapter 1, we have seen the three hybridisation forms of orbitals in carbon, sp^3, sp^2, and sp, that form single, double, and triple bonds, respectively. We also highlighted how the number of p orbitals in these hybridisations differs: more p orbitals mean a higher energy level and size. In the latter case, the sizes of the three hybridisation forms are shown in Figure 2.8 and decrease in the order $sp^3 > sp^2 > sp$. This means that the electron pairs in the sp orbital are closer to the positively charged nuclei. As we have seen with elements in the Periodic Table such as the group 17 halogen series, smaller sized atoms are more electronegative than larger atoms. Hence the sp orbital is more electronegative than sp^2 and, in turn, sp^2 is more electronegative than sp^3.

Orbital Size and Electronegativity – Key Facts

- Orbital size of hybridised orbitals: $sp^3 > sp^2 > sp$.
- Electronegativity: $sp > sp^2 > sp^3$.

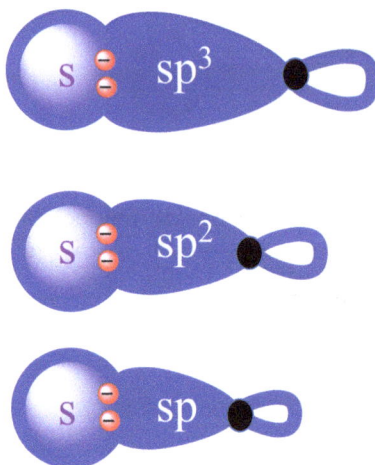

Figure 2.8 Orbital sizes of hybridised orbitals. In head-to-head overlapping with an s orbital of another element, note that the distance from the shared electrons to the atomic nuclei decreases in the order $sp^3 > sp^2 > sp$. The larger the atomic size, the less electronegative the atom becomes and hence the electronegativity decreases in the order $sp > sp^2 > sp^3$.

2.2 Intermolecular Forces

In covalent bonding, we have seen two or more atoms chemically bonded to form a molecule and this chemical bonding is based on the sharing of electrons. Based on the electronegativity difference between atoms, the forces that bring atoms together in a molecule – *intramolecular forces of attraction* – could vary. We have also highlighted that in extreme cases of electronegativity differences between atoms such as group 1 (metal) *versus* group 17 (nonmetal) elements, chemical bonding through electron transfer or ionic bonding occurs. Hence the *intramolecular forces of attraction* in ionic bonding are greater than in covalent bonding. We also have metallic bonding, although this is not relevant to our topic in organic chemistry and it will not be addressed here.

The term *intermolecular forces* refers to the attraction between molecules, and they govern how tightly molecules are packed together. These forces, although weaker than intramolecular forces, determine the physical properties of molecules such as boiling point, melting point, and density. The various types of intermolecular forces are described in the following sections.

2.2.1 London Dispersion Forces or van der Waals Forces

London dispersion forces or van der Waals forces represent the weakest intermolecular forces. They represent an attraction between two non-polar molecules (Figure 2.9) but exist in all types of molecules whether they are polar or non-polar, covalent, or ionic compounds.

In diatomic molecules, which we said have truly covalent bonds with equal sharing of electrons between atoms (*e.g.* Cl_2, Figure 2.9), we assume that the electrons are equally distributed around the nuclei within their shell. There is a probability, however, that the electrons may be momentarily denser at some regions and create a *temporary dipole*. Thus, any non-polar molecule has the capacity to be polarised (partially negative and partially positive ends) and form a dipole, and this dipole in return can induce the formation of charge separation in the neighbouring atom. Molecules through this momentary dipole formation can thus attract each other through forces that we call London dispersion forces or van der Waals forces.

Since the formation of London dispersion forces or van der Waals forces depends on the probability of electrons being temporarily polarised (denser in some areas), the higher the number of electrons in a molecule the stronger are the London dispersion forces. Thus bromine, with more electrons than chlorine, is expected to show a stronger London dispersion force than chlorine. For non-polar molecules that come together (attract each other) with these weak London

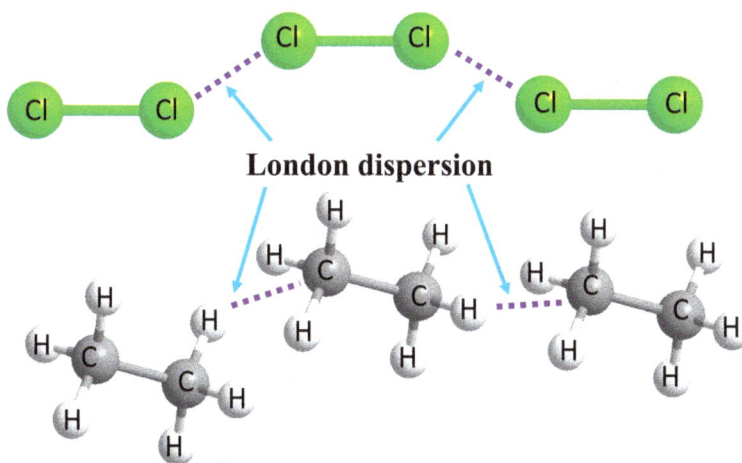

Figure 2.9 London dispersion forces or van der Waals forces of attraction between molecules.

dispersion forces, the molecular or electronic size can govern their physical properties. As shown in Figure 2.9, hydrocarbon molecules also attract each other through London dispersion forces.

London Dispersion Forces – Key Facts

- Exist in all molecules – polar or non-polar.
- Formed due to temporary instantaneous polarisation of electrons (temporary dipole) in a molecule.
- A temporary dipole in one molecule induces an opposing polarity in an adjacent molecule.
- Larger molecular size means larger electronic clouds that can give a higher degree of instantaneous polarisation, *i.e.* the larger the molecule the stronger are the London dispersion forces.

2.2.2 Dipole–Dipole Interactions

We have already explained that a molecular dipole exists when covalent bonding occurs between two elements that differ greatly in their electronegativity. We used the examples of water (H_2O), ammonia (NH_3), and hydrogen chloride (HCl). These molecules have a charge distribution and we used $\delta+$ and $\delta-$ to express dipole bonds and the molecular dipole environment. Figure 2.10 shows this charge distribution for HCl. The partially positively charged part of the HCl molecule (the hydrogen end) interacts with the partially negatively charged part of the neighbouring molecule (the Cl end). This type of *dipole–dipole interaction* brings the two molecules much closer together than the London dispersion forces. As a result, HCl occurs as a liquid instead of a gas (note that Cl_2 is a gas).

A dipole–dipole interaction can also occur in carbon–oxygen bonding. As oxygen is more electronegative than carbon, the $\delta+$ and $\delta-$ distribution to make a dipole molecule is evident in acetone (Figure 2.11).

Dipole–Dipole Interaction – Key Facts

- Is a feature of intermolecular interaction where there is a permanent dipole – polar bonds.
- Each molecule has partially charged ends ($\delta+$ and $\delta-$) that align with the opposite partial charge of another molecule.
- The interaction force is greater than the London dispersion force.
- Polar compounds with this interaction have a higher melting point and boiling point than non-polar compounds.

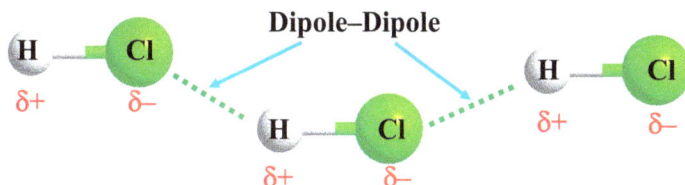

Figure 2.10　Dipole-dipole interaction between molecules of HCl.

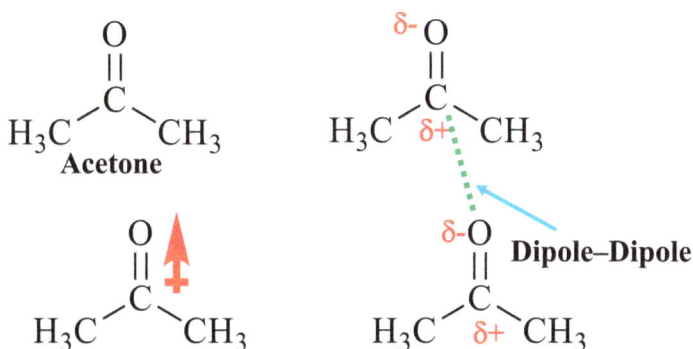

Figure 2.11　Dipole-dipole interaction in acetone.

2.2.3　Hydrogen Bonding

Hydrogen bonding is an example of a dipole–dipole interaction. It is considered as a special kind of dipole–dipole interaction and occurs when a hydrogen atom is bonded to oxygen, nitrogen, or fluorine. Figures 2.12 and 2.13 show hydrogen bonding in water, hydrogen bromide, and organic molecules such as alcohols. These three atoms (O, N, and F) are highly electronegative and make a good charge separation or polar bond with hydrogen. Hence the partially negative centre of F or O interacts with the partially positive end of hydrogen and this dipole–dipole interaction is called *hydrogen bonding*. Molecules such as water that exhibit hydrogen bonding as an intermolecular attraction force have high boiling points and melting points. In various sections of this book, we will address how hydrogen bonding is relevant to the physical properties of drug molecules and also their absorption and biological effects. Hydrogen bonding is also relevant in the structural integrity and biochemistry of biological macromolecules such as proteins and DNA.

Hydrogen Bonding – Key Facts

- Is a very strong dipole interaction – an example of dipole–dipole interaction.
- A feature of molecules where hydrogen is covalently bonded to nitrogen, oxygen, or fluorine.
- Stronger than dipole–dipole or London dispersion forces.

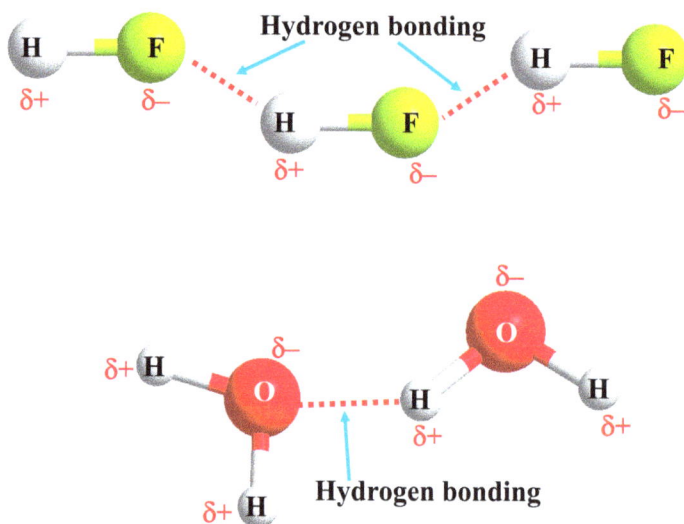

Figure 2.12   Hydrogen bonding in H_2O and HF.

2.2.4   Ionic Forces

The fourth type of intermolecular force of interaction is ionic forces that can bring oppositely charged species together while groups with the same charges repel each other. Positively charged groups called *cations* include ionised metals such as Na^+, K^+, and Ca^{2+} and ammonium ions (NH_4^+). In organic compounds, we will learn how nitrogen-containing compounds called amines form charged species due to nitrogen extending its valency to four. On the other hand, negatively charged species, called *anions*, include Cl^-, Br^-, and OH^-. The various functional groups forming charged species are discussed in Chapter 5 and their practical applications in the binding of drug molecules with biological targets are discussed in Chapter 12.

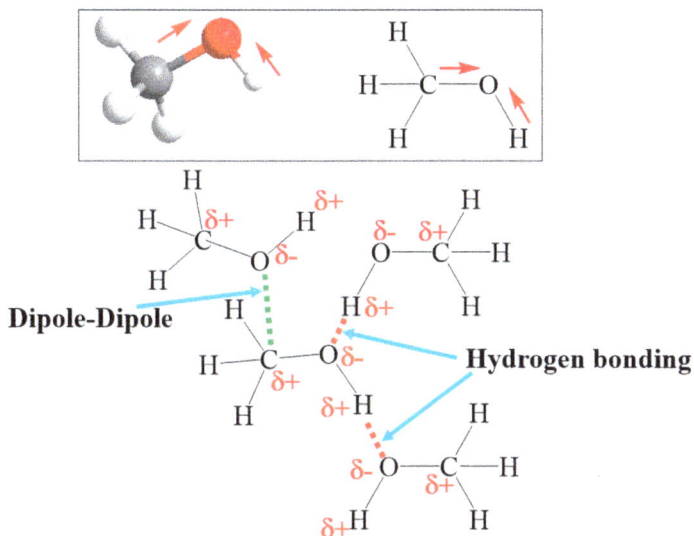

Figure 2.13 Hydrogen bonding in methanol.

2.3 Summary

In Chapter 1, we investigated the main feature of organic compounds, covalent bonding. This bonding has been further extended in this chapter to covalent non-polar and covalent polar bonds. The polarity of covalent bonds depends on the electronegativity of the elements or how far apart they are in the Periodic Table (horizontally). Nitrogen, oxygen, and group 17 elements (F, Cl, I, *etc.*) are more electronegative than carbon and hence form polar bonds with carbon. The bonding between hydrogen and these electronegative elements leads to a strong polarised bond. The common feature of a polar bond is a dipole, which is represented by partial charge or polarised electronic distribution as $\delta+$ and $\delta-$. The overall dipole of the molecule is the sum of the polarised bond and the direction and magnitude of the vectors. Hence molecules with polar bonds could have a net zero dipole or no molecular dipole.

The strongest intermolecular attraction in a polarised covalent bond is *via* hydrogen bonding, which is a special type of dipole–dipole interaction. The London force attractions are the weakest form of attraction and occur in non-polar bonds, *i.e.* the order of intermolecular attraction is ionic interaction > hydrogen bonding > dipole > London dispersion. A stronger intermolecular attraction means higher melting or boiling points.

2.4   Problems

1. By using carbon dioxide (CO_2) and carbon tetrachloride (CCl_4) as examples, explain why a molecule may not be a dipole in the presence of polar bonds.
2. Explain the polarity of hybridised orbitals based on atomic size.
3. Explain the dipole–dipole interaction between molecules of ethanol.
4. Hydrogen bonded to which elements leads to hydrogen bonding?
5. Show how ethanol has both dipole–dipole and hydrogen bonding interactions.
6. Which of the following is the strongest type of intermolecular bond: London dispersion forces, permanent dipole-to-dipole attractions, or hydrogen bonding?
7. Which intermolecular bond is caused by the temporary uneven distribution of electrons: London dispersion forces, permanent dipole-to-dipole attractions, or hydrogen bonding?
8. Crystals of NaCl dissolve in which of the following: hexane, benzene, water?
9. Assign the compounds shown in Table 2.1 to the appropriate group: ionic, polar covalent, non-polar covalent.
10. Ethanol is a liquid. When it evaporates, which bond in the molecule (C–C and C–H or C–O or O–H) breaks down?
11. What happens to the boiling point of alcohols that contain the O–H group compared with the same number of carbon and hydrogen atoms in a molecule without oxygen?

Questions 12–17 are based on Figure 2.14. Identify the compound that matches the following in Figure 2.14:

12. Has no polar covalent bonds.
13. Has a polar single bond to hydrogen.

Table 2.1   Question 9 is based on this table.

Compound	Ionic	Polar covalent	Non-polar covalent
HCl			
CH_4			
KI			
NH_3			
H_2O			
H_2			
N_2			
$CH_3CH_2CH_2CH_3$			

14. Has polar single bond to carbon.
15. Has polar double bond.
16. Has a polar triple bond.
17. Has a non-polar triple bond.
18. For the compounds shown in Figure 2.15, show partial charge separations to indicate how dipoles are created.
19. The dipole moment of organic molecules is a vector sum of polar bonds. Show this for the five compounds shown in Figure 2.16.
20. What is the order of strength of the following intermolecular forces: London force, hydrogen bonding, dipole–dipole interaction? Show your answer by using the three compounds shown in Figure 2.17. Comment on their physical properties.

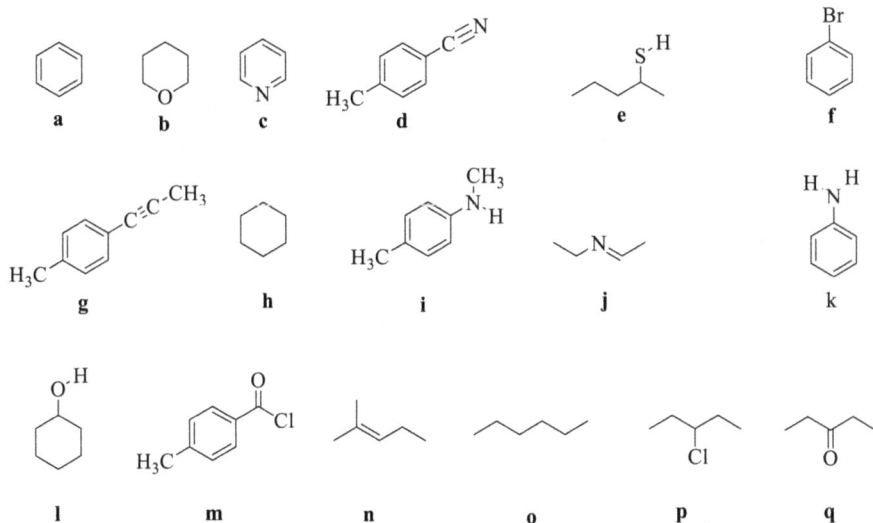

Figure 2.14 Questions 12–18 are based on structures **a–q** of this figure.

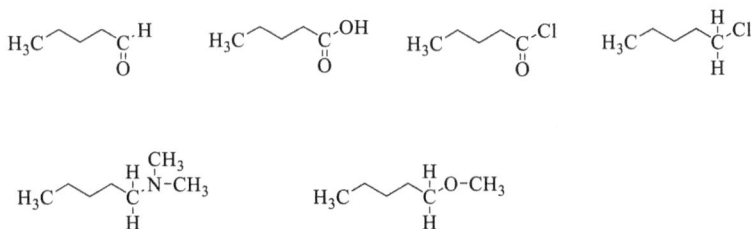

Figure 2.15 Question 18 is based on this figure.

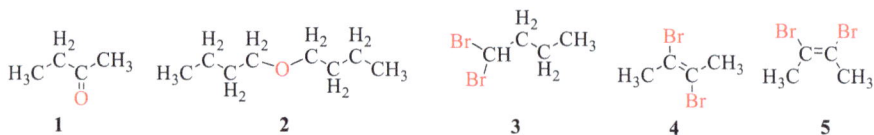

Figure 2.16 Question 19 is based on this figure.

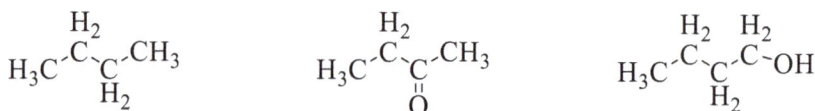

Figure 2.17 Question 20 is based on this figure.

2.5 Solutions to Problems

1. See Figure 2.7.
2. See Figure 2.8. The larger the atomic size, the less electronegative it is and hence the electronegativity decreases in the order sp $>$ sp^2 $>$ sp^3.
3. See Figure 2.13.
4. O, N, or F.
5. See Figure 2.13.
6. Order of intermolecular bonding strength: hydrogen bonding $>$ permanent dipole-to-dipole attractions $>$ London dispersion forces.
7. London dispersion forces.
8. Water – NaCl is formed through ionic bonding and is soluble in water.
9. See Table 2.2.
10. None – evaporation is a physical state change and does not involve bond breakage.
11. Alcohols form hydrogen bonds, and this makes the molecules pack tightly together. Hence they boil at a relatively higher temperature than those compounds without this hydrogen bonding.
12. **a, g, h, n,** and **o**.
13. **e, i, k,** and **l**.
14. **b, c, e, f, i, j, k, l, m,** and **p**.
15. **c, j, m,** and **q**.
16. **d**.
17. **g**.
18. See Figure 2.18.

Table 2.2 Answer to question 9.

Compound	Ionic	Polar covalent	Non-polar covalent
HCl		×	
CH_4			×
KI	×		
NH_3		×	
H_2O		×	
H_2			×
N_2			×
$CH_3CH_2CH_2CH_3$			×

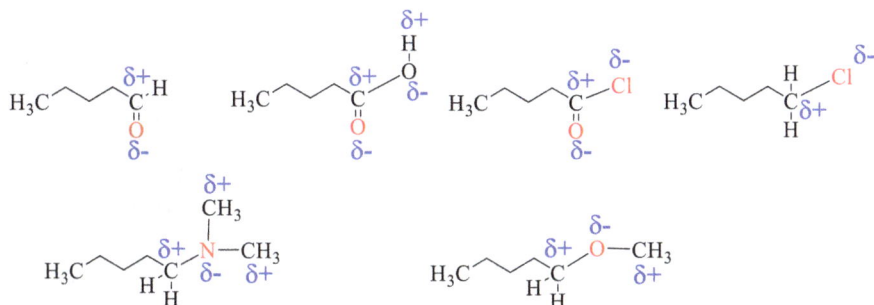

Figure 2.18 Answer to question 18.

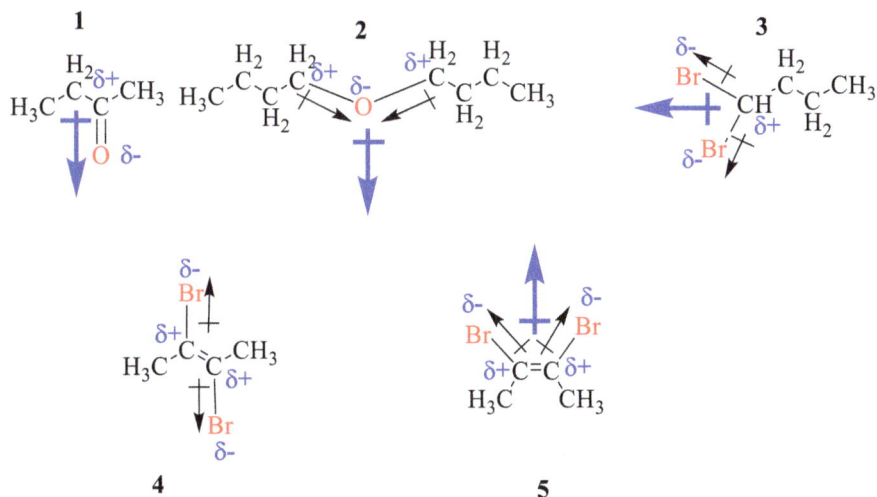

Figure 2.19 Answer to question 19.

19. The net dipole moment of the molecule is shown by the blue vector arrows (Figure 2.19). Note that an equal magnitude of vectors in the opposite direction for a compound cancels each other out, *i.e.* no net magnetic moment.

Butanol   Butanone   Butane

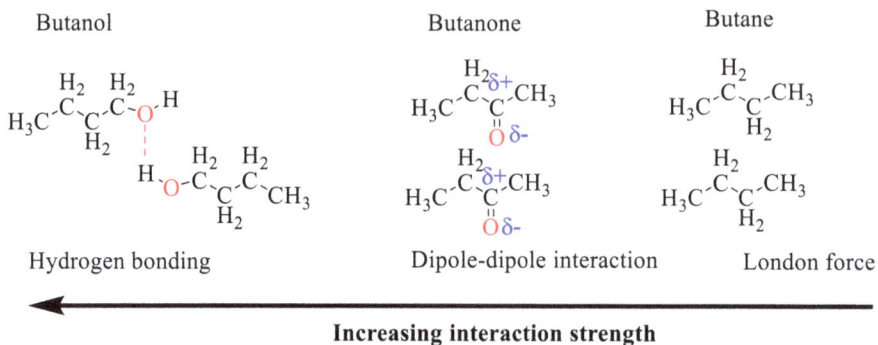

Hydrogen bonding   Dipole-dipole interaction   London force

Increasing interaction strength

Figure 2.20   Answer to question 20.

20. See Figure 2.20 for the type of interaction and order of strength.
    Butanol (*n*-butanol) with a strong hydrogen bonding interaction
    between molecules is a liquid with a boiling point of 117.7 °C.
    Butanone (but-1-one) with a lesser dipole–dipole bonding inter-
    action strength is still significant as it also occurs as a liquid with
    a boiling point of 77.6 °C. Butane (*n*-butane) with only London
    forces of attraction occurs as a gas.

3 Types of Organic Compounds, Nomenclature, and Basic Reactions: Alkanes and Cycloalkanes

Learning Objectives

After completing this chapter, you are expected to be able to:

- Describe the chemical bonding that makes up alkanes.
- Be able to name alkanes and cycloalkanes.
- Explain halogenation reactions of alkanes.

3.1 Definitions and General Characteristics of Alkanes

As outlined in Chapter 1, chemical compounds that contain carbon that is covalently bonded to other elements are generally called *organic compounds*. We will be looking at various types of organic compounds in this book, starting from simple *hydrocarbons* – compounds constructed just from hydrogen and carbon atoms. Within the hydrocarbon group, the simplest compounds are *alkanes*, which are defined as follows:

Basic Chemistry for Life Science Students and Professionals: Introduction to Organic Compounds and Drug Molecules
By Solomon Habtemariam
© Solomon Habtemariam 2023
Published by the Royal Society of Chemistry, www.rsc.org

- They are hydrocarbons – constructed from carbon and hydrogen atoms – and no other elements.
- They carry only C–C single bonds, *i.e.* there are no double or triple bonds in their molecules.
- All carbons are sp^3 hybridised, which defines their single-bond nature.
- The general formula of such hydrocarbons is C_nH_{2n+2}, where n is the number of carbon atoms in the molecule.
- They incorporate the maximum number of hydrogen atoms that can possibly be added in the C–C bonds – *they are fully saturated.*
- They used to be called *paraffins* – to mean without affinity. They are generally considered unreactive.

3.2   The Homologous Series of Alkanes

Let us consider the first four compounds in the homologous series, *i.e.* $n = 1$, $n = 2$, $n = 3$, and $n = 4$ in the C_nH_{2n+2} rule for alkanes. This gives us the molecular formulae CH_4, C_2H_6, C_3H_8, and C_4H_{10}. We call these compounds methane, ethane, propane, and butane, respectively. One common feature of their naming is that they all end with the suffix '*ane*'. Their presentation is shown in Table 3.1. As the carbon number increases by one, CH_2 is added to go to the next compound in the series.

Let us consider butane, which is written as $CH_3CH_2CH_2CH_3$. The repeating CH_2 group can be condensed to $(CH_2)_2$, as writing many CH_2 groups in a row can be cumbersome. Hence butane can also be written as $CH_3(CH_2)_2CH_3$ and, if we consider a larger alkane with 40 carbon atoms, its condensed structural formula can be written as $CH_3(CH_2)_{38}CH_3$.

One common physical property of the first four alkanes in the homologous series is that they occur as gases. As these compounds are very non-polar and small in molecular size, the only attraction force that holds their molecules together is the London dispersion intermolecular force of attraction (see Chapter 2). As a result, they are dispersed in space (not tightly packed together) and occur as gases.

As the number of carbon atoms increases in the homologous series, there may be different ways of arranging the atoms in the molecule. Let us consider butane, which we drew as a linear chain in Table 3.1. For the same formula (C_4H_{10}) that is derived from the C_nH_{2n+2} rule, we can also have a branched form called isobutane or 2-methylpropane (Figure 3.1).

Table 3.1 Examples of alkanes and their structural presentation using different models.

Alkane	Lewis model	Ball-and-stick model	Space-filling model	Skeletal model

Methane	H
	  |
	H–C–H
	  |
	H			

Ethane	H H | | H–C–C–H | | H H			—
Propane	H H H | | | H–C–C–C–H | | | H H H			
Butane	H H H H | | | | H–C–C–C–C–H | | | | H H H H			

n-Butane   Isobutane
                      (2-Methylpropane)

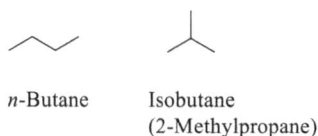

Figure 3.1 Isomers of butane.

To avoid confusion when naming butane, *n*-butane is used to refer to the linear chain form. The notation '*n*' means 'normal', and the branched form is called a structural isomer of *n*-butane. We will address more of the structural isomers in the following sections.

Alkanes from pentane to decane (Table 3.2) are all liquids and, as expected, their boiling point increases with increase in molecular size. This is explained by the correlation between the London dispersion intermolecular attraction force and the size of the molecule.

Table 3.2   Some unbranched alkanes and their boiling points.[a]

Name	Molecular formula	Structural formula	Boiling point/$^{\circ}$C
Pentane	C_5H_{12}	$CH_3(CH_2)_3CH_3$	36
Hexane	C_6H_{14}	$CH_3(CH_2)_4CH_3$	69
Heptane	C_7H_{16}	$CH_3(CH_2)_5CH_3$	98
Octane	C_8H_{18}	$CH_3(CH_2)_6CH_3$	126
Nonane	C_9H_{20}	$CH_3(CH_2)_7CH_3$	151
Decane	$C_{10}H_{22}$	$CH_3(CH_2)_8CH_3$	174

[a]Note that the boiling point increases with increase in molecular size. The boiling point data were sourced from the Hazardous Substances Data Bank (HSDB), which is available *via* Pub-Chem (https://pubchem.ncbi.nlm.nih.gov/). The unbranched structure of these compounds can be specifically indicated by using the prefix *n-* for normal-, as in *n*-pentane, *n*-hexane, *n*-heptane, *etc.*

Thus, the smallest molecular sizes of alkanes (with up to four carbon atoms) are gases, then larger alkanes occur as liquids, with the boiling point increasing with increase in molecular size, and eventually the largest alkanes (with more than 20 carbon atoms) are solids. Alkanes as hydrocarbons are *hydrophobic (water-hating) compounds*, and they are soluble in organic solvents.

Alkanes – Key Facts

- Hydrocarbons – only hydrogen and carbon atoms in their molecule.
- Single covalent bonds.
- No double or triple bonds – they are saturated.
- Structural formula C_nH_{2n+2}.

Looking at the three-dimensional structures of decane (Figure 3.2), it is easy to see the zigzag pattern, which is due to the tetrahedral nature of the sp^3 orbitals in carbon (see Chapter 1).

Continuing with the two structural isomers that we considered for butane, the number of alternative ways of arranging atoms in the molecule increases with increase in molecular size. Thus, hexane has a straight-chain isomer (*n*-hexane) and four other isomers (see Figure 3.3). We will consider their naming in the following section.

3.3   The IUPAC Nomenclature System for Alkanes

As we have already learned from the previous sections, butane may be used as a general name for *n*-butane and isobutane, and many other alkanes are also known by common names. The International Union

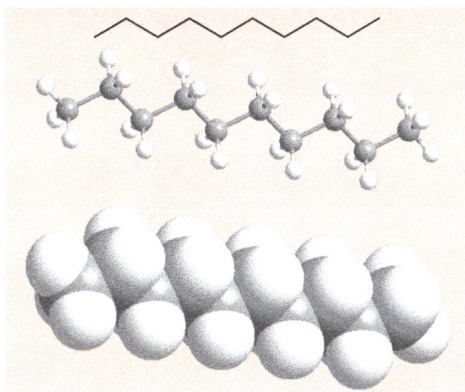

Figure 3.2 Structure of decane. Note the zigzag pattern of the structure.

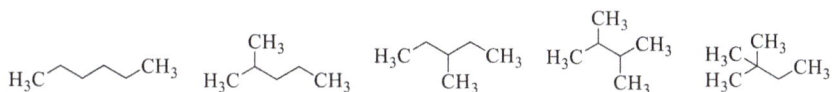

Figure 3.3 Isomers of hexane.

of Pure and Applied Chemistry (IUPAC) nomenclature is designed to adopt a systematic approach to naming compounds using rules. Let us consider naming the compound shown in Figure 3.4.

1. As shown in Figure 3.4, we must first identify the longest continuous chain of carbon atoms in the molecule. In this case, the longest chain is based on seven carbons, so the compound is a sort of *heptane*. All alkanes have the suffix '*ane*'.
2. We then identify the groups attached to the chain identified in step 1. In this case, the substituent is methyl. A methane-based attachment is methyl, ethane-based is ethyl, propane-based is propyl, *etc.*
3. We now need to number the long chain starting from one end and making sure that the branching gets the lowest number. In the example shown in Figure 3.4, numbering the compound from left to right gives a smaller number for the branching. Hence the name of the compound is 3-methylheptane.

Let us consider a similar compound that carries an additional attachment of a methyl group at the carbon-2 position as shown in Figure 3.5. In this case, we use the designation dimethyl and name it 2,3-dimethylheptane. One can use the designations tri, tetra, penta, *etc.*, for repeating substituents on the long continuous chain.

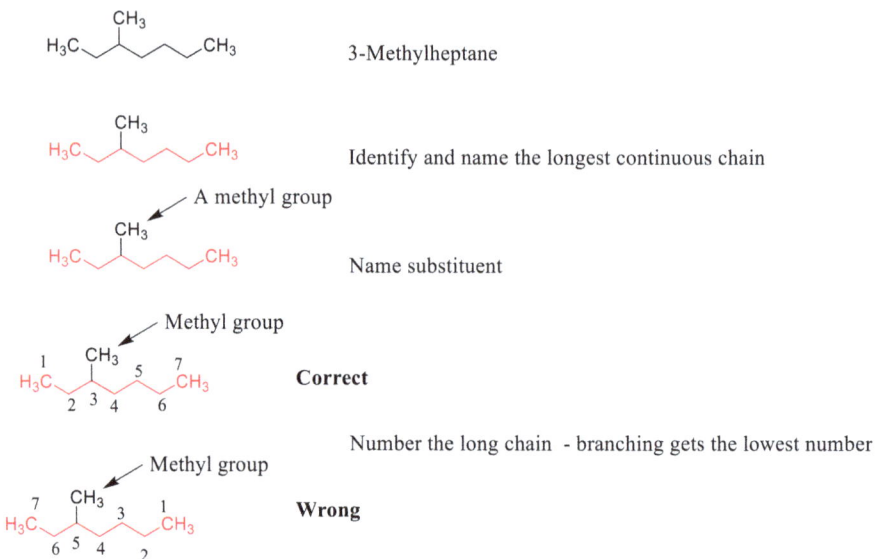

3-Methylheptane

Identify and name the longest continuous chain

A methyl group

Name substituent

Methyl group

Correct

Number the long chain - branching gets the lowest number

Methyl group

Wrong

Figure 3.4 Steps taken in the naming of alkanes: 3-methylheptane.

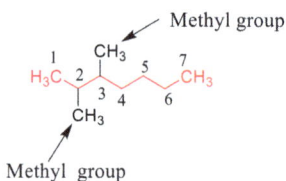

Figure 3.5 Naming alkanes: 2,3-dimethylheptane.

A similar compound that carries an attachment of an ethyl group at the carbon-2 position is shown in Figure 3.6. In this case, we use alphabetical orders of substituents – ethyl comes before methyl, so we name the compound 4-ethyl-3-methylheptane.

3.4   Cycloalkanes

Table 3.3 lists some common low molecular weight cycloalkanes. Starting from the smallest unit, cyclopropane, we add one CH_2 unit at a time to move to the next compound in the homologous series. You have probably already noticed that cycloalkanes are two hydrogens short compared with their corresponding alkane, *e.g.* propane *versus* cyclopropane. This means that the general formula for cycloalkanes is C_nH_{2n}, where *n* is again the number of carbon atoms in the molecule.

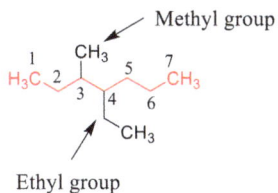

Figure 3.6 Naming alkanes: 4-ethyl-3-methylheptane.

Table 3.3 Examples of cycloalkanes.

Name	Molecular formula	Line structure	Ball-and-stick model
Cyclopropane	C_3H_6		
Cyclobutane	C_4H_8		
Cyclopentane	C_5H_{10}		
Cyclohexane	C_6H_{12}		
Cycloheptane	C_7H_{14}		

Hence, for one ring to form, we have a loss of two hydrogen atoms from the alkane's formula (C_nH_{2n+2}).

The IUPAC nomenclature rules set out for alkanes also apply to cycloalkanes. We name the cycloalkanes based on the number of carbons involved – if six carbon atoms are present, we start with cyclohexane of some sort. Naming the substituents and making the branching number as low as possible are also the same as in the nomenclature for alkanes. See the examples shown in Figure 3.7.

3.5 Sources of Alkanes

The major sources of alkanes are the petrochemical industry and natural gas. Natural gas mainly contains methane (80–95%) whereas petroleum is a mixture of gases, gasoline, fuel oil, lubricating oil, asphalt, *etc.* These components can be separated by distillation at their respective boiling points (fractional distillation). In addition to hydrocarbons, petroleum also contains small amounts of oxygen-, sulfur- and nitrogen-containing compounds. As the focus of this book is mainly on introducing organic chemistry to life science professionals and students, we do not need to go into the details of how alkanes are extracted from these sources.

3.6 Reactions of Alkanes

Going back to the old name for alkanes, 'paraffin' is based on the Latin words '*parum*', referring to too little or barely, and '*affin*', meaning related. Hence their traditional name refers to the rather small affinity they possess for other bodies. Alkanes are generally considered as compounds that do not react with traditional chemical reagents such as acids and bases. One exception is that alkanes react rapidly with oxygen.

Let us consider the reaction of methane (CH_4) with oxygen:

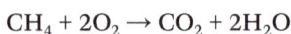

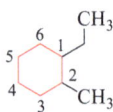

$$CH_4 + 2O_2 \rightarrow CO_2 + 2H_2O$$

1-Ethyl-2-methylcyclohexane   1-Ethyl-2,4-dimethylcyclohexane   1,2,4-Trimethylcyclohexane

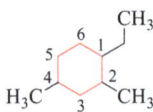

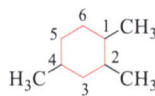

Figure 3.7 Examples of cycloalkanes and their nomenclature.

$$\text{H-}\overset{\displaystyle H}{\underset{\displaystyle H}{\text{C}}}\text{-H} + \text{Cl-Cl} \longrightarrow \text{H-}\overset{\displaystyle H}{\underset{\displaystyle H}{\text{C}}}\text{-Cl} + \text{HCl}$$

or simply

$$CH_4 + Cl_2 \longrightarrow CH_3Cl + HCl$$

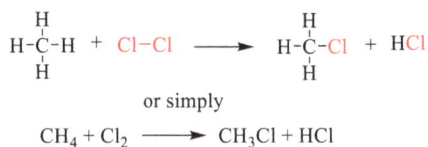

Figure 3.8 Chlorination of methane.

This is a combustion reaction or burning. For complete combustion to occur, there should be a good flow of oxygen or plenty of air. Burning methane also gives rise to soot, *i.e.* particulate carbon, so not all of the methane undergoes complete combustion. The variety of possible products obtained shows that the combustion of methane is a very complicated reaction. It is now known to proceed *via* the formation of *free radicals*.

Chapters 1 and 2 presented several examples of covalent bonding, and discussed how electrons are shared between atoms to make molecules. Electrons like to be paired up and make the atom or the molecule remain in the lowest energy level or most stable form. We will now be looking at scenarios where electrons exist unpaired and form intermediate species called free radicals.

Free radicals are fragments of molecules that contain an *unpaired electron*. Since *electrons love to pair up*, free radicals are highly *reactive*. As combustion is a complicated reaction, let us use the simple example of the chlorination reaction of alkanes such as methane (CH_4), which involves free radicals. The reaction can be summarised as shown in Figure 3.8, although we will see in the following sections how complicated the reaction is.

This is what we call a *substitution reaction* (see Chapter 11), in which one atom in a molecule is swapped with another. In this case, chlorine is swapped with hydrogen. The reaction, however, requires an energy input and occurs when the reaction mixture is exposed to ultraviolet (UV) light. Thus, methane with initiation from UV light can undergo a reaction with halogens such as chlorine in three stages as follows:

1. *Initiation* is a stage where energy from UV light is used to generate free radicals: chlorine radicals. This means that the covalent bond that makes up the homonuclear diatomic molecule of chlorine (Cl_2) is broken to generate two chlorine atoms, each carrying an unpaired electron:

$$Cl_2 \xrightarrow{\text{UV}} 2Cl^{\bullet}$$

2. *Propagation* refers to the chain of reactions that follows once a free radical is generated. This includes

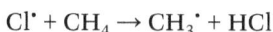

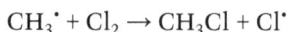

$$Cl^{\bullet} + CH_4 \rightarrow CH_3^{\bullet} + HCl$$

$$CH_3^{\bullet} + Cl_2 \rightarrow CH_3Cl + Cl^{\bullet}$$

3. *Termination* is the last step that ends the reaction and occurs when two radical species react with each other to form a stable non-radical product:

$$CH_3^{\bullet} + Cl^{\bullet} \rightarrow CH_3Cl$$

In the above example, the chlorination of methane or the substitution reaction with a methane and chlorine mixture in the presence of UV light yields chloromethane (CH_3Cl) as the final product. Reactions that involve free radicals, however, also yield numerous other side products. For example, the product of the above reaction, chloromethane, can react with other radicals in the system, including chlorine free radicals:

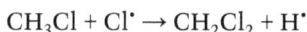

$$CH_3Cl + Cl^{\bullet} \rightarrow CH_2Cl_2 + H^{\bullet}$$

As a termination reaction, two methyl radicals can also combine to form ethane (C_2H_6):

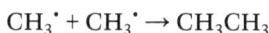

$$CH_3^{\bullet} + CH_3^{\bullet} \rightarrow CH_3CH_3$$

The reaction can go through further propagation and termination reactions as follows:

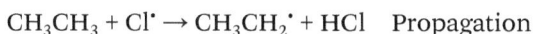

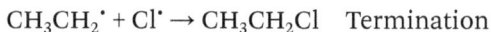

$$CH_3CH_3 + Cl^{\bullet} \rightarrow CH_3CH_2^{\bullet} + HCl \quad \text{Propagation}$$

$$CH_3CH_2^{\bullet} + Cl^{\bullet} \rightarrow CH_3CH_2Cl \quad \text{Termination}$$

Hence, although free radical-based chlorination of methane gives mainly chloromethane (CH_3Cl), it is a 'messy' reaction with so many other products also being formed. In the examples above, ethane and dichloromethane are formed. What about butane (C_4H_{10})? A trace amount of butane, $CH_3CH_2CH_2CH_3$, can also be formed from the free radical-based substitution reaction involving methane and chlorine:

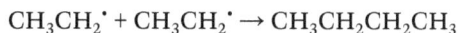

$$CH_3CH_2^{\bullet} + CH_3CH_2^{\bullet} \rightarrow CH_3CH_2CH_2CH_3$$

The above examples involve a chlorination reaction where we introduced a chlorine atom into the molecules of alkanes. The reaction is similar with other halogen series elements such as F, I, and Br. Hence we simply call the reaction a halogenation reaction, which includes chlorination, bromination, iodination, *etc.*

In summary, alkanes are not reactive except for the combustion reaction with oxygen that we effectively exploit in our households, such as its use for heating and cooking and other forms of energy generation. When exposed to UV light, alkanes, as we have seen for methane, can undergo a substitution reaction with halogens. The reaction is difficult to control, however, with so many other side products being formed.

Free radicals are relevant in biology. They are involved in cellular signalling processes and are also components of arsenals of our host defence mechanism against invading pathogens and parasites. They are produced continuously in our body through various mechanisms, including the mitochondrial electron chain reaction that we use to generate energy. Their level must, however, be checked by numerous antioxidant mechanisms in the body so that they do not damage tissues through their messy reactions with key biological molecules. When the balance between their formation and elimination is not maintained and we have excessive levels of free radicals, diseases such as arthritis, diabetes, and cancer can develop. This is an exciting topic for scientists in the fields of both biology and chemistry to understand pathological processes in diseases and to discover new drugs/medicines.

3.7 Summary

In this chapter, we have learned the following:

- Alkanes are organic compounds with the general formula C_nH_{2n+2}.
- Cycloalkanes are alkanes with a cyclic structure and have the general formula C_nH_{2n}.
- Alkanes and cycloalkanes are saturated compounds – there is no double bond in their molecules.
- We use the IUPAC nomenclature system for naming alkanes:
  - Longest chain – the parent name has the suffix 'ane' and a prefix of Greek numbering, meth, eth, prop, *etc.*, *i.e.* methane, ethane, propane, butane, *etc.*
  - Branching or substituents are named alkyl: methyl, ethyl, propyl, *etc.*
  - Numbering the parent chain (left to right or right to left) is done by making sure that the branching gets the lowest number.
  - Substituents are given in the name in alphabetical order – ethyl before methyl, *etc.*

- o Identical substituents are named di, tri, tetra, *etc.*, *e.g.* 2,2-dimethylpentane.
- o The same principle applies for naming cycloalkanes – we use the suffix 'ane', the prefix 'cyclo' and the Greek numbering prop, but, pent, *etc.*, in the middle, *e.g.* cyclopentane.

- Alkanes and cycloalkanes are generally not reactive except for the combustion reaction.
- One common reaction of alkanes and cycloalkanes is the halogenation reaction – introducing a halogen atom into the molecule.

- o Examples are chlorination – introducing chlorine; bromination – introducing bromine; iodination – introducing iodine; *etc.*
- o The reaction goes through free radical generation by irradiation with UV light.
- o Free radical generation, propagation, and termination constitute a multi-step process.
- o Reaction through free radicals is messy and produces several side products.
- o Free radicals are unstable and highly reactive species, which has implications in the development of several disease conditions.

3.8 Problems

Questions 1–7 are based on Figure 3.9. Name the common substituents on the alkane parent chain.

1. _____
2. _____
3. _____
4. _____
5. _____
6. _____
7. _____

Questions 8–12 are based on the structures in Figure 3.10. Name the compounds shown.

8. _____
9. _____
10. _____
11. _____
12. _____

Questions 13–17. Name the structures of the cycloalkanes shown in Figure 3.11.

13. _____
14. _____
15. _____
16. _____
17. _____
18. Show the chlorination of cyclohexane *via* irradiation with UV light. Indicate the three stages of the free radical reactions.

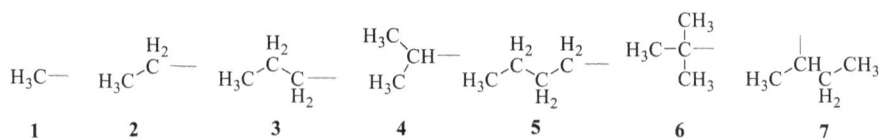

Figure 3.9 Questions 1–7 are based on this figure.

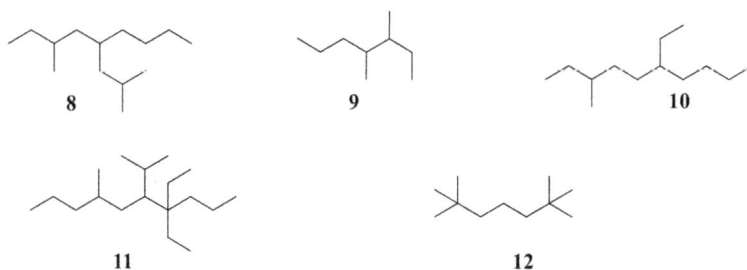

Figure 3.10 Questions 8–12 are based on this figure.

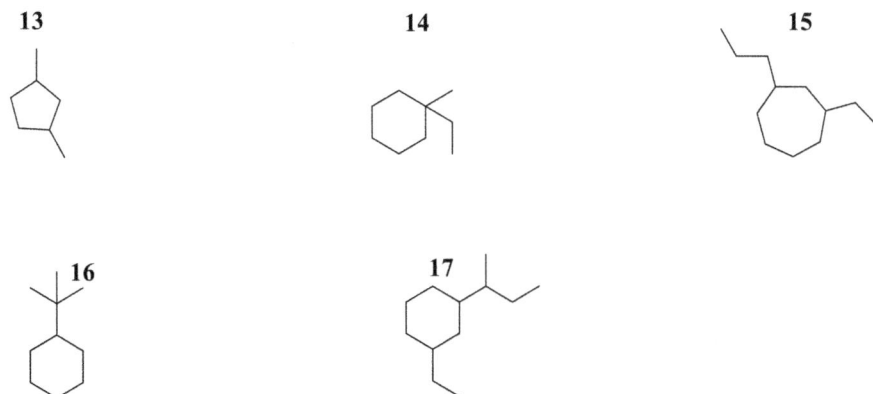

Figure 3.11 Questions 13–17 are based on this figure.

3.9 Solutions to Problems

1. Methyl.
2. Ethyl.
3. Propyl.
4. Isopropyl.
5. Butyl.
6. *t*-Butyl (*tert*-butyl).
7. *s*-Butyl (*sec*-butyl).
8. 3-Ethyl-5-(2-methylpropyl)nonane.
9. 3,4-Dimethylheptane.
10. 6-Ethyl-3-methyldecane.
11. 4,4-Diethyl-5-isopropyl-7-methyldecane.
12. 2,2,6,6-Tetramethylheptane.
13. 1,3-Dimethylcyclopentane.
14. 1-Ethyl-1-methylcyclohexane.
15. 1-Ethyl-3-propylcycloheptane.
16. *tert*-Butylcyclohexane.
17. 1-*sec*-Butyl-3-ethylhexane.
18. Other side products are also formed but the main ones are shown in Figure 3.12.

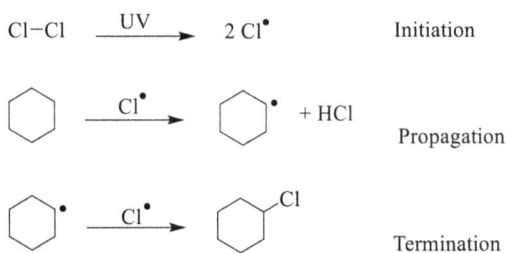

Figure 3.12 Answer to question 18.

4 Types of Organic Compounds, Nomenclature, and Basic Reactions: Alkenes, Cycloalkenes, and Other Unsaturated Hydrocarbons

Learning Objectives

After completing this chapter, you are expected to be able to answer the following questions:

- What are the distinguishing features of alkenes?
- How do we name alkenes from their structures and *vice versa*?
- What are geometrical isomers?
- What are the sources of alkenes – natural and synthesised?
- What are cycloalkenes?
- What are the main reactions of alkenes and how do we predict the yields?
- What are aromatic hydrocarbons?
- What are alkynes and how do we name them?

Basic Chemistry for Life Science Students and Professionals: Introduction to Organic Compounds and Drug Molecules
By Solomon Habtemariam
© Solomon Habtemariam 2023
Published by the Royal Society of Chemistry, www.rsc.org

4.1 Alkenes

4.1.1 Definition

Like alkanes, alkenes are hydrocarbons, hence their molecular composition is based only on carbon and hydrogen atoms. All alkenes contain at least one carbon–carbon double bond (C=C). Since one double bond means a loss of two hydrogen atoms from the corresponding alkanes, alkenes have the general formula C_nH_{2n}. Note that alkanes have the general formula C_nH_{2n+2}, where n represents the number of carbon atoms in the molecule. As alkenes do not have the maximum possible number of hydrogen atoms that can be bonded with carbon, we call them *unsaturated*. In the literature, alkenes are also known as *olefins*.

4.1.2 The Homologous Series of Alkenes

Like alkanes, there is a series of alkenes with each one being one CH_2 group larger than the previous compound in the series. However, unlike alkanes, there is no analogue of methane (CH_4), and the smallest alkene is C_2H_4 followed by C_3H_6, C_4H_8, C_5H_{10}, *etc.* They all have the suffix '*ene*': ethene, propene, butene, pentene, hexene, *etc.* Let us consider the first two in the homologous series (Table 4.1).

Both ethene and propene are low molecular weight non-polar compounds that occur as gases. There is only one possible way of placing the double bond in the molecule, hence they do not have isomers. Let us now consider the next compound in the homologous series,

Table 4.1 Alkenes: ethene and propene.

Name	Old name	Structure	Ball-and-stick model	State
Ethene	Ethylene	H H H H		Gas
Propene	Propylene	H H H C-H H H		Gas

butene, where we have the possibility of placing the double bond at the terminal carbon (end of the chain) or between the two middle carbon atoms (Figure 4.1).

But-1-ene and but-2-ene are two isomers (see Chapter 6) of butene and, by numbering the carbons, we can name the compounds in such a way that we indicate the position of the double bond in the molecule. Note that we number the carbons by making sure that *the double bond gets the lowest possible number*. See the possibility in Figure 4.2, where, if we number the carbons from right to left, we would have the incorrect name but-3-ene instead of but-1-ene.

There is also another isomer of butene, 2-methylpropene (old name isobutylene). Hence we now have three structural isomers of butene (Figure 4.3).

For but-2-ene, we have another type of isomer to consider (see Figure 4.4). Since there is no rotation around the C=C double bond, the methyl groups can be on the same side of the molecule (*Z*- or *cis*-) or opposite sides (*E*- or *trans*-). Hence, based on the geometry of groups attached to the C=C double bond, we also have isomers called *geometrical isomers* (Figure 4.4).

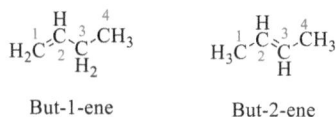

But-1-ene   But-2-ene

Figure 4.1 Possible structures of butene. The two structural isomers based on the position of the double bond are shown.

Figure 4.2 Example of incorrect numbering. In IUPAC nomenclature, we can number carbons in the molecule from left to right or right to left, making sure that the double bond gets the lowest possible numbering.

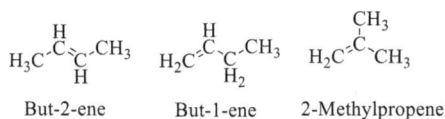

But-2-ene   But-1-ene   2-Methylpropene

Figure 4.3 Isomers of butene.

E or *trans* isomer
(*E*)-But-2-ene

Z or *cis* isomer
(*Z*)-But-2-ene

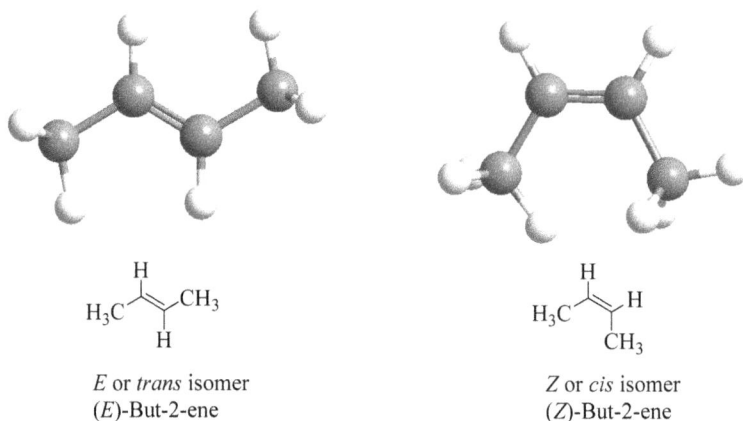

Figure 4.4 Geometrical isomers of but-2-ene.

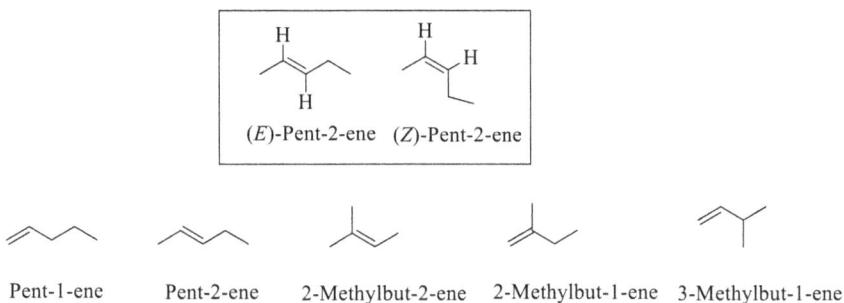

(*E*)-Pent-2-ene   (*Z*)-Pent-2-ene

Pent-1-ene   Pent-2-ene   2-Methylbut-2-ene   2-Methylbut-1-ene   3-Methylbut-1-ene

Figure 4.5 Isomers of pentene. As explained for but-2-ene, pent-2-ene also
has two forms of geometrical isomers.

As the number of carbons increases in the homologous series, the number of possible isomers also increases. For pentene, we have the structural isomers shown in Figure 4.5.

In Chapter 6, the various types of isomerism and their significance in biology are described. The physical properties of alkenes are similar to those of alkanes. The compounds of smallest molecular size occur as gases and larger compounds are liquids with increasing boiling points as the molecular size increases. Pentene is a liquid with a boiling point of 29.9 °C, heptene is a liquid with a boiling point of 93.6 °C, and dec-1-ene is a liquid with a boiling point of 170.5 °C. Eventually, the increase in molecular size results in a solid format, the melting point of which also depends on molecular size. The 20-carbon alkene dodec-1-ene, however, still occurs as a liquid with a boiling point of 213.8 °C. Hence most of the common alkenes are gases and liquids. Since alkenes are non-polar, they are not soluble in water. As *hydrophobic compounds*, they are soluble in organic solvents.

4.1.3 Nomenclature of Alkenes

The IUPAC nomenclature system for alkenes follows the same principle as that described for alkanes in Chapter 3. Hence we start by identifying the longest possible carbon chain that contains the double bond:

- When we assign the longest possible chain, it must contain the double bond within the chain. Note that a longer chain that does not contain the double bond may be found in some compounds. With this in mind, first identify the longest possible chain.
- We number the carbons by making sure that the double bond gets the lowest possible number.
- In much of the literature, you may find alkene names written with the location of the double bond given *before* the parent name, *e.g.* 1-pentene, 2-nonene, 4-heptene, *etc.* The accepted IUPAC naming, however, is now pent-1-ene, non-2-ene, hept-4-ene, *etc.*
- If there is more than one double bond in the molecule, the suffixes *diene*, *triene*, *tetraene*, *etc.*, are used. These also in the older literature are mostly written as 1,4-pentadiene, 1,5,7-decatriene, *etc.*, but here we use the current IUPAC nomenclature, penta-1,4-diene, deca-1,5,7-triene, *etc.*
- The entry of substituents and alphabetical order in the naming are similar to those described for alkanes (Chapter 3), *e.g.* 2,3,4-trimethyldeca-1,5,7-triene.

Study these IUPAC rules by using the named structures in Figure 4.6.

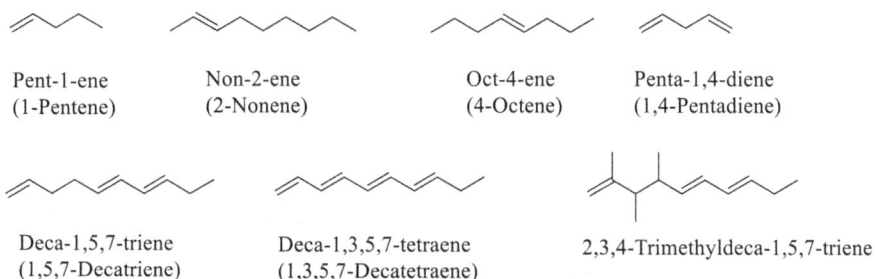

Pent-1-ene   Non-2-ene   Oct-4-ene   Penta-1,4-diene
(1-Pentene)   (2-Nonene)   (4-Octene)   (1,4-Pentadiene)

Deca-1,5,7-triene   Deca-1,3,5,7-tetraene   2,3,4-Trimethyldeca-1,5,7-triene
(1,5,7-Decatriene)   (1,3,5,7-Decatetraene)

Figure 4.6 Nomenclature of alkenes. The IUPAC names are used. Older names which are still in use in the literature are given in parentheses.

Alkenes – Key Facts

- Unsaturated hydrocarbons with a –C=C– double bond in the molecule.
- Named by using the suffix 'ene'.
- In the naming, first identify the longest chain that contains the double bond – naming substituents similarly to alkanes.
- Similar physical properties to those of alkanes – generally non-polar.
- Increased boiling or melting point with increase in molecular size.
- Can have a *cis* or *trans* configuration of isomers.

4.1.4 Sources of Alkenes

4.1.4.1 Natural Sources

As with alkanes, the major source of alkenes is the petrochemical industry. Alkenes also commonly occur in Nature in plants, animals, and microorganisms. The terpenoid class of compounds (see Chapter 13) includes isoprene, farnesene, and lycopene, which is a powerful antioxidant compound found in tomatoes (Figure 4.7).

Alkenes can also be obtained in the laboratory through chemical reactions. The two main methods for the synthesis of alkenes are described below.

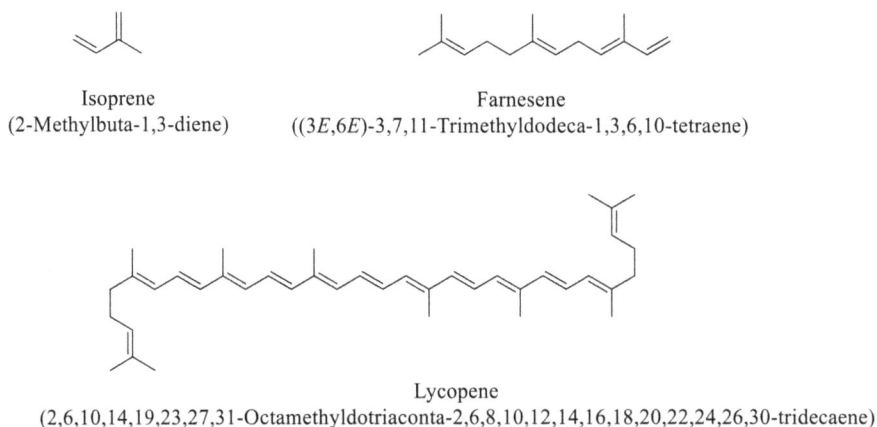

Isoprene
(2-Methylbuta-1,3-diene)

Farnesene
((3*E*,6*E*)-3,7,11-Trimethyldodeca-1,3,6,10-tetraene)

Lycopene
(2,6,10,14,19,23,27,31-Octamethyldotriaconta-2,6,8,10,12,14,16,18,20,22,24,26,30-tridecaene)

Figure 4.7 Structures of some natural alkenes. While these compounds are known by their trivial names, their IUPAC naming (in parentheses) can be used to indicate the position of the double bond and identify the geometrical isomers (omitted for lycopene owing to its structural complexity).

4.1.4.2   A Dehydrohalogenation Reaction Such As Loss of HCl from an Alkyl Chloride

The dehydrohalogenation reaction is an example of an *elimination reaction* (see Chapter 11) since one compound yields more than one product by removing certain smaller fragments of the molecule. As shown in Figure 4.8, chlorine and hydrogen are extracted from two adjacent carbon atoms to give a product with a C=C double bond – an *alkene*. The reaction requires a strong base such as potassium hydroxide in ethanol and heat. The extraction of chorine and hydrogen in this reaction is also called a *dehydrochlorination* reaction.

4.1.4.3   Loss of H_2O From an Alcohol (Dehydration Reaction)

In the presence of acids such as sulfuric acid (H_2SO_4) and with heating, alcohols can also yield alkenes by losing water (Figure 4.9).

4.1.4.4   Reaction Yields in the Synthesis of Alkenes from Alkyl Halides and Alcohols

Let us now consider scenarios of the above-mentioned alkene formation by using 2-chlorobutane as an example. In this elimination reaction, chlorine is removed from carbon-2 (C-2) while hydrogen can

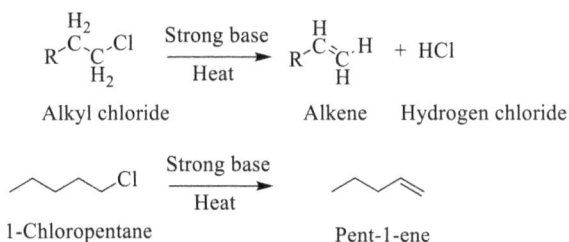

Figure 4.8   Dehydrochlorination reaction. This is a type of elimination reaction that removes hydrogen halide from alkyl halides.

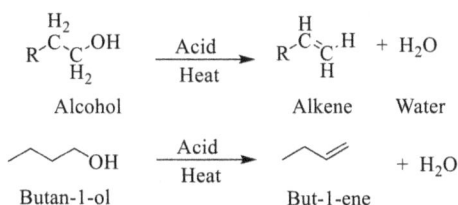

Figure 4.9   Dehydration of alcohols to form alkenes.

be removed from either C-1 or C-3. This would yield two products, but-1-ene and but-2-ene (Figure 4.10).

From the reaction shown in Figure 4.10, it can be seen that the two alkene products are not produced in a 50:50 ratio as the predominant product is but-2-ene. The same trend is also observed in the synthesis of alkenes *via* the dehydration reaction of alcohols (*e.g.* butan-2-ol), where but-2-ene is the predominant product (Figure 4.11).

Sources of Alkenes – Key Facts

- Occur naturally – mainly from the petrochemical industry.
- Plants and animals also have alkenes as metabolites, *e.g.* carotenes.
- Chemical synthesis *via* dehydrohalogenation of alkyl halides.
- Chemical synthesis *via* dehydration of alcohols.
- The reaction yield of dehydrohalogenation and dehydration reactions can be predicted based on the stability of the products.

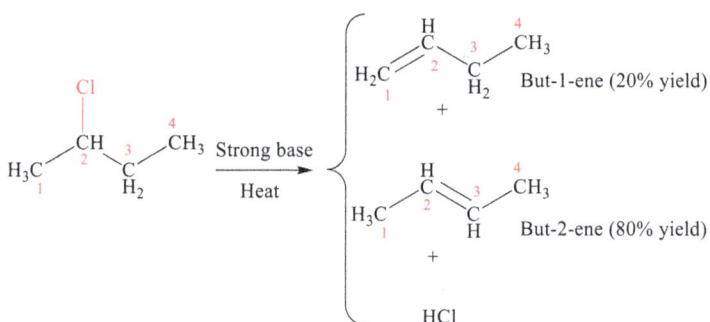

Figure 4.10   Dehydrochlorination of 2-chlorobutane. Note that the two products are not produced in the same yield.

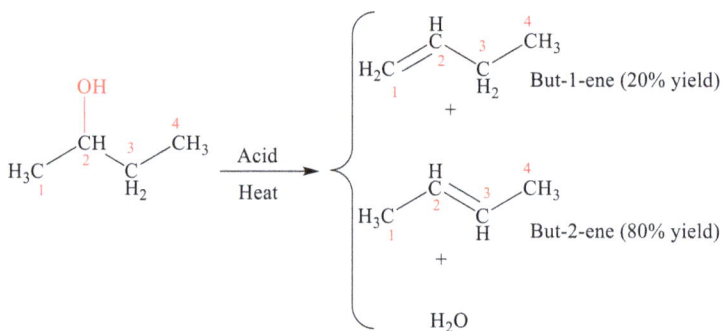

Figure 4.11   Dehydration reaction of butan-2-ol. Note that one product has a higher yield than the other.

Reactions always favour the most stable product, which in this case is but-2-ene in comparison with but-1-ene. The double bond with the most alkyl substituents (alkyl groups attached to it) is considered to be the most stable product. Hence but-2-ene with two alkyl substituents by the double bond is more stable than but-1-ene with one alkyl substituent. As a result, but-2-ene is the predominant product in the elimination/dehydration reactions in alkene synthesis (Figure 4.12).

Hence both dehydration and dehydrochlorination reactions in the formation of alkenes follow the same basic rule to dictate the reaction yield. This, in organic chemistry, is called *Zaitsev's rule* after the scientist Alexander Zaitsev, who published this observation in 1875. The most substituted alkenes are the most stable, as shown in Figure 4.13. In this regard, we can introduce two common types of substitution relevant to the double bonds of alkenes. We can distinguish the location of two substituents by using the term *geminal* when they appear on the same carbon and *vicinal* when they occur on two atoms adjacent to each other. For two carbons carrying a double bond, the substituents in a *cis–trans* configuration are in a vicinal relationship.

Stability of Alkenes – Key Facts

- Reactions always favour the most stable product.
- The double bond with the most alkyl substituents (alkyl groups attached to it) is considered the most stable product.
- In the synthesis of alkenes from alcohols or alkyl halides, we investigate the number of alkyl substituents on the C=C double bond to determine which product is more stable or predominant.
- In disubstituted cases, *trans* or *geminal* substitution is more stable than *cis* substitution.

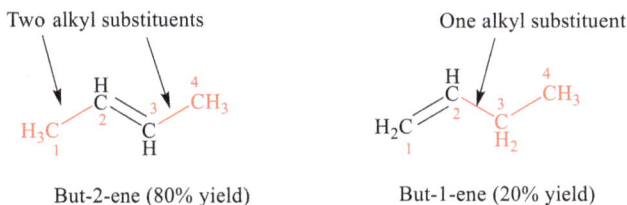

Figure 4.12 Stability of alkenes. Alkenes with more alkyl substituents are more stable.

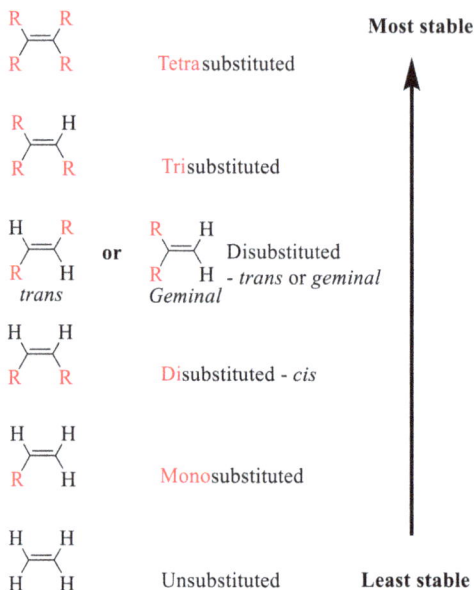

Figure 4.13 The stability of alkenes increases with increasing substitution. The R group represents an alkyl group such as methyl, ethyl, butyl, *etc.* Note that the *cis* configuration has two alkyl groups crowded on the same side of the double bond and hence is less stable than the *trans* isomer. Geminal refers to two atoms or groups attached to the same atom. The two R groups in *cis* or *trans* forms are vicinal to each other.

4.2 Cycloalkenes

When discussing cycloalkanes, we established that a one-ring system requires the loss of two hydrogen atoms from the alkane counterpart. In the example shown in Figure 4.14, cyclohexane has two hydrogens fewer than hexane. With alkenes, cyclisation to make cycloalkenes similarly leads to a product with two hydrogens fewer than the linear chain counterpart. When numbering carbons in the ring system of cycloalkenes, the double bond is between carbon-1 and carbon-2.

Once the double bond has been located and numbered, the substituents and attachment may be further numbered by making sure that they get the smallest possible numbering. For compounds containing more than one double bond in their structures, we follow the same rule as for alkenes. Hence the name 1,3-cyclopentadiene in the older literature is now replaced with cyclopenta-1,3-diene (Figure 4.15).

Just as we have methyl, ethyl, propyl, *etc.*, substituents in alkanes, alkenes, and their cyclic counterparts, we can also have alkene

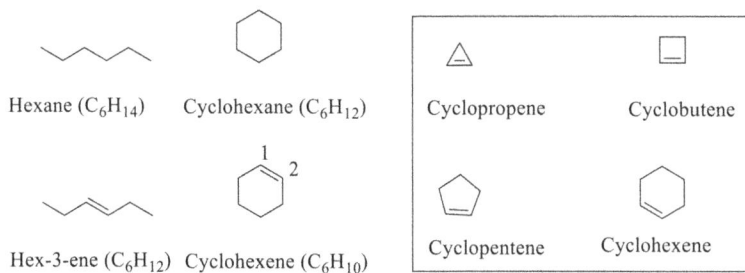

Hexane (C_6H_{14})   Cyclohexane (C_6H_{12})

Cyclopropene   Cyclobutene

Hex-3-ene (C_6H_{12})   Cyclohexene (C_6H_{10})

Cyclopentene   Cyclohexene

Figure 4.14 Basic structures of cycloalkenes and their structural difference from alkanes and cycloalkanes.

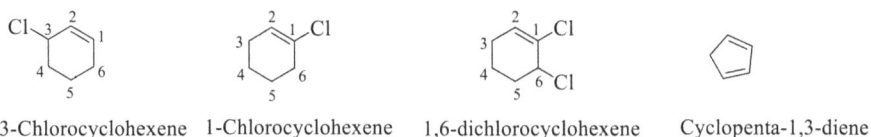

3-Chlorocyclohexene 1-Chlorocyclohexene 1,6-dichlorocyclohexene Cyclopenta-1,3-diene

Figure 4.15 Naming of cycloalkenes.

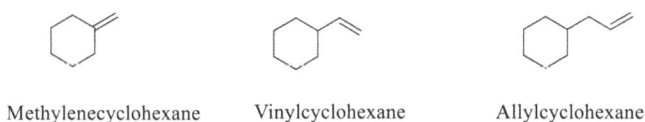

Methylenecyclohexane   Vinylcyclohexane   Allylcyclohexane

Figure 4.16 Common names based on alkene substituents.

substituents. These are mostly important when they occur in cyclic structures and include methylene ($=CH_2$), vinyl ($-CH=CH_2$), and allyl ($-CH_2-CH=CH_2$) groups. Compounds are named based on these substituents as shown in Figure 4.16.

Cycloalkenes and alkenes occur in Nature in various structural forms; some examples (see Figure 4.17) include limonene, which is a fragrant compound in citrus fruits, zingiberene in ginger, and caryophyllene in cloves and other essential oils. The orange-coloured pigment β-carotene, which is a principal component of carrots, is a provitamin – provitamin A.

4.3 Reactions of Alkenes and Cycloalkenes

The reactions of alkenes and cycloalkenes are mainly addition reactions in which two molecules can combine to form a larger molecule of a product. Several structural groups can be added to alkenes to give the general products shown in Figure 4.18.

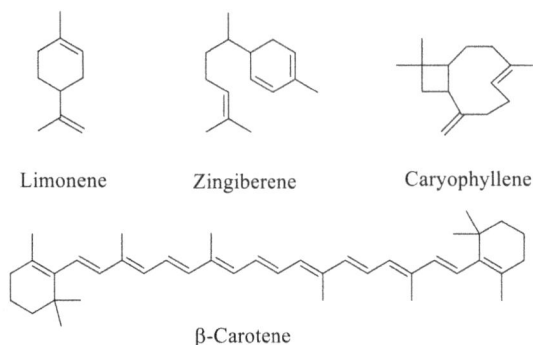

Figure 4.17   Some examples of natural alkenes and cycloalkenes.

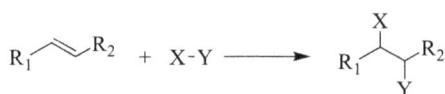

Figure 4.18   General addition reaction of alkenes (and similarly cycloalkenes). Upon addition of X and Y to either side of the C=C double bond, we change the sp^2 hybridisation to the sp^3 form of a saturated carbon system.

4.3.1   Hydrogenation Reaction

In a *hydrogenation reaction*, two hydrogen atoms are added to the double bond to give alkanes or cycloalkanes. Hence the hydrogenation of alkenes or cycloalkanes is also called a reduction reaction as we increase the number of hydrogen atoms in the molecule.

Hydrogenation reactions (Figure 4.19) are employed at high pressure and use catalysts to increase the reaction yields by facilitating contact between the hydrogen atoms and alkenes. Common catalysts are metals, such as platinum (Pt), palladium (Pd), and nickel (Ni). Instead of alkenes, a vast array of other chemicals carrying double bonds can also be hydrogenated. A good example is the hydrogenation of fatty acids, which is employed extensively within the food industry.

4.3.2   Halogenation Reaction

In the *halogenation of alkenes*, chlorine or bromine is added to give alkyl halides. It is also called chlorination, bromination, or simply halogenation (Figure 4.20).

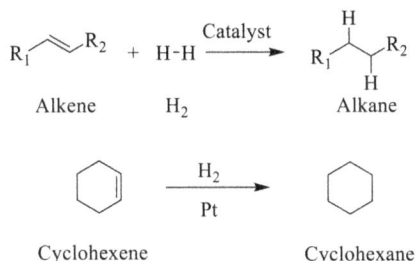

Alkene H_2 Alkane

Cyclohexene   Cyclohexane

Figure 4.19 Hydrogenation reaction. Both alkenes and cycloalkenes undergo hydrogenation reactions. Metal catalysts such as platinum (Pt) are used to increase the rate of reaction.

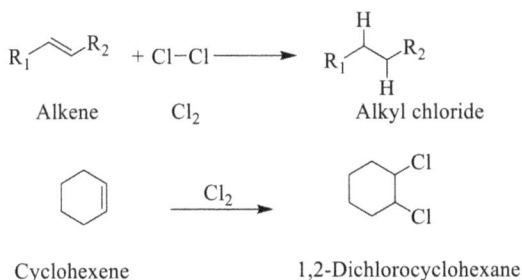

Alkene Cl_2 Alkyl chloride

Cyclohexene   1,2-Dichlorocyclohexane

Figure 4.20 Chlorination of alkenes and cycloalkenes.

4.3.3 Addition of Hydrogen Halides

In the *addition of hydrogen halides* such as HCl to alkenes and cycloalkenes, alkyl halides are also formed. There is, however, a complication with the products depending on which carbon in the double bond receives the hydrogen or the halide. Let us consider the addition of HCl to propene as shown in Figure 4.21.

In the reaction (Figure 4.21), the yields of the products are not the same. As a rule, the hydrogen from hydrogen chloride goes to the carbon that carries more hydrogen atoms. This is called *Markovnikov's rule*: 'In the addition of hydrogen halides to unsymmetrical alkenes, the hydrogen attaches to the carbon that already has the greatest number of hydrogen atoms'. Vladimir Vasilyevich Markovnikov in 1869 described the addition of HCl to unsymmetrical alkenes in terms of the electron-rich component (chlorine) added to the carbon atom with fewer hydrogen atoms bonded to it, and the electron-deficient component (hydrogen) added to the carbon atom with more hydrogen atoms attached to it. This is depicted in Figure 4.22.

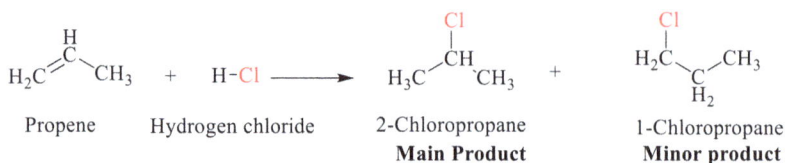

Figure 4.21 Addition of hydrogen chloride to propene.

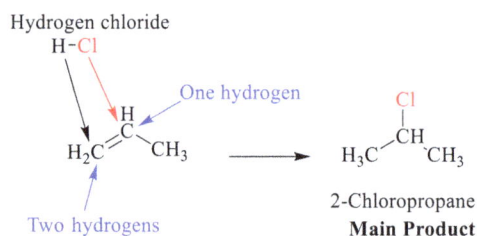

Figure 4.22 Application of Markovnikov's rule in the addition of hydrogen chloride to propene.

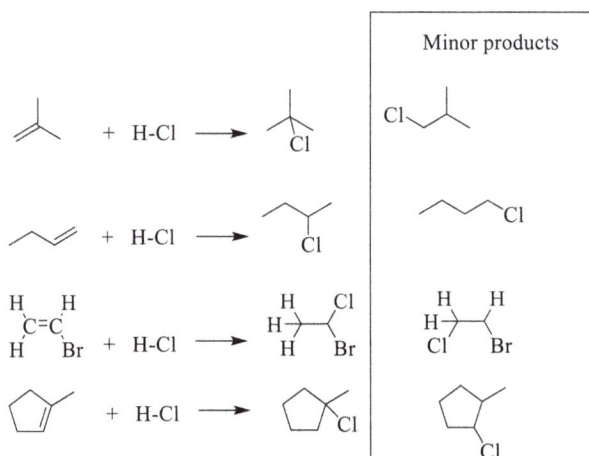

Figure 4.23 Examples of the Markovnikov addition of alkyl halides to alkenes and cycloalkenes. The predominant products are shown – the expected minor products are shown in the box.

As an exercise, observe the reactions shown in Figure 4.23 and the predominant yield.

One exception to the *Markovnikov addition* of hydrogen halides to alkenes is the addition reaction with hydrogen bromide. This is called *anti-Markovnikov addition* and occurs because of the presence of peroxide in hydrogen bromide – it is also called the peroxide effect (Figure 4.24).

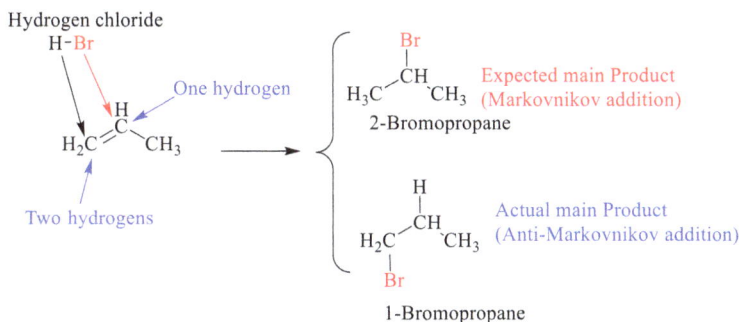

Figure 4.24 Anti-Markovnikov addition – addition of HBr to alkenes.

4.3.4 Addition of Water

The addition of water to alkenes and cycloalkenes can also proceed through Markovnikov addition (Figure 4.25). The reaction is catalysed by acids and hence is called acid-catalysed hydration of alkenes.

By using the peroxide effect of the anti-Markovnikov addition that we explained above for hydrogen bromide, it is also possible to obtain alcohols from alkenes and cycloalkenes through anti-Markovnikov addition. Through a two-step reaction using diborane, $(BH_3)_2$, followed by hydrogen peroxide (H_2O_2) under basic (OH^-) conditions, only one anti-Markovnikov addition product can be formed (Figure 4.26).

4.3.5 Polymerisation of Alkenes

A *polymerisation* reaction of alkenes involves a small alkene molecule as a monomer used to build up or make a long-chain molecule. This results in the opening of the double bond to give a saturated polymer as shown in Figure 4.27.

Polymerisation of alkenes is achieved by using a catalyst to form a dimer, then a trimer, and so on. This process has many industrial applications. For example, polyethene (more commonly called polyethylene or polythene) is a polymer made from ethene and the polymer length can be based on several thousand units of the ethene monomer. Polyethylene is used for making plastic bags, bottles, toys, electrical insulation, *etc.* Other similar products include polypropylene and polyvinyl chloride (Figure 4.28), which are used to manufacture bottles, luggage, pipes, *etc.* Natural and synthetic rubber and plastics are also examples of products formed by the polymerisation of alkenes.

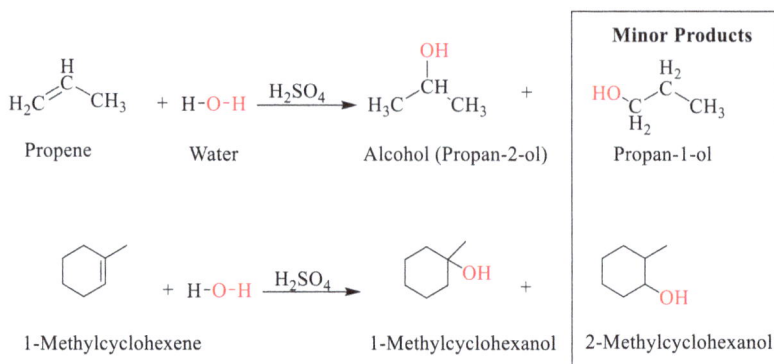

Figure 4.25   Acid-catalysed hydration of alkenes and cycloalkenes. This also follows the Markovnikov addition where the hydrogen goes to the carbon with the greater number of hydrogen atoms.

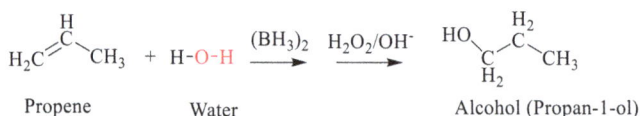

Figure 4.26   Anti-Markovnikov hydration of alkenes using the peroxide effect.

Reaction of Alkenes and Cycloalkenes – Key Facts

- Mostly an addition reaction to make a saturated compound.
- Addition of hydrogen – hydrogenation.
- Addition of halogens – halogenation.
- Hydrogen halides and water addition follow Markovnikov's rule – hydrogen attaches to the carbon that already has the greatest number of hydrogen atoms. The exception is the addition of HBr.
- Anti-Markovnikov addition using the peroxide effect can be used in the synthesis of alcohols.
- Polymerisation of alkenes gives polymeric materials such as plastics.

4.4   Aromatic Hydrocarbons

Another important group of hydrocarbons are aromatic compounds or *arenes*, which contain a benzene ring system in their structure. These kinds of compounds are quite common in Nature and are addressed in various parts of this book. Good examples of aromatic skeletons are

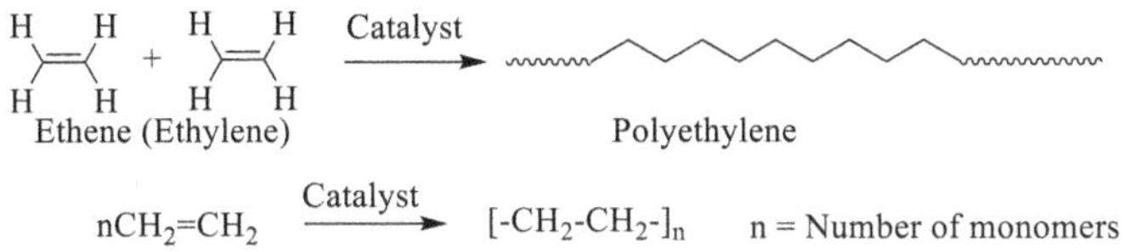

Ethene (Ethylene)   Polyethylene

$$nCH_2=CH_2 \xrightarrow{\text{Catalyst}} [-CH_2\text{-}CH_2\text{-}]_n \quad n = \text{Number of monomers}$$

Figure 4.27 Polymerisation of alkenes. The zigzag line indicates a long alkyl chain; or the repeating units simply indicated by *n* to show the number of monomers. In the polymerisation of ethene under high temperature and pressure, thousands of monomeric units make polyethylene materials such as plastics.

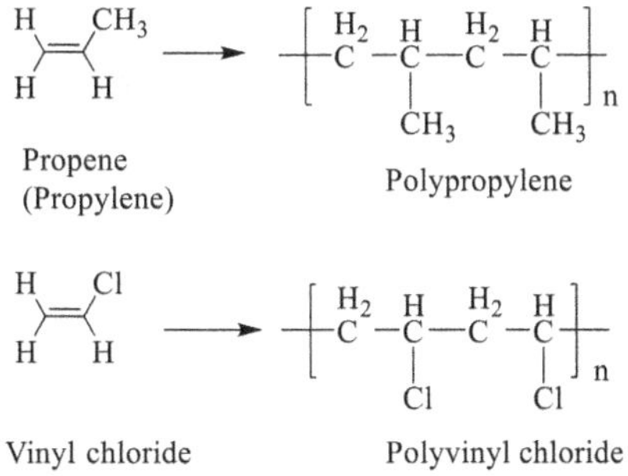

Propene
(Propylene)   Polypropylene

Vinyl chloride   Polyvinyl chloride

Figure 4.28 Synthesis of polypropylene and polyvinyl chloride. Long polymeric chains of repeating units (*n*) are made of monomers such as propene and vinyl chloride.

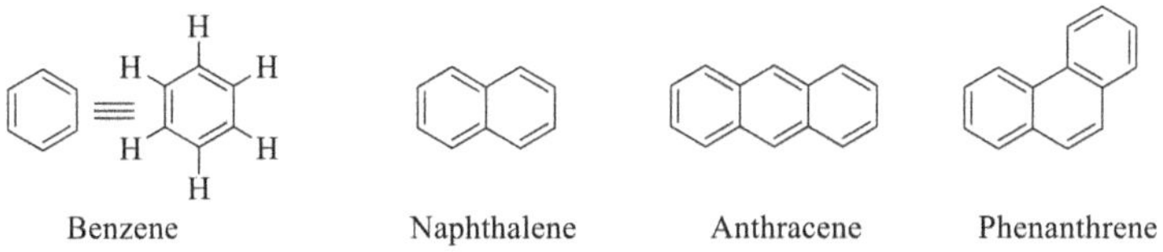

Benzene   Naphthalene   Anthracene   Phenanthrene

Figure 4.29 Benzene and polynuclear aromatic compounds.

shown in Figure 4.29. They include polynuclear aromatic compounds such as naphthalene, anthracene, and phenanthrene.

The orbital hybridisation model of bonding in benzene is special in that all six carbon atoms in the ring system are sp^2-hybridised carbons. In addition to the six σ bonds that firmly hold the carbons in the ring, the six π electrons (from the unhybridised p orbitals) circulate above and below the plane of the ring. A unique feature of benzene is also that the six π electrons (three pairs for each double bond) are delocalised over the entire ring system (Figure 4.30):

Each π electron in benzene is therefore shared by all six carbon atoms and the six delocalised π electrons can be represented by

Delocalised

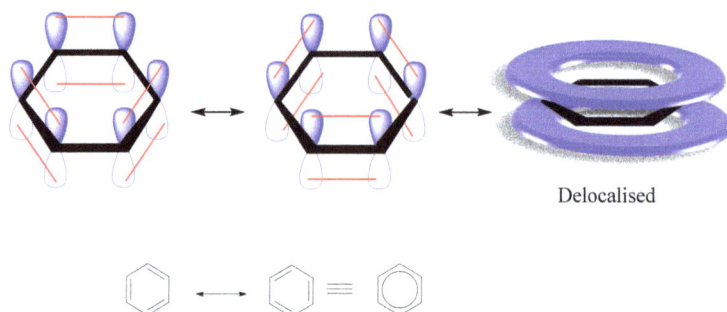

Figure 4.30 Molecular orbitals and resonance structure of benzene. The arrow (↔) is called a resonance arrow and indicates that the two structures differ from each other only in the way in which the electrons are arranged. The molecule is therefore viewed as a hybrid between the two forms. For the benzene structure at the bottom, a circle drawn in the middle shows this reality although such a model does not show the shared electron pairs, especially when we try to show the movement of electrons during chemical reactions.

a circle above and below the plane of the benzene δ bonds. This unique property of the benzene ring system is structurally presented in Figure 4.30.

4.5 Alkynes

Alkynes are another group of hydrocarbons with at least one carbon–carbon triple bond (–C≡C–). The general molecular formula of alkynes is therefore C_nH_{2n-2}. The molecular geometry and the sp hybridisation in carbon are discussed in Chapter 1. The presence of a triple bond in a molecule is indicated in the name by the suffix '*yne*' and the first compound in the homologous series is ethyne (also called acetylene). This is followed by propyne. But after that the position of the triple bond in the molecules must be indicated by appropriate numbering (see Figure 4.31). Hence the triple bond may not necessarily be at the terminal carbon.

The nomenclature of complex alkynes follows the same rules as those for alkenes. We must first number the carbons in the longest continuous chain by making sure that the triple bond gets the lowest possible number. If there is a double bond in addition to the triple bond, the parent name is based on the alkyne (yne) with the double bond entered with its location as a substituent (*e.g.* 3-en-). A few examples are shown in Figure 4.32.

But-1-yne   But-2-yne   Pent-1-yne   Pent-2-yne
(1-Butyne)   (2-Butyne)   (1-Pentyne)   (2-Pentyne)

Hex-1-yne   Hex-2-yne   Hex-3-yne
(1-Hexyne)   (2-Hexyne)   (3-Hexyne)

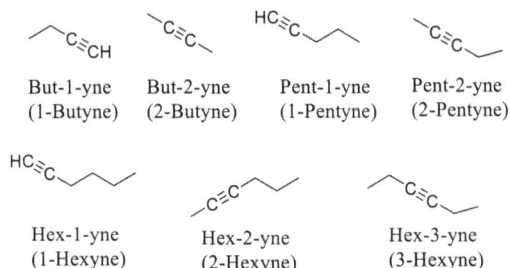

Figure 4.31 Examples of alkynes. Note the geometry in the sp-hybridized C≡C triple bonds: a linear or 180° bond angle geometry is evident. The old names or synonyms are given in parentheses.

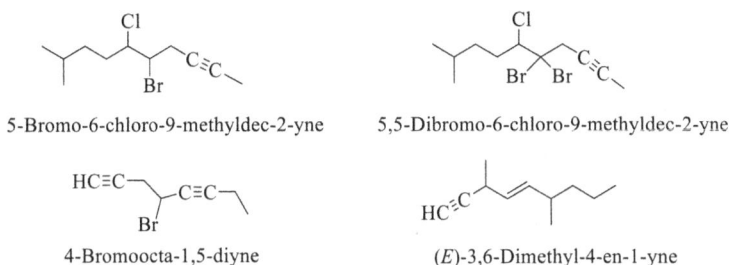

5-Bromo-6-chloro-9-methyldec-2-yne   5,5-Dibromo-6-chloro-9-methyldec-2-yne

4-Bromoocta-1,5-diyne   (*E*)-3,6-Dimethyl-4-en-1-yne

Figure 4.32 Nomenclature of alkynes. Note that in (*E*)-3,6-dimethyl-4-en-1-yne, the parent name is an alkyne (not alkene) and the geometry of the alkene is shown as *trans* (*E*).

Alkynes are examples of unsaturated compounds and the principal reaction in which they are involved is the addition reaction, just as for alkenes and cycloalkenes. Hence they undergo reactions such as catalytic hydrogenation to give alkanes. Other reactions of alkenes such as hydration (addition of water) are also possible with alkynes. The reaction of alkynes therefore involves the breaking of the C≡C bond to form a C=C double bond, which also breaks down sequentially to form a C–C single bond (Figure 4.33).

Alkynes – Key Facts

- Unsaturated hydrocarbons with a C≡C triple bond.
- Naming takes the suffix '*yne*', *e.g.* hex-2-yne.
- If a double bond and a triple bond occur in the same molecule, the naming in the suffix is '*yne*', *i.e.* it is called an alkenyne (*e.g.* hex-4-en-1-yne).
- They undergo addition reactions.

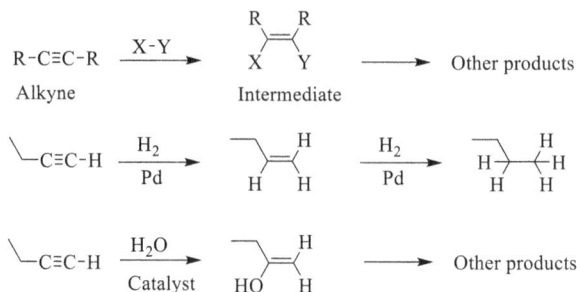

Figure 4.33 Reactions of alkynes. The hydrogenation reaction of alkynes is similar to that of alkenes and the reaction goes all the way to the formation of alkanes. In the hydration reaction, different products are formed depending on which carbon atom the –OH and hydrogen atoms go to. The products can also have other forms that are not discussed here.

4.6 Summary

In this chapter, we have learned the following:

- Alkenes are unsaturated hydrocarbons with at least one double bond in their molecules.
- Alkenes are named based on the IUPAC nomenclature rules.
- Geometrical isomers (*cis–trans* or *E* and *Z*) are important features of alkenes.
- Alkenes can be obtained from alcohols through a dehydration reaction.
- Alkenes can be obtained from alkyl halides (*e.g.* alkyl chlorides) through a dehydrohalogenation reaction (*e.g.* dehydrochlorination).
- The yield of dehydration and dehydrohalogenation reactions depends on the stability of the alkene products. Alkenes with more alkyl substituents on the double bond are more stable.
- Cycloalkenes are alkenes in a cyclic structure. They have two fewer hydrogen atoms for a one-ring system than the corresponding alkenes, *e.g.* hexene (C_6H_{12}) with 12 hydrogen atoms *versus* cyclohexene (C_6H_{10}) with 10 hydrogen atoms in the molecules.
- The main reactions of alkenes and cycloalkenes are addition reactions as follows:

  o Hydrogenation reactions – addition of hydrogen atoms.
  o Halogenation reactions – addition of halogen atoms (chlorine, bromine, iodine, *etc.*).

    o Hydrohalogenation reactions – addition of hydrogen halides (*e.g.* HBr, HCl).

    o Hydration reactions – addition of water.

    o Polymerisation reactions – synthesis of polymers (*e.g.* polyethylene) from alkenes.

- In the addition of hydrogen halides (except HBr) and water, the major yield is obtained when the hydrogen atom goes to the carbon with the greatest number of hydrogen atoms – *Markovnikov addition.*
- In the addition of HBr, the Markovnikov rule is not obeyed owing to the peroxide effect – *anti-Markovnikov addition.*
- Anti-Markovnikov addition can be employed for addition reactions in alkenes by using the peroxide effect.
- Benzene, naphthalene, anthracene, and phenanthrene are arene skeletons.
- The benzene ring system is highly stabilised by its resonance forms – delocalisation of π electrons.
- Alkynes are hydrocarbons with C≡C triple bonds.
- Alkynes are compounds with a C≡C triple bond that undergoes an addition reaction.

4.7 Problems

Questions 1–4 are based on Figure 4.34. Name structures **1–4**.

    1. _____

    2. _____

    3. _____

    4. _____

Questions 5–9: Draw the structures of the following alkenes:

    5. 2,5,7-Trimethyldec-2-ene.

    6. Hept-3-ene.

    7. 4,5,6,7-Tetraethylnon-3-ene.

    8. 3-Ethyl-3-methylnon-1-ene.

    9. 7-Bromo-2,5-dimethylnon-2-ene.

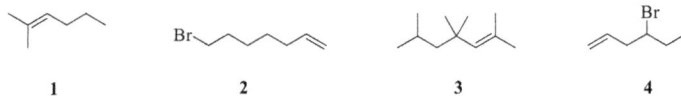

Figure 4.34 Questions 1–4 are based on this figure.

Questions 10–14: Draw the structures of the following compounds:

10. 1,4-Dichlorobenzene.
11. 1,3-Dibromo-2,4-diethylbenzene.
12. 1,3,5-Trimethylbenzene.
13. 1,3-Dimethylcyclohexene.
14. 1,3-Dimethylcyclopentene.

Questions 15–18 (see Figure 4.35): Indicate the geometry of the double bond by assigning *E* and *Z* notations to the names.

15. _____
16. _____
17. _____
18. _____

Questions 19–22: The compounds shown in Figure 4.36 have more than one double bond in their structure. Name the compounds – do not consider *cis–trans* isomers for your answer.

19. _____
20. _____
21. _____
22. _____

Questions 23 and 24: For hexa-1,3,5-triene, draw the structures of the two geometrical isomers.

23. _____
24. _____

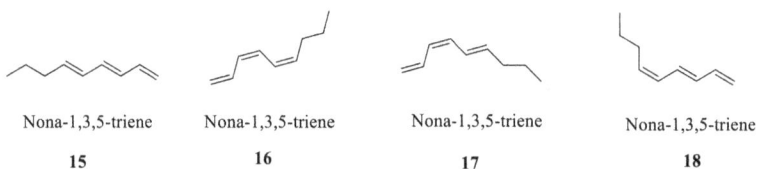

| Nona-1,3,5-triene | Nona-1,3,5-triene | Nona-1,3,5-triene | Nona-1,3,5-triene |
| 15 | 16 | 17 | 18 |

Figure 4.35 Structure of geometrical isomers of nona-1,3,5-triene.

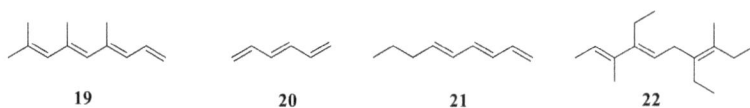

| 19 | 20 | 21 | 22 |

Figure 4.36 Questions 19–22 are based on this figure.

Questions 25–29 are based on Figure 4.37. Name the compounds shown.

25. _____
26. _____
27. _____
28. _____
29. _____

Questions 30–33 are based on Figure 4.38. Name the structures of alkynes **30–33** shown.

30. _____
31. _____
32. _____
33. _____

34. In obtaining alkenes through dehydration and dehydrochlorination reactions, the yield depends on the stability of the alkene product. Predict the stability order of the compounds shown in Figure 4.39.
35. Catalytic hydrogenation of alkenes gives out heat (exothermic reaction) and the more unstable alkenes give out more heat

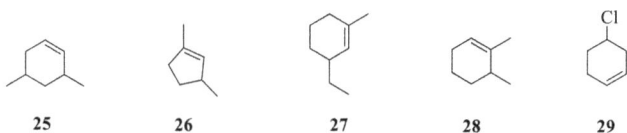

Figure 4.37 Name the compounds (**25–29**) shown in this figure.

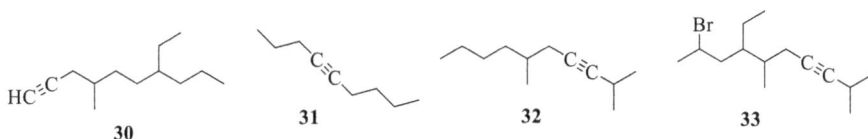

Figure 4.38 Questions 30–33 are based on this figure.

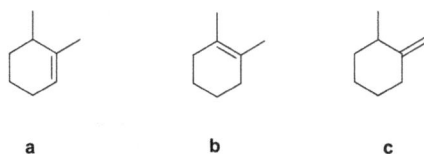

Figure 4.39 Show the order of stability of the indicated compounds.

energy than the stable compounds. This heat release is called heat of hydrogenation. What is the order of the heats of hydrogenation for but-1-ene, (Z)-but-2-ene, and (E)-but-2-ene?

36. For the compounds shown in Figure 4.40, predict the major and minor yields of the Markovnikov addition of HCl to alkenes.

37. For the compounds shown in Figure 4.41, complete the indicated hydrogenation reaction.

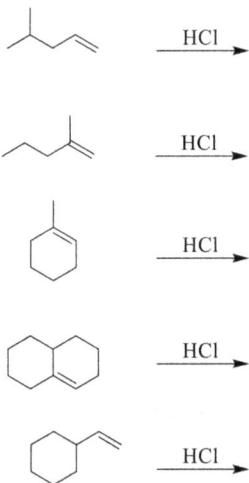

Figure 4.40 Predict the reaction products and yields for the indicated compounds.

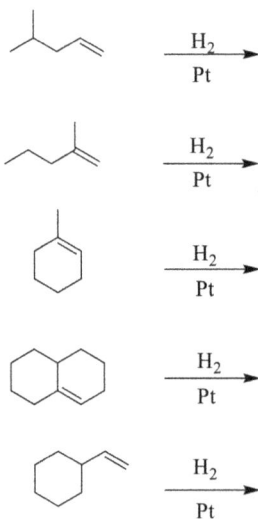

Figure 4.41 Complete the reaction.

4.8 Solutions to Problems

1. 2-Methylhex-2-ene.
2. 7-Bromohept-1-ene.
3. 2,4,4,6-Tetramethylhept-2-ene.
4. 4-Bromohex-1-ene.

For questions 5–9, see Figure 4.42.
For questions 10–14, see Figure 4.43.
For questions 15–18, based on Figure 4.35:

15. (3*E*,5*E*)-Nona-1,3,5-triene.
16. (3*Z*,5*Z*)-Nona-1,3,5-triene.

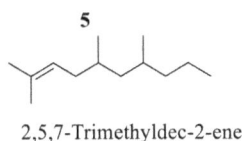

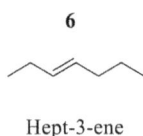

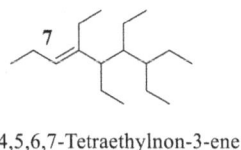

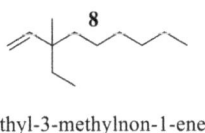

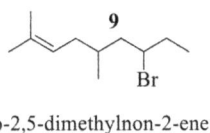

5

2,5,7-Trimethyldec-2-ene

6

Hept-3-ene

7

4,5,6,7-Tetraethylnon-3-ene

8

3-Ethyl-3-methylnon-1-ene

9

7-Bromo-2,5-dimethylnon-2-ene

Figure 4.42 Answers to questions 5–9.

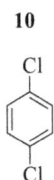

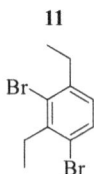

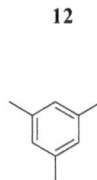

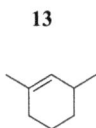

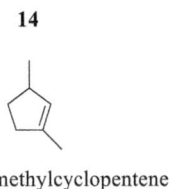

10

1,4-Dichlorobenzene

11

1,3-Dibromo-2,4-diethylbenzene

12

1,3,5-Trimethylbenzene

13

1,3-Dimethylcyclohexene

14

1,3-Dimethylcyclopentene

Figure 4.43 Answers to questions 10–14.

17. $(3Z,5E)$-Nona-1,3,5-triene.
18. $(3E,5Z)$-Nona-1,3,5-triene.

For questions 19–22, based on Figure 4.36:

19. 4,6,8-Trimethylnona-1,3,5,7-tetraene.
20. Hexa-1,3,5-triene.
21. Nona-1,3,5-triene.
22. 4,7-Diethyl-3,8-dimethyldeca-2,4,7-triene.

For questions 23 and 24, see Figure 4.44.
For questions 25–29 based on Figure 4.37, you should assign numbering by giving priority first to the longest possible chain containing the double bond in the ring system and then identify the location of the branching – lowest possible number for both the double bond and branching/substituents.

25. 3,5-Dimethylcyclohexene.
26. 1,3-Dimethylpentene.
27. 3-Ethyl-1-methylcyclohexene.
28. 1,6-Dimethylcyclohexaene.
29. 4-Chlorocyclohexene.

For questions 30–33, based on Figure 4.38:

30. 7-Ethyl-4-methyldec-1-yne.
31. Non-4-yne.
32. 2,6-Dimethyldec-3-yne.
33. 9-Bromo-7-ethyl-2,6-dimethyldec-3-yne.

34. Stability of compounds shown in Figure 4.39: **b** > **a** > **c**. A greater degree of substitution means greater stability.
35. This question is about the stability of alkenes, which is in the order (E)-but-2-ene, which is more stable than (Z)-but-2-ene, then (Z)-but-2-ene, which is more stable than but-1-ene. Hence (E)-but-2-ene has the lowest heat of hydrogenation.

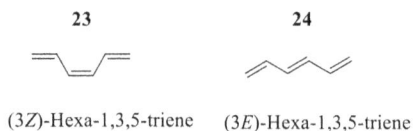

23	24
$(3Z)$-Hexa-1,3,5-triene	$(3E)$-Hexa-1,3,5-triene

Figure 4.44 Structures of hexa-1,3,5-triene.

36. For the question based on Figure 4.40, the complete reactions are shown in Figure 4.45.
37. For the question based on Figure 4.41, the complete reactions are shown in Figure 4.46.

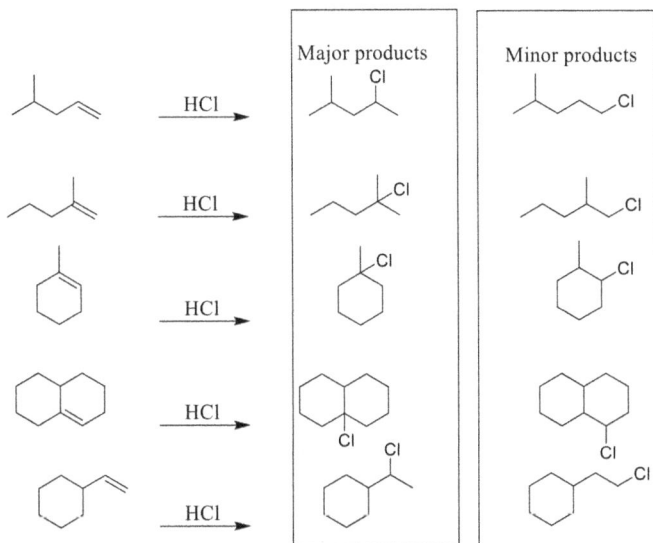

Figure 4.45   Answer to question 36.

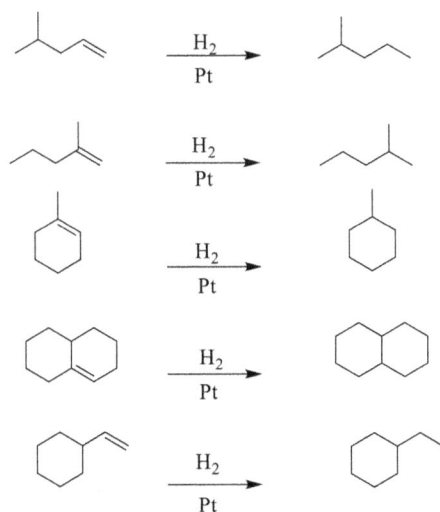

Figure 4.46   Hydrogenation reaction – answer to question 37.

5 Types of Organic Compounds, Nomenclature, and Basic Reactions: Functional Groups

Learning Objectives

After completing this chapter, you are expected to be able to:

- Identify functional groups in organic molecules.
- Be able to name organic compounds based on the accepted nomenclature for the functional group.
- Understand the order of polarity of organic compounds based on their structural groups.
- Explain the physical and chemical properties of organic compounds based on the functional groups they possess.
- Describe common reactions and the interconversion of functional groups.
- Be able to predict the solubility of organic compounds and what approach to take to increase their solubility in water.

Basic Chemistry for Life Science Students and Professionals: Introduction to Organic Compounds and Drug Molecules
By Solomon Habtemariam
© Solomon Habtemariam 2023
Published by the Royal Society of Chemistry, www.rsc.org

5.1 General Overview of Functional Groups

Molecules of organic compounds generally have two parts – the hydro-carbon part and the functional groups. The hydrocarbon part con-sists of only hydrogen and carbon and does not react readily (except to burning). The functional groups are the reactive part that contains elements other than carbon and hydrogen. An overview of the hydro-carbon part and the functional groups is presented in Figure 5.1.

As shown in Figure 5.1, functional groups are polar groups that are reactive. Reactions with these groups make some changes that mostly do not affect the non-reactive hydrocarbon part of the molecule. In Chapter 2, the polar bonds in organic compounds due to the covalent bonding of the carbon atom (and also hydrogen) with electronega-tive elements such as halogens, oxygen, and nitrogen were explained.

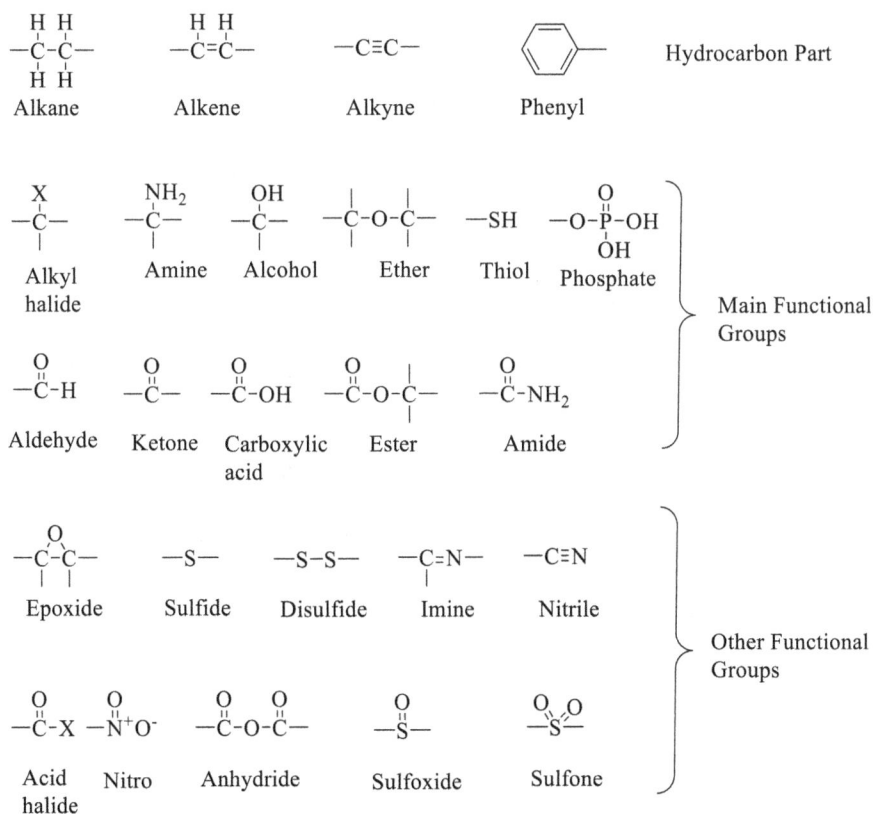

Figure 5.1 Structural overview of the hydrocarbon part and functional groups of compounds.

In this chapter, we consider some of the main functional groups that we encounter in biological systems and the life sciences.

5.2   Alcohols

5.2.1   Definition and Nomenclature

Alcohols are organic compounds that contain a hydroxyl (–OH) functional group. If we return to the general formula of hydrocarbons that we defined as alkanes, C_nH_{2n+2}, we replace one hydrogen with OH to obtain alcohols. In their nomenclature, their names end in '-*ol*', *e.g.* methan*ol*, ethan*ol*, propan*ol*, butan*ol*, pentan*ol*, hexan*ol*, *etc.* For alcohols based on three (propanol) or more carbons, the location of the hydroxyl group in the molecule needs to be specified. Examples of four carbon-based alcohols (butanols) are shown in Figure 5.2.

An alcohol may be considered as primary (1°), secondary (2°), or tertiary (3°) based on the nature of the carbon to which the hydroxyl group is attached (Figure 5.2). As shown in this example, the hydroxyl-bearing carbon attached to one alkyl chain is primary, to two carbons or chains secondary, and to three carbons tertiary. Note that the first alcohol in the homologous series, methanol, does not have any carbon attachment.

The naming of alcohols follows the same IUPAC rule discussed in the previous chapters and in this case a suffix '*ol*' applies to indicate the alcohol functional group. We must first identify the longest chain that contains the hydroxyl group and we assign the numbering by making sure that the alcohol-bearing carbon gets the lowest possible number (Figure 5.3). Cases where the alcohol functional group is not given priority in this numbering is when there are ketone, aldehyde, or carboxyl groups, which are discussed in the following sections. Alcohols with multiple hydroxyl groups can be named using the parent alkyl name followed by di, tri, *etc.*, before the suffix '-*ol*' (Figure 5.3).

It should be noted that a hydroxyl group may be part of other groups in compounds that we do not consider as alcohols. For example,

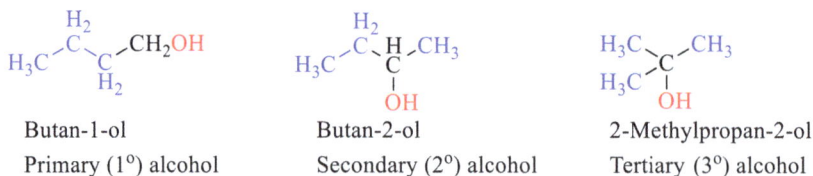

| Butan-1-ol | Butan-2-ol | 2-Methylpropan-2-ol |
| Primary (1°) alcohol | Secondary (2°) alcohol | Tertiary (3°) alcohol |

Figure 5.2   Classification of alcohols as primary, secondary, and tertiary.

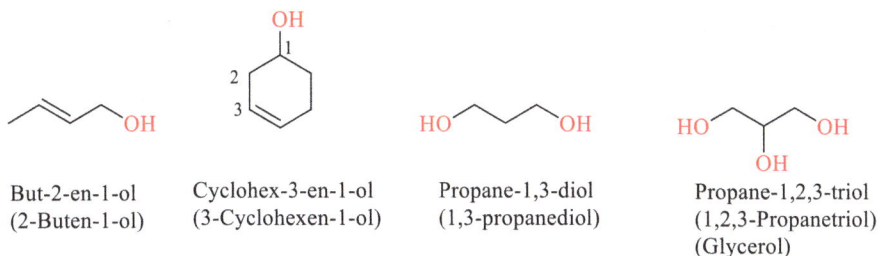

But-2-en-1-ol
(2-Buten-1-ol)

Cyclohex-3-en-1-ol
(3-Cyclohexen-1-ol)

Propane-1,3-diol
(1,3-propanediol)

Propane-1,2,3-triol
(1,2,3-Propanetriol)
(Glycerol)

Figure 5.3 Examples of alcohol nomenclature. Synonyms or other common names (shown in parentheses) also exist, for example, for propane-1,3-diol, the older name 1,3-propanediol is also used.

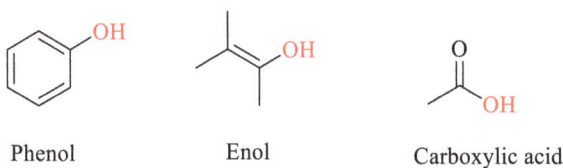

Phenol

Enol

Carboxylic acid

Figure 5.4 Structures of phenol, enol, and the carboxyl functional group. These are examples where a molecule is not considered an alcohol even though a hydroxyl group is present.

phenols are compounds with an aromatic ring system to which at least one hydroxyl group is attached. These are an important group of compounds commonly found in food and medicinal plants, and are discussed in Chapter 13. They have higher acidity owing to the tight coupling of the aromatic ring with the oxygen and a relatively loose bond between the oxygen and hydrogen. When a hydroxyl group is attached to double bond-carrying carbons such as alkenes, we call them *enols*. The reactivity of enols is different from that of alcohols. We also have a functional group that is called *carboxyl*, in *carboxylic acids* (Figure 5.4), discussed in the following sections.

5.2.2 Common Sources of Alcohols

Methanol, ethanol, and glycerol are good examples of alcohols that are extensively utilised in many areas. They are common natural products that can also be obtained chemically. Ethanol (also called ethyl alcohol) as a fermentation product of fruit (such as grape) juices has been used as a beverage since prehistoric times. Beverages containing ethanol are also produced from grains such as corn (maize), wheat, rye, and barley, common examples being different kinds of beer and spirits. Ethanol can also be produced from a variety of natural sources. Various starch- and sugar-based crops and also cellulose feedstocks may be used in the fermentation of plants to produce ethanol. The production of ethanol using crop residues and wood, which are not used as common foods, is considered as a sustainable and renewable means of ethanol biorefining. Most of the ethanol production, however, is from food sources such as corn, sugar beet, and wheat. This biorefining includes processes such as extraction of the carbon source or sugars, the fermentation process, distillation and dehydration or removal of water from the distillate. The goal of future research and development in this field is to utilise agricultural residues not destined for human consumption, such as straw, non-food lignocellulose (plant dry matter or mass) materials, and waste. Glycerol is another natural product that can be sourced from Nature, and it has various industrial uses, *e.g.* as a solvent, as a moisturising agent in the cosmetics industry, and others such as a plasticiser, antifreeze, and water-soluble lubricant.

Numerous chemical compounds of natural and synthetic origin contain alcohol functional groups. Good examples are fragrant essential oils in plants that are extensively used in the perfumery industry. Linalool is an alcohol that is found in lavender oil and others such as rose and basil oils. Geraniol is commonly found in citronella, lemongrass, and lavender oils, menthol in peppermint oil, and farnesol in the oils of various herbs. These compounds (Figure 5.5) can be obtained from plants through a distillation process as they are volatile molecules owing to their very small molecular size and their relatively non-polar nature.

Many vitamins (*e.g.* retinol or vitamin A), cholesterol, steroids, and hormones also contain the alcohol functional group (Figure 5.6).

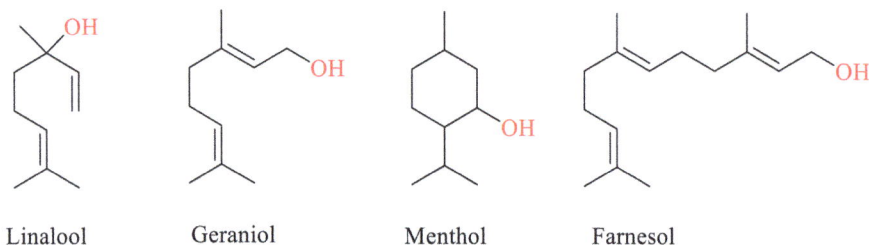

Linalool   Geraniol   Menthol   Farnesol

Figure 5.5 Examples of some natural fragrant molecules containing the alcohol functional group. Note that common names are used for these compounds; their IUPAC names are as follows: linalool = 3,7-dimethylocta-1,6-dien-3-ol, geraniol = (2*E*)-3,7-dimethylocta-2,6-dien-1-ol, menthol = 5-methyl-2-propan-2-ylcyclohexan-1-ol, and farnesol = (2*E*,6*E*)-3,7,11-trimethyldodeca-2,6,10-trien-1-ol.

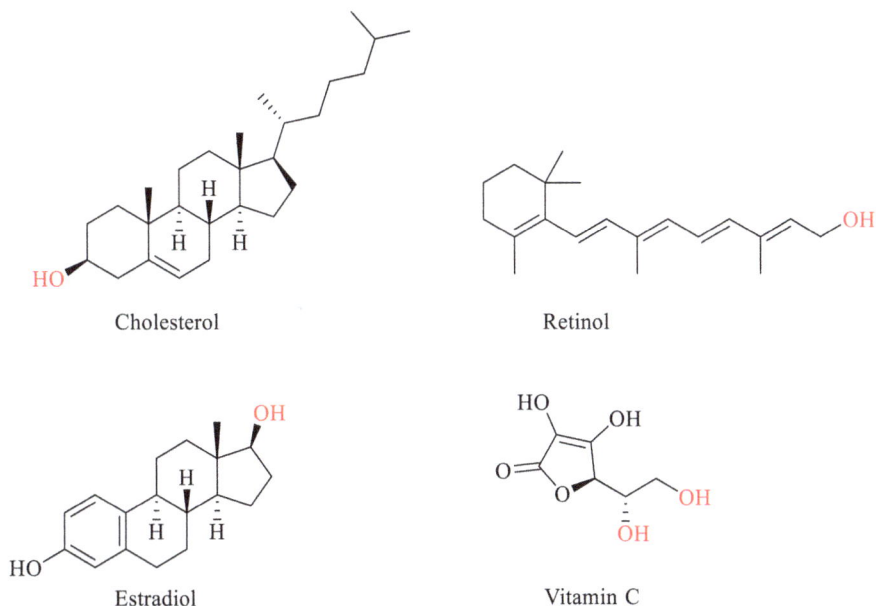

Cholesterol   Retinol

Estradiol   Vitamin C

Figure 5.6 Hormones and vitamins with an alcohol functional group. Also
note the enol functional group in vitamin C and phenol in estradiol. The IUPAC names for these compounds are complicated
and beyond the scope of this book. Their common names are
used in the literature. Note also that retinol has all the double
bonds in *trans* (*E*) isomer form.

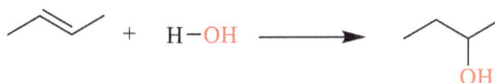

Figure 5.7 Reaction of alkenes with water to yield alcohols. This reaction
is also called hydration of alkenes and is commonly performed
using acid catalysts.

As discussed in Chapter 4, alcohols, especially those with higher
molecular weight, can be obtained by the hydration of alkenes (Figure
5.7). Note the *Markovnikov* and *anti-Markovnikov rules* of addition that
we discussed in Chapter 4. There are also various reactions in organic
chemistry that yield alcohols. The reduction of ketones, aldehydes,
and carboxylic acids is discussed in the following sections.

5.2.3 Properties of Alcohols

In Chapter 2, we discussed electronegativity and covalent bonding
between carbon and oxygen (C–O) or between oxygen and hydrogen
(O–H). The O–H bond is highly polarised with a δ– and δ+ electronic

distribution for the oxygen and hydrogen atoms, respectively. This results in intermolecular hydrogen bonding (Figure 5.8) and, as a result, alcohols have higher boiling points than the corresponding alkanes. In fact, methanol is a liquid whereas methane, ethane, and butane are gases at room temperature. For the same reason, alcohols also form hydrogen bonds with water molecules and therefore they are soluble in water (Figure 5.8).

The solubility of alcohols, however, depends on the size of the hydrocarbon part of the alcohol that is not involved in hydrogen bonding. As the non-polar hydrophobic region increases, the solubility in water also decreases, *i.e.* alcohols with a small molecular size are miscible in water, but the solubility decreases as the size of the alkyl group increases (Figure 5.9).

The general physical characteristics of some common alcohols including solubility in water and boiling points are presented in Table 5.1.

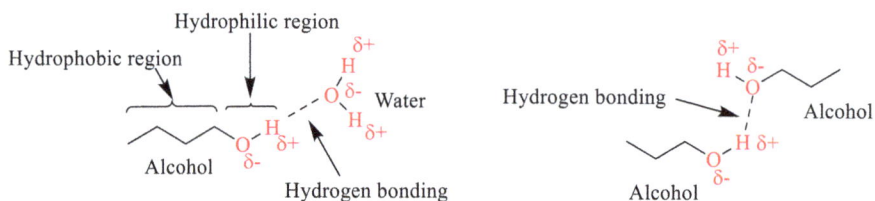

Figure 5.8   Hydrogen bonding between two alcohol molecules and between alcohol and water molecules.

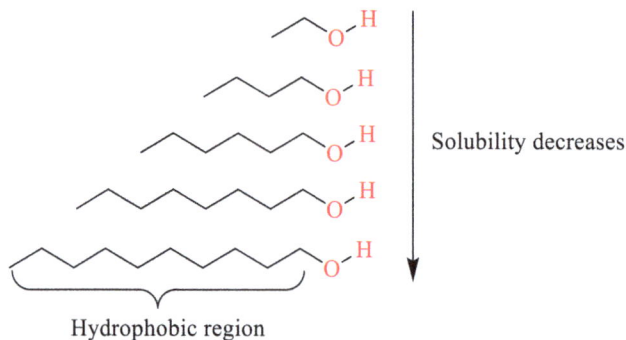

Figure 5.9   The solubility of alcohols in water decreases with increase in the size of the hydrocarbon or hydrophobic part. As an exercise, you may name the alcohols shown in the figure by replacing '-e' in the parent alkane name (*e.g.* ethane) with the suffix '-ol' (*e.g.* ethanol).

Alcohols – Key Facts

- An OH group attached to an sp³-hybridised or saturated carbon structure (*e.g.* alkane) – alcohol.
- Not all functional groups carrying an OH group are considered an alcohol:

  o A carbonyl carbon attached to an OH group is called carboxylic acid.

  o An OH group attached to a C=C double bond carbon (*e.g.* in alkenes) is called enol.

  o A benzene ring carbon attached to an OH group makes phenol.

- Hydrogen bonding is a feature of alcohols:

  o Alcohols have higher boiling points than the corresponding alkanes and alkenes.

  o Smaller sized alcohols are water soluble.

  o For larger molecules, the hydrophobic region of alcohols wins: they are soluble in organic solvents.

- Grouped into primary, secondary, and tertiary. Check: how many carbons are bonded to the carbon carrying the OH group?
- A compound is not named an alcohol if the molecule has other functional groups such as ketone, aldehyde, nitrile, or carboxyl groups.

5.2.4 Reactions of Alcohols

Alcohols can undergo a range of chemical reactions and here we consider just a few examples. They react readily with hydrogen halides (HCl, HBr, or HI) to form alkyl halides:

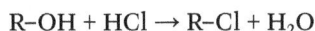

$$R\text{–}OH + HCl \rightarrow R\text{–}Cl + H_2O$$

All primary, secondary, and tertiary alcohols can react with the above-mentioned strong acids to replace OH with a halogen atom. This is a good example of a substitution reaction (see Chapter 11) and, for clarity, the reaction can be divided into several stages. The halide ion represented by X^- (Br^-, Cl^-, or I^-) with an excess electron (nucleophile) has a greater capacity to donate an electron pair and form a chemical bond (more nucleophilic) than a hydroxyl ion (OH^-). The strong acid that generates X^- then initiates a good leaving group that

Table 5.1 Some common alcohols and their physical properties.

IUPAC name	Formula	Common name	b.p.[a]/°C	Solubility in water[a]/g L^{-1} at 25 °C
Methanol	CH_3OH	Methyl alcohol	6.7	Miscible
Ethanol	CH_3CH_2OH	Ethyl alcohol	78.24	Miscible
Propan-1-ol	$CH_3CH_2CH_2OH$	*n*-Propyl alcohol	97.2	Miscible
Propan-2-ol	$(CH_3)_2CHOH$	Isopropyl alcohol	82.3	Miscible
Butan-1-ol	$CH_3(CH_2)_3OH$	*n*-Butyl alcohol	117.6	63.2
Butan-2-ol	$(CH_3)CH(OH)CH_2CH_3$	*sec*-Butyl alcohol	99.5	181
2-Methylpropan-1-ol	$(CH_3)_2CHCH_2OH$	Isobutyl alcohol	108.7	66.5–90.9
2-Methylpropan-2-ol	$(CH_3)_3COH$	*tert*-Butyl alcohol	82.3	Miscible
Pentan-1-ol	$CH_3(CH_2)_4OH$	*n*-Pentyl alcohol	137.5	22
3-Methylbutan-1-ol	$(CH_3)_2CHCH_2CH_2OH$	Isopentyl alcohol	132.5	26.7
2,2-Dimethylpropan-1-ol	$(CH_3)_3CCH_2OH$	Neopentyl alcohol	114	35
Hexan-1-ol	$CH_3(CH_2)_5OH$	*n*-Hexanol	157	5.9
Heptan-1-ol	$CH_3(CH_2)_6OH$	*n*-Heptyl alcohol	175.8	1.67
Octan-1-ol	$CH_3(CH_2)_7OH$	*n*-Octyl alcohol	194.7	—
Nonan-1-ol	$CH_3(CH_2)_8OH$	*n*-Nonyl alcohol	215	—
Decan-1-ol	$CH_3(CH_2)_9OH$	*n*-Decyl alcohol	229	—

[a]Boiling point (b.p.) and solubility values can vary slightly in different databases. Those given in this table are sourced from the Hazardous Substances Data Bank (HSDB), available *via* PubChem (https://pubchem.ncbi.nlm.nih.gov/).

can be replaced with X$^-$ (Figure 5.10). In such a reaction, the movement of electrons is shown by arrows. OH$^-$ is a strong base and is a poor leaving group. On the other hand, water (H_2O) is a weak base but an excellent leaving group. The reaction goes forwards since X$^-$ is more reactive to donate an electron than OH$^-$. Consider the examples shown in Figure 5.10 that follow the same principle of alcohols reacting with hydrogen halides (HBr, HCl, or HI). Note that the H–F bond is stronger than the H–I bond and the tendency to give a proton (H$^+$) or acidity decreases in the order HI > HBr > HCl > HF. Thus, HI is more reactive than HF in the substitution reaction with alcohols. More examples of these and the reactivity of alcohols are discussed in Chapter 11.

Alcohols behave like acids and react with active metals such as sodium to give a sodium salt (alkoxide) and hydrogen gas:

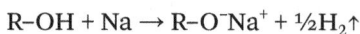

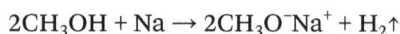

$$R–OH + Na \rightarrow R–O^-Na^+ + \tfrac{1}{2}H_2\uparrow$$

$$2CH_3OH + Na \rightarrow 2CH_3O^-Na^+ + H_2\uparrow$$

Methanol + sodium → sodium methoxide + hydrogen gas

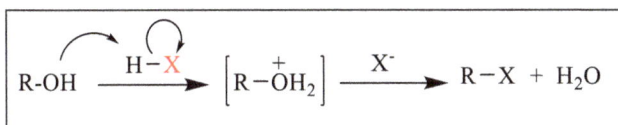

$$R\text{-OH} \xrightarrow{H-X} \left[R-\overset{+}{O}H_2\right] \xrightarrow{X^-} R-X + H_2O$$

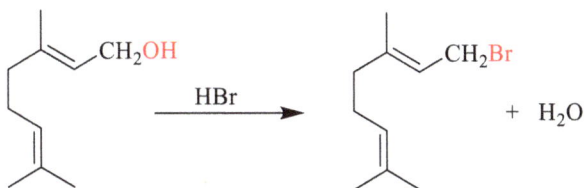

Geraniol (1° Alcohol)

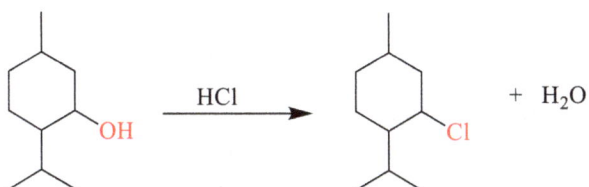

Menthol (2° Alcohol)

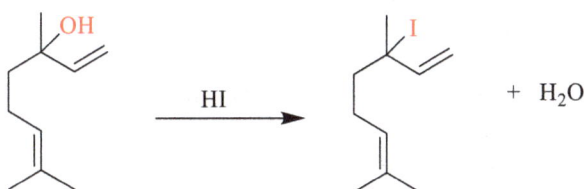

Linalool (3° Alcohol)

Figure 5.10 Reactions of alcohols with hydrogen halides. The reaction shown in the box at the top is what we call nucleophilic substitution (detailed in Chapter 11). The alkyl halides act as acids and hence their reactivity decreases in the order HI > HBr > HCl > HF. The reaction goes through multiple steps: a very fast reversible reaction of the alcoholic oxygen accepting the proton from the acid to make a good leaving group, water; water leaving the molecule through a slow reaction (rate-limiting step); and a fast reaction of the halide ion replacing water. At this stage, consider that alcohols as a base react with hydrogen halides as acids to yield alkyl halides and water.

5.2.5   Methylation of Alcohols – Ethers

Ethers are organic compounds that contain the functional group R–O–R, where R is either an alkyl or aryl (phenyl, Figure 5.1) group. If one of the alkyl groups is simply methyl, the –OCH_3 group is called methoxy. The alkyl–oxygen group, also called *alkoxy*, is therefore methoxy in this case. The simplest ether is dimethyl ether, and the chain length can increase, *e.g.* diethyl ether, dipropyl ether, dibutyl ether, *etc.* The ether could also be asymmetric, *e.g.* ethyl methyl ether, methyl propyl ether, *etc.* These are all common names conveniently used throughout the literature. The preferred IUPAC name for ethyl methyl ether is methoxyethane. Hence the IUPAC nomenclature dictates dimethyl ether to be named as methoxymethane, and diethyl ether is named as ethoxyethane. For long alkyl chains carrying a methoxy group, the naming takes the long alkyl name followed by the methoxy position located as a prefix, *e.g.* 2-methoxypropane (common name isopropyl methyl ether) (Figure 5.11)

Even though the electronegativity of oxygen in ethers leads to a polar bond compared with the corresponding alkanes, they do not have a polarised –OH bond such as alcohols possess. As a result, the boiling points of ethers are much lower than those of the corresponding alcohols. Hence they have much weaker intermolecular forces than alcohols. They also have a far higher lipid solubility than alcohols. Being a gas and with a high lipid solubility, diethyl ether is useful in general anaesthesia. It is also highly flammable, similarly to methane and other small alkanes.

Ethers can also occur as a cyclic structure with a ring system containing an oxygen single bond and are hence called *cyclic ethers*. Since the ring contains more than one type of atom (elements other than carbon) it is called *heterocyclic*. This could be an ether constructed from three atoms (two carbons and one oxygen), which we call an oxirane or epoxide, or a four-atom ring called oxetane, *etc.* There are several ways of naming cyclic ethers but the most accepted is now (IUPAC nomenclature system) based on denoting the rings from three to ten as *ir, et, ol, in, ep, oc, on,* and *ec*, respectively, after the prefix 'ox'.

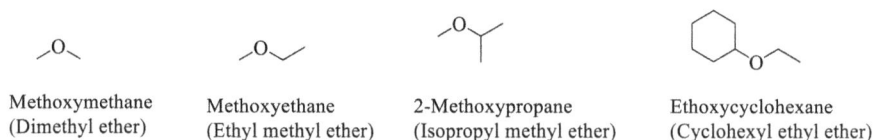

| Methoxymethane | Methoxyethane | 2-Methoxypropane | Ethoxycyclohexane |
| (Dimethyl ether) | (Ethyl methyl ether) | (Isopropyl methyl ether) | (Cyclohexyl ethyl ether) |

Figure 5.11   Nomenclature of ethers. IUPAC names and common names (in parentheses) are shown.

The suffix for a saturated alkyl chain or cycloalkane skeleton is 'ane' (Figure 5.12).

Many alternative naming systems also exist for the above-mentioned saturated cyclic ethers. For example, oxacyclopropane, oxacyclobutane, oxacyclopentane, oxacyclohexane, *etc.*, are commonly used in the literature. Let us call all these names *synonyms*, some of which are shown in Figure 5.13.

In the IUPAC nomenclature system, the unsaturated alkyl chain does not have a uniform order of naming except for the prefix 'ox'. The three- to ten-membered compounds are called oxirene, oxete, oxole, oxin, oxepin, oxocin, oxonin, and oxecin, respectively. The position of

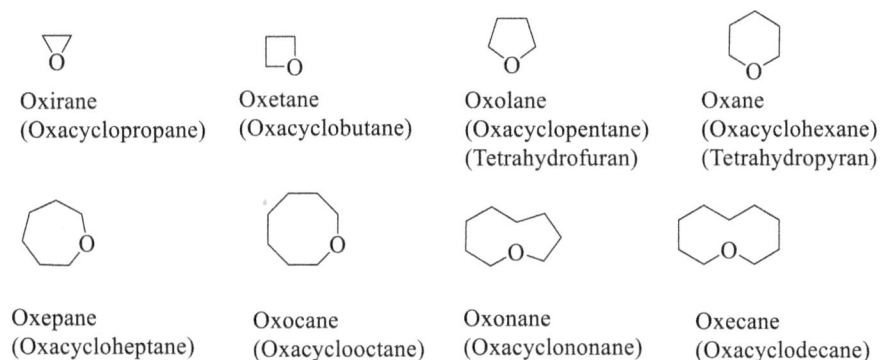

Oxirane   Oxetane   Oxolane   Oxane
(Oxacyclopropane) (Oxacyclobutane)   (Oxacyclopentane)   (Oxacyclohexane)
                                              (Tetrahydrofuran)   (Tetrahydropyran)

Oxepane   Oxocane   Oxonane   Oxecane
(Oxacycloheptane)   (Oxacyclooctane)   (Oxacyclononane)   (Oxacyclodecane)

Figure 5.12   IUPAC nomenclature for cyclic ethers. There are also several common names, some of which are shown in parentheses. Common names such as tetrahydrofuran instead of the IUPAC name oxolane are favoured in the academic literature.

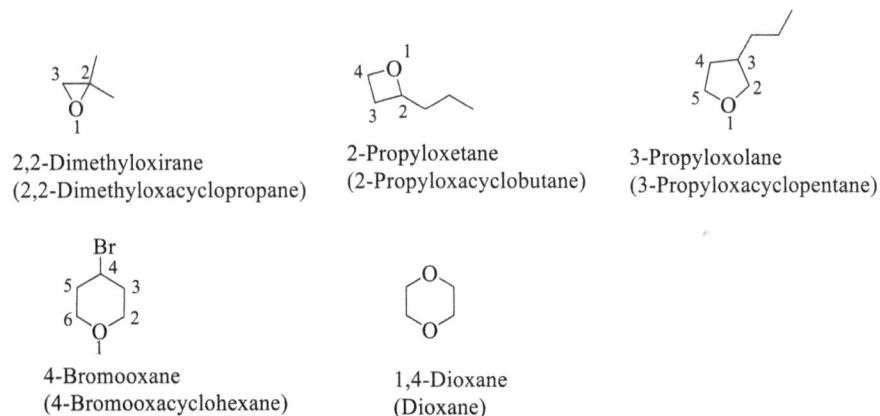

2,2-Dimethyloxirane   2-Propyloxetane   3-Propyloxolane
(2,2-Dimethyloxacyclopropane) (2-Propyloxacyclobutane)   (3-Propyloxacyclopentane)

4-Bromooxane   1,4-Dioxane
(4-Bromooxacyclohexane)   (Dioxane)

Figure 5.13   Examples of some saturated cyclic ethers. Common names are also shown in parentheses.

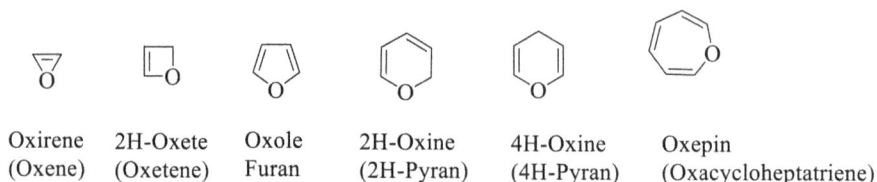

| Oxirene | 2H-Oxete | Oxole | 2H-Oxine | 4H-Oxine | Oxepin |
| (Oxene) | (Oxetene) | Furan | (2H-Pyran) | (4H-Pyran) | (Oxacycloheptatriene) |

Figure 5.14   IUPAC nomenclature for unsaturated cyclic ethers. Furan, also a name accepted by IUPAC, is the favoured name for oxole. Common names are shown in parentheses.

the unsaturated carbon can also be indicated, as shown for 2*H*-oxete, 2*H*-oxine, and 4*H*-oxine (Figure 5.14).

Many other alternative names also occur and, in this case, furan and pyran, for example, are popular names for the five- and six-membered oxygen heterocycles, respectively.

The transfer of a methyl group to organic compounds is called *methylation*. This is conveniently done in alcohols to convert the –OH group to –OCH$_3$. The conversion of hydroxyl groups in alcohols to methoxy derivatives or methyl ethers is one way of making them lipophilic. As part of our body's metabolic process, it is also widely used to detoxify drugs and other molecules. Our liver contains enzymes that perform this methylation task, whereas in the laboratory methylation is a common experimental method used to modify the structures of compounds. Enzymes called *O*-methyltransferases catalyse the methylation of alcohols and are found in plants, animals, and many other living organisms.

Several general and selective approaches to methylating hydroxyl groups are available. Common methyl donors used in chemistry laboratories include iodomethane, dimethyl sulfate, dimethyl carbonate, and tetramethylammonium chloride. Details of these reactions are beyond the scope of this book.

Ethers and Cyclic Ethers – Key Facts

- Represented by R–O–R.
- Far less polar than alcohols – no hydrogen bonding.
- Small ethers, *e.g.* diethyl ether, are highly lipophilic and are used in anaesthesia.
- Methylation of alcohols (*e.g.* in the liver) is one means of detoxification of drugs and other agents or metabolic processing in the body.

5.2.6 Acetylation of Alcohols

The *acetylation* of alcohols is also called an *esterification* reaction with acetic acid or another suitable reagent. This reaction forms an *acyl functional group*, which is discussed in detail in Section 5.3.

5.2.7 Phenols

As with alcohols, phenols also have a hydroxyl (–OH) group attached to a carbon atom but they are based on an aromatic (phenyl, Figure 5.1) ring system. They are one of the most common and diverse groups of natural products, found in cereals, fruits, vegetables, and beverages. They are also common industrial products and by-products. Common structural groups and their nomenclature are shown in Figure 5.15.

Phenol
(Hydroxybenzene)

Benzene-1,2-diol
(Catechol)

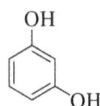

Benzene-1,3-diol
(Resorcinol)

Benzene-1,4-diol
(Hydroquinone)

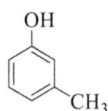

3-Methylphenol
(*Meta*-Cresol)

4-Chlorophenol
(*Para*-Chlorophenol)

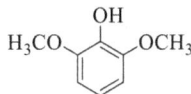

2,6-Dimethoxyphenol
(Syringol)

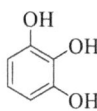

Benzene-1,2,3-triol
(Pyrogallol)

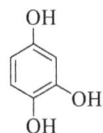

Benzene-1,2,4-triol
(Hydroxyhydroquinone)

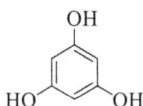

Benzene-1,3,5-triol
(Phloroglucinol)

Naphthalen-1-ol
(1-Naphthol)

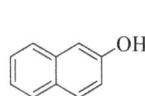

Naphthalen-2-ol
(2-Naphthol)

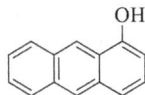

Anthracen-1-ol
(1-Hydroxyanthracene)

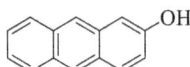

Anthracen-2-ol
(2-Hydroxyanthracene)

Figure 5.15 Examples of and IUPAC nomenclature for phenolic compounds. Common names are shown in parentheses.

Lower molecular weight phenols are common in fragrant herbs and essential oils (Figure 5.16). Thymol is a classic example of a fragrant molecule extracted from thyme (*Thymus vulgaris*) as an essential oil. Carvacrol is another phenol that is common in many herbs and medicinal plants, such as oregano (*Origanum vulgare*). Eugenol is an essential oil component in herbs and spices such as clove oil, nutmeg, and cinnamon. In addition to uses in food flavouring, it has numerous clinical applications including in dentistry preparations for its antiseptic and anti-inflammatory properties. Isoeugenol is also an essential oil component that is present in ylang–ylang (*Cananga odorata*).

Based on complex phenolic structures, we have numerous examples of drugs, structural components of plants such as lignin, and a range of compounds available in fruits and vegetables that are considered as antioxidants. These are discussed in detail in Chapter 13 and some representative compounds are mentioned here. Catechin as a principal component of tea is a powerful antioxidant that displays a range of biological effects. Resveratrol as a component of red wine is known for its health benefits, and cyanidin and related compounds are antioxidant compounds in fruits and are also responsible for the red to blue coloration of fruits and flowers. The polymeric forms of these compounds also occur in Nature and have various functions, including medicinal uses. Because these compounds have several phenolic moieties in their structures (Figure 5.17), they are also called *polyphenolic* compounds (or *polyphenols*).

One important feature of phenols is the resonance stabilisation of the phenoxide anion through delocalisation of electrons into the aromatic ring system. Let us first consider the lone pair of electrons

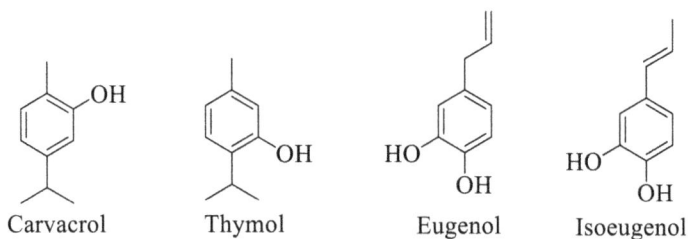

Figure 5.16 Fragrant molecules with a phenolic structure from herbs and essential oils. These compounds are known in the literature by their common names and their IUPAC names are as follows: carvacrol = 2-methyl-5-propan-2-ylphenol, thymol = 5-methyl-2-propan-2-ylphenol, eugenol = 2-methoxy-4-prop-2-enylphenol, and isoeugenol = 2-methoxy-4-[(*E*)-prop-1-enyl] phenol.

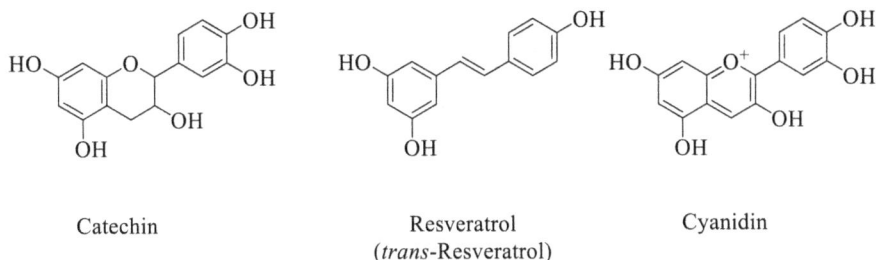

Catechin   Resveratrol   Cyanidin
                       (*trans*-Resveratrol)

Figure 5.17 Examples of plant phenolic compounds. Catechin is common in tea, resveratrol in grapes and wines, and cyanidin in flower pigments and fruits.

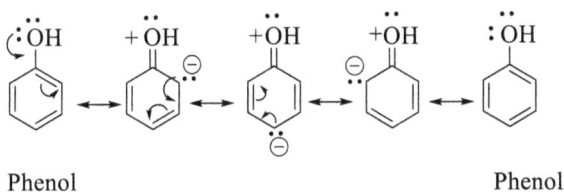

Phenol   Phenol

Figure 5.18 Resonance forms of phenoxide ion.

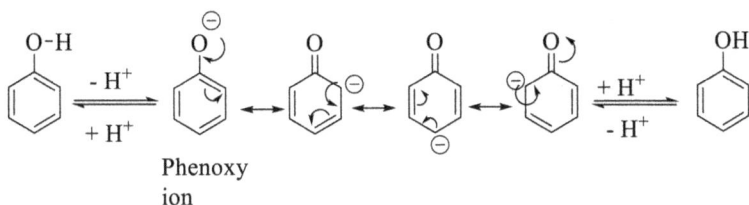

Phenoxy
ion

Figure 5.19 Acidity of phenols and resonance forms through electron delocalisation.

(valence electrons, which are not shared with another atom) of oxygen, which have a tendency to form a bond with carbon and make the oxygen atom positively charged. The resulting charge or negative charge of excess electrons can be stabilised through electron delocalisation into the ring system to form what are called resonance structures (Figure 5.18).

In the same way, we can also consider phenols as acids that liberate a hydrogen ion (H^+) and form a phenoxide ion. The ion is also stabilised by resonance through delocalisation of electrons into the ring system as shown in Figure 5.19.

The above examples suggest that phenol groups have an electron excess at the *ortho* (*o*) and *para* (*p*) positions, whereas the *meta* (*m*)

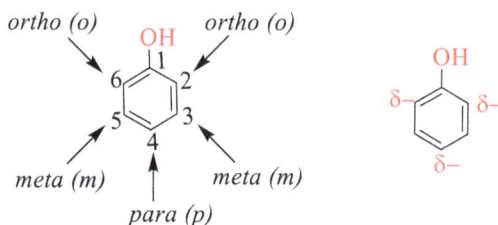

Figure 5.20 Electron excess positions on the phenol structure.

position is relatively unaffected. This can be presented at a partially negative charge centre as shown in Figure 5.20.

As a result, if phenols are subjected to an addition reaction with an electrophile (electron-loving group), the *ortho* and *para* positions are where the addition occurs.

Phenols – Key Facts

- Hydroxyl group attached to an arene or benzene ring system.
- More acidic than alcohols.
- Far more reactive than alcohols.
- Resonance-stabilised phenoxy ion, electron-rich *ortho* and *para* positions.
- React with electrophiles (electron-loving groups), favourable at *ortho* and *para* positions.
- Polyphenols are very common in Nature and are mostly antioxidants.

5.2.8 Combustion of Alcohols

Remember that alcohols have a hydrocarbon skeleton and are flammable: you may remember the tradition of setting fire to the Christmas pudding! In the laboratory, alcohols such as ethanol and methanol are used with caution because of their potential hazard due to combustion and a clear label with a flammable hazard warning sign must be displayed on their containers (Figure 5.21).

5.3 Carboxylic Acids

5.3.1 General Features

Carboxylic acids are a group of organic compounds in which the terminal carbon is bonded to an oxygen (O) atom by a double bond and also a hydroxyl group (−OH) that we already mentioned for alcohols.

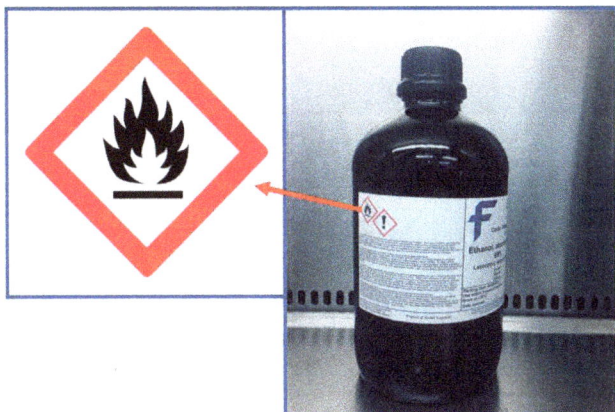

Figure 5.21   Alcohols such as ethanol are flammable. Note the hazard warning sign on the ethanol bottle (see the enlarged image); this is common for many organic solvents in use in the laboratory and highlights the risk of combustion.

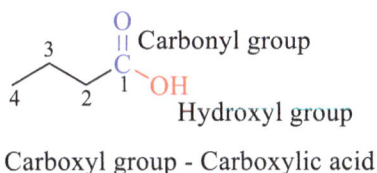

Carboxyl group - Carboxylic acid

Figure 5.22   The carboxyl structural group.

The C=O group is called a *carbonyl group* and together with the *hydroxyl group* make a *carboxyl* group (–COOH) (Figure 5.22).

The carboxyl carbon is conveniently numbered as carbon-1 and their IUPAC nomenclature dictates the use of the suffix *-oic acid*. From the alkane nomenclature (*e.g.* meth*ane*), we omit the final *-e* in the name and replace it with *-oic acid* (*e.g. methanoic acid*). The first 10 acids in the homologous series together with their boiling points and common names are listed in Table 5.2. Both in common names and in chemical reactions, the positions of carbons with respect to the carbonyl carbon of the carboxylic acid (C-1) may be represented as α, β, γ, δ, *etc.* Thus 3-methylbutanoic acid is also called β-methylbutyric acid (see Figure 5.23).

In the above examples, other functional groups such as the amino group (see Section 5.5) can also be named by using Greek letters rather than the IUPAC nomenclature. For example, γ-aminobutyric acid is a neurotransmitter in the brain and is mostly known by this common name in the literature rather than its IUPAC name.

Table 5.2   IUPAC names and common names of the first 10 carboxylic acids in the homologous series.

IUPAC name	Formula	Common name	Boiling point/°C[a]
Methanoic acid	HCO_2H	Formic acid	101
Ethanoic acid	CH_3CO_2H	Acetic acid	117.9
Propanoic acid	$CH_3CH_2CO_2H$	Propionic acid	141.1
Butanoic acid	$CH_3(CH_2)_2CO_2H$	Butyric acid	163.5
Pentanoic acid	$CH_3(CH_2)_3CO_2H$	Valeric acid	186.5
Hexanoic acid	$CH_3(CH_2)_4CO_2H$	Caproic acid	205.8
Heptanoic acid	$CH_3(CH_2)_5CO_2H$	Enanthic acid	222.2
Octanoic acid	$CH_3(CH_2)_6CO_2H$	Caprylic acid	239
Nonanoic acid	$CH_3(CH_2)_7CO_2H$	Pelargonic acid	254.5
Decanoic acid	$CH_3(CH_2)_8CO_2H$	Capric acid	268.7

[a]Note that the boiling point increases with increase in molecular size (see Section 5.3.3). Boiling point values can vary slightly in different databases and those given in this table were sourced from the Hazardous Substances Data Bank (HSDB), available *via* PubChem (https://pubchem.ncbi.nlm.nih.gov/).

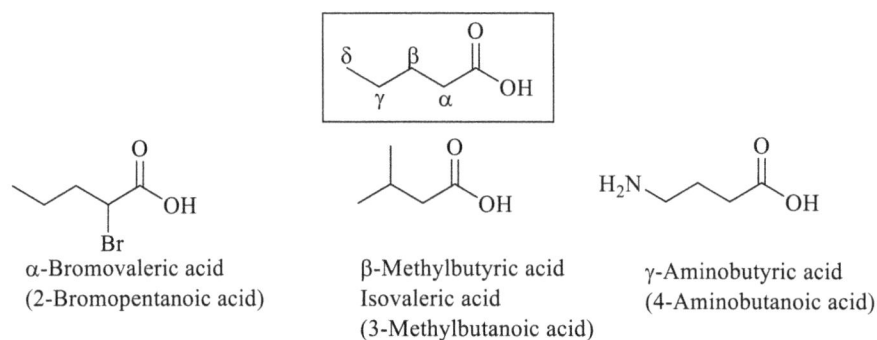

α-Bromovaleric acid
(2-Bromopentanoic acid)

β-Methylbutyric acid
Isovaleric acid
(3-Methylbutanoic acid)

γ-Aminobutyric acid
(4-Aminobutanoic acid)

Figure 5.23   Common naming system of carboxylic acids. The IUPAC names of the compounds are shown in parentheses.

5.3.2   Natural Occurrence

Carboxylic acids are abundantly found in Nature. Butter made from cattle, sheep, and goat milk contains carboxylic acids in the form of fatty acids. The most common fatty acids in butter are short-chain organic acids such as butyric acid (*butyrum* in Latin means butter). Propanoic, hexanoic, and decanoic acids are also found in milk and butter products. Formic acid (methanoic acid) is found in most ants and some species use it as a defence or to incapacitate their prey. Acetic acid (ethanoic acid) is a component of vinegar, which contains about 4% acetic acid, and is present in pickled food. Although acetic acid is produced industrially by synthesis (carbonylation of methanol using carbon monoxide), its main source for the food industry is from natural sources through fermentation using acetic acid bacteria such as the *Acetobacter* genus and *Clostridium acetobutylicum*. Following the fermentation process to generate ethanol, subsequent oxidation yields a distinctive sour-tasting and pungent-smelling product, acetic acid. Fatty acids as components of fats and oils and also cellular structures as part of cell membranes are discussed in Chapter 9.

The bacteria growing in milk convert the sugar lactose into lactic acid (sour milk marker) and its build-up results in milk proteins that coagulate due to a decrease in pH. Citric acid, as the name implies, is found in citrus fruits. Both lactic acid and citric acid are also metabolic products in the body. The generation of energy from food products through a catabolic process starting from sugars involves various carboxylic acids in the metabolic process. Most of these key biosynthesis intermediates in cellular energy production are shown in Figure 5.24.

Carboxylic acids are also common in aromatic compounds. Benzoic acid, salicylic acid, and caffeic acid (Figure 5.25) are examples of ubiquitous natural products that are found abundantly in food cereals, fruits, vegetables, and medicinal plants.

In aromatic compounds, the carbon carrying the carboxyl group (α-carbon) is conveniently numbered as carbon-1. The locations of other substituents can be identified by numbering or naming the

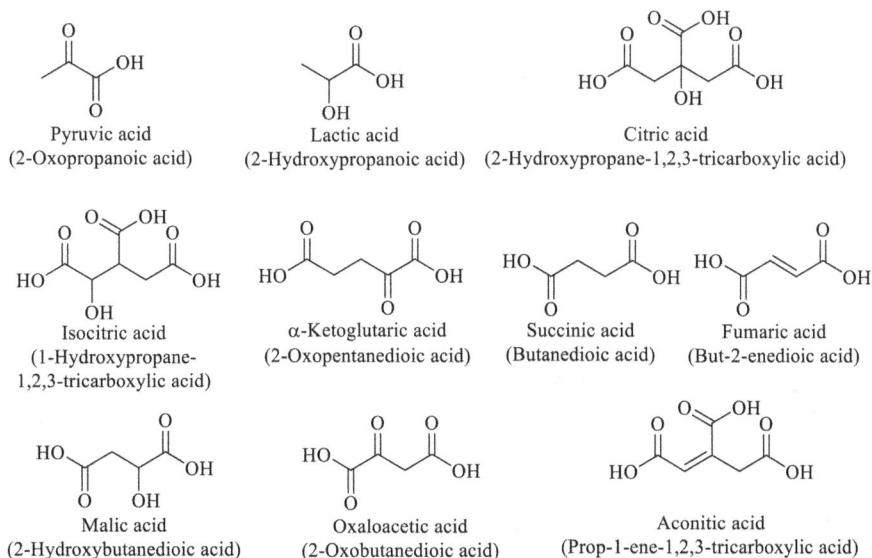

Pyruvic acid
(2-Oxopropanoic acid)

Lactic acid
(2-Hydroxypropanoic acid)

Citric acid
(2-Hydroxypropane-1,2,3-tricarboxylic acid)

Isocitric acid
(1-Hydroxypropane-1,2,3-tricarboxylic acid)

α-Ketoglutaric acid
(2-Oxopentanedioic acid)

Succinic acid
(Butanedioic acid)

Fumaric acid
(But-2-enedioic acid)

Malic acid
(2-Hydroxybutanedioic acid)

Oxaloacetic acid
(2-Oxobutanedioic acid)

Aconitic acid
(Prop-1-ene-1,2,3-tricarboxylic acid)

Figure 5.24 Common organic acids involved in a cellular energy generation system. Their IUPAC names are shown in parentheses.

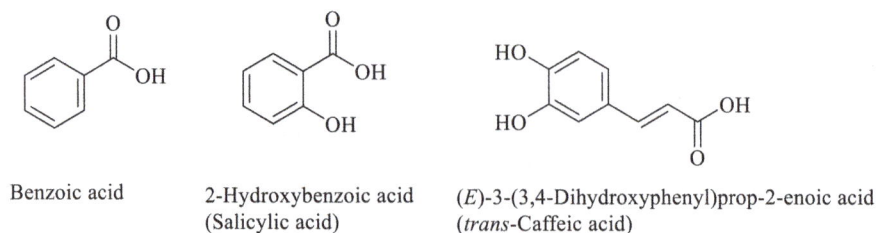

Benzoic acid | 2-Hydroxybenzoic acid (Salicylic acid) | (*E*)-3-(3,4-Dihydroxyphenyl)prop-2-enoic acid (*trans*-Caffeic acid)

Figure 5.25 Examples of aromatic carboxylic acids. Benzoic acid, salicylic acid, and caffeic acid are common in plants. They have applications in food and medicinal preparations. Note that salicylic acid and cinnamic acid are common names that are more widely used in the literature than their IUPAC names.

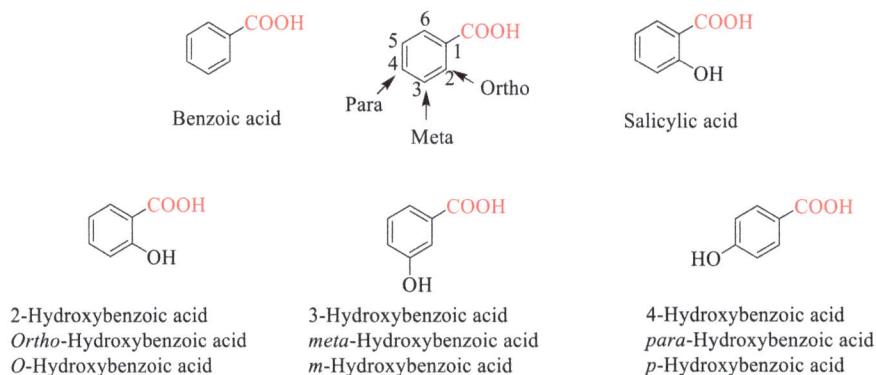

Benzoic acid

Para | Ortho | Meta

Salicylic acid

2-Hydroxybenzoic acid
Ortho-Hydroxybenzoic acid
O-Hydroxybenzoic acid

3-Hydroxybenzoic acid
meta-Hydroxybenzoic acid
m-Hydroxybenzoic acid

4-Hydroxybenzoic acid
para-Hydroxybenzoic acid
p-Hydroxybenzoic acid

Figure 5.26 Nomenclature of aromatic carboxylic acids. The *ortho* (*o*), *meta* (*m*), and *para* (*p*) designations are commonly used in the nomenclature of aromatic acids.

traditional *ortho* (*o*), *meta* (*m*), and *para* (*p*) positions. Thus salicylic acid and its analogues can be named as shown in Figure 5.26.

5.3.3   Properties of Carboxylic Acids

The presence of carbonyl and also hydroxyl groups in carboxylic acids means that they are highly polar. The two sets of polar groups and the formation of intermolecular hydrogen bonds are shown in Figure 5.27.

As a result, the boiling points of carboxylic acids (Table 5.2) are far higher than those of the corresponding alkanes, alkenes, and alcohols and other compounds such as ketones and aldehydes. As shown in Figure 5.27, they also form dimeric structures due to hydrogen bonding. Furthermore, molecules with a carboxylic acid functional group

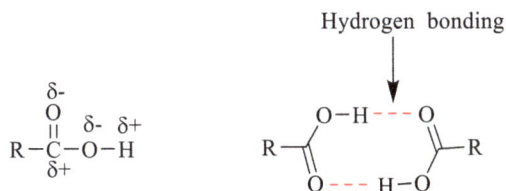

Figure 5.27 Carboxylic acids form dimers through hydrogen bonding.

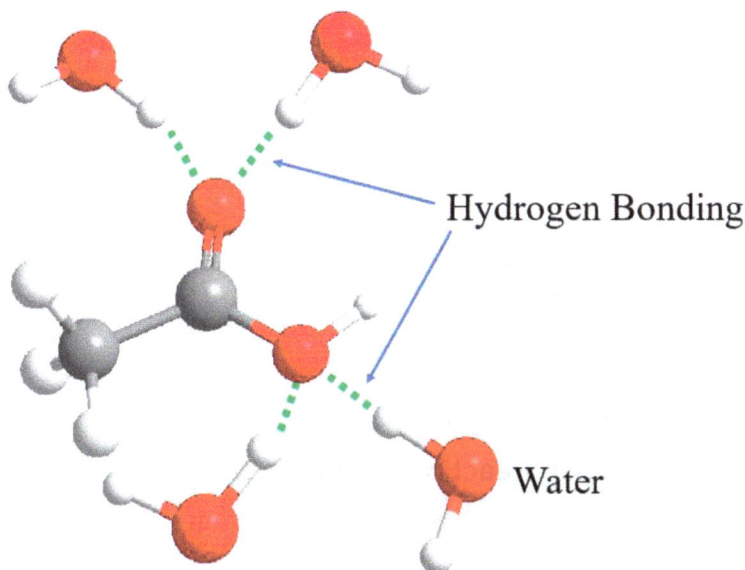

Figure 5.28 Intermolecular hydrogen bonding between ethanoic acid and water.

can form hydrogen bonds with many water molecules (Figure 5.28). Accordingly, shorter chain carboxylic acids (1–4 carbons) are highly miscible in water. As with alcohols, increasing the hydrocarbon chain leads to an increase in hydrophobicity and hence a decrease in water solubility.

The other main characteristic feature of carboxylic acids is their acidity, and their pH is typically between 2 and 4. Although weaker than mineral acids such as hydrochloric acid (HCl) and sulfuric acid (H_2SO_4), their acidity is higher than those of any other functional groups including alcohols.

The polar carbonyl bond in aromatic carboxylic acids such as benzoic acid has a tendency for the bond (C=O) electrons to move towards the oxygen atom. The resulting negatively charged oxygen creates an

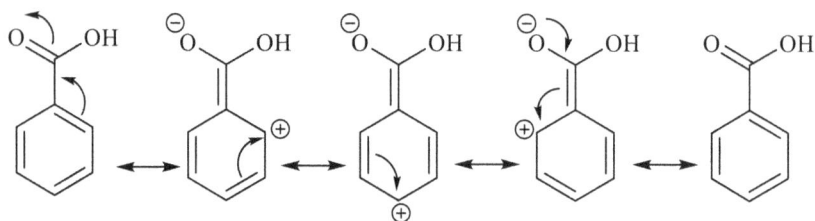

Figure 5.29 Resonance structure of benzoic acid.

aromatic π resonance delocalisation to form stable ions as shown in Figure 5.29.

In chemical reactions involving a carboxylic acid group attached to an aromatic structure (see benzoic acid in Figure 5.29), note that the *ortho* and *para* positions represent an electron-deficient (positive) site compared with the *meta* position. This is the opposite of what we observe for the amines (see Section 5.5). Hence aromatic carboxylic acids interact preferentially with electron-rich chemical groups at *ortho* and *para* positions.

5.3.4   Reactions of Carboxylic Acids

5.3.4.1   Acid–Base Reactions to Form Salts

Carboxylic acids react with a strong base to give a salt and water. When we name the corresponding salt, we first name the cation (the positively charged group) followed by the name of the acid where we drop *-ic acid* and replace it with *-ate*.

Examples of salts of carboxylic acids are as follows (see also Figure 5.30):

- CH_3CO_2Na: sodium acetate (sodium ethanoate)
- $CH_3CH_2CH_2CO_2NH_4$: ammonium butyrate (ammonium butanoate)
- $(CH_3CH_2COO)_2Mg$: magnesium propanoate.

Aromatic acids also undergo similar reactions to form salts (Figure 5.30).

Benzoic acid is readily soluble in organic solvents such as acetone, chloroform, and alcohols but is poorly or only slightly soluble in cold water. On the other hand, sodium benzoate is a salt and is readily soluble in water. Sodium benzoate is used as a preservative in foods, medicines, and cosmetic products for its properties of preventing spoilage

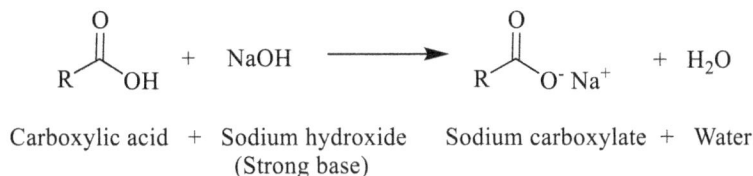

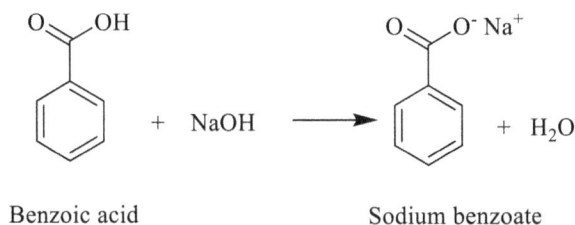

Figure 5.30 Reaction of a carboxylic acid with sodium hydroxide to form a salt (sodium carboxylate). Note that salts are ionised in water.

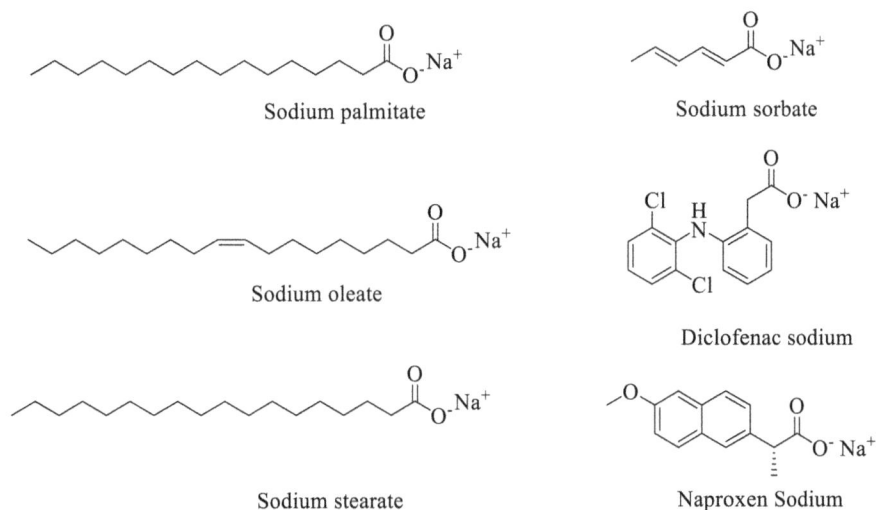

Figure 5.31 Examples of sodium salts of organic acids.

by bacteria, yeasts, and moulds. In addition to benzoic acid, salts of organic acids such as sorbates and propionates have been used extensively as food/medicine/cosmetic preservatives for their antimicrobial activities.

Salt formation is used extensively in the preparation of active ingredients and additives in foods, medicines, and cosmetic products. Fatty acids, which are soluble only in organic solvents (and not water), are converted to salt forms in the preparation of soaps (see Figure 5.31).

Preservatives (*e.g.* sorbate; see Figure 5.31) and drugs with a carboxylate functional group are converted to their salt form to improve their physicochemical properties such as achieving better stability and formulation features.

Many drug molecules containing carboxylic acid functional groups are converted to their salt form to increase their solubility in aqueous media and improve their formulation properties (*e.g.* stability and ease of administration). The anti-inflammatory drugs diclofenac and naproxen are examples of organic acids converted to their sodium salt form (Figure 5.31) in their formulation. In this connection, at least 50% of pharmaceutical products are expected to be formulated in their salt forms. Note that the fatty acids in plant oils (oleic acid, palmitic acid, and stearic acid) are also converted to their salt form to make soap. Salt formation can also be achieved by manipulating other functional groups such as amines (see Section 5.5).

5.3.4.2   Reactions with Active Metals

Carboxylic acids also react with active metals such as sodium or magnesium to produce salts and hydrogen.

$$\text{Metal} + \text{carboxylic acid} \rightarrow \text{salt} + \text{hydrogen}$$

$$Na + CH_3CH_2COOH \rightarrow CH_3CH_2COONa + \tfrac{1}{2}H_2$$

$$Mg + 2CH_3CH_2COOH \rightarrow (CH_3CH_2COO)_2Mg + H_2$$

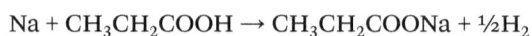

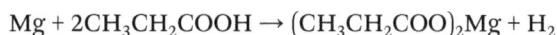

Conversion of Carboxylic Acids to Salts – Key Facts

Making salts of carboxylic acids is the best way to increase solubility in water. In doing so, some drug molecules that are not water soluble can be converted to their salt forms to increase their absorption from the gastrointestinal system. The stability of drug molecules and their pharmacokinetic profile can also be altered by making a salt form of the carboxylic acid functional group.

5.3.4.3   Reduction Reactions

By using reducing agents, carboxylic acids can be reduced to either aldehydes or primary alcohols. A variety of reducing agents such as metal hydrides, most commonly lithium aluminium hydride ($LiAlH_4$) and diborane (B_2H_6), may be used as strong reducing agents to produce alcohols (Figure 5.32). Obviously, the reaction goes through the aldehyde intermediates, but the rapid reactions quickly proceed to the final product, an alcohol. There are milder reagents that yield

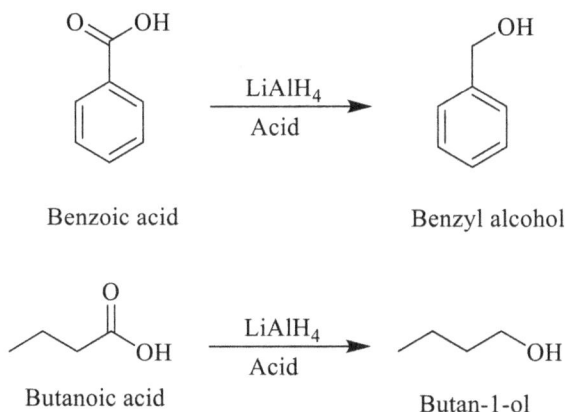

Benzoic acid → LiAlH₄ / Acid → Benzyl alcohol

Butanoic acid → LiAlH₄ / Acid → Butan-1-ol

Figure 5.32 Reduction reaction of organic acids. By using a reducing agent, organic acids can be converted to alcohols through aldehyde intermediates. The use of a strong reducing agent may lead instantly to alcohol formation without seeing the aldehyde intermediates.

aldehydes from acids, and there are also other ways of making aldehydes from carboxylic acids that are not discussed here.

5.3.4.4 Esterification Reactions

Carboxylic acids react with alcohols to produce esters. Alcohols are normally used as excess solvents to dissolve carboxylic acids and the reversible reaction in the presence of acid catalysts yields esters. A good example is the synthesis of aspirin from salicylic acid. Although acetylation using acetic acid and traditional acids such as sulfuric acid (H_2SO_4) or *p*-toluenesulfonic acid (TsOH or tosylic acid) is used, acetylation using acetic anhydride is the easiest method for the synthesis of aspirin (Figure 5.33).

For those who need to synthesise aspirin and related esters in the laboratory, other reagents are also available. *Note that reversing the hydroxyl polar bond by ester or acetylation will reduce the polarity. This means that you are making acids lipophilic by converting them to esters.* In the above example, we used acetic anhydride, which is another functional group, an *acid anhydride*. This is a functional group in which two acid molecules bond through an oxygen bridge by losing hydrogen. The reaction is, however, effectively carried out by using a more reactive *acid chloride* functional group as shown in Figure 5.34.

Salicylic acid   Acetic acid   Aspirin

Salicylic acid   Acetic anhydride   Aspirin   Acetic acid

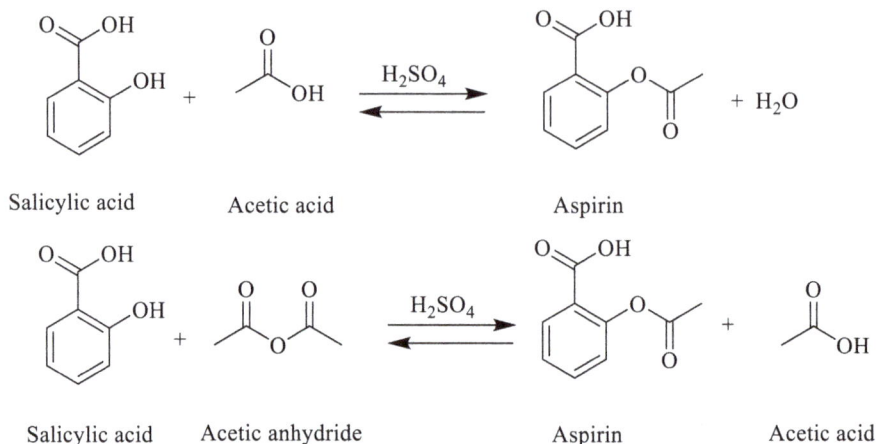

Figure 5.33 Example of the esterification reaction of organic acids. The reversible reaction (which can also be represented using the symbol ⇄ or ⇌ is shown.

Ethanoic acids   Ethanoic anhydride   Water

Ethanoic acid   Ethanoyl chloride   Ethanoic anhydride

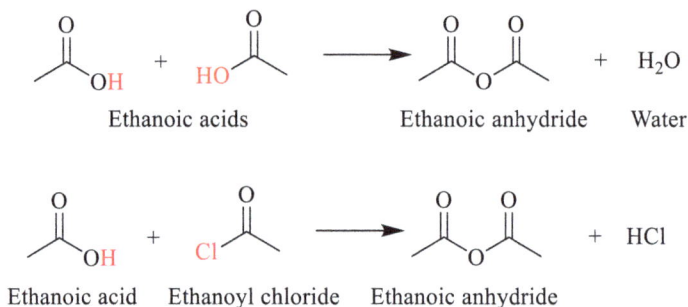

Figure 5.34 Synthesis of an acid anhydride. Loss of water or dehydration of ethanoic acid can yield ethanoic anhydride. Note that acid chlorides are more reactive than carboxylic acids (see Section 5.3.4.5).

5.3.4.5 Acid Chlorides (Acyl Chlorides)

Acid chlorides (*acyl chlorides*) such as ethanoyl chloride are functional groups that are used effectively to facilitate reactions involving carboxylic acids, *i.e.* acyl chlorides are far more reactive than carboxylic acids. The traditional reagent for this conversion of carboxylic acids to acid chlorides is thionyl chloride ($SOCl_2$, Figure 5.35).

Carboxylic acids also react with several other functional groups, including thiols and amines. These are beyond the scope of this book, however, and are not discussed here.

Benzoic acid   Benzyl chloride

Benzyl chloride   Ethanoic acid   Acid anhydride

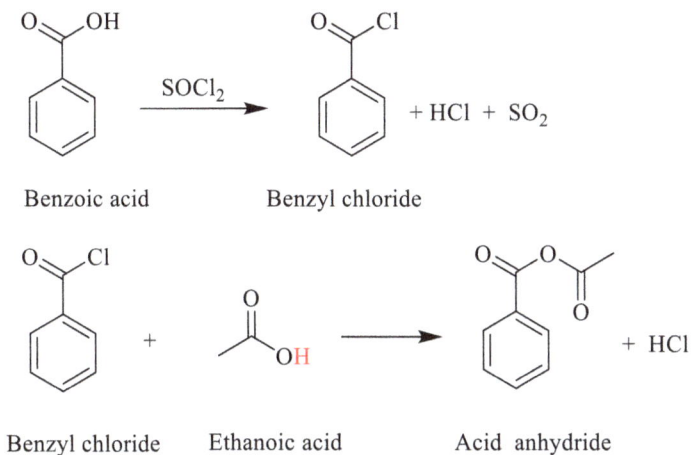

Figure 5.35   A more reactive acid chloride instead of an organic acid is used in the chemical reaction. Benzoic acid is converted to a more reactive benzyl chloride by reacting it with thionyl chloride ($SOCl_2$).

Carboxylic Acids – Key Facts

- Organic compounds with a carboxyl group – a carbonyl carbon (C=O) attached to a hydroxyl group.
- Very common in Nature, *e.g.* fatty acids and aromatic acids.
- Nomenclature – suffix -oic acid (*e.g.* butanoic acid).
- Salt form with metal named with suffix -ate (*e.g.* sodium butanoate).
- Acyl halide is a structure in which a carbonyl is attached to –Cl, –Br, *etc.* and is named with suffix -yl chloride, *etc.* (*e.g.* butanoyl chloride).
- The anhydride forms of acids are named with suffix -ic anhydride (*e.g.* butanoic anhydride).
- An ester with an alkyl or aryl group is named with the suffix -ate (*e.g.* methyl butanoate).
- Characteristics – acidic and high boiling point due to hydrogen bonding.
- For aromatic acids, the reaction site in the benzene ring is based on resonance structures. *Ortho* and *para* positions are electron-deficient centres.

5.4 Ketones and Aldehydes

5.4.1 General Features

Just like the carboxylic acids that were discussed in the previous section, ketones and aldehydes also have a carbonyl (C=O) functional group. If one of the other elements bonded to this carbonyl carbon is hydrogen, the compound is called an aldehyde. This occurs when carbonyl carbon, like the carboxylic acids, is a terminal carbon in the chain. On the other hand, if carbonyl carbon does not have hydrogen and instead has either alkyl or aryl groups on both sides, it is a ketone functional group.

The IUPAC nomenclature **uses the** suffix '*al*' for aldehyde and '*one*' for ketones (Figure 5.36).

Note that the homologous series of ketones starts from propanone, so there is no counterpart to methanal and ethanal (Figure 5.36). When other functional groups such as alcohols are present, the naming of the compound gives precedence to ketone or aldehyde, as exemplified by 3-hydroxybutanal and 4-hydroxypentan-2-one. In compounds where both ketone and aldehyde groups exist, the aldehyde take precedence in the naming and the ketone is indicated as oxo, *e.g.* 4-oxopentanal. A compound with two aldehyde functional groups can be named as a dial (*e.g.* pentanedial), three as a trial, and so on. Similarly, a compound with two ketone groups can be named as a dione (*e.g.* pentane-2,4-dione), three as a trione, and so on. If ketone and aldehyde groups occur together with a carboxylic acid, the carboxylic acid takes precedence in the naming, *e.g.* 4-oxopentanoic acid.

5.4.2 Occurrence

Both ketone and aldehyde functional groups are very common in Nature. Low molecular weight fragrance molecules such as essential oils of herbs contain ketones and aldehydes (Figure 5.37). They have numerous applications in the perfumery industry and in the flavouring of foods and beverages. They also have medical applications. Up to 90% of cinnamon oil is composed of cinnamaldehyde. Representing aldehydes, vanillin is a major component of vanillin bean and citral is the main component of lemongrass oil. Representing ketones of essential oils, carvone is a component of spearmint and caraway oil, and camphor is a component of the camphor tree. The structures of these representative fragrance molecules are shown in Figure 5.37.

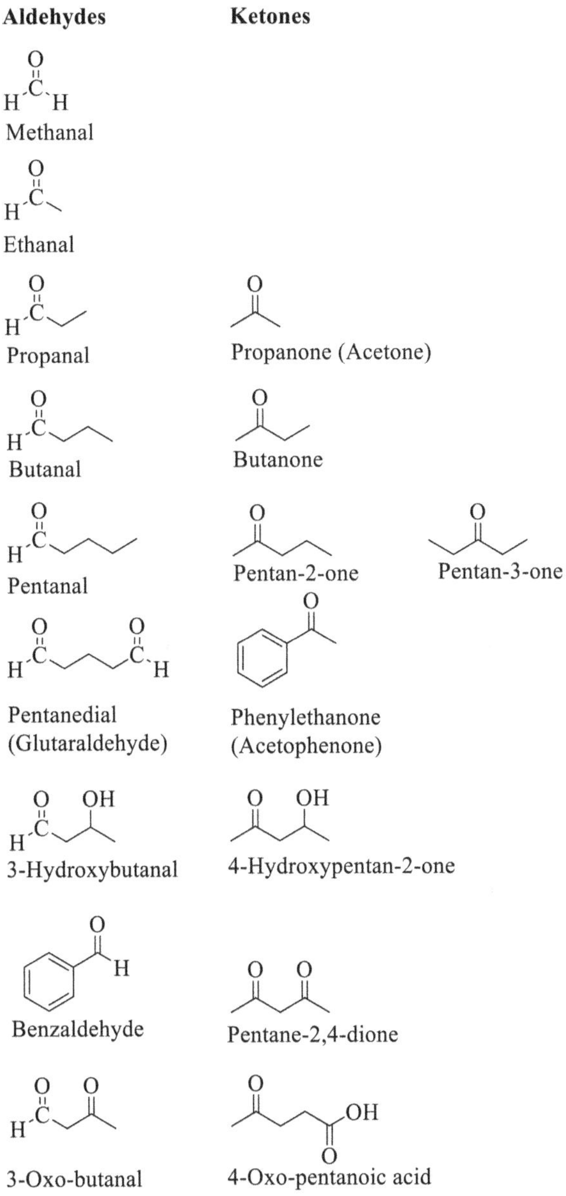

Aldehydes

Ketones

O
‖
H–C–H
Methanal

O
‖
H–C–
Ethanal

O
‖
H–C–
Propanal

O
‖
Propanone (Acetone)

O
‖
H–C–
Butanal

O
‖
Butanone

O
‖
H–C–
Pentanal

O
‖
Pentan-2-one

O
‖
Pentan-3-one

O   O
‖   ‖
H–C–   C–H

Pentanedial
(Glutaraldehyde)

O
‖
Phenylethanone
(Acetophenone)

O   OH
‖
H–C–
3-Hydroxybutanal

O   OH
‖
4-Hydroxypentan-2-one

O
‖
H
Benzaldehyde

O   O
‖   ‖
Pentane-2,4-dione

O   O
‖   ‖
H–C–
3-Oxo-butanal

O
‖
OH
‖
O
4-Oxo-pentanoic acid

Figure 5.36 Nomenclature of ketones and aldehydes.

Numerous drug molecules and hormones carry ketone and aldehyde functional groups. Good examples (see Figure 5.38) are steroidal hormones such as testosterone, progesterone, and aldosterone and anti-inflammatory steroidal drugs such as dexamethasone and

| Cinnamaldehyde | Vanillin | Citral | Carvone | Camphor |

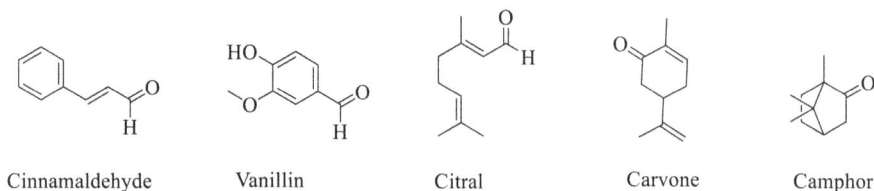

Figure 5.37 Examples of volatile acids and aldehydes in herbs and spices. The common names that are popularly used in the literature are shown.

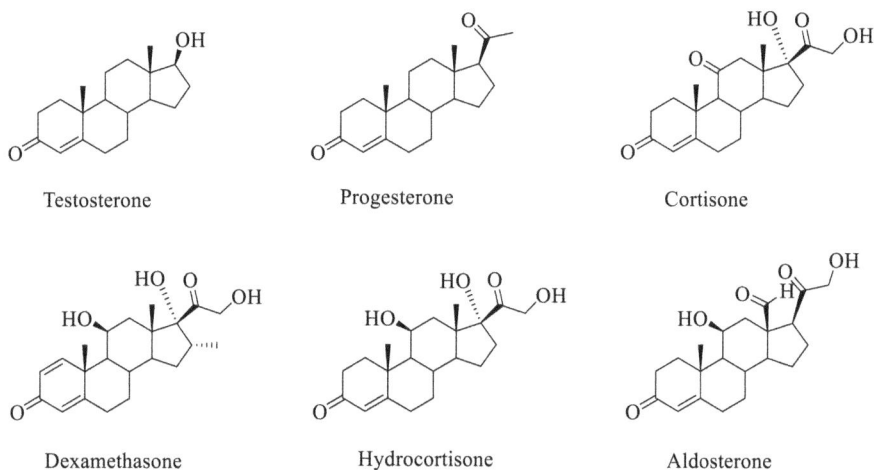

| Testosterone | Progesterone | Cortisone |

| Dexamethasone | Hydrocortisone | Aldosterone |

Figure 5.38 Ketone and aldehyde functional groups in drugs and hormones. The IUPAC names are far too complex for our discussion here and we rather use the common names that are popular in the literature.

hydrocortisone. Note that these compounds also have hydroxyl functional groups.

Aldehydes and ketones can be obtained through oxidation of alcohols and various other reactions. By using appropriate oxidising agents, primary alcohols can give rise to aldehydes and secondary alcohols can be oxidised to give ketones (Figure 5.39).

It should be borne in mind that aldehydes and ketones undergo a range of reactions including addition reactions and reduction reactions to give alcohols as the reverse reaction of obtaining them from alcohols. They could further oxidise or participate in other types of reactions. One of the most important reactions of aldehydes and ketones is with primary amines (see Section 5.5) to form the *imine functional group* (Figure 5.40).

$$H_3C\overset{}{\diagup}CH_2OH \xrightarrow{\text{Oxidation [O]}} H_3C\overset{}{\diagup}\underset{O}{\overset{}{C}}\text{-H}$$

Propan-1-ol   Propanal

$$H_3C\overset{OH}{\underset{}{\diagup}}CH_3 \xrightarrow{\text{Oxidation [O]}} H_3C\overset{O}{\underset{}{\diagup}}CH_3$$

Propan-2-ol   Propanone

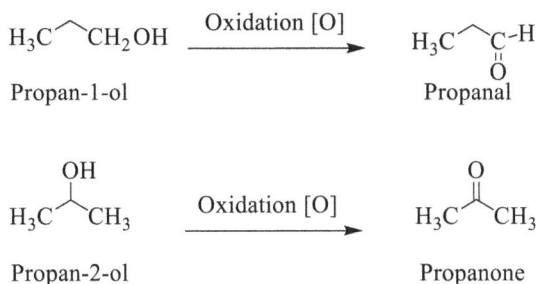

Figure 5.39 Formation of aldehydes and ketones through oxidation of alcohols.

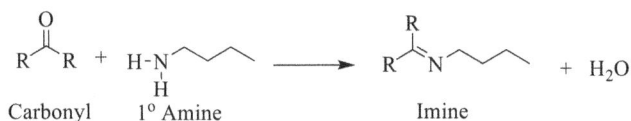

$$\underset{\text{Carbonyl}}{R\overset{O}{\underset{}{\diagdown}}R} + \underset{1°\text{ Amine}}{H\text{-}\underset{H}{\overset{}{N}}\diagup\diagdown} \longrightarrow \underset{\text{Imine}}{R\overset{R}{\underset{}{\diagdown}}N\diagup\diagdown} + H_2O$$

Figure 5.40 Reaction of a carbonyl and a primary amine to form an imine. Note that water is eliminated in this reaction.

5.5 Amines

5.5.1 General Features and Nomenclature

Amines are a diverse group of organic compounds that contain nitrogen in their structure. In a simplistic presentation, the hydrogen in ammonia is replaced with carbon to make the homologous series based on an alkane skeleton (Figure 5.41).

The homologous series of amines starting from methane is methylamine (also called aminomethane), ethylamine (aminoethane), propylamine, butylamine, *etc.* (Table 5.3). These are based on replacing one hydrogen in the alkane with NH_2 and hence can be represented by the general formula $C_nH_{2n+1}NH_2$. These are for saturated hydrocarbons that can be represented by an R group carrying an NH_2 functional group. They are expressed as RNH_2 and are called *primary amines*.

The requirement for primary amines is the presence of an NH_2 functional group in organic compounds, hence the hydrocarbon can be of an alkene type or of any other functional group. The hydrocarbon chain can also either be alkyl or have an aromatic structure just like the neurotransmitters dopamine and norepinephrine and the psychoactive compound amphetamine (Figure 5.42).

Note that the locations of the amine group and double bonds can be identified as shown for but-2-en-1-amine. The IUPAC nomenclature

Lone pair electrons – Not shared with another atom

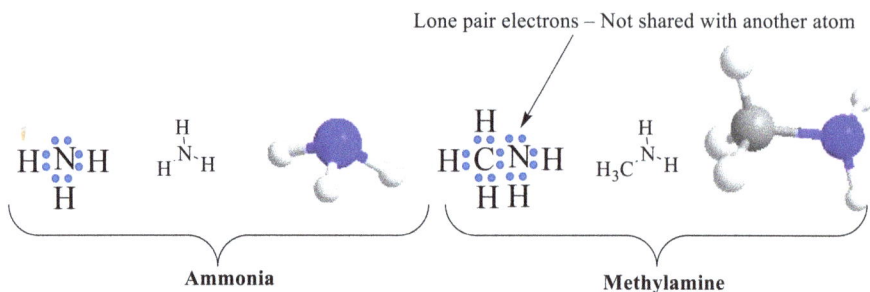

Ammonia   **Methylamine**

Figure 5.41 Methylamine as the first amine in the homologous series.

Table 5.3 The first 10 amines in the homologous series.

Structural formula	Common name	IUPAC name
CH_3NH_2	Methylamine	Methanamine
$CH_3CH_2NH_2$	Ethylamine	Ethanamine
$CH_3(CH_2)_2NH_2$	Propylamine	Propan-1-amine
$CH_3(CH_2)_3NH_2$	*n*-Butylamine	Butan-1-amine
$CH_3(CH_2)_5NH_2$	*n*-Pentylamine	Pentan-1-amine
$CH_3(CH_2)_6NH_2$	*n*-Hexylamine	Hexan-1-amine
$CH_3(CH_2)_7NH_2$	*n*-Heptylamine	Heptan-1-amine
$CH_3(CH_2)_8NH_2$	*n*-Octylamine	Octan-1-amine
$CH_3(CH_2)_9NH_2$	*n*-Nonylamine	Nonan-1-amine
$CH_3(CH_2)_{10}NH_2$	*n*-Decylamine	Decan-1-amine

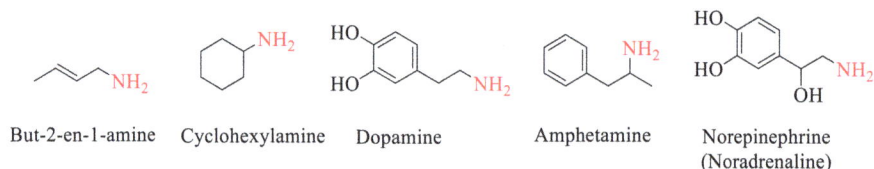

But-2-en-1-amine   Cyclohexylamine   Dopamine   Amphetamine   Norepinephrine
                                                                     (Noradrenaline)

Figure 5.42 Some examples of amines. All carry the NH_2 group and are therefore primary amines. Note that dopamine, amphetamine, and norepinephrine are common names that are conveniently used in the literature.

for alkylamines (Figure 5.43) is based on naming the alkane first and indicating the location of the amine group in the alkyl chain (Table 5.3). In a branched system, the nomenclature is also based on the naming of alkanes. When all the substituents on the nitrogen atom are the same group, we can use the prefix 'di' or 'tri'. For unsymmetrical substitution, we apply the name of the longest parent chain and the smaller units are entered as N-substituents as shown in Figure 5.43.

In aromatic compounds, the carbon carrying the amine group is conveniently numbered as carbon-1 (Figure 5.44). As discussed for

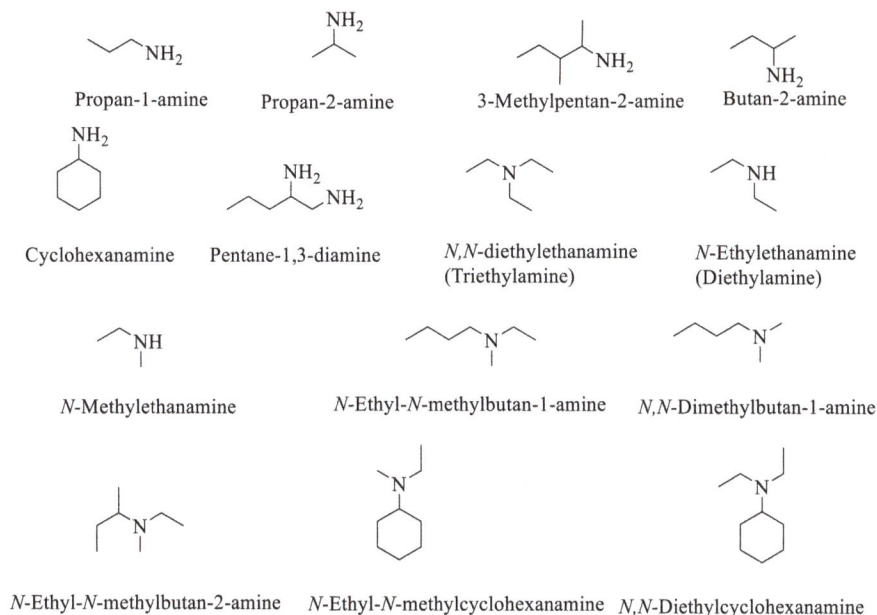

Figure 5.43   IUPAC nomenclature for alkylamines.

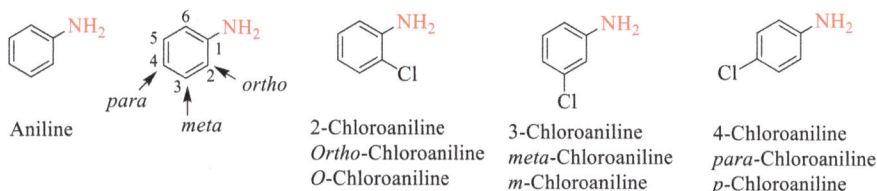

Figure 5.44   Nomenclature of arylamines.

carboxylic acids, the locations of other substituents can be identified by numbering or the traditional *ortho* (*o*), *meta* (*m*), and *para* (*p*) positions to the amine group.

All the above examples of amines, which are represented by the general formula RNH$_2$ where R is either alkyl or aryl, are called primary (1°) amines. Secondary (2°) amines have two organic substituents (alkyl, aryl, or both) and are represented by the general formula R$_2$NH, and tertiary (3°) amines have three organic substituents, *i.e.* all the hydrogen atoms of ammonia are replaced with organic substituents, alkyl or aryl or both, to give the general formula of tertiary amines as R$_3$N.

Most biologically active compounds, drugs, and hormones contain amine functional groups (Figure 5.45).

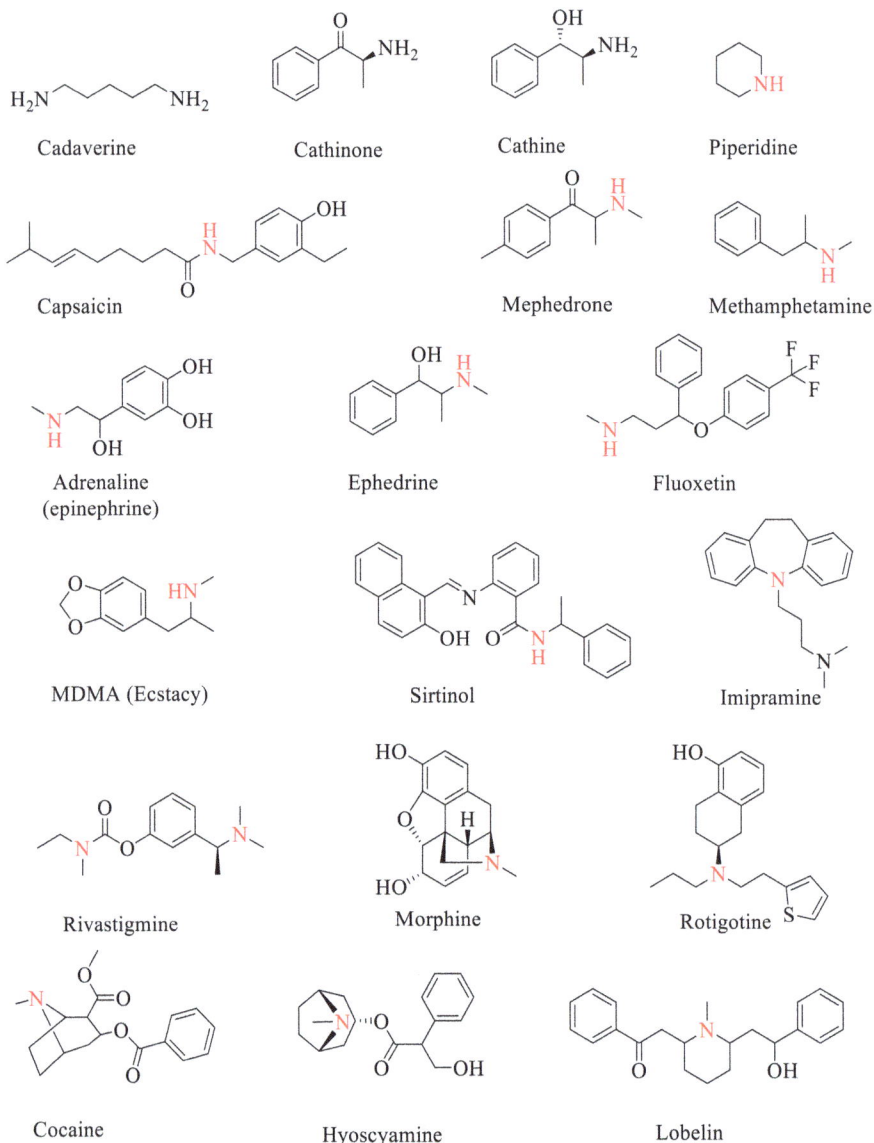

Figure 5.45 The structures of many drugs and biologically active compounds such as hormones contain the amine functional group. Note that stereochemistry is discussed in Chapter 6 and this figure is intended just to appreciate the presence of amine functional groups in many biologically active compounds.

The unique feature of nitrogen in its chemical bonding is its ability to extend its valency to four. This is shown in the ionic form of quaternary ammonium compounds, which have the general formula R_4N^+. This is also the salt form of amines and hence they are water soluble. Quaternary amines can be prepared by reacting amines with acids:

$$RNH_2 + H^+ \rightarrow RNH_3{}^+$$

$$RNH_2 + HCl \rightarrow RNH_3{}^+Cl^-$$

Many natural and synthetic drugs are used in their quaternary amine form. The neurotransmitter acetylcholine and the neuroactive compounds hemicholinium and hexamethonium are examples of quaternary amines (Figure 5.46). In the naming of quaternary ammonium salts, we use aminium as the suffix followed by the anion (*e.g.* bromide, chloride, hydroxide, *etc.*), *e.g.* ethanaminium chloride (Figure 5.46).

In summary, amines are categorized by the number of alkyl groups attached to the nitrogen atom as follows:

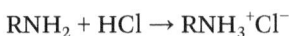

Ethanaminium chloride *N,N,N*-Triethylethanaminium hydroxide *N*-Ethyl-1-propanaminium bromide

N,N-Diethyl-*N*-methyl-1-propanaminium bromide *N*-ethyl-*N,N*-dimethylcyclohexanaminium hydroxide

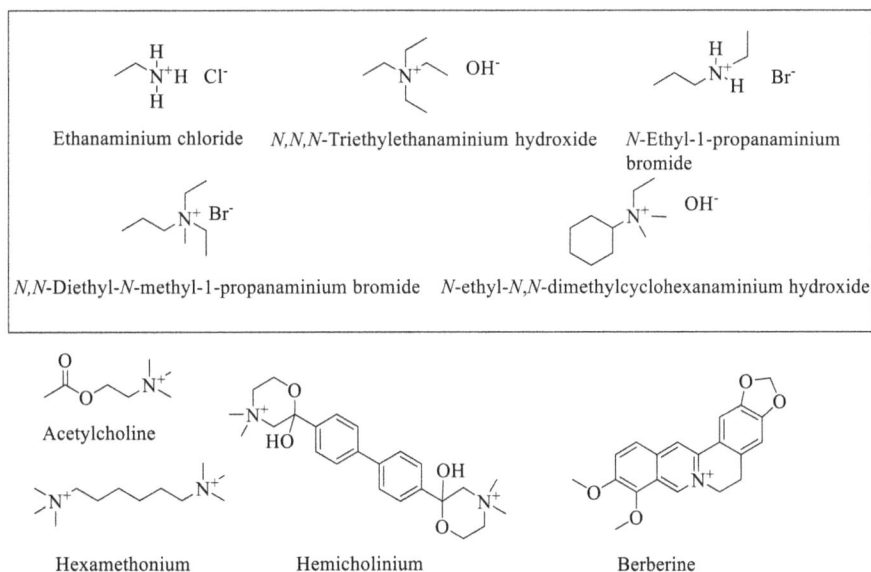

Acetylcholine

Hexamethonium Hemicholinium Berberine

Figure 5.46 Examples of drugs with a quaternary amine structural group. The box at the top shows the naming of quaternary ammonium salts. Bear in mind that there are many competing names for quaternary amine salts. Some examples of cationic drugs are illustrated, and more examples are discussed in Chapter 13. Acetylcholine is a neurotransmitter and hexamethonium, hemicholinium, and berberine are drugs that modify neurotransmission.

- 1° (primary amine) RNH_2
- 2° (secondary amine) R_2NH
- 3° (tertiary amine) R_3N
- 4° (quaternary amine salt) R_4N^+

5.5.2   Properties of Amines

All amines can undergo hydrogen bonding with water. The bond between carbon and nitrogen in all amines (C–N) and the bond between nitrogen and hydrogen (N–H) in primary and secondary amines are polarised. Accordingly, amines can undergo a hydrogen bonding interaction with water (Figure 5.47). Thus, smaller molecular sized amines are water soluble. Ammonia, despite being a gas, is also able to form hydrogen bonds with water and is soluble in water. As with alcohols, the solubility of amines in water decreases as the molecular size increases. Hence amines with a hydrophobic hydrocarbon chain with the order of six carbon atoms and above are not soluble in water. Note that the electronegativity of oxygen is higher than that of nitrogen. As a result, alcohols undergo stronger hydrogen bonding interactions than amines. The boiling point of amines decreases in the order primary > secondary > tertiary. Note that tertiary amines do not have a hydrogen atom attached to the nitrogen atom that could undergo hydrogen bonding. As explained above, quaternary amines are salts and are readily soluble in water.

The nitrogen atom in amines has a pair of unshared electrons (lone pair electrons) and tends to break away from the nitrogen nucleus

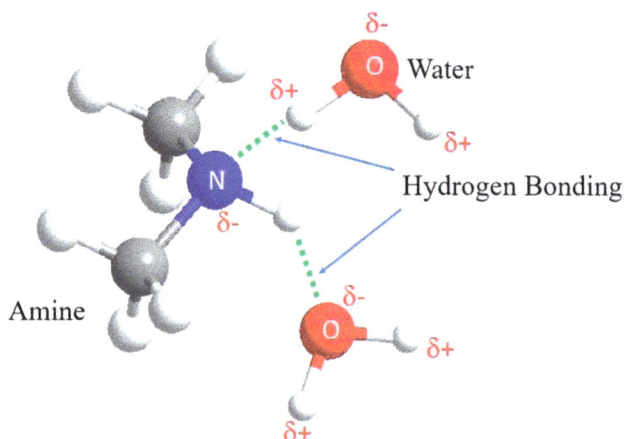

Figure 5.47   Intermolecular hydrogen bonding of amines with water.

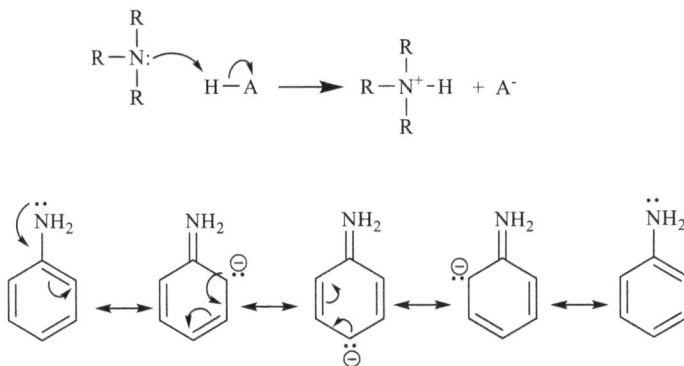

Figure 5.48   Reactivity of amines and the resonance structure of aniline. Note the electron excess site at the *ortho* and *para* positions.

and form a bond with a hydrogen atom. This means that amines, just like ammonia, are basic. This is also the reason why they react readily with acids to give the quaternary ammonium salt form. The reactivity of amines as a base (basicity) can be presented as shown in Figure 5.48. The tendency of the lone pair electrons in nitrogen to make a bond is also involved in the aromatic π resonance delocalisation system, as shown for aniline (phenylamine or benzamine) in Figure 5.48.

Since the lone pair electrons responsible for the basicity of amines are involved in resonance in an aromatic system (as shown in Figure 5.48 for aniline), aliphatic (in a chain) amines are more basic than aromatic amines. In chemical reactions involving the NH_2 group attached to an aromatic structure (see the example of aniline), note that the *ortho* and *para* positions have an electron-rich (partial negative) site compared with the *meta* position. This is the opposite of the carboxyl group discussed in Section 5.3.3.

There are numerous nitrogen-containing compounds that occur in Nature and as synthetic compounds. These compounds, called alkaloids, are useful as drug molecules and are discussed in Chapter 13.

5.5.3   Reactions of Amines

5.5.3.1   Addition Reactions

As explained above, amines react with acids (*e.g.* H_2SO_4, HNO_3, and HCl) to form salts. This involves the addition of a hydrogen ion (H^+) to make a new bond *via* the lone pair electrons of the nitrogen atom in amines (primary, secondary, or tertiary). The reaction yields quaternary amines, which are water soluble.

5.5.3.2   Acylation or Substitution Reactions

Just like alcohols (–OH group), primary and secondary amines (RNH_2 and R_2NH) can undergo an acylation reaction (Figure 5.49). This is a substitution reaction in which the hydrogen atom bonded to the nitrogen atom in amines is replaced with an acyl group. Note that an acyl group is derived from an acid, such as RCOOH with the removal of –OH, such as RC(=O)Cl. The most reactive acyl group is represented by acyl chloride, which was described under carboxylic acids (see Section 5.3.4.5).

In the acylation reaction (Figure 5.49), hydrogen chloride is vigorously formed but is consumed by the amine to form ammonium chloride salt. Hence the products will be largely amide and ammonium chloride salt.

5.5.3.3   Alkylation Reactions

Alkylation refers to the addition of an alkyl group to an organic molecule, *i.e.* from the alkyl donor called an alkylating agent to an acceptor such as an amine. Alkyl halides (RI, RBr, RCl, and RF, where R is an alkyl group) can be added directly to amines to make ammonium salts (Figure 5.50).

Note that there are numerous other reactions of amines that are beyond the scope of this book.

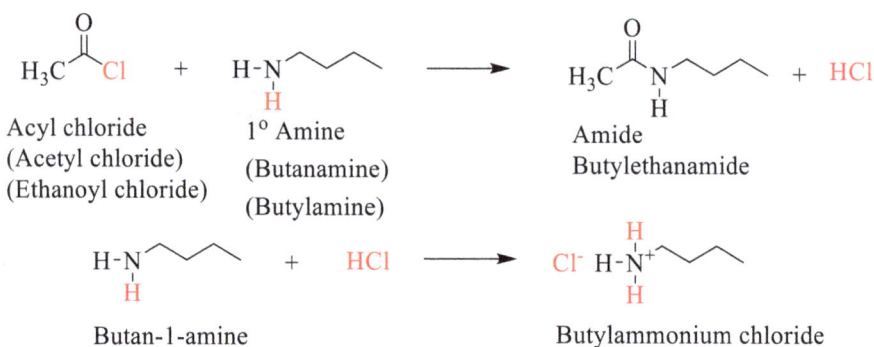

Figure 5.49   Acylation of amines.

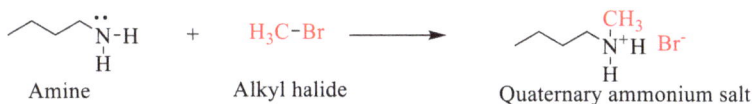

Figure 5.50 Alkylation of amines.

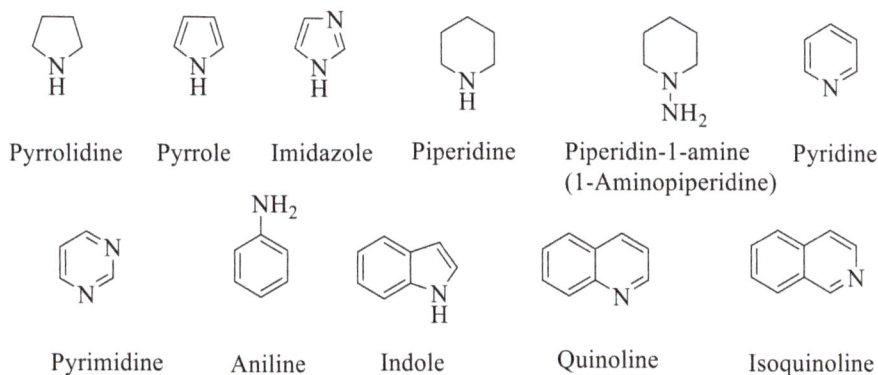

Figure 5.51 Examples of heterocyclic skeletons of nitrogen-containing compounds.

5.5.4 Aromatic and Heterocyclic Amines

As we have seen for cyclic ethers, nitrogen can also be incorporated in a ring system. Heterocyclic compounds – with atoms other than carbon in the cyclic structure – contain *heteroatoms* in a ring system. Nitrogen, oxygen, and sulfur are common elements that are present in heterocyclic compounds. In plants and other living organisms, these kinds of amines are called alkaloids and are major products that we aim to exploit as potential drugs. Some of the structural skeletons in these groups are shown in Figure 5.51.

The role of these compounds and structural groups as a function of other biologically active compounds are addressed elsewhere in this book (see Chapter 13). Heterocyclic amines also include compounds formed during the cooking process of muscle meats from beef, pork, and fish. High cooking temperatures or over-cooked meats are considered major sources of these dangerous products. The compounds themselves are not considered toxic but their by-products during the cooking process (*N*-hydroxylated, *N*-hydroxysulfated, or otherwise *N*-hydroxy-substituted products) are carcinogenic.

Amines – Key Facts

- Nitrogen-containing compounds.
- Many drug molecules have nitrogen in their molecules.
- Exist in primary (RNH_2), secondary (R_2NH), and tertiary (R_3N) forms.
- The ammonium cation, quaternary form (R_4N^+), is a water-soluble salt.
- The assignment of $1°$, $2°$, $3°$, and $4°$ amines is different from that of alcohols:

    o In alcohols, we investigate how many carbons are bonded to the carbon carrying the OH group.
    o In amines, we investigate how many carbons are bonded to the nitrogen atom.

5.6   Alkyl Halides and Aryl Halides

While discussing the various groups of organic compounds, we have already mentioned alkyl halides, which are also called *haloalkanes*. In our alkane examples of either linear or branched-chain structures, halogen atoms (fluorine, chlorine, bromine, or iodine) may replace one or more hydrogen atoms to give alkyl halides. Hence we may have primary (1°), secondary (2°), or tertiary (2°) alkyl halides. As shown in the structures in Figure 5.52, alkyl halides are commonly named with the suffix '*-ide*' reflecting the halogen component (fluoride, chloride, bromide, or iodide), *e.g.* methyl chloride, ethyl chloride, propyl chloride, and so on. In the IUPAC nomenclature system, however, the prefix is the halogen (fluoro, chloro, bromo, or iodo) and is followed by the name of the alkyl chain (Figure 5.52), *e.g.* chloromethane, chloroethane, chloropropane, *etc.* Examples of the IUPAC naming system are shown in Figure 5.52.

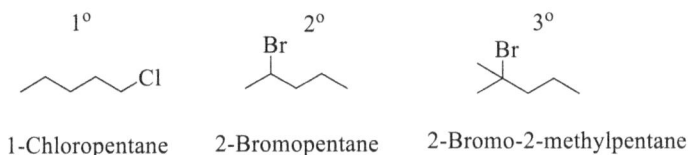

Figure 5.52   IUPAC nomenclature for alkyl halides.

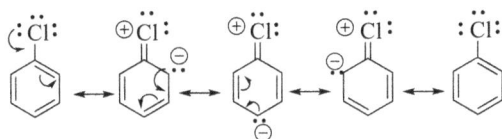

Figure 5.53   Resonance structure of chlorobenzene.

Owing to the electronegativity of halogens and the polar C–X bond (where X is the halogen atom), alkyl halides are involved in various chemical reactions. The relevant reactions involving alkyl halides have been discussed in different sections elsewhere and are not repeated in detail here. A couple of good examples that have already been discussed are substitution reactions to give alcohols and an elimination reaction to yield alkenes. In a substitution reaction, the halogen (called a leaving group) leaves as a halide ion (X^-) and is replaced with an –OH group. In the presence of a strong base, we have also seen how alkyl halides yield alkenes (Chapter 4).

As with alkyl halides, we also have aryl halides or haloarenes. In this case, the halogen atoms are bonded to the carbon atoms in the aromatic ring system. Just like phenols where the lone pair electrons of oxygen are involved in electron delocalisation by resonance in the aromatic ring system, aryl halides show the trend of excess electrons at the *ortho* and *para* positions (Figure 5.53). This trend is similar with the –NH$_2$ group and is opposite to that of the carboxyl (–COOH) group. This means that aryl halides can react with electrophilic (electron-loving) groups particularly at the *ortho* and *para* positions of the benzene ring.

5.7   Amides

Esters as products of a reaction between an alcohol and a carboxylic acid were discussed in Section 5.3.4.4. If we take amines as equivalents of alcohols, amides are equivalents of esters. The amide functional group consists of a carbonyl group bonded to a nitrogen and an ester has a carbonyl group bonded to oxygen. Hence amides can be represented by the general formula R–CO–NR$_2$ as shown in Figure 5.54.

Just like amines, the nitrogen in primary (1°) amides may be attached to a single carbon, two carbons in a secondary (2°) amide, and three carbons in a tertiary (3°) amide. In naming amides, the attachment of alkyl or other groups with nitrogen in secondary and tertiary amines is indicated by the prefix N- as shown in Figure 5.55.

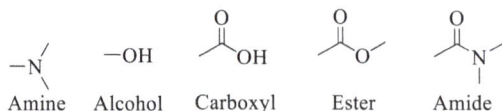

Figure 5.54 Comparison of the amide bond with other functional groups. As a functional group, an amide can also be called a *carboxamide*.

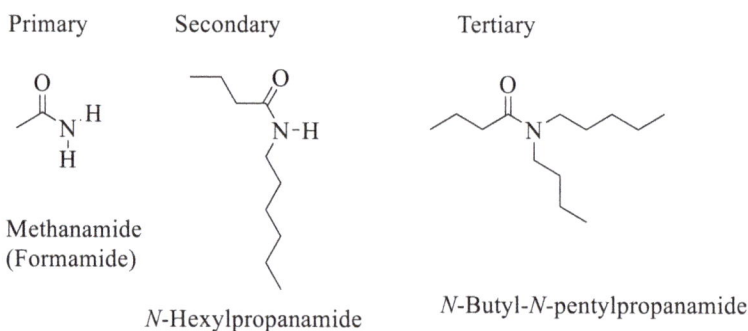

Figure 5.55 Examples of primary, secondary, and tertiary amine structures.

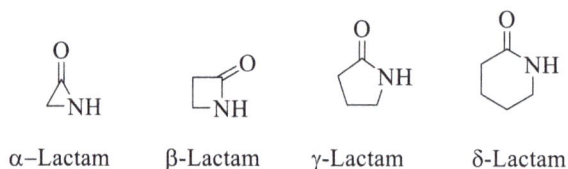

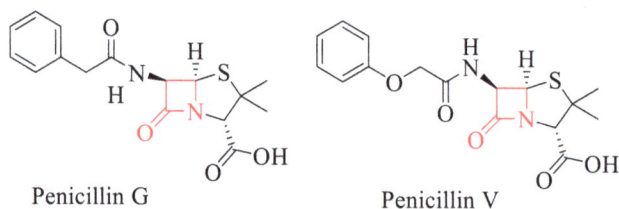

Figure 5.56 Heterocyclic rings with an amide bond.

Amides can also exist as heterocyclic rings and the three-to six-membered rings are called α-lactam, β-lactam, γ-lactam, and δ-lactam rings, respectively (Figure 5.56). The best examples are penicillin antibiotics, the structures of which constructed from the β-lactam skeleton play a key role in their antibacterial effect.

As with amines, amides can form hydrogen bonds with water and the low molecular weight amides obtained are expected to be water

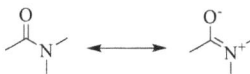

Figure 5.57 Resonance forms of the amide bond.

soluble. Amides of larger molecular size with an extended hydrophobic alkyl or aryl group would be lipophilic and dissolve in organic solvents instead of water. Since both nitrogen and oxygen atoms that possess lone pair electrons occur in amides, their delocalisation can establish a stable charged species as shown in Figure 5.57.

5.8 Other Functional Groups

In addition to those already discussed in this chapter, we also encounter various other functional groups in drugs and biological molecules. For nitrogen-containing functional groups, we have discussed primary, secondary, tertiary, and quaternary amines. We also have the following functional groups.

The *imine functional group* is a general structural group containing a carbon–nitrogen double bond. It is represented by $R_2C=NR$, where R represents alkyl chains or hydrogen, as shown in Figure 5.58. The nitrogen atom could bear either a hydrogen atom or an alkyl chain and the carbon atom could bear R groups with either both being alkyl groups or one of them being hydrogen.

The *nitrile group* is represented by RCN and has a characteristic carbon–nitrogen triple bond ($C\equiv N$). Nitrile compounds are named by using the suffix nitrile, such as in hexanenitrile, propanenitrile, *etc.* (Figure 5.59). There is no need to indicate the position of the nitrile group as it always occurs at the terminal end just like carboxylic acids. Hence the nitrile carbon is numbered C-1.

In addition to the amide group that we have already discussed, functional groups containing both nitrogen and oxygen atoms include nitro (RNO_2), carbamate [$RO(C=O)NR_2$], and urea [$R_2N(C=O)NR_2$] (Figure 5.60).

Sulfur-containing functional groups play a key role in biological systems both in the structures of proteins and enzymes and also in biological reactions. In this case, we have the thiol (RSH), thioether or sulfide, and disulfide functional groups (Figure 5.61). In drug molecules, we also have sulfur-containing structures such as sulfoxide (RSOR) and sulfone (RSO_2R) functional groups (Figure 5.61). Owing to

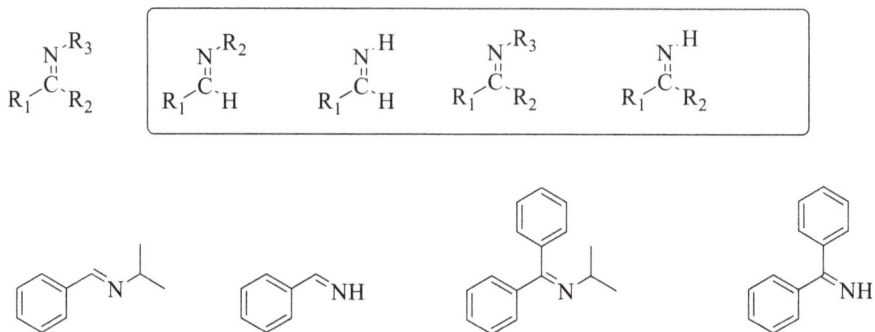

Figure 5.58 The imine functional group. The box shows variations in the substituents of alkyl groups at both the carbon and nitrogen ends of the C=N bond.

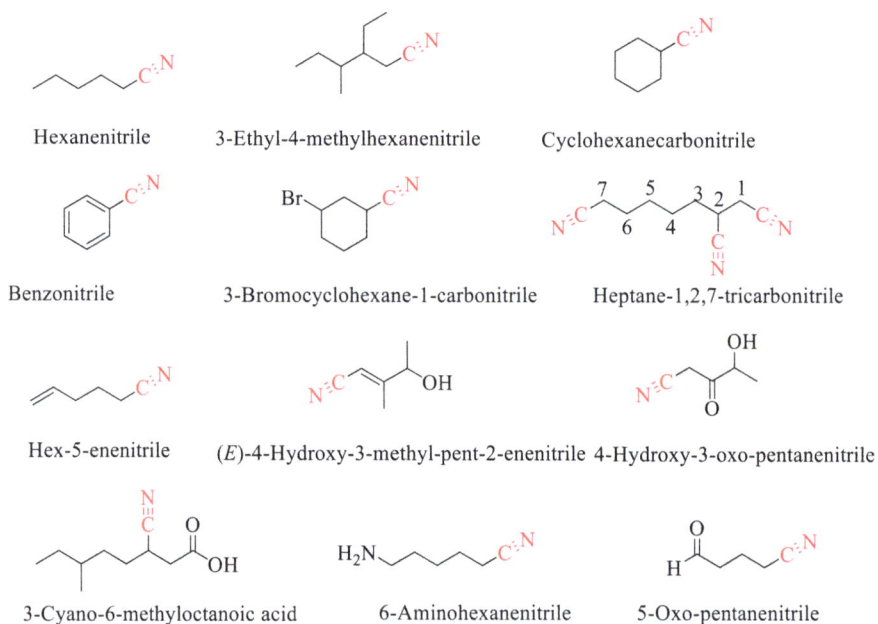

Hexanenitrile	3-Ethyl-4-methylhexanenitrile	Cyclohexanecarbonitrile
Benzonitrile	3-Bromocyclohexane-1-carbonitrile	Heptane-1,2,7-tricarbonitrile
Hex-5-enenitrile	(E)-4-Hydroxy-3-methyl-pent-2-enenitrile	4-Hydroxy-3-oxo-pentanenitrile
3-Cyano-6-methyloctanoic acid	6-Aminohexanenitrile	5-Oxo-pentanenitrile

Figure 5.59 The nitrile functional group and nomenclature. See how the carbonitrile suffix is used where the nitrile functional group appears conjugated to (or attached to) a ring system and multiple nitrile functional groups occur in the molecule. When the nitrile group occurs with alkene, alcohol, ketone, aldehyde, or amine groups, the name takes the nitrile suffix. However, the carboxyl group has a higher priority than the nitrile group.

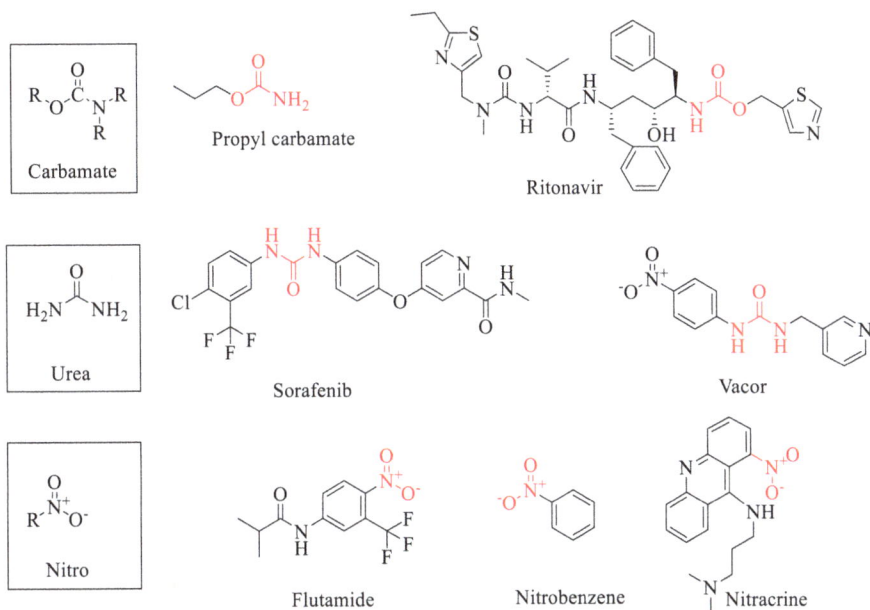

Figure 5.60 Examples of drugs containing carbamate, urea, and nitro structural groups.

the reactivity of the thiol functional group, reactions involving disulfide bridge formation and reactions with drug molecules are major topics of interest in medicinal chemistry. In terms of reactivity, thiols are the sulfur analogues of alcohols. Hence sulfides are similar to ethers but have oxygen replaced with sulfur. In a similar way, we can have an ester analogue called a thioester – an ester where the oxygen is replaced with sulfur.

Many biological molecules that include genetic material (*e.g.* DNA) contain the *phosphate functional group* (Figure 5.62). The phosphate functional group is also an integral part of many biological molecules such as adenosine triphosphate (ATP), proteins, and enzymes. Several structural forms are also possible, such as acyl phosphate where a carbonyl is bonded to a phosphate group – hence it is an analogue of acyl chloride. Note that the phosphate functional group has ionisable hydroxyl groups that make the molecule water soluble. Many organic compounds and biological molecules may further contain a *sulfonate functional group*. Taurine, for example, is a common biological molecule in animal tissues and is also incorporated in the structures of bile salt (Figure 5.62).

R–S⟨H	R–S–R	O∥R–S–R	O∥ O∥R–S–R	R–S–S–R
Thiol	Sulfide	Sulfoxide	Sulfone	Disulfide

Glutathione   Cysteine   N-Acetylcysteine

Cystine   Methionine   Probucol

Esomeprazole   Sulindac   Mesoridazine

Furosemide   Bumetanide   Torsemide

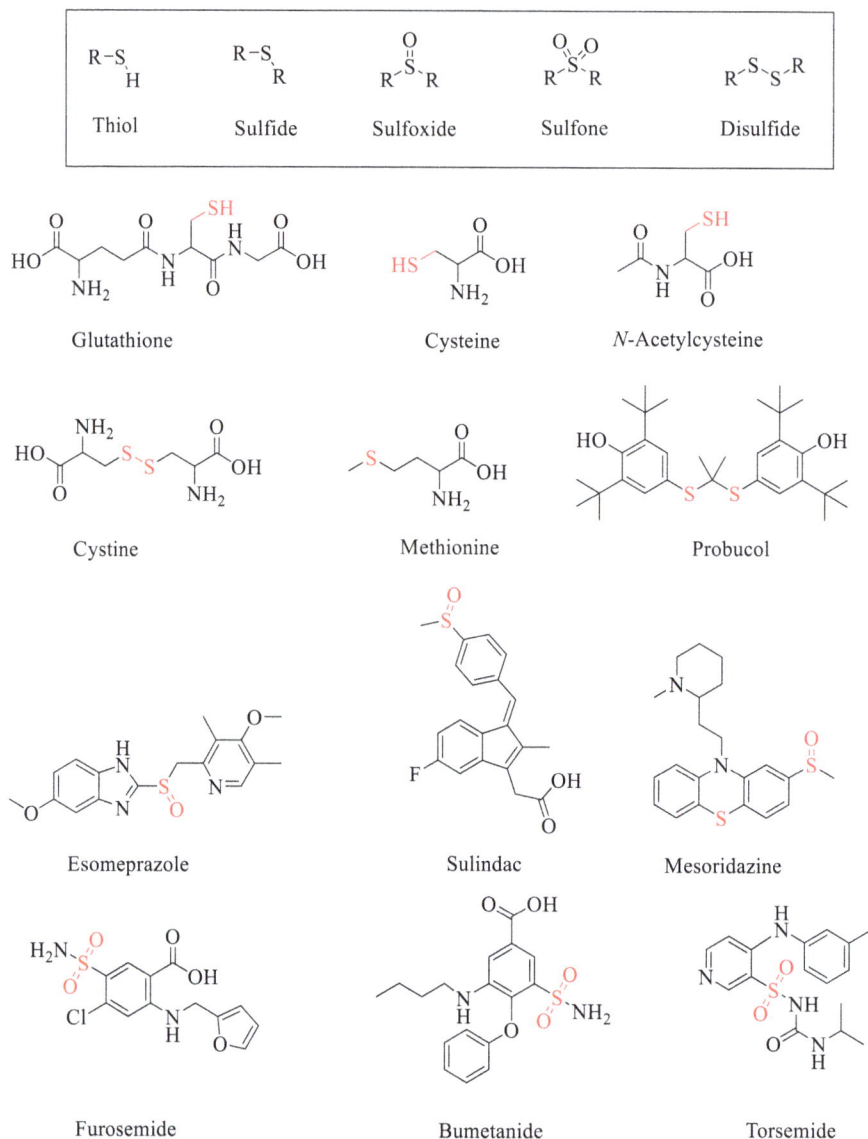

Figure 5.61 Sulfur-containing functional groups.

5.9 Summary

In previous chapters, we studied structural classes based on carbon–carbon bonding in hydrocarbons such as alkanes, alkenes, and alkynes. We also investigated cyclic structures such as cycloalkanes, cycloalkenes, and arenes. In this chapter, the focus was to highlight

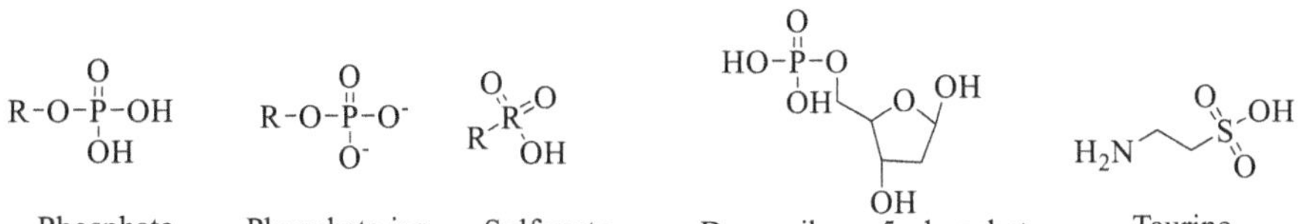

Phosphate | Phosphate ion (Phosphite) | Sulfonate | Deoxyribose-5-phosphate | Taurine

Figure 5.62 Phosphate and sulfonate functional groups. Note that the phosphate functional group has an ionisable -OH group at normal physiological pH.

polar bonds that we call functional groups. The various functional groups that we have learned about include the following:

Oxygen-containing functional groups:

- Alcohols (ROH): primary, secondary, and tertiary alcohols. Check how many carbons are bonded to the carbon carrying the –OH group.
- Ethers (ROR).
- Aldehydes (RCHO).
- Ketones (RCOR).
- Carboxylic acids (RCOOH): a carbonyl carbon bonded to a hydroxyl group. Always occurs at the terminal carbon.
- Esters (RCOOR).
- Acid anhydrides (RCOOCOR): two carboxylic acids combine to form an anhydride *via* a loss of water.

Alkyl halide functional groups:

- RF, RCl, RBr, and RI.

Nitrogen-containing functional groups:

- Amine: primary (RNH_2), secondary (R_2NH), tertiary (R_3N), and quaternary (R_4N^+). Check how many carbons are bonded to the nitrogen.
- Imine ($R_2C{=}NR$): carbon–nitrogen double bond. Nitrogen has either hydrogen or carbon bonding.
- Nitrile (RCN), also called the cyano group, with a nitrogen–carbon triple bond ($-C{\equiv}N$).

Both nitrogen- and oxygen-containing functional groups:

- Amide ($RCONR_2$): nitrogen can be bonded to either hydrogen or carbon.
- Carbamate [$RO(C{=}O)NR_2$].
- Nitro (RNO_2).
- Urea [$R_2N(C{=}O)NR_2$].

Sulfur-containing functional groups:
- Thiol (RSH).
- Thioether or sulfide (RSR).
- Sulfoxide (RSOR).
- Sulfone (RSO$_2$R).

Naming compounds with more than one functional group:
- When alcohols and amine groups exist in a molecule, the alcohol takes the name with suffix 'ol', *e.g.* 4-aminohexan-2-ol.
- For halogen, an alcohol, amine, ether, aldehyde, ketone, and a carboxylic acid, the name takes the acid with suffix 'oic acid' and the others are presented as substituents.
- When an OH and ketone groups occur, the ketone is used for naming and 'hydroxy' is used as a substituent.
- If ketone and aldehyde functional groups occur together, the naming takes the aldehyde.

5.10 Problems

Questions 1–3 are based on Figure 5.63. Classify the compounds as 1°, 2°, or 3° alcohols.

1. Primary alcohol:_____
2. Secondary alcohol:_____
3. Tertiary alcohol:_____

Questions 4–6 are based on Figure 5.64. Classify the compounds as 1°, 2°, or 3° amines.

4. Primary amine:_____
5. Secondary amine:_____
6. Tertiary amine:_____
7. Complete the reaction shown in Figure 5.65 where alcohols are converted to alkyl halides by reaction with strong acids.

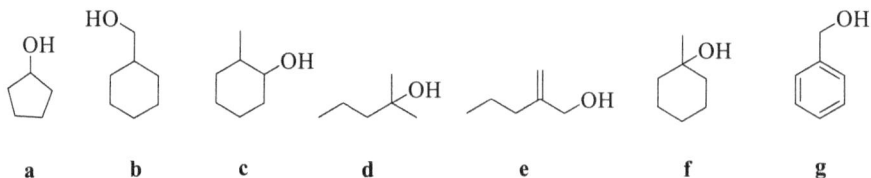

Figure 5.63 Classification of alcohols – questions 1–3 are based on structures **a–g**.

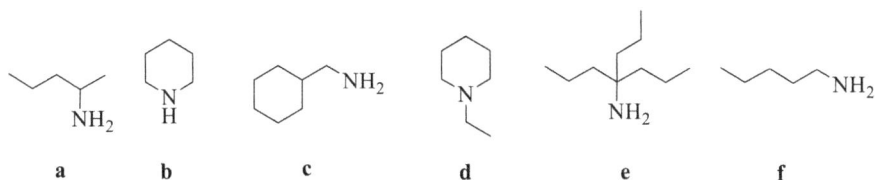

a	b	c	d	e	f

Figure 5.64 Classification of amines – questions 4-6 are based on structures **a-f**.

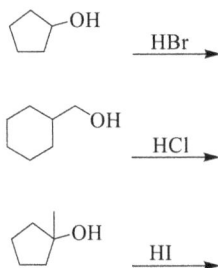

Figure 5.65 Reaction of alcohols with hydrogen halides – question 7.

8. Decanoic acid is poorly soluble in water. Show the reaction that you undertake to make it soluble in water.
9. Decan-1-amine is poorly soluble in water. Show the reaction that you undertake to make it soluble in water.

Questions 10–18 are based on Figure 5.66. Name the indicated compounds.

10. _____
11. _____
12. _____
13. _____
14. _____
15. _____
16. _____
17. _____
18. _____

Questions 19–21 are based on Figure 5.67.

19. Name the compounds: **a,**_____; **b,**_____; **c,**_____; **d,**_____.
20. Arrange the compounds in order of their polarity: __ > __ > __ > ___.

21. Arrange the compounds in order of their boiling point: __ > __ > __ > ___.

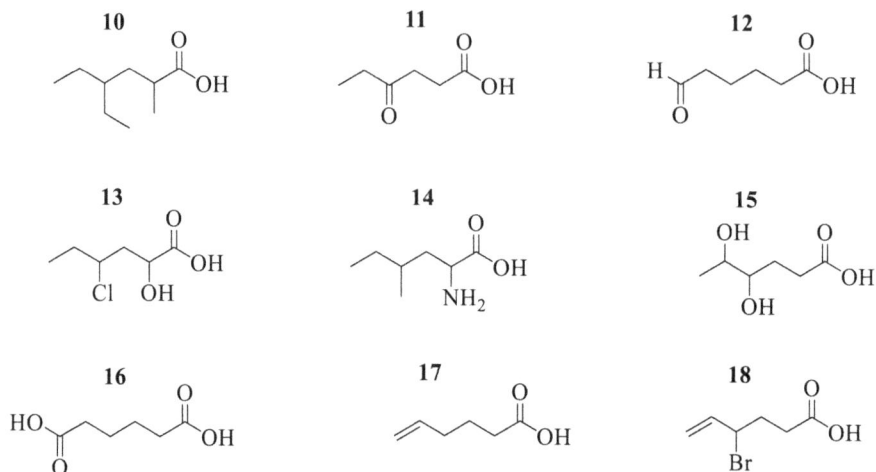

Figure 5.66   Name the compounds – questions 10–18.

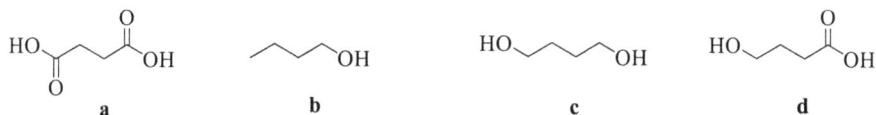

Figure 5.67   For questions 19–21, refer to structures **a-d**.

22. Chlorine is more electronegative than oxygen, but the boiling point of ethanol is 78.2 °C whereas that of chloroethane is 12.5 °C. Explain.
23. Draw the chemical structures of the following amides:
    a 4-Ethylhexanamide.
    b 4-Ethyl-5-hydroxyhexanamide.
    c Decanamide.
    d 3-Methylbenzamide.
    e Benzamide.
    f N-Phenyldecanamide.
    g N-Ethyldecanamide.
24. Show the reaction of benzylamine with chloromethane.

Questions 25–38 are based on Figure 5.68. Which compound/drug has the following functional group?

25. Amide: _____
26. Alcohol: _____

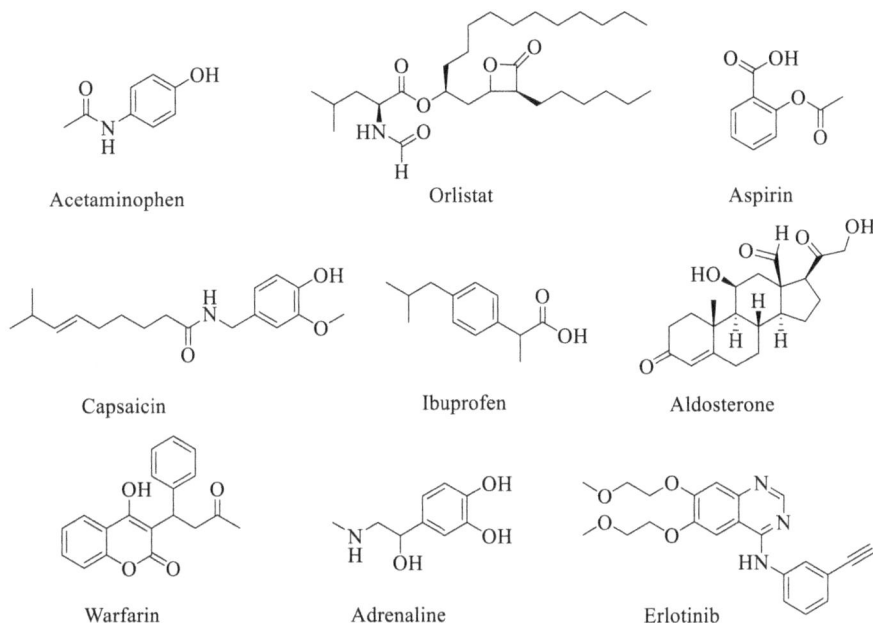

Figure 5.68 For questions 25–38.

27. Ether: _____
28. Alkene: _____
29. Ester (acyclic): _____
30. Catechol: _____
31. Carboxylic acid: _____
32. Imine: _____
33. Phenol: _____
34. Aldehyde: _____
35. Cyclic carboxylic ester (lactone): _____
36. Amine: _____
37. Ketone: _____
38. Alkyne: _____
39. The order of the boiling points of butanol isomers is shown in Figure 5.69. Explain.

Questions 40–49 are based on Figure 5.70. Identify the following structural groups in the molecule of the anticancer drug taxol.

40. Carboxylic acid: _____
41. Aldehyde: _____
42. Benzene/arene: _____
43. Amine: _____

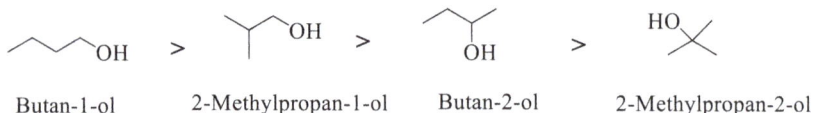

Figure 5.69 Boiling point of butanol isomers – question 39.

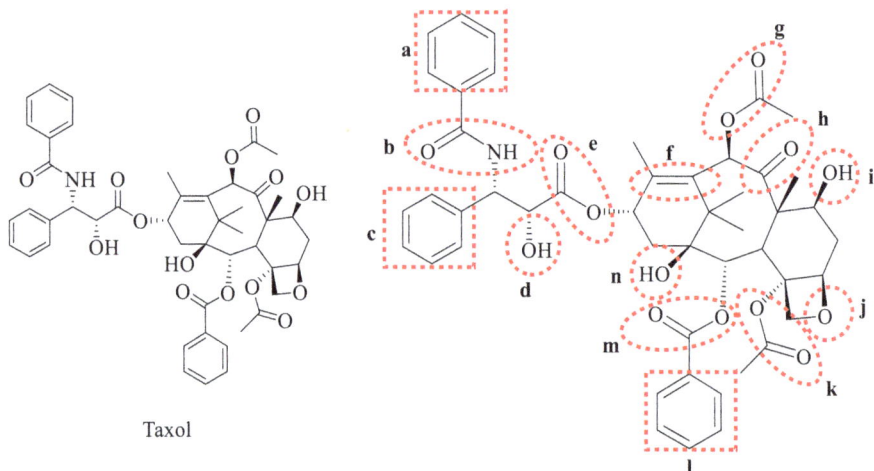

Taxol

Figure 5.70 For questions 40–49, identify the structural or functional groups labelled **a–n**.

44. Amide:_____
45. Alcohol:_____
46. Alkene:_____
47. Ether of cycloether:_____
48. Ketone:_____
49. Ester:_____

Questions 50–54. In the structure of morphine (Figure 5.71), identify the functional group associated with the five ring systems.

50. Ring A: _____
51. Ring B: _____
52. Ring C: _____
53. Ring D: _____
54. Ring E: _____
55. Show why carboxylic acids have higher boiling points and water solubilities than the corresponding alcohols.
56. In chemical reactions of aromatic carboxylic acids, which positions in the benzene ring react with the electron-rich group?

Morphine

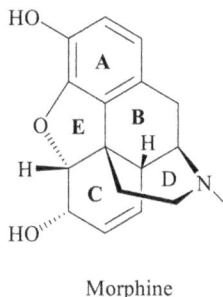

Figure 5.71 Structure of morphine – questions 50–54.

57. In chemical reactions of aromatic amines, which positions in the benzene ring react with the electron-deficient group?
58. Show how the reaction of aryl halides with electrophilic groups favours the *ortho* and *para* positions of the benzene ring.

5.11 Solutions to Problems

1. Primary alcohol: **b, e, g.**
2. Secondary alcohol: **a, c.**
3. Tertiary alcohol: **d, f.**
4. Primary amine: **a, c, e, f.**
5. Secondary amine: **b.**
6. Tertiary amine: **d.**
7. See Figure 5.72.
8. We can make the acid react with a base such as NaOH to make a salt which is water soluble:

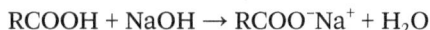

$$RCOOH + NaOH \rightarrow RCOO^-Na^+ + H_2O$$

9. Amine as a base reacts with acids such as HCl to form a salt (quaternary amine):

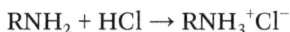

$$RNH_2 + HCl \rightarrow RNH_3^+Cl^-$$

Questions 10–18 are based on Figure 5.66.
10. 4-Ethyl-2-methylhexanoic acid.
11. 4-Oxohexanoic acid.
12. 6-Oxohexanoic acid.
13. 4-Chloro-2-hydroxyhexanoic acid.
14. 2-Amino-4-methylhexanoic acid.
15. 4,5-Dihydroxyhexanoic acid.

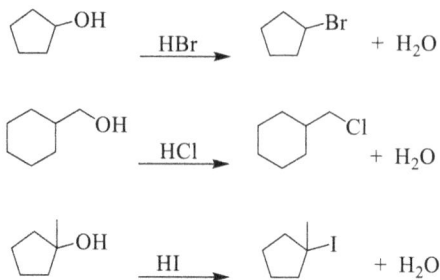

Figure 5.72 Answer to question 7.

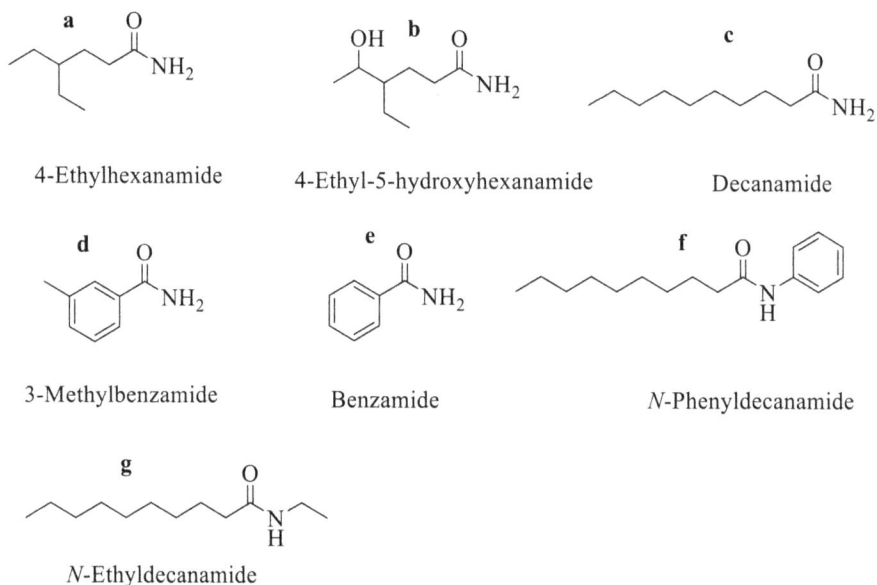

4-Ethylhexanamide   4-Ethyl-5-hydroxyhexanamide   Decanamide

3-Methylbenzamide   Benzamide   *N*-Phenyldecanamide

N-Ethyldecanamide

Figure 5.73 Answer to question 23.

16. Hexanedioic acid.
17. Hex-5-enoic acid.
18. 4-Bromohex-5-enoic acid.
    See Figure 5.67 for questions 19–21.
19. Names of compounds: **a**, butanedioic acid; **b**, butan-1-ol; **c**: butane-1,4-diol; **d**, 4-hydroxybutanoic acid.
20. Compounds in order of their polarity: **a** > **d** > **c** > **b**.
21. Compounds in order of their boiling point: **a** > **d** > **c** > **b**.
22. Hydrogen bonding in ethanol makes a stronger intermolecular bond than just the dipole interaction in chloromethane.
23. See Figure 5.73.

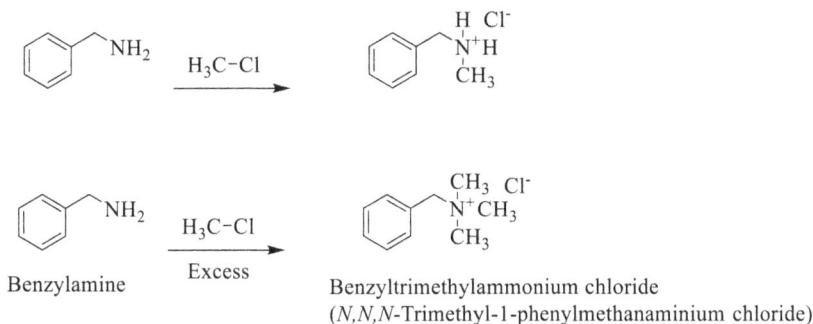

Figure 5.74 Answer to question 24.

24. See Figure 5.74.
    See Figure 5.68 for questions 25–38.
25. Amide: acetaminophen, capsaicin, orlistat.
26. Alcohol: adrenaline, aldosterone.
27. Ether: capsaicin, erlotinib.
28. Alkene: capsaicin, aldosterone.
29. Ester (acyclic): aspirin, orlistat.
30. Catechol (1,2-dihydroxybenzene): adrenaline.
31. Carboxylic acid: aspirin, ibuprofen.
32. Imine: erlotinib.
33. Phenol: acetaminophen, adrenaline, capsaicin.
34. Aldehyde: aldosterone.
35. Cyclic carboxylic ester (lactone): orlistat, warfarin.
36. Amine: adrenaline.
37. Ketone: aldosterone.
38. Alkyne: erlotinib.
39. All have the same molecular formula and alcohol functional group. The –OH group that undergoes hydrogen bonding freely would have a higher boiling point than that with a shielded –OH group. Thus, the primary alcohol butan-1-ol has a higher boiling point than the slightly shielded primary alcohol 2-methylpropan-1-ol and, in turn, this has a higher boiling point than the secondary alcohol butan-2-ol. The tertiary alcohol 2-methylpropan-2-ol has the lowest boiling point.
    See Figure 5.70 for questions 40–49.
40. Carboxylic acid: none.
41. Aldehyde: none.
42. Benzene/arene: **a, c, l**.
43. Amine: none.

44. Amide: **b**.
45. Alcohol: **d, i, n**.
46. Alkene: **f**.
47. Ether of cycloether: **j**.
48. Ketone: **h**.
49. Ester: **e, g, k, m**.
    See Figure 5.71 for questions 50–54.
50. Ring A: phenol.
51. Ring B: cyclohexene.
52. Ring C: cyclohexenol.
53. Ring D: *N*-methylpiperidine (amine is also accepted).
54. Ring E: furan ring (partially saturated).
55. Strong intermolecular bond formation – see Figures 5.27 and 5.28.
56. *Ortho* and *para* positions – see Figure 5.29.
57. *Ortho* and *para* positions – see Figure 5.48.
58. Electron delocalisation by resonance – see Figure 5.53.

6 Isomerism in Organic Compounds and Drug Molecules: Chemistry and Significance in Biology

Learning Objectives

After completing this chapter, you are expected to be able to:

- Explain the difference between chain isomers, positional isomers, functional isomers, and tautomerism.
- Identify and name structural isomers from the molecular formula.
- Identify geometrical isomers in cyclic and acyclic structures.
- Locate chiral centres in the structures of organic compounds.
- Be familiar with the significance of isomerism in drug therapeutics.
- Determine the optical purity of drug samples.

6.1 Introduction

In Chapters 3 and 4 (alkanes and alkenes), we studied compounds that are composed of the same number of atoms but differ in the way in which the atoms are arranged either in the order of atoms attached to each other or in spatial arrangement. The word isomer, originating from the Greek words '*isos*' and '*meros*', referring to equal parts,

Basic Chemistry for Life Science Students and Professionals: Introduction to Organic Compounds and Drug Molecules
By Solomon Habtemariam
© Solomon Habtemariam 2023
Published by the Royal Society of Chemistry, www.rsc.org

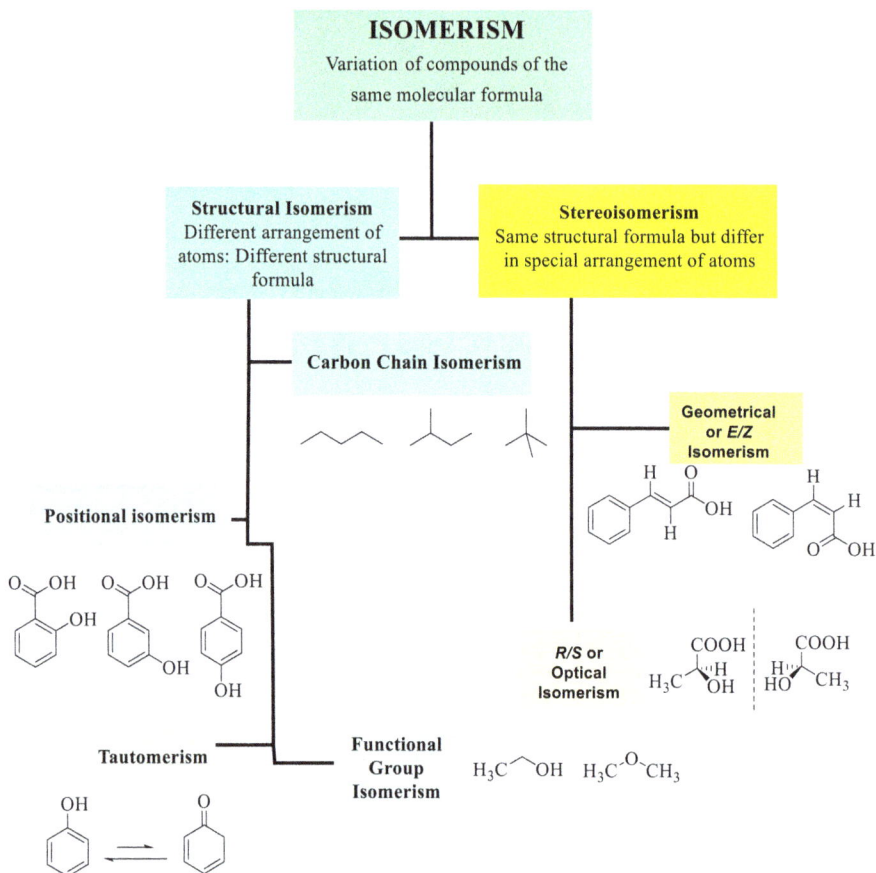

Figure 6.1 Overview of isomerism.

represents this feature in such compounds. In organic chemistry, the Greek meaning refers to equal parts in atomic composition and yet differing from each other, or not the same in either physical or chemical properties. These various chemical compounds based on the same molecular formula are called *isomers*. In the following sections, we describe the various types of isomerism and a brief overview is presented in Figure 6.1.

6.2 Constitutional or Structural Isomers

Organic compounds with the same molecular formula, and hence the same atomic composition, can differ based on how the atoms are connected to each other. The resulting different structures are called *structural* or *constitutional isomers*. A good example that we have already studied is the structural difference in alkanes with the same hydrogen and carbon composition. In this case, a linear or branched structure can be constructed for carbon chains with four or more carbons in a molecule, *i.e.* hydrocarbons with 1–3 carbon atoms do not have structural isomers. For butane (C_4H_{10}) there are two isomers and pentane has three (Figure 6.2).

As the number of carbon atoms in the chain increases, so does the number of possible structural isomers. Since the difference in these compounds is based on the possible ways of branching that can be constructed from the molecular formula, they are also called *branch isomers* or *carbon chain isomers*. Thus hexane has five (Figure 6.3) and heptane has nine possible structural or chain (branch) isomers (Figure 6.4).

With increasing number of carbon atoms in the alkane hydrocarbon chain, the number of possible chain isomers also increases, as

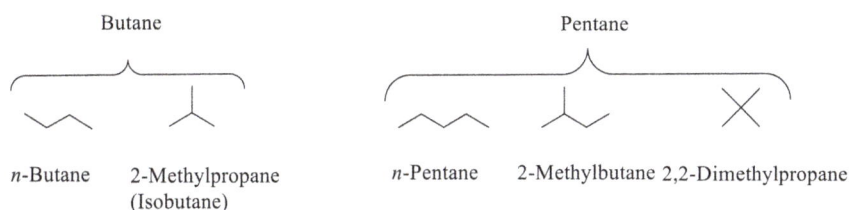

Butane

n-Butane   2-Methylpropane (Isobutane)

Pentane

n-Pentane   2-Methylbutane   2,2-Dimethylpropane

Figure 6.2 Structural isomers of butane and pentane.

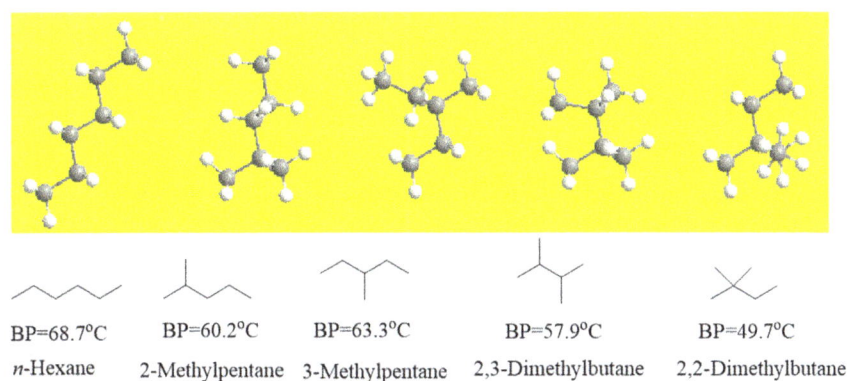

BP=68.7°C   BP=60.2°C   BP=63.3°C   BP=57.9°C   BP=49.7°C

n-Hexane   2-Methylpentane   3-Methylpentane   2,3-Dimethylbutane   2,2-Dimethylbutane

Figure 6.3 Structural or chain isomers of hexane. Note the lower boiling point (BP) for isomers with a compact structure. The BP data were taken from the Hazardous Substances Data Bank (HSDB), which is available *via* PubChem (https://pubchem.ncbi.nlm.nih.gov/).

n-Heptane   2-Methylhexane   3-Methylhexane   2,2-Dimethylpentane   3,3-Dimethylpentane

2,3-Dimethylpentane   2,4-Dimethylpentane   3-Ethylpentane   2,2,3-Trimethylbutane

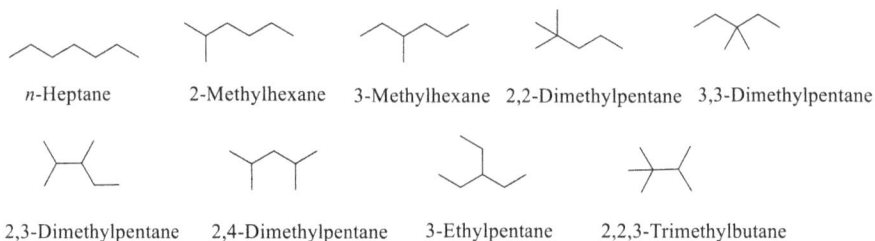

Figure 6.4 Structural or chain isomers of heptane.

Table 6.1 Number of possible structural isomers for alkanes.

No of carbons in the molecule	1	2	3	4	5	6	7	8	9	10	11	12
No of structural isomers		1	1	1	2	3	5	9	18	35	75	159	355

shown in Table 6.1. Note that alkanes are hydrocarbons with the general formula C_nH_{2n+2} (see Chapter 3).

One consequence of structural isomerism is the differences in physical properties such as boiling and melting points. Mostly, branching to make the molecular structure more compact leads to a decrease in either the boiling or melting point. In the case of pentane, *n*-pentane is a liquid with a boiling point of 34 °C whereas its isomer, 2-methylbutane, is a more volatile liquid with a boiling point of 28 °C. The more compact isomer of pentane, 2,2-dimethylpropane, even appears as a gas with a boiling point of just 9.5 °C. The physical properties of hexane isomers are also shown in Figure 6.3, where branching to make the molecule more compact results in a decrease in boiling point. Also, one can expect variations in other physical properties such as the density and melting point of isomers of alkanes, with a general trend of a decrease when the molecular structures appear in compact forms.

In alkenes (Chapter 4), we also showed that different chemical structures can be constructed from the same molecular formula based on the position of the double bond in the molecule. Thus hexene has structural isomers as shown in Figure 6.5. In this case, as the carbon chain and/or the number of double bonds increases, the possible number of structural isomers also increases. Also, note that the general formula for alkenes fits for cycloalkanes (Chapter 3) as the loss of two hydrogen atoms from alkanes makes either a double bond (alkene) or a ring system. Hence a molecular formula of C_5H_{10} for pentene includes five isomeric cyclic structures in addition to five aliphatic chain forms (Figure 6.5).

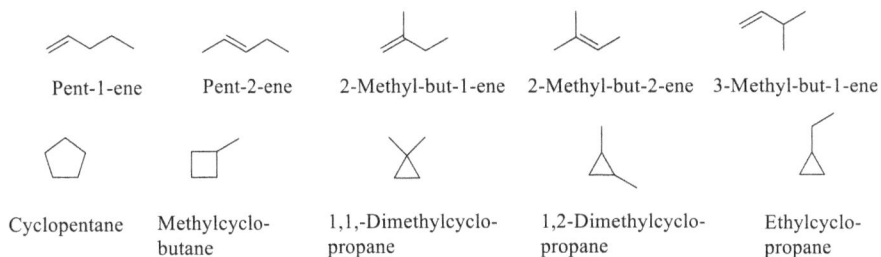

Figure 6.5 Structural isomers of C_5H_{10} (pentene and cyclopentane). Note that the *cis–trans* isomers are not considered here.

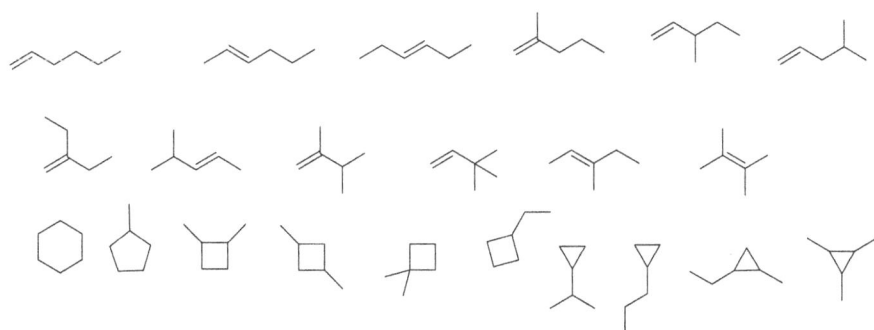

Pent-1-ene   Pent-2-ene   2-Methyl-but-1-ene   2-Methyl-but-2-ene   3-Methyl-but-1-ene

Cyclopentane   Methylcyclo-butane   1,1,-Dimethylcyclo-propane   1,2-Dimethylcyclo-propane   Ethylcyclo-propane

Figure 6.6 Structural isomers of C_6H_{12} (hexene). Note that the *cis–trans* isomers are not considered here.

Similarly, a molecular formula of C_6H_{12} for hexene also has structural isomers of both acyclic and cyclic structures as shown in Figure 6.6. You should also consider that structural isomers based on double bond positions in the molecule have implications for the variation in physical properties.

When the hydrocarbon skeleton carries a more reactive group such as oxygen (see functional groups in Chapter 5), the possible structural isomers would have even more pronounced physical and chemical properties. For example, consider a butane skeleton carrying one oxygen atom with a molecular formula of $C_4H_{10}O$. Four isomers of these are based on an alcoholic functional group while three can be drawn based on an ether functional group (Figure 6.7). Organic compounds with an alcohol functional group also differ from each other based on the position of the hydroxyl group in the molecules. Hence they are also called *positional isomers*. On the other hand, three positional isomers also occur for $C_4H_{10}O$ based on the ether functional group (Figure 6.7). Hence we can expect further variations or possible numbers of positional isomers as the number or type (oxygen, nitrogen, sulfur, *etc.*) of atoms in the molecule increases.

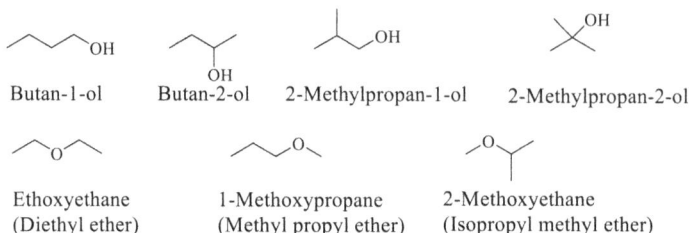

Butan-1-ol   Butan-2-ol   2-Methylpropan-1-ol   2-Methylpropan-2-ol

Ethoxyethane   1-Methoxypropane   2-Methoxyethane
(Diethyl ether)   (Methyl propyl ether)   (Isopropyl methyl ether)

Figure 6.7   Isomers of molecular formula $C_4H_{10}O$. The difference between alcohols and ethers is an example of functional group isomerism. Ethoxyethane and 1-methoxypropane can be considered as positional isomers. On the other hand, the difference between butan-1-ol (alcohol) and diethyl ether (ether) is an example of functional isomerism.

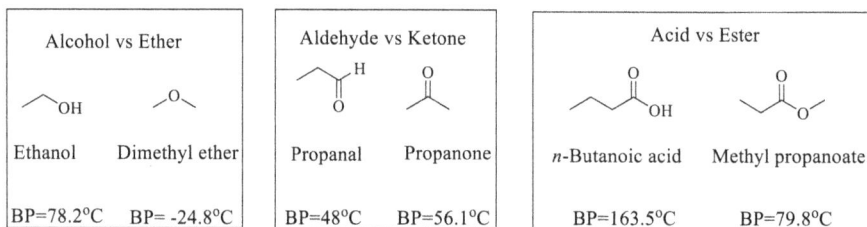

Alcohol vs Ether	Aldehyde vs Ketone	Acid vs Ester

Ethanol   Dimethyl ether

Propanal   Propanone

n-Butanoic acid   Methyl propanoate

BP=78.2°C   BP= -24.8°C

BP=48°C   BP=56.1°C

BP=163.5°C   BP=79.8°C

Figure 6.8   Examples of functional group isomerism. The boiling point (BP) data were taken from the Hazardous Substances Data Bank (HSDB), which is available *via* PubChem (https://pubchem.ncbi.nlm.nih.gov).

Since ethers differ greatly from alcohols in their chemical properties, the difference in these isomers is far greater than that for the structural isomers we looked at for alkanes and alkenes. Such isomerism (*e.g.* based on alcohol *versus* ether) is called *functional group isomerism.*

In Figure 6.8, a pair of structural isomers based on functional group isomerism is shown. Whereas ethanol is a liquid with a boiling point of 78.2 °C, dimethyl ether is a gas with a boiling point of −24.8 °C. Similarly, whereas *n*-butanoic acid is a polar molecule with a boiling point of 163.5 °C, its ester isomer, methyl propanoate, has a boiling point of 79.8 °C. The reactivities of functional group isomers also differ greatly.

When considering the various structural isomers, one should also consider cyclic structures if the hydrogen count in the molecule is less than what we expect for alkanes (for example, in alkenes). For the molecular formula $C_5H_{10}O$, consideration of branching, functional, and positional isomerism provides the structural isomers shown in Figure 6.9. These include functional groups of ketone, aldehyde, alcohol, ether, cyclic and heterocyclic structures.

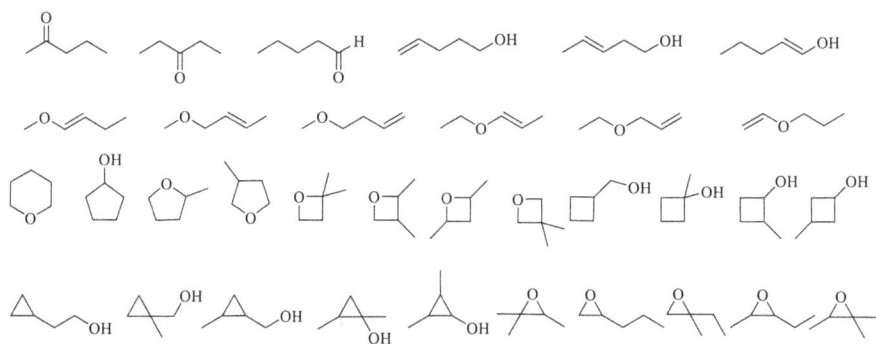

Figure 6.9 Structural isomers of $C_5H_{10}O$. Note that there are other possible isomers that are not shown – can you work out the structures of the missing ones?

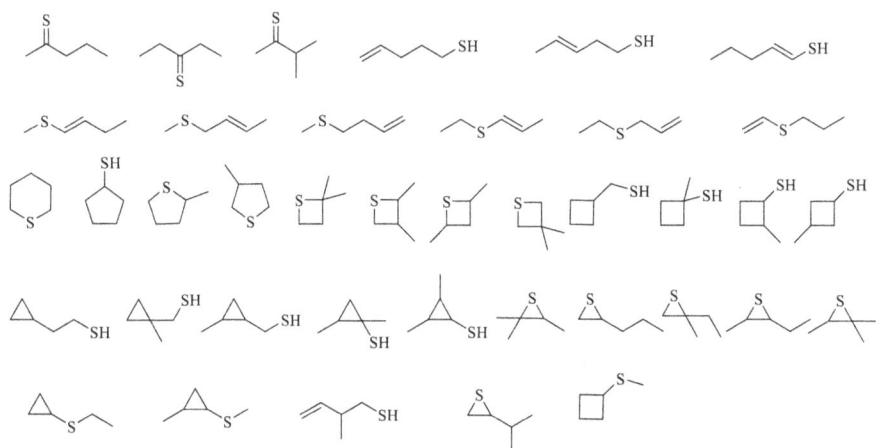

Figure 6.10 Structural isomers of $C_5H_{10}S$.

Both positional and functional group isomerism can apply for elements other than oxygen present in the hydrocarbon skeleton. Structural isomers for compounds with molecular formula $C_5H_{10}S$ are shown in Figure 6.10.

Halogen series such as chloroalkanes also give various isomers through either positional- or branching-based structural isomers. Figure 6.11 shows examples for C_4H_9Cl. One can also consider a range of organic compounds that contain other elements such as nitrogen and phosphorus.

Some chemical compounds may not be structurally stable and may convert to another form. This could also be facilitated by using experimental conditions that favour one particular structural form. For

1-Chlorobutane   2-Chlorobutane   1-Chloro-2-methylpropane   2-Chloro-2-methylpropane

Figure 6.11   Structural isomers of C_4H_9Cl.

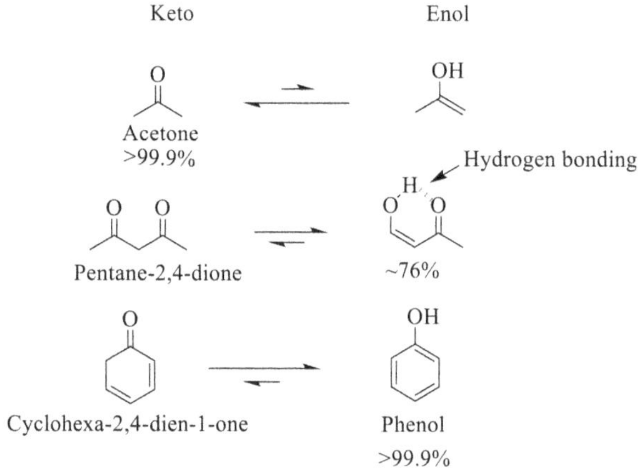

Figure 6.12   Keto–enol tautomerism. The longer arrow indicates the predominant form.

example, ketones and enols are interconverted to each other with the resulting isomerism called *tautomerism*. For acetone, for example, the more stable form is the *keto* tautomer, which is estimated to constitute over 99.9%, the *enol* tautomer being a very minor component (Figure 6.12). When there is a possibility of stabilisation through hydrogen bonding, the enol form can exist at a higher percentage, and this is shown in Figure 6.12 for pentane-2,4-dione. This hydrogen bond formation and stabilisation also depend on what solvent system is used. If we dissolve pentane-2,4-dione in benzene, the predominant form is the enol tautomer, whereas in water the keto tautomer predominates. In some cases, however, the enol tautomer is more predominant than the keto form, as shown for phenol with the enol form existing at over 99.9% (Figure 6.12). This is due to the stable aromatic ring system in the phenol. Several other factors, which are beyond the scope of this book, also affect the isomeric content of the tautomeric forms.

In terms of positional isomerism, one example in drug molecules can be explained using aromatic structures. For example, consider salicylic acid, a precursor in the synthesis of aspirin (Figure 6.13). The structure is based on a benzoic acid skeleton with a hydroxyl group at

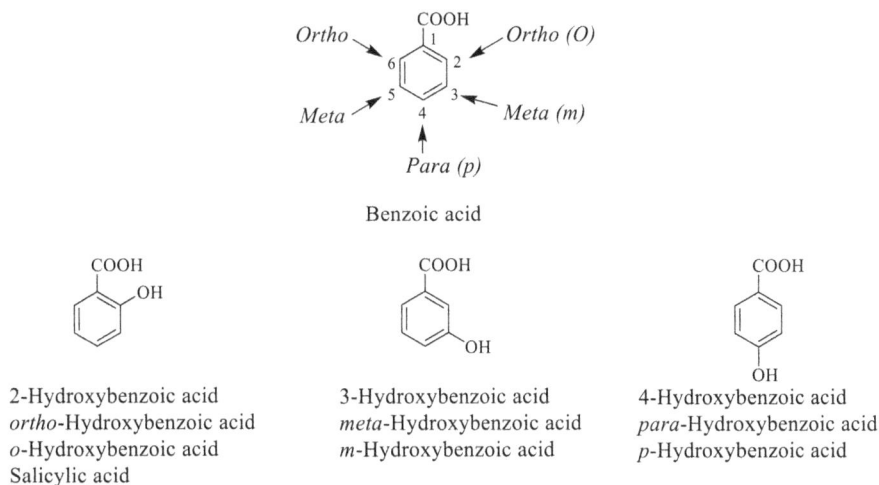

Benzoic acid

2-Hydroxybenzoic acid
ortho-Hydroxybenzoic acid
o-Hydroxybenzoic acid
Salicylic acid

3-Hydroxybenzoic acid
meta-Hydroxybenzoic acid
m-Hydroxybenzoic acid

4-Hydroxybenzoic acid
para-Hydroxybenzoic acid
p-Hydroxybenzoic acid

Figure 6.13 Positional isomers in an aromatic structure. With respect to the carboxyl functional group, the hydroxyl group can be placed at either *ortho*, *meta*, or *para* positions within the aromatic ring. Note that these isomers have distinctly different physical and chemical properties.

carbon position 2 (C-2) of the carboxyl group, which is also called the *ortho* (next carbon) position. There is also the possibility of placing the hydroxyl group at the *meta* position (or C-3) or *para* position (C-4), so we have three isomers or positional isomers.

Similarly, functional group isomers can also occur in aromatic structures with various substitution patterns. Consider the molecular formula C_7H_8O, which represents a common drug ingredient, benzyl alcohol. As shown in Figure 6.14, its functional isomers are methyl-phenol, which can have three positional isomers (*ortho*, *meta*, and *para*), and methoxybenzene.

Structural Isomers – Key Facts

- Same atomic composition but differ in the way in which the atoms are connected to each other.
- Branch or chain isomers – differ in C–C arrangements in a chain.
- Functional group isomers – isomers have different functional groups (*e.g.* alcohols *versus* ethers).
- Tautomerism – keto–enol tautomerism.

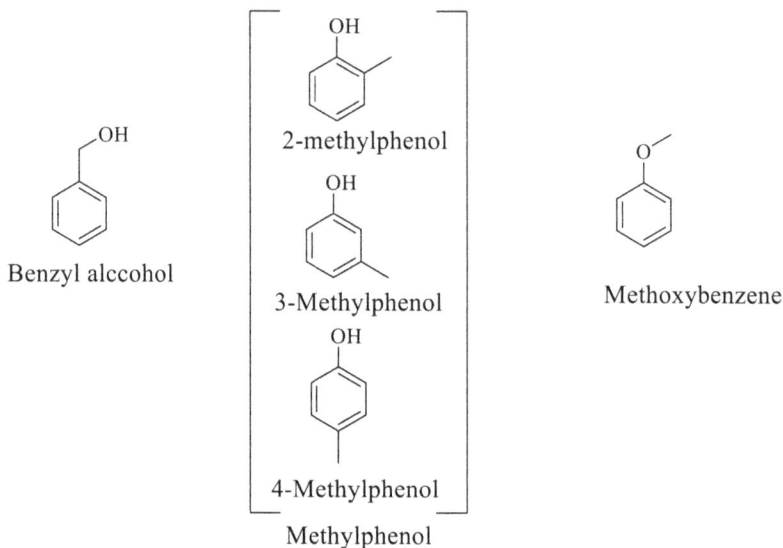

OH

Benzyl alcohol

OH

2-methylphenol

OH

3-Methylphenol

OH

4-Methylphenol

Methylphenol

Methoxybenzene

Figure 6.14 Functional group isomers of C_7H_8O. Note that methylphenol has three positional isomers. Benzyl alcohol and methoxybenzene are functional group isomers.

6.3   Stereoisomerism

Derived from the Greek word '*stereos*' meaning solid, stereochemistry in organic chemistry is concerned with the three-dimensional properties of molecules. In Chapter 4, we studied alkenes and how they differ from each other based on the spatial orientation of atoms arranged around the double bonds. These are what we call geometrical isomers. We also have another type of stereoisomerism called optical isomers or *R* and *S* isomers. Since drugs interact with their targets through specific interactions within a defined spatial surface area, both constitutional isomerism and stereoisomerism must be considered when designing therapeutic agents.

6.3.1   Geometrical Isomerism or *Cis–Trans* Isomerism

Also known as *cis–trans* or *E–Z* isomerism, geometrical isomerism arises due to restricted rotation around a bond or somewhere in the molecule. In a single C–C bond or a bond between two sp^3-hybridised carbon atoms, there is free rotation around the bond. Hence what is spatially on the top side of the bond could be on the bottom side due to free rotation. Consider 1,2-dichloroethane in Figure 6.15, where

Free rotation around C-C single bond

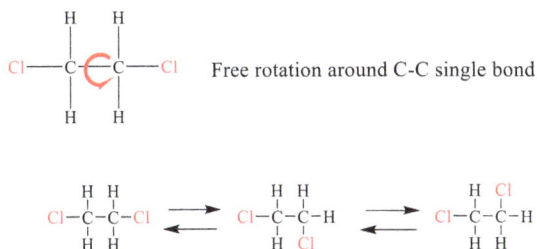

Figure 6.15 Free rotation of a C–C single bond.

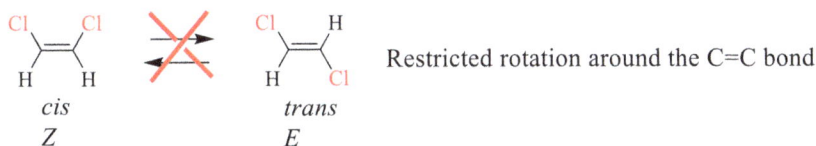

Restricted rotation around the C=C bond

cis

Z

trans

E

Figure 6.16 Geometrical isomers of 1,2-dichloroethene. The rigid structure of the double bond means that the two geometrical isomers are not interconvertible. Hence the compound exists as either *cis*-1,2-dichloroethene or *trans*-1,2-dichloroethene. The 'X' on the arrows indicates that the two forms are *not* interconvertible.

one can place the chorine atom attached to either carbon at any position of the three possible sites.

Introducing a double bond between the two carbon atoms, however, restricts the rotation. This is a feature of bonding between two sp^2-hybridised carbons. In this case, the two chlorine atoms on either side of the double bond could be on either the same side or the opposite side to each other. This is exemplified by 1,2-dichloroethene (Figure 6.16).

In addition to restricted rotation around the C=C bond, we also have restricted rotation in a ring system even in a saturated system (without a double bond). At the very best, the carbon–carbon single bonds in a ring system rotate partially, but it is not possible to interconvert between the *cis* and *trans* forms. Hence two substituents on adjacent carbon atoms could be on the same or opposite face of the molecule. We normally indicate whether the substituents are located either above or below the carbon ring. Using a bold wedge indicating above and a dashed wedge indicating below the ring plane, the *cis–trans* configuration between two atoms in the ring system is shown in Figure 6.17. The *cis–trans* isomerism in a ring system, however, is more complicated as the ring system could have several conformations (as discussed later).

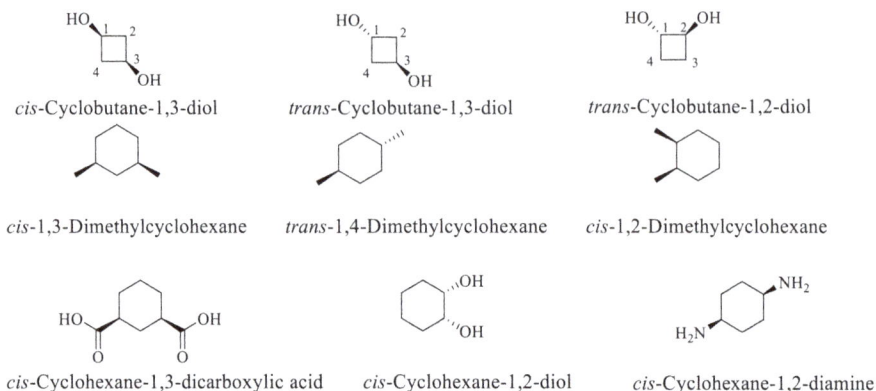

cis-Cyclobutane-1,3-diol   *trans*-Cyclobutane-1,3-diol   *trans*-Cyclobutane-1,2-diol

cis-1,3-Dimethylcyclohexane   *trans*-1,4-Dimethylcyclohexane   *cis*-1,2-Dimethylcyclohexane

cis-Cyclohexane-1,3-dicarboxylic acid   *cis*-Cyclohexane-1,2-diol   *cis*-Cyclohexane-1,2-diamine

Figure 6.17 *Cis–trans* isomerism in a ring system. Bold and dotted lines indicate positions above and below the plane, respectively.

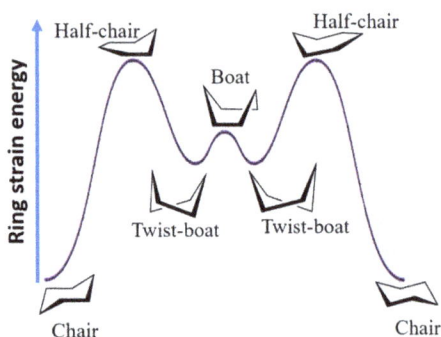

Figure 6.18 Energy diagram for cyclohexane conformations. The relative energy levels of different conformers are shown.

6.3.2 Ring Conformations

For sp^3-hybridised carbon atoms such as in alkanes, we expect to see a bond angle of 109.5°. A ring system, however, constrains this and cyclopropane, which has an equilateral triangular shape with angles of about 60° at the three corners, suffers from eclipsing and angle strain. As the carbon chain length in the ring system increases, starting from cyclopentane, it would have angle strain only if it adopts a planar conformation. Cyclohexane is the best example where these strains can be totally removed through non-planar conformations (Figure 6.18).

In a planar structure of cyclohexane, assume that the bond angle is 120°, which is larger than the tetrahedral 109.5°, and every C–C bond is eclipsed. The angle and eclipsing strain (torsional strain) make this structure a high-energy or unstable form. In terms of energy, this ring strain is estimated as 20 kcal mol^{-1}. The most stable conformation is the strain-free *chair conformer*, where four carbons are in the same plane while the other two poke above and below the plane. The name implies the resemblance of this conformer to a chair. Hence the two chair conformers have no eclipsing, are non-strained, and have the tetrahedral nature of sp^3-hybridised carbon atoms fully met. It is this lack of strain that makes it the lowest energy level. As shown in Figure 6.18, several other conformers with different degrees of ring strain also exist. These include the half-chair conformer with a ring strain of about 10.8 kcal mol^{-1}, the boat conformer with a ring strain of about 7 kcal mol^{-1}, and the twist-boat conformer with a ring strain of about 5.5 kcal mol^{-1}.

In the chair conformation of cyclohexane, six of the 12 hydrogen atoms are located about the periphery of the carbon ring and are called equatorial, whereas the other six are either above or below the plane of the ring system and are called axial protons. Axial protons appear parallel to the *symmetry axis* of the plane. Figure 6.19 shows the chair conformers of cyclohexane in a ball-and-stick model.

Even though the two chair forms of cyclohexane are interconvertible and exist in equal proportions, the presence of other substituents may influence which one predominates. As a rule, note that steric hindrance of the axial position favours substituents on chair conformers to occupy equatorial positions. For example, a methyl substituent (methylcyclohexane) favours a chair conformer in which the methyl group is located at the equatorial position (see Figure 6.20). In a similar way, when more than one substituent is present on the cyclohexane skeleton, equatorial substitution of both units or at least the bulkier substituent on the equatorial position predominates, as shown in Figure 6.20.

Another way of presenting *cis–trans* isomerism in a ring system is by using the Haworth projection model (Figure 6.21). More examples are presented for sugars in Chapter 8.

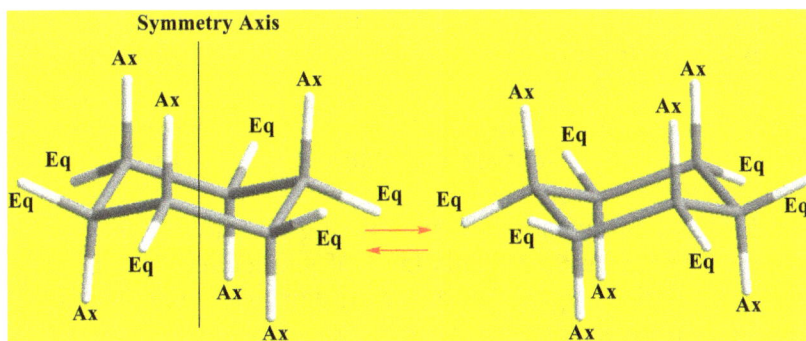

Figure 6.19 The two chair conformation structures of cyclohexane. Axial (Ax) and equatorial (Eq) hydrogens are shown.

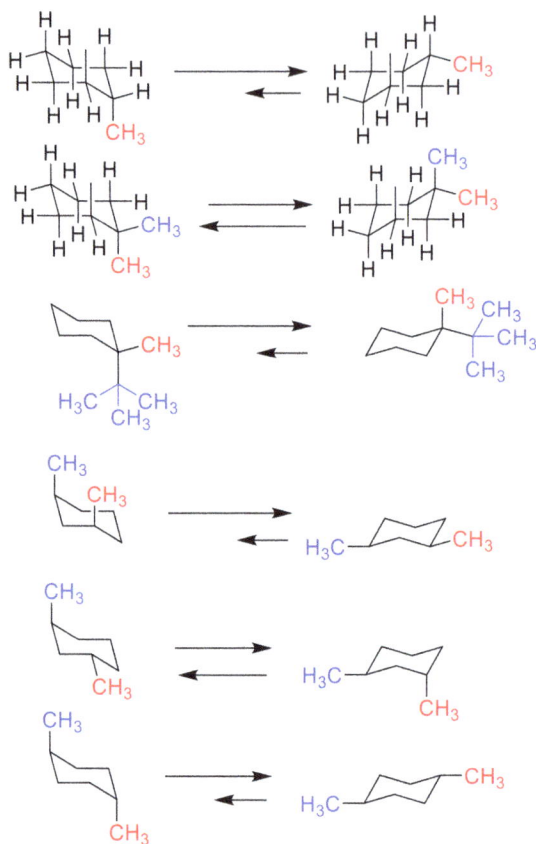

Figure 6.20 Conformations of cyclohexane derivatives. Note that the conformer with the alkyl chain at the equatorial position is predominant. Also, the longer or bulkier alkyl chain at the equatorial position is favoured. Note that hydrogen atoms are not shown in some of the structures. The longer arrow indicates the predominant form.

An important feature of *cis–trans* isomerism relevant to the action of drugs comes from the stereochemistry at the ring junctions. Two rings may be fused in a *trans* or *cis* manner, leading to the three-dimensional structure of the substituents at the junction being either close to each other or far apart. Considering that the most stable conformation of the cyclohexane ring, as discussed above, is in a chair form, decalin has two stable forms of ring junction: *cis*-decalin and *trans*-decalin (Figure 6.22). This kind of stereochemistry is important for the steroidal type of hormones and drugs that are constructed from fused multicyclic rings (Figure 6.22).

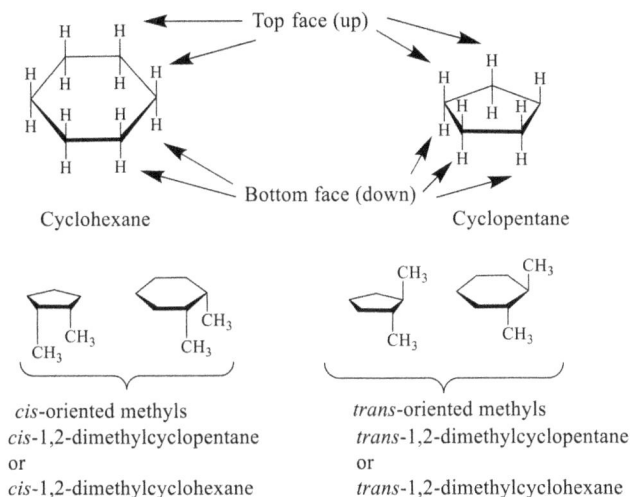

cis-oriented methyls
cis-1,2-dimethylcyclopentane
or
cis-1,2-dimethylcyclohexane

trans-oriented methyls
trans-1,2-dimethylcyclopentane
or
trans-1,2-dimethylcyclohexane

Figure 6.21 Presentation of *cis–trans* isomerism in a ring system using the Haworth projection model.

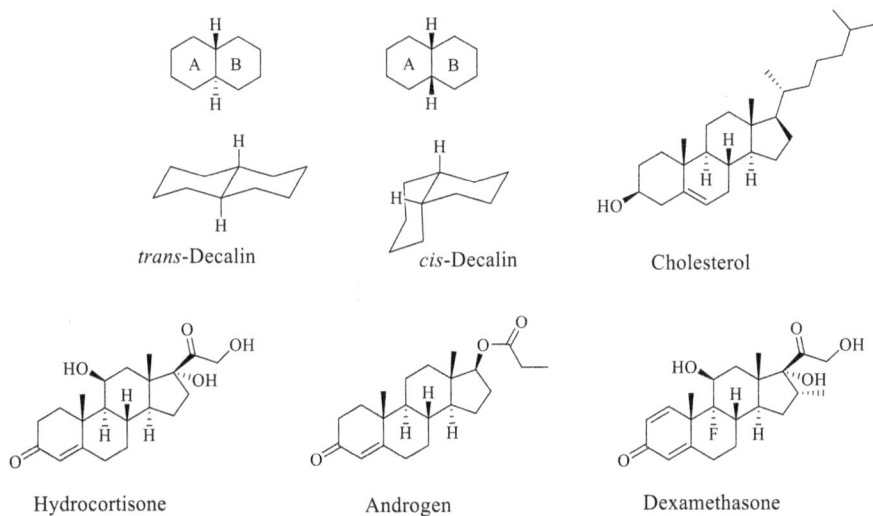

trans-Decalin   cis-Decalin   Cholesterol

Hydrocortisone   Androgen   Dexamethasone

Figure 6.22 *Cis-trans* isomerism at ring junctions. Note its occurrence in steroidal hormones and drugs and also in cholesterol. Also compare the proximity of the two hydrogen atoms in decalin at the ring junction, *i.e.* close to each other in the *cis*-decalin isomer and far apart in the *trans*-decalin isomer.

> **Geometrical Isomers – Key Facts**
>
> - *Cis–trans* or *E–Z* isomerism.
> - A feature of the carbon–carbon double bond – restricted rotation.
> - *Cis* (*Z*), same side; *trans* (*E*), opposite side.
> - Also occur in a ring system of sp^3-hybridised carbons, *e.g.* cyclohexane substituents.

6.3.3 Optical Isomers or *R* and *S* Isomers

6.3.3.1 General Structural Features

The other type of stereoisomerism is for molecules that rotate the plane of polarised light in the opposite direction but of the same magnitude. They are called *optical isomers* or D and L, *R* and *S*, or + and − isomers. This type of isomerism is related to the term *chirality*, which refers to an object not superimposable on its mirror image. This occurs when there is no symmetry within the molecule, hence the object is called *asymmetric*.

The word *chiral* is derived from the Greek '*cheir*', referring to the hand. Chirality in organic chemistry was first introduced in 1848 by the French chemist Louis Pasteur, who observed the two isomers of sodium ammonium tartrate crystals. The crystal shapes of the two isomers, left or right handedness, differ based on which two forms could be separated by hand. However, if there is symmetry in an object, it lacks chirality, and the object or the molecule is called *achiral*. Today, chirality is defined by analogy with one's right and left hands, which are mirror images and not superimposable on each other. Before we go into details of how the two optical isomers differ from each other and the significance of *R–S* isomerism in both chemistry and biology, let us define chirality in organic compounds.

The most common source of chirality in organic molecules is due to a carbon bonded to four different groups, *i.e.* a tetrahedral carbon atom with four single bonds with all the groups attached to that carbon differing from each other. This carbon atom is called the *chiral centre*. A molecule may have one or more chiral centres and, in addition to carbon, other elements including sulfur, phosphorus, and nitrogen can also form chiral centres. Let us consider compounds with one chiral centre. Figure 6.23 shows a structural model based on a carbon bonded to four different groups. This can give us two mirror

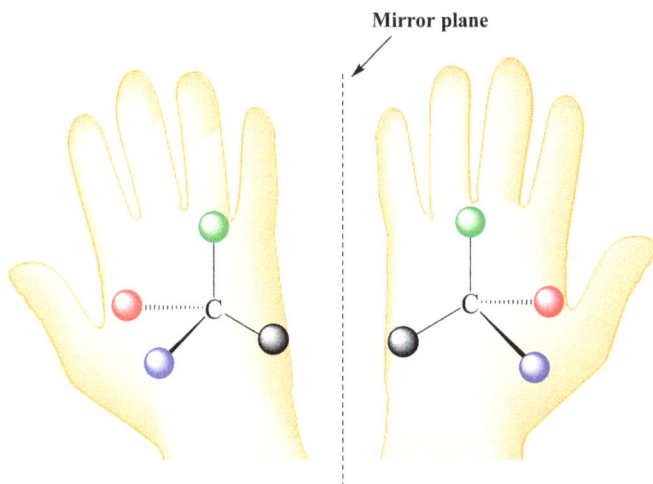

Figure 6.23 Enantiomers are non-superimposable mirror images. As the left hand is not superimposable on the right hand, mirror images of chiral compounds are not superimposable. Note that the chiral carbon centre is bonded with four different groups represented by different colours.

images that are not superimposable on each other, and we call them *enantiomers*.

One way of describing these enantiomers is by the R and S convention. Any compound can be denoted as R or S in reference to the chiral centre on the basis of the four different groups attached to the asymmetric or chiral centre. The simple procedure for R and S designation is as follows:

- We establish a priority list for each of the four substituents/groups based on the atomic number of the element attached to the chiral centre. Atoms with a high atomic number have higher priority and the order for the common elements is as follows:

  Atomic number: $^1H < {}^6C < {}^7N < {}^8O < {}^{16}S < {}^{17}Cl < {}^{35}Br < {}^{53}I$.
  Priority, example: $-H < -CH_3 < -NH_2 < -OH < SH < -Cl < -Br < -I$.

- If the atoms bonded to the chiral centre have the same order (say both are carbon atoms), the priority level is established on the next set of atoms. For example, $-CH_3 < -CH_2CH_3 < -CH_2OH$.
- If a double bond occurs, consider it as if it is bonded to similar atoms *via* a single bond (Figure 6.24). The same rule applies for triple bonds, as shown in Figure 6.24.
- Number from the priority 1 (highest) to 4 (lowest) of the four substituents of the chiral centre.

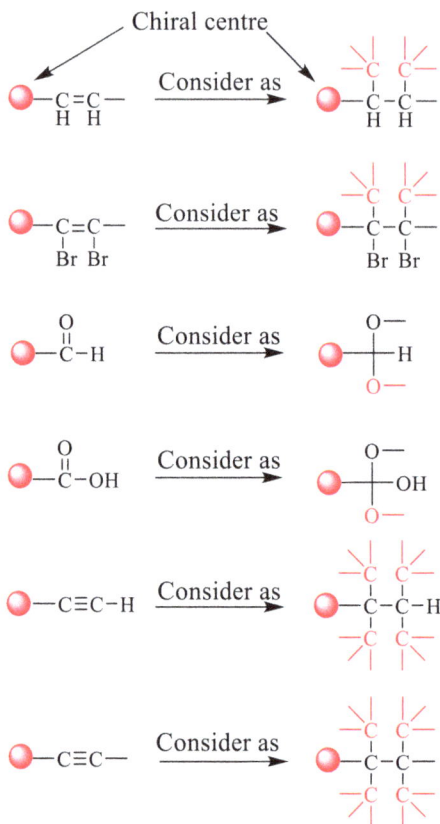

Figure 6.24 Priority setting in *R* and *S* designation. For the carbon of a double or triple bond attached to a chiral centre, consider it as if it is with the equivalent single bonds attached to the same atoms as shown in the examples.

- Put the lowest priority group (4) away from your view.
- The three groups projecting towards you (1, 2, and 3) may align in either clockwise order (*R*) or counterclockwise order (*S*) (see Figure 6.25).

The priority setting also applies in cyclic structures, as shown in Figure 6.26.

Based on the above examples, a molecule with one chiral centre has two $(2^1 = 2)$ possible stereoisomers that we called enantiomers (mirror images). If a molecule has two chiral centres, the number of expected stereoisomers is four $(2^2 = 4)$. Hence the number of possible isomers for a molecule is 2^n, where n is the number of chiral centres. When a molecule has more than one chiral centre, not all the stereoisomers

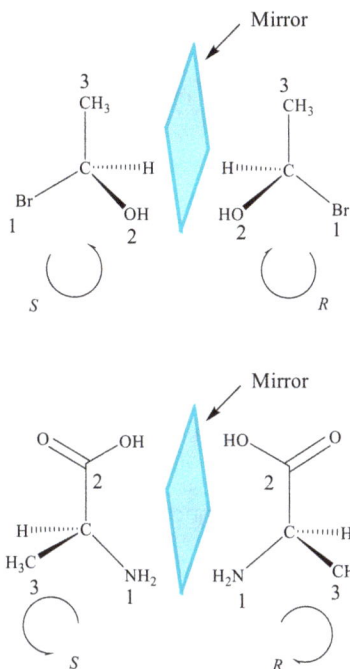

Figure 6.25 The *R* and *S* designation through priority setting of the four substituents at the chiral centre. Always place the lowest priority group, the hydrogen in this figure, away from your view.

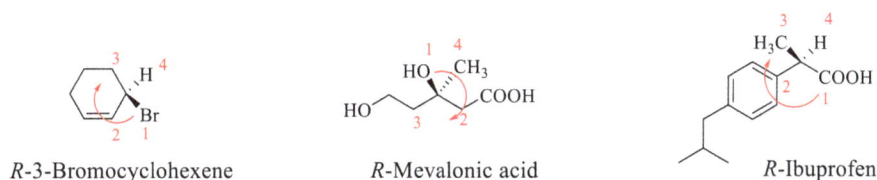

R-3-Bromocyclohexene   *R*-Mevalonic acid   *R*-Ibuprofen

Figure 6.26 Priority setting in *R* and *S* configuration assignment. Note that the lowest priority group is placed away from your view.

are mirror images of each other. Those which are superimposable, or mirror images, are enantiomers whereas the non-mirror image stereoisomers are *diastereomers*. Let us consider a compound with molecular formula $C_4H_8O_3$, a sugar that may be called either erythrose or threose based on the stereochemistry of the two chiral carbons (Figure 6.27). The two chiral centres in the *R,R* (D-erythrose) and *S,S* (L-erythrose) configurations are mirror images or enantiomers of erythrose, whereas the *S,R* (D-threose) and *R,S* (L-threose) configurations are mirror images or enantiomers of threose (Figure 6.27).

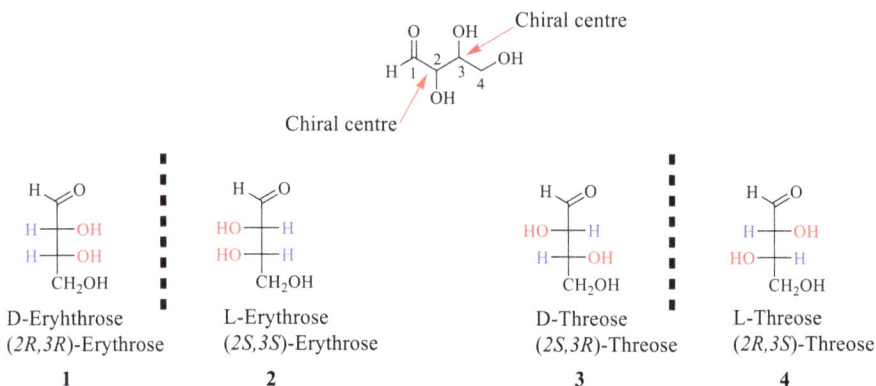

Figure 6.27 Enantiomers and diastereomers. Note that structures **1** and **2** are enantiomeric pairs of erythrose; whereas **3** and **4** are enantiomeric pairs of threose. The other mixes of pairs, **1** and **3**, **1** and **4**, **2** and **3**, and **2** and **4**, are diastereomers.

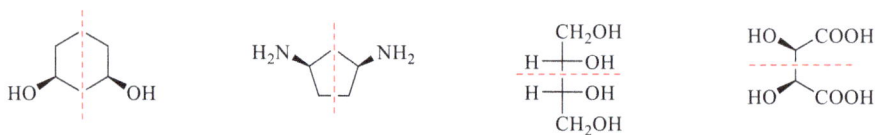

Figure 6.28 Molecules with an internal plane of symmetry are achiral even if they may have chiral centres. All compounds in this figure show an internal plane of symmetry and are called *meso* compounds. These compounds are achiral.

Some molecules with a chiral centre may not give the expected stereoisomers owing to internal symmetry, *i.e.* if a mirror is placed in the middle of the molecule, one half is already a mirror image of the other half. Molecules with this kind of internal symmetry are *achiral* (Figure 6.28), and such an achiral compound in the presence of chiral carbon in the molecule is called a *meso* compound.

In tartaric acid, with two chiral centres, only three stereoisomers exist as one pair has internal symmetry, which is called the *meso* form. As shown in Figure 6.29, the 2*S*,3*R* and 2*R*,3*S* forms of tartaric acid with internal symmetry are identical with each other and are achiral. This means that a compound in these forms (2*S*,3*R* and 2*R*,3*S*) with two chiral centres is actually an achiral compound called a *meso* compound.

Review the structures shown in Figure 6.30 and try to identify which pairs are enantiomers and diastereomers, and which are *meso* compounds.

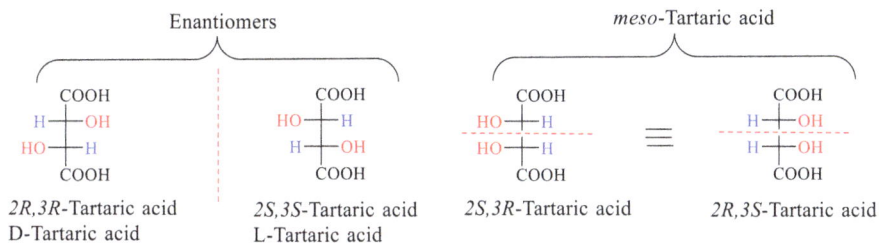

Enantiomers   *meso*-Tartaric acid

| 2*R*,3*R*-Tartaric acid
D-Tartaric acid | 2*S*,3*S*-Tartaric acid
L-Tartaric acid | 2*S*,3*R*-Tartaric acid | 2*R*,3*S*-Tartaric acid |

Figure 6.29 Stereoisomers of tartaric acid. Tartaric acid has three stereo-isomers instead of the expected four as the internal symmetry for one of the pairs on the right-hand side of the figure makes it *meso*-tartaric acid, which is achiral. The D and L are enantiomers whereas D and *meso* or L and *meso* are diastereomers.

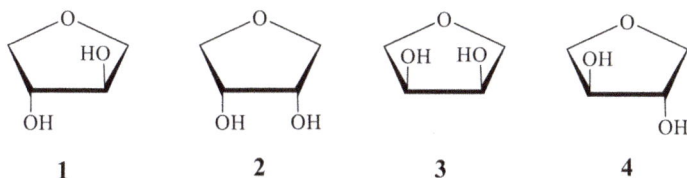

1   2   3   4

Figure 6.30 Identification of enantiomers, diastereomers, and *meso* compounds. Compounds **1** and **4** are enantiomers whereas other combinations, **1** and **2**, **1** and **3**, **2** and **4**, **3** and **4**, and **2** and **3**, are diastereomers. Compounds **2** and **3** with an internal plane of symmetry are *meso* compounds and hence are achiral.

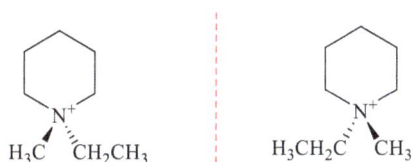

Figure 6.31 Quaternary amines can make a chiral centre based on nitrogen if the four substituents are different.

Since nitrogen can extend its valency to four, or simply quaternise (positively charged) to make four single bonds, it can also make a chiral centre like carbon. As explained for carbon, a nitrogen atom chiral centre must have four different groups attached to it (Figure 6.31).

6.3.3.2 Optical Activity of Enantiomers

A feature of enantiomers is their *optical activity* – they rotate plane-polarised light in an opposite direction. Light, being an example of electromagnetic radiation, has electric field and magnetic field components that are perpendicular to each other and oscillate in all directions perpendicular to the direction of travel (Figure 6.32).

On the other hand, plane-polarised light oscillates only in one direction or parallel planes. The direction of oscillation of the two fields that are perpendicular to each other is contained within a single plane. Chiral compounds rotate the plane of this polarisation to either the left or right, and an instrument called a *polarimeter* measures the extent and direction of this rotation. The instrumental setup is shown in Figure 6.33.

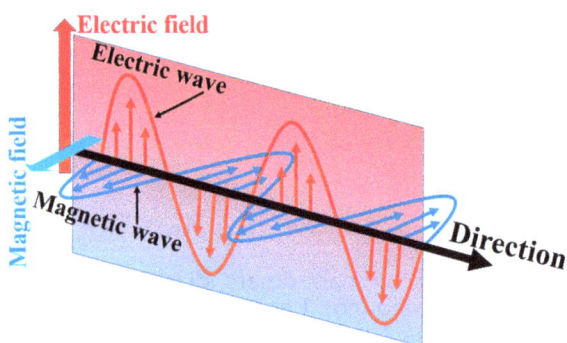

Figure 6.32 Electromagnetic radiation.

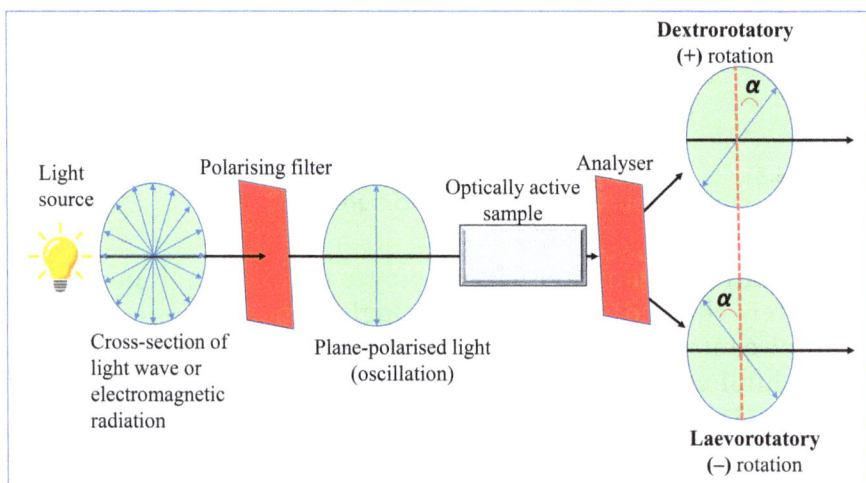

Figure 6.33 Schematic representation of optical activity measurements using a polarimeter.

The deflection of this light is measured as the angle (alpha, α) to the direction either on the right, called *dextrorotatory* (+), or left, called *laevorotatory* (−). For the measurement of optical activity, the sample must be dissolved in a solvent and the solution placed in a special glass tube. The degree of rotation is dependent on the concentration of the sample and the size (length) of the sample tube. At a concentration of the sample expressed in g mL^{-1} and a tube length of 1 dm, the measurement is called *specific rotation*, which is expressed with a note of the temperature condition.

The general equation for the expression of the specific rotation of a chiral compound in an optical activity measurement is presented as follows:

$$[\alpha]_{\lambda}^{t} = \frac{\alpha}{c \times l}$$

where $[\alpha]$ = specific rotation, t = temperature, λ = wavelength, α = optical rotation in degrees, c = concentration in g mL^{-1}, and l = optical pathlength of the sample tube in decimetres (dm). It is also common to indicate the solvent used to dissolve the sample and the common monochromatic light wavelength used is 589 nm [the sodium (Na) D line], which is simply indicated as 'D'. Hence the equation can be expressed as

$$[\alpha]_{D}^{t}(\text{solvent}) = \frac{\alpha}{c \times l}$$

As a general note, the degree of optical rotation for a given compound depends not only on which enantiomer is used, but also on the pathlength, solvent, temperature, and wavelength of light used. As an example, suppose that a solution of 0.2 g of a chiral compound is in 5 mL of water and the optical rotation measured in a 20 cm cell (sample tube) at 25 °C with the sodium D line was −5°. Let us now calculate the specific rotation:

$$[\alpha]_{D}^{25°C}(\text{water}) = \frac{-5}{0.04 \text{ mL}^{-1} \times 2 \text{ dm}} = \frac{-5}{0.08} = -62.5$$

Note: 0.2 g in 5 mL is 0.04 g mL^{-1} and 20 cm = 2 dm; the units of specific rotation are ° mL g^{-1} dm^{-1}.

If enantiomers are mixed in equal amounts, the optical rotation of the mixture would be 0°. A 50:50 mixture of R and S or + and − enantiomeric forms is called a *racemic mixture*. Suppose that a compound is expected to have an optical rotation of −100°. If the optical activity measurement shows less than the expected value, say a reading of −80°, it means that it is not pure or contains some of the other enantiomer. Its optical purity can be expressed as 80%. Optical purity is important for drug molecules and is expressed by the general equation

$$\text{Optical purity} / \% = \frac{[\alpha]_{\text{sample}}}{[\alpha]_{\text{pure enantiomer}}} \times 100$$

The difference in the percentage values of the two forms of the enantiomers is called the *enantiomeric excess* (ee), which is also a measure of optical purity. Hence the enantiomer may exist in pure form (enantiomerically pure), in a 50:50 ratio (racemate), or with one enantiomer in enantiomeric excess. Since the two enantiomers have an identical rotation value in opposite directions, the enantiomeric excess can be calculated from the ratio in the mixture on a weight basis. For example, if we have 7 g of (+)-adrenaline and 3 g of (−)-adrenaline, the enantiomeric excess can be calculated as

$$ee = \frac{7-3}{7+3} \times 100 = 40\%$$

The enantiomeric excess can also be calculated if one knows the expected optical rotation for the enantiomerically pure compound and that observed for the mixture. *i.e.*

$$ee = \frac{[\alpha]_{\text{observed}}}{[\alpha]_{\text{pure enantiomer}}}$$

If the enantiomerically pure compound in the above example is present with an enantiomeric excess of 40% and the expected specific rotation for (+)-adrenaline is +53°, then

$$ee = 40\% = \frac{[\alpha]_{\text{observed}}}{+53°}$$

Hence

$$[\alpha]_{\text{observed}} = 0.4 \times +53 = +21.2°$$

which is what is expected to be measured for the mixture.

The enantiomeric excess can also be calculated if we know the percentage of the major enantiomer in the mixture.

Understanding Optical Purity or Enantiomeric Excess – Key Facts

- The best way to understand optical purity or ee is by visualising your samples at a molecular level.
- If you have 100 molecules in a pot, a racemic mixture (ee = 0%) means that the clockwise rotation by 50 molecules is cancelled out by the counterclockwise rotation of the other 50 molecules.
- If you have an ee value of 40% in favour of the *S* isomer, it means that the rotation by 40 molecules of the *S* isomer of the 100 molecules in the pot was not cancelled out. Hence the remainder (60%) is 30 molecules each of the *R* and *S* forms in the mixture, which were cancelled out. Hence the two enantiomers are present in a ratio of 70% *S* form (40 + 30) and 30% *R* form.

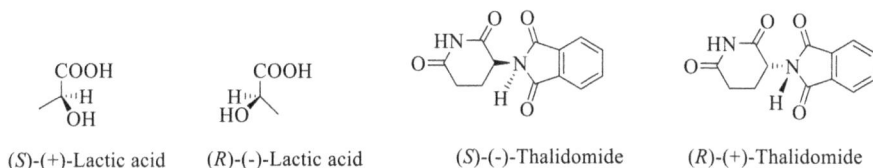

(*S*)-(+)-Lactic acid   (*R*)-(-)-Lactic acid   (*S*)-(-)-Thalidomide   (*R*)-(+)-Thalidomide

Figure 6.34   The designation of *R* and *S* is different from the – and + assignment of optical rotation. A given compound with an *R* designation may have a negative rotation, whereas another *R* compound may have a positive rotation.

It should be noted that the *R*–*S* configuration is based on priority assignment of the four substituents of the chiral centre; while the – and + notation for a compound refers to the direction of rotation of plane-polarised light measured using a polarimeter. Hence for one compound, an *R* assignment may give –, whereas for another compound an *R* assignment could correspond to the + designation based on the specific rotation measurement. See the examples in Figure 6.34.

So far, we have discussed how to identify chirality based on the chiral centre such as a tetrahedral (sp³-hybridised) carbon atom bonded to four different groups (asymmetric carbon), or for other elements such as nitrogen and sulfur similarly bonded to four different groups. We also outlined that the presence of a chiral centre does not necessarily make the molecule chiral as an internal plane of symmetry (molecular symmetry) makes the molecule achiral. Readers pursuing further study or a career in chemistry-related fields will learn that some organic compounds may show optical activity even in the absence of

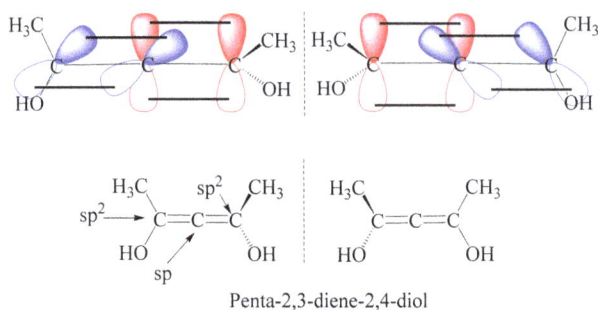

Penta-2,3-diene-2,4-diol

Figure 6.35 Optical activity in the absence of asymmetric carbon – penta-2,3-diene-2,4-diol. This compound is expected to show optical activity. The central carbon is sp hybridised with two p orbitals involved in π bonding with two sp^2-hybridised carbons. There is restricted or no rotation around these double bonds.

a chiral centre in their molecules. This is mostly a feature of allenes, which are compounds with three or more adjacent carbon atoms in a molecule bonded with double bonds. Figure 6.35 shows the orientation of the π bonds with the central carbon in penta-2,3-diene-2,4-diol, which has two p orbitals perpendicular to each other, *i.e.* the central carbon with a double bond on both sides is an sp-hybridised carbon (just like alkynes, Chapter 4) with two π orbitals appearing perpendicular to each other. The resulting two substituents on the opposite sides of the two carbons are thus perpendicular to each other. This gives non-superimposable mirror images and hence the molecule is optically active.

Another good example of optical activity without asymmetric carbon is explained by biphenyl compounds with bulky *ortho* substituents that restrict free rotation about the C–C single bond. The energy required to twist one ring through a 180° angle is very high, hence such molecules have restricted rotation resulting in a non-superimposable mirror image, or they display optical activity. This is shown in Figure 6.36 for 6,6′-dihydroxy-2,2′-biphenyldicarboxylic acid. This kind of isomerism is called *atropisomerism* and the structural requirements for it are as follows:

- Common in biaryl compounds that exhibit restricted rotation.
- Substitution of the benzene ring typically at the *ortho* position that restricts free rotation.
- Bulky group substitution restricts free rotation.
- The compound should not also have a plane of symmetry, as discussed for the tetrahedral carbon-based isomerism.

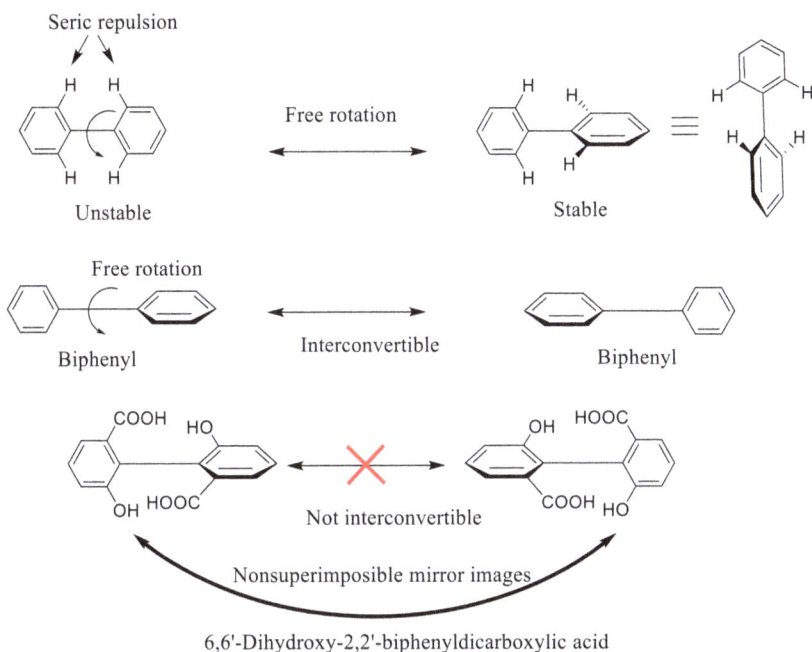

Seric repulsion

Free rotation

Unstable

Stable

Free rotation

Biphenyl

Interconvertible

Biphenyl

Not interconvertible

Nonsuperimposible mirror images

6,6'-Dihydroxy-2,2'-biphenyldicarboxylic acid

Figure 6.36 Optical activity in the absence of asymmetric carbon – a biaryl (biphenyl) compound, 6,6'-dihydroxy-2,2'-biphenyldi-carboxylic acid. When two phenyl rings are attached with a single bond (pivotal bond) they take a perpendicular plane (one vertical and the other in the horizontal plane) arrangement to achieve stability. This is because the hydrogens in the *ortho* position sterically repulse each other to dictate that the non-coplanar conformation is more stable than the coplanar conformation. The single bond can rotate and the two forms (*e.g.* biphenyl) can be interconvertible unless there are substituents that restrict such free rotation. Hence 6,6'-dihydroxy-2,2'-biphenyldicarboxylic acid has optical isomers called atropisomers.

Hence biphenyl, binaphthyl, or generally biaryl compounds with bulky *ortho* substituents can give rise to optical isomerism (atropisomerism) provided that there is no plane of symmetry in these compounds (see Figure 6.36).

Instead of the *R* and *S* configurations used in tetrahedral stereoisomers, *P* for clockwise and *M* for counterclockwise assignments are used in atropisomerism. Examples of such optical isomerism for the naturally occurring biaryl compounds knipholone and knipholone anthrone are shown in Figure 6.37. There are other cases of optical activity in organic compounds in the absence of chiral/asymmetric carbons that are not addressed here as they are beyond the scope of

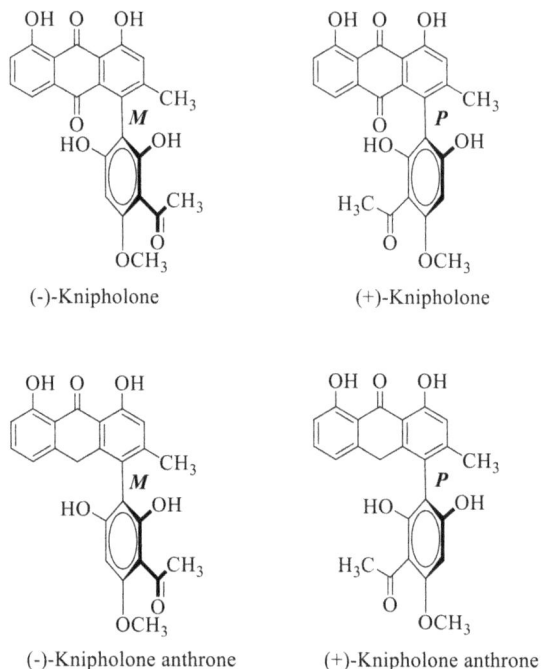

(-)-Knipholone

(+)-Knipholone

(-)-Knipholone anthrone

(+)-Knipholone anthrone

Figure 6.37 Optical activity of biaryl compounds: knipholone and knipholone anthrone. The dextrorotatory enantiomers (+)-knipholone and (+)-knipholone anthrone have the P configuration whereas the laevorotatory enantiomers (−)-knipholone and (−)-knipholone anthrone are naturally occurring compounds with the M configuration.

this book. Complex structural assignments based on atropisomerism are also beyond the scope of this book.

6.3.3.3 Physical Properties of Optical Isomers

As outlined above, what makes enantiomers differ from each other is only their optical activity. Provided that they are not placed in chiral environments, enantiomers otherwise exhibit identical physical properties. Hence enantiomers display similar boiling points and melting points. They also exhibit similar acidity (if they are acidic) or basicity (if they are basic). On the other hand, diastereomers differ from each other in their chemical and physical properties. Owing to the close similarity of their properties, enantiomers are difficult to separate from each other once they are in a mixture. Techniques for their separation, including chromatographic methods and chemical methods, are available but are not addressed here as they are beyond the scope of this book.

6.4 Biological Significance of Chirality and Stereoisomerism

Many chemical compounds of pharmaceutical importance may not have a chiral centre in their molecules, or even if there are one or more chiral centres they may be marketed as racemic mixtures. This only means, however, that the two enantiomers of the racemic mixture may be either equally potent or at least no toxic side effect is detected for the enantiomer that may not be effective. The therapeutic effect of drug molecules may be due to specific binding with a receptor, enzyme, ion channel, specific macromolecule (such as DNA or cell membrane components), or other biological targets. Drugs are also absorbed from the gastrointestinal tract through interaction with various regions of the gut and transported in the blood by binding with some blood components such as plasma proteins. The metabolism and clearance of drugs also require interaction with various enzymes and other biological molecules in the body. Hence one should expect that enantiomers have the potential to differ from each other in the way in which they interact with biological targets, thereby potentially differing in their *pharmacodynamic* and *pharmacokinetic* profiles. Figure 6.38 depicts a three-point attachment of enantiomers with their target and how one fits to a target whereas the other one may not fit.

Chirality and stereoisomers are fundamentally applicable to every biological event in living organisms. It is astonishing to note the difference in odour for carvone enantiomers (Figure 6.39) based on the difference of one chiral centre (enantiomers). Whereas the *R* form gives the characteristic odour of spearmint oil, the *S* enantiomer features an odour of caraway seed oil. Although we have to work hard to

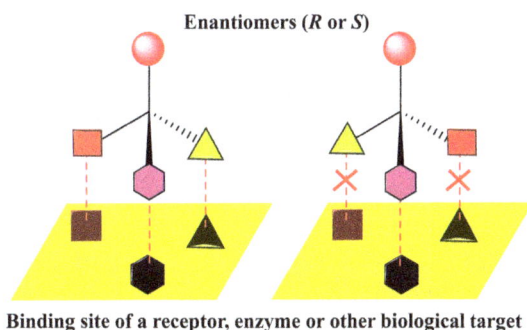

Figure 6.38 Attachment of a drug molecule with its target – a three-point binding model. The model shows one enantiomer like a hand-and-glove fit, whereas the other may not fit.

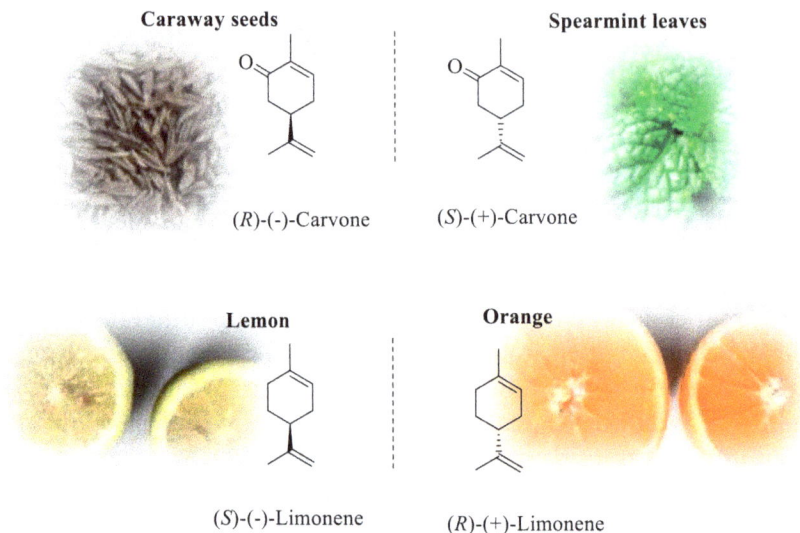

Caraway seeds   **Spearmint leaves**

(R)-(-)-Carvone   (S)-(+)-Carvone

Lemon   **Orange**

(S)-(-)-Limonene   (R)-(+)-Limonene

Figure 6.39   Enantiomers perceived by the olfactory system to have different odours. The odours of carvone and limonene are shown for the enantiomeric pairs.

distinguish these two compounds in the laboratory, our nose, equipped with odour receptors, can distinguish between over 10 000 different smells/scents. For this to happen, there must be different ways of binding these odorous chemicals with receptors. As such, receptors themselves are chiral, and their specific interaction with enantiomers can be distinguished with a biological response of smell detection. Another good example is the small fragrant molecule limonene, which occurs naturally as two enantiomers with R and S forms. Whereas (R)-limonene has a characteristic smell of oranges, (S)-limonene is perceived by the nose to smell like lemons (Figure 6.39).

Insects have a well-developed system of chemical communication throughout their developmental cycle. This includes the use of distinct chiral compounds, *pheromones*, that attract the opposite sex for mating. Some other chiral compounds with a distinct smell are also used by living organisms (including plants) to deter undesirable guests. We often use these kinds of chemicals to deter undesirable insects or direct them to the chemical bait for their removal/destruction. Hence chirality has many applications in the agrochemical industry and in disease management (*e.g.* malaria) where insects act as intermediate hosts.

As with our sense of smell, the sense of taste amazingly responds to chirality. For glucose as a sugar, the D and L forms are equally sweet,

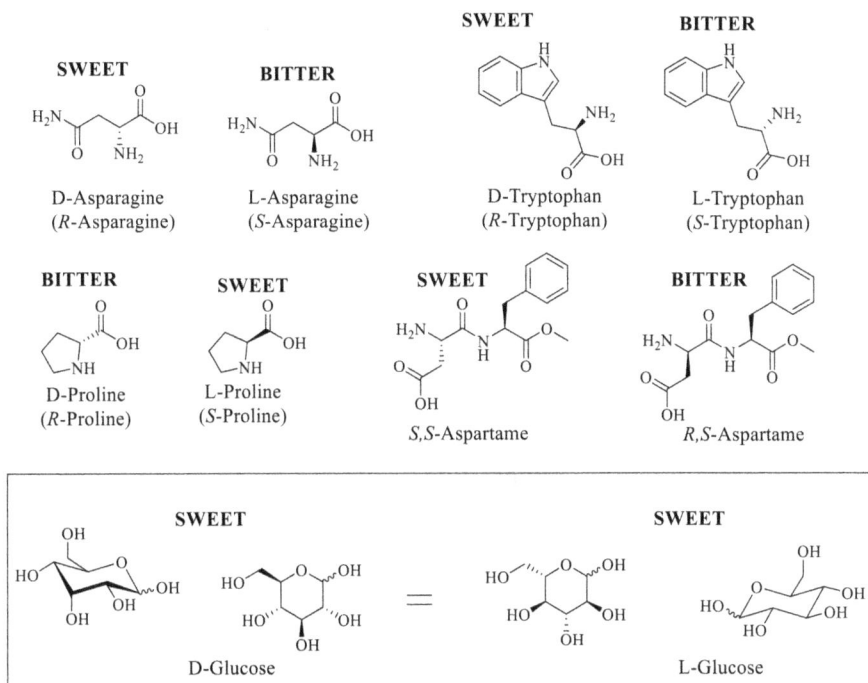

Figure 6.40 Chirality in the taste of sweet and bitter. Note that the stereo-chemistry difference due to chirality results in a different taste of amino acids and this leads to the identification of aspartame with a sweet isomer being about 160 times sweeter than sugar.

but the D forms of amino acids are mostly considered sweet whereas the L forms are mostly bitter or tasteless (Figure 6.40). Tryptophan is a good example, with the D (*R*) form being severalfold sweeter than sugar, whereas the L (*S*) form is bitter. Asparagine is another example where the D (*R*) form is sweet and the L (*S*) form is bitter. Although the distinction is less for some amino acids such as phenylalanine and tyrosine, there is still a taste difference between the D and L forms in favour of sweetness for the D forms. There are, however, exceptions, with proline as a good example where the D form (D-proline) is bitter and L-proline is on the sweet side of the scale. On the other side, the amino acids serine and alanine exhibit similar taste characteristics on the sweeter side of the scale for their D and L forms. A good example of chirality in sweetness is the synthetic sweetener aspartame, which is a peptide made from the reaction of the carboxy group of L-aspartic acid with the amino group of methyl L-phenylalaninate (methyl ester of phenylalanine). The striking difference between chirality in this molecule is that one form [(*R,S*)-aspartame] is bitter whereas another form [(*S,S*)-aspartame] is over 160 times sweeter than table sugar (Figure 6.40). In terms of the binding of aspartame with the sweet receptors, the L,L (*S,S*) isomer with a different orientation of the benzene ring in space gives a sweet taste, the D,L (*R,S*) isomer, which still interacts with receptors, gives a bitter taste, and the other two combinations do not match the binding site of the receptor.

The difference in the biology of enantiomers is better represented by reviewing the efficacy and toxicity of drug molecules (see Table 6.2).

Often, one enantiomer is biologically active whereas the other may be less active or inactive altogether. The differential activity of adrenaline (epinephrine) stereoisomers was established by the beginning of the twentieth century. In our body, the D- or *R*-(−) enantiomer of adrenaline is produced in the adrenal medulla as a hormone and among its diverse effects is constriction of blood vessels and an increase in blood pressure, in addition to increasing the activity of the

Table 6.2 Summary of pharmacological effects of enantiomeric drugs.

Stereochemistry (*R*-form)	Stereochemistry (*S*-form)	Pharmacology
R-(-)-Adrenaline	*S*-(+)-Adrenaline	*R*-(−)-Enantiomer is about twice as potent than the racemate (±)-adrenaline; *S*-(+)-enantiomer is about 12–15-fold weaker than the natural *R*-(−)-enantiomer as a vasoconstrictive agent; receptor binding is stronger for the *R* isomer than the *S*-enantiomer.
R-(-)-Noradrenaline	*S*-(+)-Noradrenaline	*R*-(−)-Enantiomer is a more effective vascular agent than the *S*-enantiomer; receptor binding is stronger for the *R*-isomer than the *S*-isomer.
R-(-)-Methamphetamine	*S*-(+)-Methamphetamine	*S*-(+)-Enantiomer is more potent than the *R*-(−)-enantiomer; *S*-(+)-form completely metabolised and at a faster rate than the *R*-(−)-isomer.

Table 6.2 (continued)

Stereochemistry (*R*-form)	Stereochemistry (*S*-form)	Pharmacology
R-(-)-Amphetamine	S-(+)-Amphetamine	S-(+)-Enantiomer is about twice as potent than R-(−)-amphetamine; the S-(+) isomer has a shorter onset of action as well as a shorter half-life than the R-(−)-isomer.
(S)-(+)-Ketamine	(R)-(-)-Ketamine	S-Enantiomer is more potent in treating major depressive and bipolar disorders than the R-isomer.
R-(-)-Flurbiprofen	S-(+)-Flurbiprofen	Used as a racemate but its effect is due to only the S-(+)-enantiomer able to inhibit prostaglandin synthesis by inhibiting the key enzyme (cyclooxygenase).
R-(-)-Ketoprofen	S-(+)-Ketoprofen	Used as a racemate but its effect is due to only the S-(+)-enantiomer able to inhibit prostaglandin synthesis by inhibiting the key enzyme (cyclooxygenase).
R-(-)-Ibuprofen	S-(+)-Ibuprofen	S-(+)-Enantiomer is the active form but the R-(−)-enantiomer is slowly converted to the active form in the body.
R-(-)-naproxen	S-(+)-naproxen	S-(+)-Enantiomer is 28 times more active than the R-(−)-enantiomer in inflammatory enzyme (cyclooxygenase) inhibition.

(continued)

Table 6.2 (continued)

Stereochemistry (R-form)	Stereochemistry (S-form)	Pharmacology
R-(+)-Warfarin	S-(-)-Warfarin	The S-enantiomer is 2–5 times more active as an anticoagulant than the R-isomer. The racemate is used as an antidepressant while the S-(+)-isomer is effective in treating migraine headaches and chronic pain.
R-(-)-Fluoxetine	S-(+)-Fluoxetine	R-Fluoxetine is metabolised about four times slower than S-fluoxetine.
R-(+)-Thalidomide	S-(-)-Thalidomide	R-(+)-Isomer (the good) was used for morning sickness in pregnant women while the (S)-(−)-isomer was proven to be teratogenic.
R-(-)-Albuterol	S-(+)-Albuterol	R-(−)-Form is a tracheal muscle relaxant in asthma therapy while the S-(+)-enantiomer is weakly active with unpredictable side effects.
R-(-)-Fenfluramine	S-(+)-Fenfluramine (Dexfenfluramine)	The S-(+)-enantiomer is an appetite suppressor while the R-(−)-form causes drowsiness. The S-(+)-enantiomer still has other side effects however.

heart. It is known that (R)-(−)-adrenaline is about twice as potent as the racemate (±)-adrenaline, whereas (S)-(+)-adrenaline is about 12–15-fold weaker than the natural (R)-(−)-adrenaline as a vasoconstrictive agent. Similarly, noradrenaline (norepinephrine) is a neurotransmitter produced in neuronal cells with similar effects to adrenaline;

(*R*)-(−)-noradrenaline is a more effective vascular agent than the *S* isomer. The differential biological activity of adrenaline and noradrenaline is related to the inability of the *S* isomer to bind effectively to the receptor. In biological terms, the enantiomer or stereoisomer with lower activity or affinity for a given target (*e.g.* receptor) is called a *distomer*.

The D isomers of amphetamine (dextroamphetamine) and methamphetamine exhibit a higher central nervous system (CNS) stimulant activity than the L isomers. Note that the D and L notations refer to the direction of the rotation of plane-polarised light. In terms of binding with their receptors as a measure of stimulant effect, the *S* enantiomer of methamphetamine, which is dextrorotatory, is about five times more potent than the *R* enantiomer (laevorotatory). On the other hand, (*S*)-(+)-methamphetamine is completely metabolised in the body and at a faster rate than (*R*)-(−)-methamphetamine. The stimulant activity of (*S*)-(+)-amphetamine is about twice as high as that of (*R*)-(−)-amphetamine. In other conditions such as psychotic syndrome, however, (*R*)-(−)-amphetamine is known to be as effective as the *S*-(+) enantiomer. It is worth noting that these drugs are available commercially in their racemate forms. Ketamine as an antidepressant agent is also available commercially in its racemate form [(±)-ketamine] or as a mixture of (*S*)-(+)-ketamine and (*R*)-(−)-ketamine. The (*S*)-ketamine enantiomer is, however, now acknowledged to be potent in patients with major depressive and bipolar disorders. Experimental data in rats show the superiority of (*R*)-(−)-ketamine over the *S* enantiomer in abolishing depression-related disorders, but whether this effect is relevant in humans is in need of further research.

Sometimes, obtaining the pure form of the enantiomers as drugs can be difficult or too expensive and the racemate may be used even if one enantiomer is superior in efficacy to the other. This depends, of course, on the other enantiomer not having a known side effect. Flurbiprofen, ketoprofen, and ibuprofen are analgesic and anti-inflammatory drugs that are sold as the racemate forms [equal amounts of the *R*-(−) and *S*-(+) enantiomers]. It is only the *S*-(+) enantiomer that is effective, however, and there has been active research in recent years on synthesising and/or purifying the active enantiomer. They act by inhibiting a proinflammatory enzyme called cyclooxygenase, and through this action they also inhibit platelet aggregation just like aspirin and hence possess an antithrombotic effect. On the positive side, (*R*)-(−)-ibuprofen is slowly metabolised (up to 90%) in the body to be converted to the active form or (*S*)-(+)-ibuprofen. In a similar fashion, naproxen is an analgesic and anti-inflammatory agent that acts by inhibiting the cyclooxygenase enzyme. Only the S-(+) enantiomer of naproxen is marketed, however, since its potency as an anti-inflammatory agent is about 28 times greater than that of (R)-(−)-naproxen. Although the S enantiomer of warfarin is 2–5 times more active as an anticoagulant (blood-thinning agent) than the R isomer, the racemate form [(±)-warfarin, trade name Coumadin] is used in therapy. It is the most widely used medication for the treatment and/or prevention of thrombosis (thromboembolic conditions). Its effect is associated with inhibition of a vitamin K-dependent step in the synthesis of clotting factors II (prothrombin), VII, IX, and X by the liver. In addition to the differential biological effect of these enantiomers, they also differ in their metabolism in the body.

Fluoxetine in its racemate form [(±)-fluoxetine] is a common therapy for major depression, panic disorder, and obsessive–compulsive disorder. It is a drug that produces an antidepressant-like effect by inhibition of a neurotransmitter serotine reuptake back into neuronal cells after its release. (R)-Fluoxetine is metabolised about four times more slowly than (S)-fluoxetine. On the other hand, recent studies suggest that the S-(+) isomer of fluoxetine is useful in treating migraine headaches and chronic pain.

At the other extreme in cases of isomerism, enantiomers could be dangerously different, and caution must be exercised in separating them before we consider using them as drugs. Perhaps the most vivid example of the significance of chirality in medicine is the thalidomide story. Its racemate form was applied in the 1950s as a medicine to pregnant women to treat morning sickness. The resulting deaths and birth defects (teratogenic effect) discovered in thousands of children before the drug was taken off the market in 1961 was a painful reminder of how we should treat enantiomers differently when it comes to drug therapy. Whereas (R)-(+)-thalidomide is the enantiomer associated with the indicated therapeutic effect, (S)-(−)-thalidomide causes a teratogenic effect. Since then, thalidomide has shown a comeback in therapeutic applications in cancer and inflammatory diseases.

Albuterol (also called salbutamol) is a chiral compound with its R-(−) form active as a tracheal muscle relaxant and it is used in treating asthma. Its mechanism of action is similar to that of adrenaline, and it activates adrenaline receptors (β_2-adrenoceptors) located in the lungs, leading to muscle relaxation. On the other hand, (S)-(+)-albuterol is a distomer and is weakly active, and emerging evidence suggests that it has an unpredictable effect with negative consequences. Among the adverse effects of (S)-(+)-albuterol are hyperkalaemia and implications in white blood cells (eosinophil activation) and pro-inflammatory properties in the lung.

Fenfluramine, introduced as a racemate as an appetite suppressor (anorectic), is active due to the D isomer [*S*-(+) enantiomer], whereas the L isomer [*R*-(−) enantiomer] causes drowsiness. This D isomer, marketed as dexfenfluramine, however, still showed undesirable side effects, including the risk of pulmonary hypertension and valvular heart disease, owing to which it was withdrawn from the market (together with the racemic fenfluramine) in 1997.

Chiral Drug Molecules – Key Facts

Enantiomers of drug molecules may:
- Be of the same potency – we can use them as a racemic mixture.
- Have differential potency – consider separation. In practice, this depends on the cost of the separation process.
- Be dangerously different. One may act as a drug but the other may be toxic or have toxic side effects – must be separated!
- The difference could be in the pharmacokinetic profile of the enantiomers.

6.5 Summary

In this chapter, we have learned the following:

- For the same molecular formula, we may have different compounds based on the way in which the atoms are connected (structural isomers) or the spatial arrangement of the atoms (stereoisomers).
- In structural isomerism, a simple variation in the branching pattern (chain or branch isomers) could give rise to variations in physical and chemical properties.
- A compact molecule as opposed to a long chain is expected to have a relatively lower boiling/melting point.
- The molecular formula for alkenes also fits cycloalkane structures – both pentene and cyclopentane have the molecular formula C_5H_{10}. Hence consider isomers of both cyclic and acyclic structures.
- Positional isomers differ in the placement of a structural group or substitutions, *e.g.* butan-1-ol *versus* butan-2-ol.
- Positional isomers in an aromatic structure include the *ortho*, *meta*, and *para* positioning of a substituent with respect to the main functional group such as a carboxylic acid.

- Functional group isomers have different functional groups such as alcohol *versus* ether.
- Ketones and enols are interconvertible with each other to give isomerism called tautomerism. One form (the keto or enol tautomer) may predominate, depending on the stability of the structure.
- In the chair conformation of cyclohexane derivatives, a bulkier substituent on the equatorial position is favoured.
- In multicyclic compounds such as steroids, ring junction stereochemistry (*cis–trans*) plays a key role in their biological activities.
- Chirality refers to asymmetry or non-superimposable objects.
- For carbon, chirality occurs when it is bonded to four different groups – this carbon is called a chiral carbon.
- *R* and *S* configurations are based on priority setting (on atomic number) for the four substituents or groups attached to the chiral centre.
- The number of possible isomers for a molecule is 2^n, where n is the number of chiral centres.
- Not all the stereoisomers are a mirror image of each other – mirror images are enantiomers whereas the non-mirror image stereoisomers are diastereomers.
- A molecule with internal symmetry is called a *meso* compound – one half is a mirror image of the other half – it is achiral. Thus, a compound with a chiral centre could be achiral.
- Enantiomers rotate plane-polarised light in the opposite direction but with the same magnitude.
- Some organic compounds may show optical activity even in the absence of a chiral centre in their molecules. Allenes and biaryl compounds (atropisomerism) are good examples.
- The specific rotation of enantiomers depends on the concentration of the sample. Other factors are pathlength, solvent, temperature, and wavelength of the light used.
- A given compound with *R* designation may have a negative rotation, whereas another *R* compound may have a positive rotation.
- A racemic mixture – a 50:50 mixture of *R* and *S* or + and − enantiomers – has an optical rotation of 0°.
- Measurement of optical purity is critical for drug molecules which are chiral.
- An enantiomer or stereoisomer with lower activity or affinity for a given target (*e.g.* receptor) is called a distomer.
- Chirality has relevance in the food, agrochemical, and pharmaceutical industries.

6.6 Problems

Questions 1–4 are based on butanoic acid $(CH_3CH_2CH_2COOH)$ with the molecular formula $C_4H_8O_2$.

1. Draw functional group isomers as esters.
2. Draw one functional isomer that contains both ketone and hydroxyl functional groups.
3. Draw an isomer in a cyclic structure – ether.
4. Identify isomers with chiral centre(s).

Questions 5–7. *n*-Hexane has five chain isomers:

5. Draw their structures.
6. Identify two sets of positional isomers.
7. Which chain isomer is chiral?

Questions 8 and 9. For a molecular formula C_6H_{12}, we have both cyclic and acyclic (non-cyclic) isomers:

8. Draw the structures of acyclic isomers.
9. Indicate structures which are geometrical isomers.
10. 1,3,5-Trihydroxycyclohexane has several structural isomers. Keeping the six-membered cyclohexane ring intact, identify at least six structural isomers.

Questions 11–13. Identify the functional group isomer for the indicated compound:

11. Propanone.
12. Ethanol.
13. Butanoic acid.

Questions 14 and 15. For a compound with a molecular formula $C_4H_{10}O$:

14. Identify the alcohol functional group isomers.
15. Identify the ether functional group isomers.
16. For cyclohexane-1,4-diol, show the *cis* and *trans* configurations.
17. Give an example of functional group isomerism such as alcohol *versus* ether, aldehyde *versus* ketone, acid *versus* ester.
18. Show the keto–enol tautomerism for the compounds illustrated in Figure 6.41.

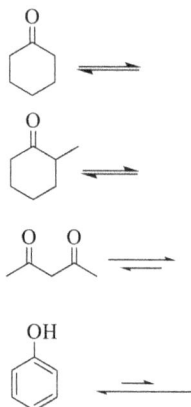

Figure 6.41 Question 18.

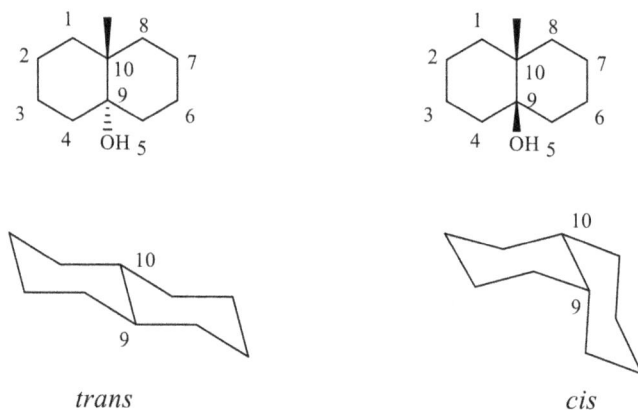

trans   *cis*

Figure 6.42 Question 19.

19. The stereochemistry of the ring junction in organic compounds such as steroids is relevant to their biological activities. In Figure 6.42, complete the *trans* and *cis* fused rings in the indicated chair conformers by placing the methyl (C-10) and hydroxyl (C-9) groups as appropriate. Comment on the difference between the two structural presentations.

Questions 20–28 are based on Figure 6.43. How many chiral centres occur in the structures of:

20. Cholesterol.
21. Nicotine.
22. Penicillin G.
23. Aspirin.

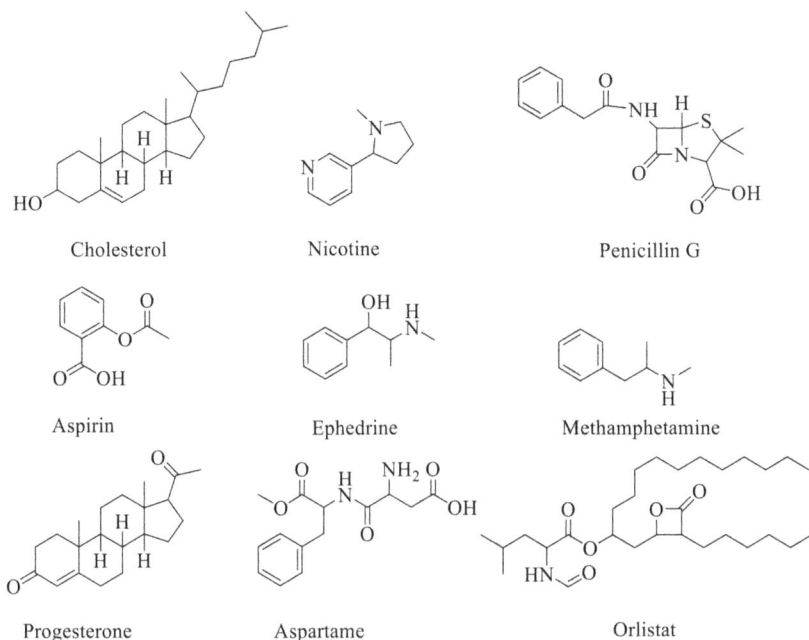

Figure 6.43 Questions 20–28.

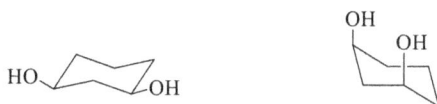

Figure 6.44 Question 29.

24. Ephedrine.
25. Methamphetamine.
26. Progesterone.
27. Aspartame.
28. Orlistat.
29. One of the conformers shown in Figure 6.44 is more stable: why? Use horizontal reverse arrows to show your answer.

Questions 30–32. A drug molecule has one chiral centre and optical activity. What would be the enantiomeric excess (ee) of the *R* isomer under the following conditions:

30. A sample of racemic mixture.
31. A sample of 70% of the *R* isomer.
32. A sample of 100% of the *R* isomer.

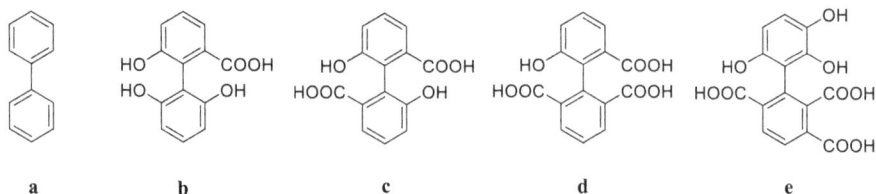

Figure 6.45   Question 37 is based on structures **a–e**.

33. A drug molecule of the *R* isomer was expected to have a specific rotation of −20° but your optical measurement recorded −5°. What is the ee of the *R* isomer and the percentage of the enantiomers?

Questions 34–36. (*R*)-Epinephrine has a specific rotation of −53.3° but your optical activity measurement recorded +20°.

34. Identify which isomer is in excess.
35. Calculate ee.
36. What would be the percentage of the *S* isomer in the sample?
37. For compounds **a–e** shown in Figure 6.45, identify those that show optical isomerism (atropisomerism).

6.7   Solutions to Problems

Questions 1–4. See Figure 6.46.

1. Structures **c–f**.
2. Structure **h**.
3. Structure **g**.
4. Structures **b** and **h**.

Answers for questions 5–7. *n*-Hexane has five chain isomers. See Figure 6.47.

5. See Figure 6.47.
6. Structures **b** and **c**; **d** and **e**.
7. None.
8. See Figure 6.48.
9. See Figure 6.48.
10. See Figure 6.49.
11. Propanal.
12. Methoxymethane.

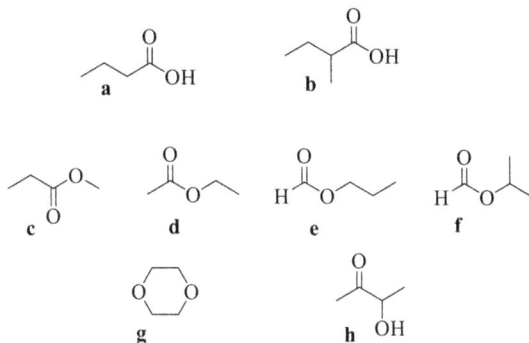

Figure 6.46 For solutions 1–4, see structures **a–h**.

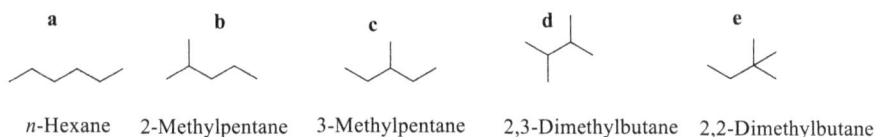

n-Hexane   2-Methylpentane   3-Methylpentane   2,3-Dimethylbutane 2,2-Dimethylbutane

Figure 6.47 For solutions 5–7, see structures **a–e**.

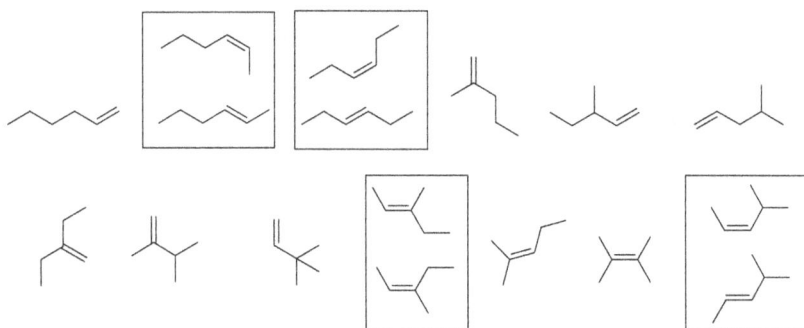

Figure 6.48 Acyclic isomers of C_6H_{12}. Geometrical isomers are shown in the boxes.

13. Methyl propanoate.
14. See Figure 6.7.
15. See Figure 6.7.
16. See Figure 6.50.
17. See Figure 6.8.
18. See Figure 6.51.
19. See Figure 6.52. Note the close proximity of the two groups in the *cis* configuration.

1,3-5-Trimethylcyclohexane

1,2,3-Trimethyl
cyclohexane

1,3,4-Trimethyl
cyclohexane

1,2,2-Trimethyl
cyclohexane

1,3,3-Trimethyl
cyclohexane

1,4,4-Trimethyl
cyclohexane

Isopropyl
cyclohexane
(Propan-2-
cyclohexane)

1-Ethyl-2-methyl
cyclohexane

1-Ethyl-3-methyl
cyclohexane

1-Ethyl-4-methyl
cyclohexane

Propyl
cyclohexane

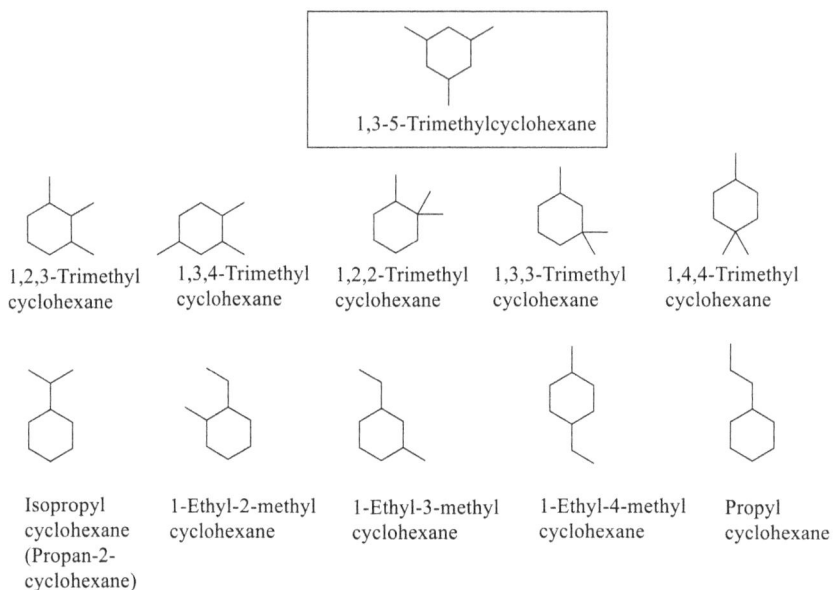

Figure 6.49   Answer to question 10.

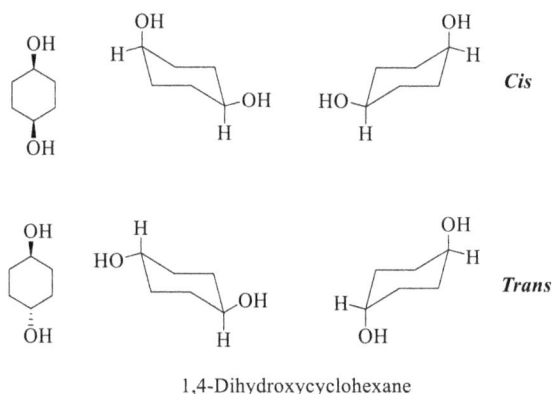

Cis

Trans

1,4-Dihydroxycyclohexane

Figure 6.50   Answer to question 16.

Answers to questions 20–29. Number of chiral centres in the structures of (see Figure 6.43):

20. Cholesterol: 8.
21. Nicotine: 1.
22. Penicillin G: 3.
23. Aspirin: none.
24. Ephedrine: 2.

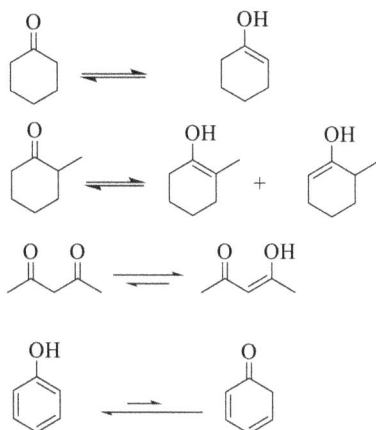

Figure 6.51 Answer to question 18.

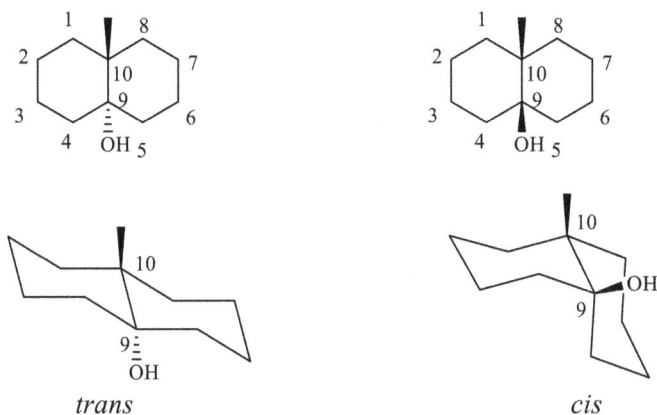

Figure 6.52 Answer to question 19.

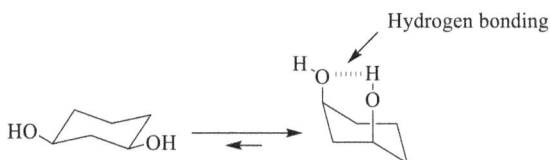

Figure 6.53 Answer to question 29.

25. Methamphetamine: 1.
26. Progesterone: 6.
27. Aspartame: 2.
28. Orlistat: 4.
29. See Figure 6.53. Structure stabilised by hydrogen bonding.

30. A racemic mixture is a 50:50 ratio of the two enantiomers, *i.e.* 50% of *R* isomer. Hence *R–S* = 0%.
31. 70% *R* isomer means the *S* isomer is 30%; 70–30 = 40% = enantiomeric excess (ee).
32. 100% purity means an ee of 100%.
33. $ee = \dfrac{\text{observed}}{\text{expected maximum}} = \dfrac{-5}{-20} = \dfrac{1}{4} = 25\%.$

   - Enantiomeric excess of 25% for *R* means the rest (75%) is for the racemate (35% each).
   - *R* isomer = 25% + 35% = 60%.
   - *S* isomer = 40%.

For questions 34–36:

   - Specific rotation for the *R* isomer is −53.3° and for the *S* isomer +53.3°.
   - The observed rotation is +20° so the *S* isomer predominates in the mixture.
   - $ee = \text{optical purity} = \dfrac{+20}{+53.3} \times 100 = 37.52\%$

      = percentage excess of *S* isomer.

   - 100 − 37.52 = 62.48% is the percentage of the racemate, half of which (31.24%) is the *S* isomer.
   - Total *S* isomer in the sample is 37.52 + 31.24 = 68.76%.

37. Compounds **c** and **e** have no symmetry and hence can have optical isomerism – atropisomers.

SECTION II
Organic Macromolecules in Cellular Structures, Metabolism, and as Drugs

7 Organic Macromolecules in Cellular Structures, Metabolism, and as Drugs: From Amino Acids to Proteins

Learning Objectives

After completing this chapter, you are expected to be able to:

- Describe the molecular structures of amino acids, peptides, and proteins.
- Distinguish the structural differences between amino acids and classify them based on their functional groups and properties.
- Explain the chemical basis of primary, secondary, tertiary, and quaternary structures of proteins.
- Identify the kind of interactions that proteins undertake based on their amino acid residues or amino acid side chains.
- Correlate the functions of proteins with their role as drugs or drug targets based on their chemical compositions.

Basic Chemistry for Life Science Students and Professionals: Introduction to Organic Compounds and Drug Molecules
By Solomon Habtemariam
© Solomon Habtemariam 2023
Published by the Royal Society of Chemistry, www.rsc.org

7.1 Overview of Proteins

Proteins are high molecular weight polymers with monomeric units that we call *amino acids*. The way in which these amino acids are assembled to make the polymeric chain and the way in which the chains fold up to make three-dimensional structures of proteins vary greatly. As a result, we have different kinds of proteins in living systems which are adapted to specific functions. Some proteins serve as *catalysts* for biological reactions of metabolic pathways of either anabolic (building up) or catabolic (breaking down) reactions. These are what we call enzymes, which are also targets for many drugs. Other proteins are involved in *transporting* materials in the body, such as haemoglobin in red blood cells transporting oxygen or lipoproteins in the blood transporting various types of lipids including fat and cholesterol. Some proteins are also adapted for transporting materials within the cells. These include those proteins of the cell membrane involved in trafficking materials in and out of cells, or those transporting materials between organelles in the cells. Such processes are evidently seen in neuronal cells where proteins are synthesised within the cell body and transported to the other end of the cell, which may be over 1 m long.

Proteins are found abundantly in spaces between cells and such proteins include collagen and fibronectin, which are part of the extracellular matrix. They have numerous functions, including *mechanical support*. Every cell has a defined shape, also mainly due to proteins that constitute the cytoskeleton system. The coordinated action of proteins in our skeletal muscles to contract and relax allows us to move, while at the cellular level *cell motility* is also a function of proteins. Unicellular organisms such as flagellates, including protozoa, bacteria, and algae, use proteins for their motility. Similarly, in mammalian systems, some cells such as sperm cells and airway epithelial cells with cilia exhibit motility due to special proteins. As with skeletal muscles, the coordinated contraction and relaxation of proteins in smooth muscle cells govern body functions from the gut to cardiovascular regulation. Proteins play a critical role in *cellular communications*, including neuronal transmission, while within the cells they serve as *signalling molecules* to control cell activity, cell growth, and differentiation. Defence against invading organisms such as pathogens is also possible owing to proteins serving as *antibodies* and mediators of inflammation.

For the above-mentioned reasons, proteins are one of the most important macromolecules to sustain life. This also means that they are major targets for drug therapy in addition to toxins. Proteins also serve as drugs. While highlighting their biological role, the focus of this chapter is to present an overview of their chemistry that would help us understand them both as drug targets and themselves serving as drugs.

Protein Functions – Key Facts

All living organisms utilise proteins for the following key functions:

- Structural support – at cellular, tissue, and organ levels.
- Biological reactions – as enzymes to catalyse anabolic and catabolic reactions.
- Signalling – in cell-to-cell communications (*e.g.* as hormones) and cell signalling.
- As defence against infection (*e.g.* antibodies).
- Transport materials and in cell motility.

They also serve as drugs and drug targets.

7.2 Introduction to Amino Acids

The chemical structure of amino acids is constructed from a basic skeleton with one central carbon, also called the α-carbon, attached to four groups: a carboxyl group, an amine group, a hydrogen atom, and an R group. Hence they differ from each other based on the composition of the R group or the side chain. Amino acids with these basic functional groups retained are also called α-amino acids: in the nomenclature of carboxylic acids that we discussed in Chapter 5, you may note that the carbon atom next to the carbonyl group is called the alpha-carbon (α-carbon). Amino acids possess both basic (amine) and acidic (carboxyl) functional groups. Their acidity in solution is thus seen as a neutral solution due to the formation of what we call the *zwitterion* (Figure 7.1).

The presence of an acidic or basic side chain (the R group) can influence the overall charge, polarity, and acidity of amino acids. Even though amino acids exist as zwitterions, we have basic and acidic amino acids owing to structural differences in the side chain (Table 7.1).

There are 20 α-amino acids that are commonly found in mammalian proteins. The side chain of these amino acids may be constructed from just a hydrogen atom in glycine, or a non-polar aliphatic or saturated alkyl chain, or an aromatic group. Some have a sulfur-containing chain, some are acidic due to the presence of a carboxyl group in

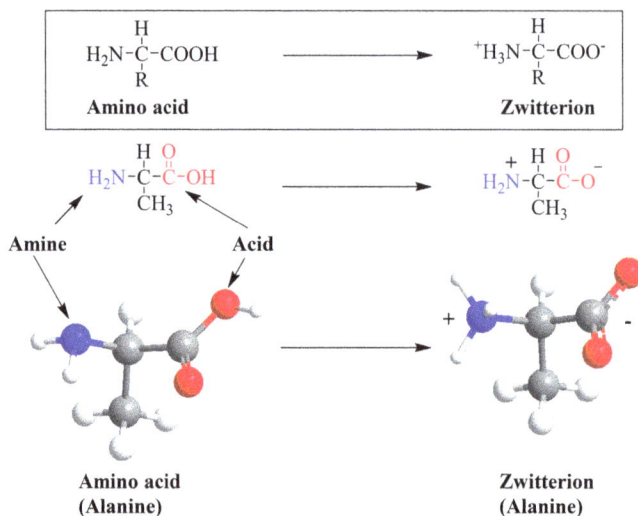

$$H_2N-\overset{\overset{\displaystyle H}{|}}{\underset{\underset{\displaystyle R}{|}}{C}}-COOH \longrightarrow {}^+H_3N-\overset{\overset{\displaystyle H}{|}}{\underset{\underset{\displaystyle R}{|}}{C}}-COO^-$$

Amino acid   Zwitterion

Amine   Acid

Amino acid   Zwitterion
(Alanine)   (Alanine)

Figure 7.1 General structure of amino acids. As shown for alanine, amino acids have amino and carboxyl functional groups. For alanine, the R group is a methyl group. Amino acids exist as zwitterions due to two functional groups: one behaves like a base (amino) and the other (carboxyl) behaves like an acid, *i.e.* the acid loses a proton, and the base accepts a proton to make a zwitterion.

the side chain, some have an amide side chain, some are basic due to the presence of an amine group in the side chain, *etc.* They are summarised in Table 7.1.

There are nine amino acids that our body cannot synthesise and hence we rely purely on the dietary supply of these *essential amino acids*. These amino acids are also called *indispensable amino acids* as their deficiency in the diet has severe clinical implications. *Conditionally essential amino acids* are those that can be formed in the body. For example, tyrosine can be synthesised in the body from phenylalanine by the action of the enzyme phenylalanine hydroxylase. In people who have a faulty phenylalanine hydroxylase enzyme due to mutation, however, tyrosine would become an essential amino acid that could only be obtained from the diet. We call such amino acids *conditionally essential*. Those amino acids which are readily formed in our body are called *non-essential amino acids*. As mentioned above, tyrosine is synthesised from phenylalanine, whereas the other *non-essential amino acids* are synthesised from glucose. They include alanine, arginine, asparagine, aspartate, cysteine, glutamate, glutamine, glycine, proline, and serine.

Table 7.1 Structures of the 20 α-amino acids found in proteins.

Amino acid	Abbreviation: Three-letter (or one-letter) code	Structure	Significance
Amino acids with aliphatic R groups			
Glycine	Gly (G)		Conditionally essential
Alanine	Ala (A)		Non-essential
Valine	Val (V)		Essential
Leucine	Leu (L)		Essential
Isoleucine	Ile (I)		Essential
Non-aromatic with hydroxyl R group			
Serine	Ser (S)		Non-essential
Threonine	Thr (T)		Essential
With sulfur-containing R group			
Cysteine	Cys (C)		Conditionally essential
Methionine	Met (M)		Essential
Acidic			
Aspartic acid	Asp (D)		Non-essential
Glutamic acid	Glu (E)		Non-essential

(*continued*)

Table 7.1 (continued)

Amino acid	Abbreviation: Three-letter (or one-letter) code	Structure	Significance
With amide R group			
Asparagine	Asn (N)		Non-essential
Glutamine	Gln (Q)		
With basic R group			
Arginine	Arg (R)		Conditionally essential
Lysine	Lys (K)		Essential
Histidine	His (H)		Essential
With R group containing aromatic rings			
Phenylalanine	Phe (F)		Essential
Tyrosine	Tyr (Y)		Conditionally essential
Tryptophan	Trp (W)		Essential
Imino acids			
Proline	Pro (P)		Conditionally essential

Ubiquitous Amino Acids – Key Facts

There are 20 α-amino acids universally present in living systems for a variety of functions:

- All amino acids have two functional groups – carboxyl and amino (amine) groups.
- The two functional groups are charged and form *zwitterions*.
- The carbon atom carrying these two functional groups also has a variable R group.
- The R groups could be charged, giving some amino acids a net positive or net negative charge.
- Common R groups may simply be alkyl or aromatic, or carry hydroxyl, sulfur, acidic, basic amide, or amino groups.
- Some amino acids are not synthesised in the body and are called essential amino acids.
- Some amino acids are made in the body and become conditionally essential if their biosynthesis process is faulty.

7.3 Uncommon Amino Acids

Beyond the 20 α-amino acids described in the previous section, both plants and animals also have unusual amino acids incorporated into selective proteins. These amino acids could be a derivative of the α-amino acids as exemplified by 5-hydroxylysine and 4-hydroxyproline (Figure 7.2). These two amino acids are the hydroxy derivatives of lysine and proline, respectively, and both are found in collagen, which is an extracellular matrix protein occurring between cells and as a main component of connective tissues. 5-Hydroxylysine is also found in plant cell-wall proteins and serves as the site of attachment of sugar residues to make glycoproteins. The conversion of these two amino acids to hydroxy derivatives occurs after the proteins have been synthesised. For these reactions, both plants and animals have hydroxylase enzymes, proline hydroxylase and lysine hydroxylase, that catalyse the hydroxylation reaction.

There are also amino acids that are not an integral part of proteins but are involved in protein metabolism. An excess amount of nitrogen in the body is normally removed from the body *via* urea after degradation of amino acids. In the cytosol (cytoplasm) of cells arginine is converted to ornithine to liberate urea, whereas in the mitochondria ornithine is converted to citrulline. Hence ornithine and citrulline are intermediates in the generation of urea or the urea cycle (Figure 7.3).

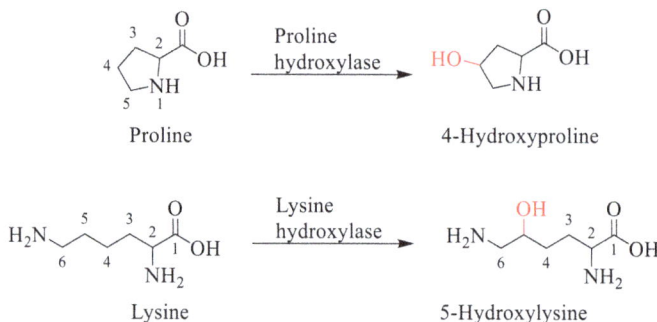

Figure 7.2 Structures of 5-hydroxylysine and 4-hydroxyproline and their biosynthesis.

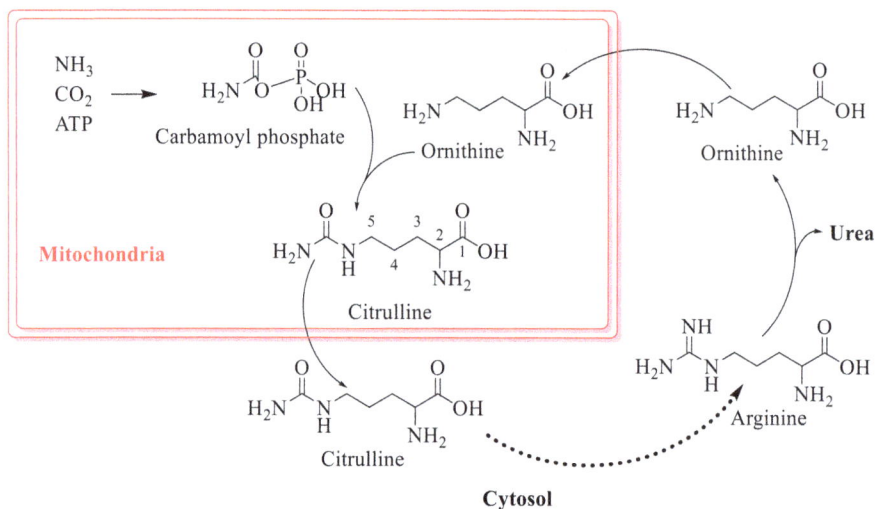

Figure 7.3 The urea cycle. The degradation of amino acids to form urea involves arginine and ornithine as intermediates. The formation of carbonyl phosphate in the mitochondria is a rate-limiting step in the process, *i.e.* the source of citrulline is the mitochondria, while the actual release of urea from arginine takes place in the cytosol (cytoplasm). The dotted arrow indicates multiple steps in the reaction.

Nitric oxide (NO) is a gas with various roles in mammalian cell signalling both within the cell and in cell-to-cell communication as a local hormone. It is produced by diverse cells, including muscle cells, blood vessel cells (endothelial cells), and neurones. It is produced through oxidation of arginine to NO and L-citrulline (Figure 7.4). There are enzymes that catalyse these reactions, collectively called nitric oxide synthases. They are important targets for drugs used in the management of a range of cardiovascular and neuronal diseases.

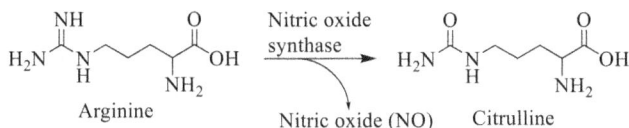

Figure 7.4 Formation of nitric oxide in a biological system. The enzyme nitric oxide synthase (NOS) catalyses the reaction in which arginine is converted to citrulline to release nitric oxide. There are two isoforms of the enzyme: the constitutively expressed NOS that produces NO to serve as a local hormone or in the regulation of normal functions (kidney and gut function, vasodilation, *etc.*), and the induced expression of the enzyme (iNOS) during inflammation/disease, which we target with drugs.

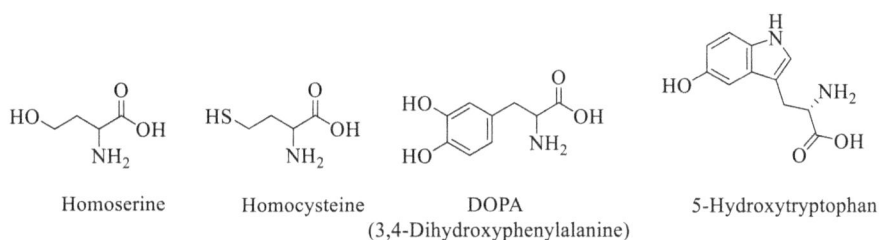

Figure 7.5 Examples of non-proteinogenic amino acids. The structures of homoserine, homocysteine, DOPA (3,4-dihydroxyphenylalanine), and 5-hydroxytryptophan are shown.

Nitric Oxide – Key Facts

- Nitric oxide (NO) is a local hormone and signalling molecule in various cells, such as endothelial and neuronal cells.
- It mediates vasodilation and some drugs work by modifying this effect, *e.g.* Viagra (sildenafil) as a treatment for erectile dysfunction enhances the NO-mediated vasodilation effect by inhibiting the enzyme phosphodiesterase type 5 (PDE 5).
- NO is produced from arginine by the enzymatic action of NO synthase (NOS).
- Two forms of NOS exist – constitutional and that induced (iNOS) under a pathological condition such as inflammation.
- iNOS is a target for many drugs.

Homoserine and homocysteine (Figure 7.5) are non-proteinoid (non-proteinogenic) amino acids, *i.e.* they are not incorporated into proteins. They are involved in the metabolism of amino acids. For example, homoserine is involved in the synthesis of methionine, threonine, and isoleucine. Homocysteine is also involved in the synthesis of amino acids, methionine, and cysteine. It is a metabolic product formed from demethylation of methionine. Since methionine is abundant in animal proteins, consumption of a high-meat diet results in the production of high levels of homocysteine. A high level of homocysteine is also considered as a pathological marker for cardiovascular diseases such as atherosclerosis and inflammatory diseases.

Plants and bacteria also synthesise many amino acids that differ from the 20 α-amino acids either in their atomic composition or their three-dimensional structures (stereochemistry – see Chapter 6). There are also numerous amino acids that are metabolic products and byproducts. For example, neurotransmitter synthesis generates several α-amino acid derivatives such as DOPA (3,4-dihydroxyphenylalanine) and 5-hydroxytryptophan (Figure 7.5).

In addition to the α-amino acids, there are also β-amino acids such as β-alanine with the amino group located at the beta position to the carboxyl carbon. β-Alanine (Figure 7.6) is not found in proteins but occurs in short-chain peptides such as vitamin B$_5$ (pantothenic acid). γ-Aminobutyric acid (GABA, Figure 7.6), as the name implies, has the amino group at the gamma position and is a neurotransmitter in the brain.

Several taxonomic families of plants, including some edible legumes, are known to produce a variety of non-protein amino acids. Some of these amino acids are toxic to humans. These include (Figure 7.7) mimosine, which is abundant in the seeds of the plants *Mimosa pudica* and *Leucaena leucocephala*, hypoglycin, found in the unripe fruits of *Blighia sapida*, canavanine, present in high yield in the seeds of jack bean (*Canavalia ensiformis*) and *Dioclea megacarpa*, and a proline analogue, azetidine-2-carboxylic acid, which is found in *Convallaria majalis*. Although these compounds show toxicity to humans, they have a special purpose in the plants that produce them as they serve as a defence against diseases such as fungal infection and pests (*e.g.* insects).

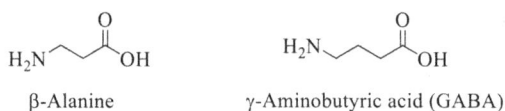

β-Alanine   γ-Aminobutyric acid (GABA)

Figure 7.6   Structures of β-alanine and γ-aminobutyric acid (GABA).

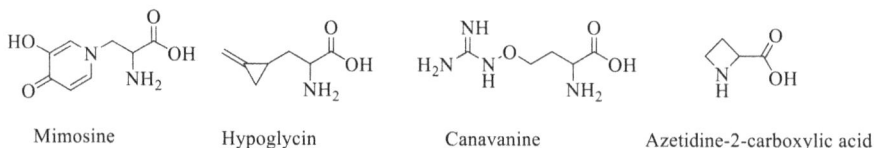

Mimosine   Hypoglycin   Canavanine   Azetidine-2-carboxylic acid

Figure 7.7   Examples of amino acids in plants that are toxic to humans.

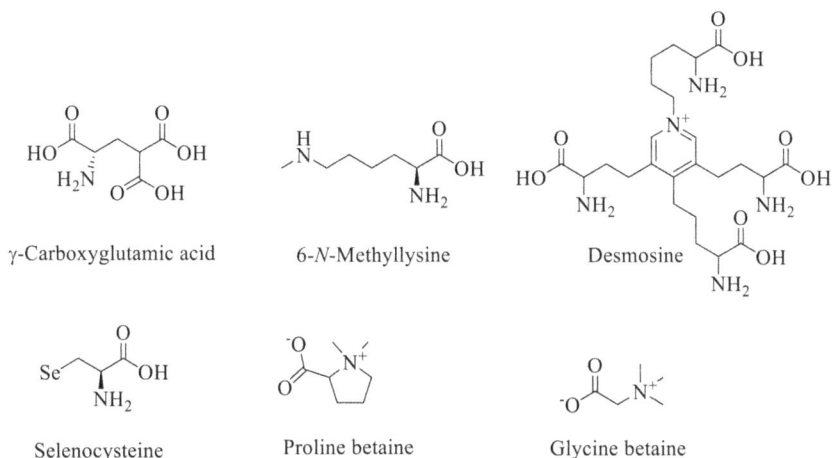

Figure 7.8 Further examples of rare amino acids.

Further examples of rare or uncommon amino acids are shown in Figure 7.8. γ-Carboxyglutamic acid is found in the blood-clotting factors or proteins (*e.g.* prothrombin, factor X, factor IX, and factor VII) and also some calcium-binding proteins. 6-*N*-Methyllysine, which is formed by the methylation of lysine, is an integral part of the muscle fibre myosin and is involved in muscle contractile activity. Desmosine is an amino acid unique to elastin (a fibrous protein of connective tissues) and thus serves as a biomarker of elastin degradation. Derived from the amino acid serine, selenocysteine is a rare selenium-containing compound, which, as its names implies, is found in selenoproteins – they are antioxidant proteins. Various proteins involved in cell signalling incorporate the phosphate group *via* phosphorylated sites or amino acids such as serine, threonine, and tyrosine. It is the reversible phosphorylation and dephosphorylation events in such proteins that allow the regulation of cellular processes such as cell growth, differentiation, and death. In plants, quaternary ammonium compounds based on amino acids called betaines (glycine and proline betaines) are common and are involved in stress adaptations.

7.4 Peptides and Proteins – Structural Considerations

7.4.1 Primary Structure

To make proteins as polymers of amino acids, two amino acids at a time come together to condense or form a *peptide bond*. The peptide bond is a covalent bond formed between the nitrogen atom of an amino group of one amino acid and the carbonyl carbon (C=O) atom of the carboxyl group of another amino acid (Figure 7.9). Hence a peptide bond is what we called an *amide bond* in Chapter 5. Since water is liberated in the process, the reaction is also called a *dehydration reaction*. Once a peptide bond has been formed between two amino acids, the resulting dipeptide still has one amine and one carboxyl group at opposite ends of the molecule. This allows the addition of more amino acids in the chain from both sides. The linear sequence of amino acids in the peptide bonds that make up a protein is called the *primary structure of a protein.* For any protein in a biological

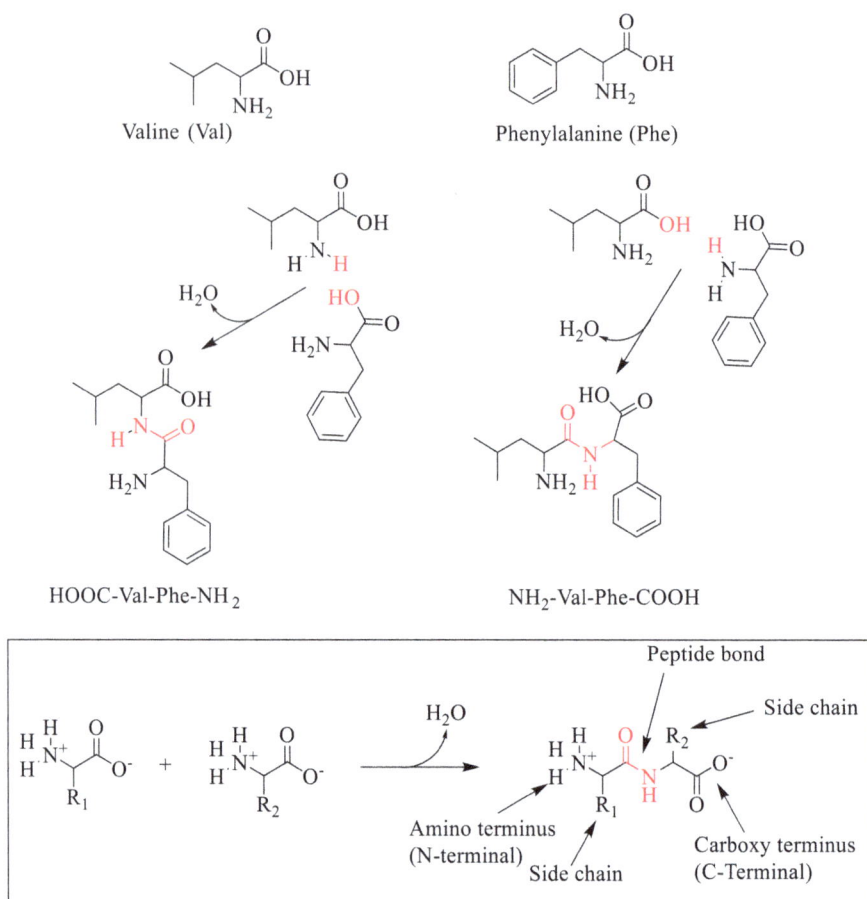

Valine (Val)

Phenylalanine (Phe)

HOOC-Val-Phe-NH$_2$

NH$_2$-Val-Phe-COOH

Peptide bond

Side chain

Amino terminus
(N-terminal)

Side chain

Carboxy terminus
(C-Terminal)

Figure 7.9   The peptide (amide bond). Note the two possibilities of making a peptide bond between valine and phenylalanine. The carboxyl (COOH) and amino (NH$_2$) ends are indicated. Since amino acids exist in zwitterion form, peptides also have carboxyl and amino ends that exist in charged form.

system, the primary structure is governed by the *genetic code.* Proteins may contain a phosphate group, sugar units, or metal groups such as iron, manganese, copper, *etc.* These additions, however, occur post-translation (modification after the protein synthesis). Since we have 20 amino acids that make up proteins, we have theoretically 20^2 (or 400) different types of combinations to consider at a time. Given that proteins also have a large number of amino acid residues, the probability of making different proteins from the 20 amino acids is extremely high. Once again, in biology, which amino acids, in what sequence or combination, or what length of the peptide chain, *etc.,* are generally determined by the genetic code and genes.

Proteins may contain thousands of amino acids. If we have a smaller number of amino acids in a chain, usually less than 50 amino acid residues, we call them peptides. In peptides, each amino acid residue is joined with another amino acid with a peptide bond to make the backbone structure in the sequence. The R groups that protrude outside are called the side chains and these are responsible for many other interactions that govern the three-dimensional structure of proteins. Consider a peptide made from eight amino acids as shown in Figure 7.10.

Primary Structure of Proteins – Key Facts

- The linear sequence of amino acids within a protein.
- Amino acids are joined together by a peptide bond, which is an amide bond.
- Peptide bond formation is an example of a dehydration reaction – loss of water.
- The primary structure of proteins is a reflection of the sequence of DNA coding in the genome.
- We can synthesise peptides in the laboratory – one should think about the different possible combinations.

7.4.2 Secondary Structure

We have already discussed how hydrogen bonding plays a part in intermolecular interactions. In the same way, hydrogen bonding, particularly between the carbonyl group of one amino acid residue and the hydrogen atom of the amide (NH) group of another amino acid, affects the way in which a peptide bond makes its secondary structure. There are two known secondary structures of proteins resulting from hydrogen bonding: the α-helices and β-pleated sheets (Figure 7.11).

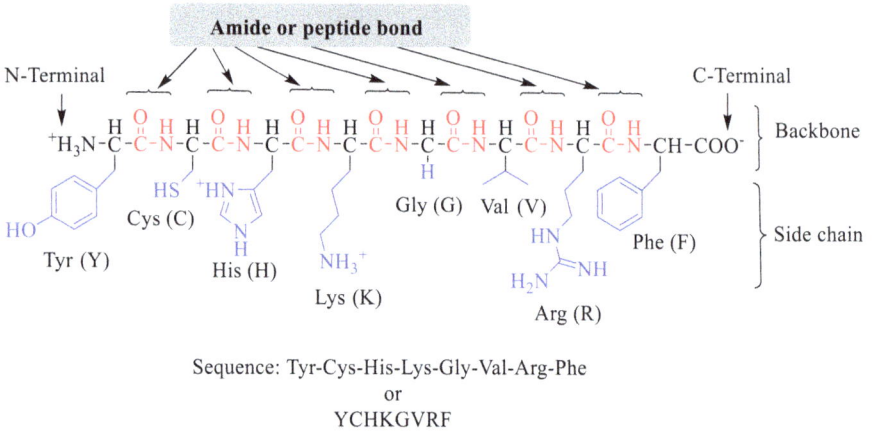

Sequence: Tyr-Cys-His-Lys-Gly-Val-Arg-Phe
or
YCHKGVRF

Figure 7.10   Structural presentation of peptide bonds for the sequence Tyr-Cys-His-Lys-Gly-Val-Arg-Phe.

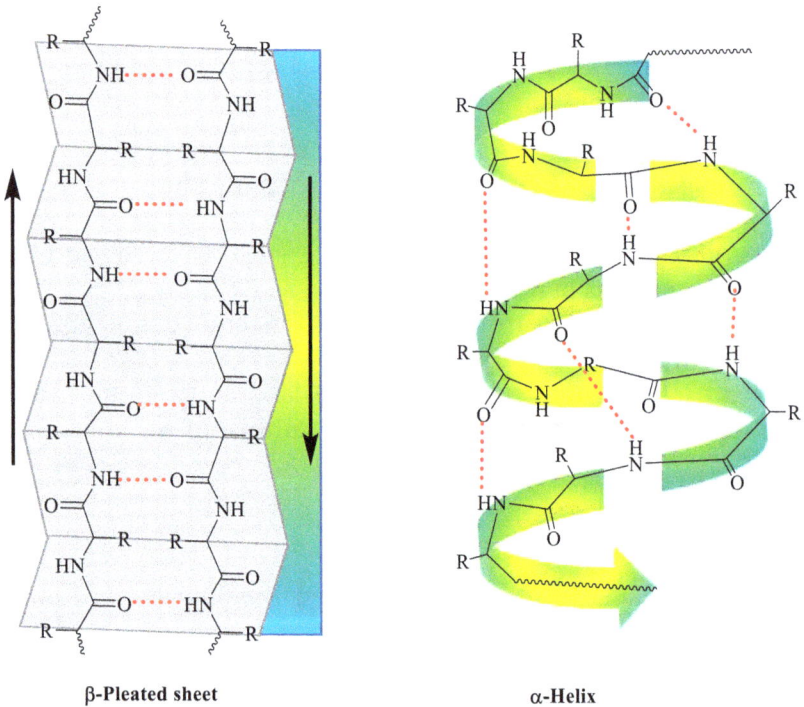

β-Pleated sheet   α-Helix

Figure 7.11   Secondary structure of proteins. Note the hydrogen bonding shown in red.

Hydrogen bonding at the backbone of amino acid residues creates a repeating pattern of arrangement of either an α-helix or a β-pleated sheet. Any given protein may have these two orientations at some regions of the peptide chain. In the case of an α-helix secondary structure, a coiled polypeptide chain makes a spring-like structure, whereas in a β-pleated sheet, the folded peptides are packed alongside each other (Figure 7.11).

Secondary Structure of Proteins – Key Facts

- A feature of hydrogen bonding between amide hydrogens and carbonyl oxygens of the peptide backbone.
- Major secondary structures are α-helix and β-sheet structures.
- Such hydrogen bonding between amino acids away from each other by about four residues in a chain can make a right-handed coil – α-helices
- Zigzag pattern of folding is a feature of β-sheets.

7.4.3 Tertiary Structure

The contribution of the side chain of amino acid residues to the over-all three-dimensional structure of proteins is what we call the *tertiary structure of the proteins*. This is also similar to the intermolecular attractions that we discussed in previous chapters and includes the following interactions.

7.4.3.1 Ionic Interactions

As shown in Figure 7.12 for aspartic acid and glutamic acid, the R groups of some amino acids have carboxyl groups that give them negatively charged sites whereas others such as lysine have an R group containing an $-NH_2$ group that can be positively charged. Hence an ionic interaction is expected at the site that carries the lysine residue and either aspartic or glutamic acid. Ionic interactions are stronger than hydrogen bonding and hence can bring oppositely charged sites close to each other.

7.4.3.2 Disulfide Bridges

A disulfide bridge is a covalent bond formed between two sulfur atoms of cysteine residues. Hence oxidation of sulfhydryl (thiol or

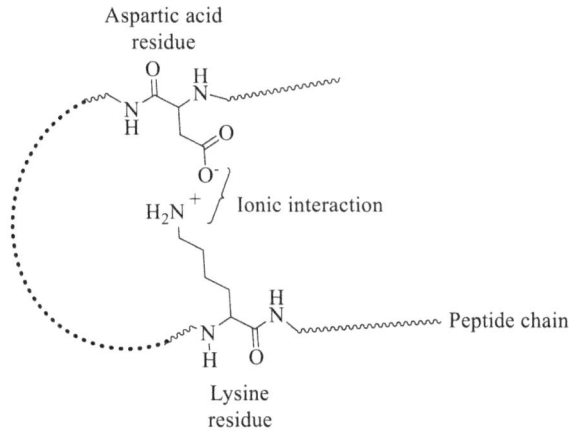

Figure 7.12 Ionic interaction between charged side chains brings amino acid residues closer. The dotted line depicts the long peptide backbone structure.

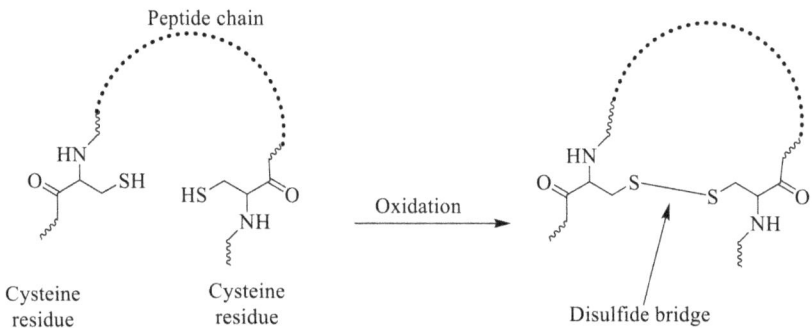

Figure 7.13 Disulfide bridge formation due to oxidation of cysteine residues. Dotted lines represent the long peptide backbone structure.

–SH) groups from two cysteine residues creates unique peptide folding at the cysteine sites (Figure 7.13).

7.4.3.3 Hydrogen Bonding

In the secondary structures of proteins, we looked at hydrogen bonding at the backbone of the peptide chain that arises from the –C=O and –NH– functional groups. For side chains of amino acids that contain either –OH, –COOH, –CONH$_2$, or –NH$_2$ groups, hydrogen bonding is also possible. Hence the number and positions of amino acids containing these functional groups at their side chain, which is a primary structure of proteins, also determine the tertiary structures. See Table 7.1 for a review of amino acids that contribute to hydrogen bonding.

7.4.3.4 van der Waals Forces

The weakest intermolecular force that we discussed in Chapter 2 is the *van der Waals* or *London dispersion force*, which plays a significant role in the three-dimensional structure of proteins by bringing together non-polar regions of amino acids. Good examples of non-polar amino acids are alanine, valine, leucine, isoleucine, and phenylalanine. In essence, hydrophobic residues of amino acids in the peptide chain aggregate to make a region of non-polar sites in the protein structure. On the other hand, amino acids with hydrophilic side chains include serine, threonine, cysteine, proline, asparagine, and glutamine. Some side chains with charges are even more polar and include aspartic and glutamic acids, which are negatively charged, and lysine, arginine, and histidine, which are positively charged. Tyrosine and proline are further members of the non-polar group. Since our body's function is mostly in an aqueous medium, polar amino acids tend to appear at the surface of the protein, whereas the hydrophobic core aggregates at the centre of the protein. Hence proteins in an aqueous medium have a hydrophobic central core and a hydrophilic surface facing the water. On this basis, most functional proteins such as enzymes and receptors have a globular or spherical shape and are called *globular proteins*: a ball-shaped structure with hydrophobic amino acids located at the centre and hydrophilic amino acids found on the surface. This makes them water soluble. On the other hand, some proteins are called *fibrous proteins* as they are made mostly from repeating sequences of amino acids to form a fibre-like elongated structure. Structural proteins such as cartilage are made from collagen protein fibres. Keratin in hair, horn, and nails is another example of fibrous proteins. Intermediate filaments such as fibrous proteins of the cytoskeleton serve as a scaffold inside the cell. Collagen, elastin, and other proteins of the extracellular matrix are also fibrous in nature. These structural features therefore are adapted to the function of proteins. Enzymes, haemoglobin, insulin, antibodies, and immunoglobins are globular types of functional proteins, whereas collagen, myosin, fibrin, actin, elastin, keratin, *etc.*, are fibrous types of structural proteins. Whereas globular types are mostly water soluble and generally sensitive to pH and temperature changes, fibrous proteins are mostly insoluble in water and less sensitive to changes in temperature and pH.

> **Tertiary Structure of Proteins – Key Facts**
>
> - Three-dimensional structures.
> - Based on the following interactions of the amino acid side chains:
>
>   o Ionic interactions.
>   o Hydrogen bonding interactions.
>   o Lipophilic or van der Waals force interactions.
>   o Covalent disulfide bridge formation between two cysteine residues.
>
> - Make distinctions between fibrous proteins (mostly water insoluble and resistant to pH change) and globular proteins (mostly water soluble and pH sensitive). Their shape is adapted to their function.

7.4.4 Quaternary Structures

Two or more peptides also come together to make a functional protein that we call the *quaternary structure of proteins*. When two peptides of the same type come together, we call the protein a *homodimer*, while two different peptides can make a *heterodimer* protein. In collagen, three different peptides make a trimeric protein, whereas in haemoglobin, two alpha- and two beta-peptides make a tetrameric structure. The quaternary structure based on the association of two or more polypeptides is held together through a variety of interactions. The ionic, hydrogen bonding, van der Waals, and hydrophobic interactions that we discussed for tertiary structures could also play a part for quaternary structures (between peptides). In addition to these non-covalent intermolecular interactions, a disulfide covalent bond may also be formed between peptides to make a firm association. A good example of disulfide bonding in quaternary structures is that linking the polypeptides of antibodies as depicted in Figure 7.14.

   As shown for the antibody structure (Figure 7.14), the association of several peptide chains or protein subunits makes a quaternary structure of a protein, which is specifically adapted to its function. Without packing of these subunits in the designed functional quaternary structure, the protein is unlikely to function properly. In the case of haemoglobin, which we said is composed of four peptides or subunits, it also has a haem group that we call a *prosthetic group*. The haem group (Figure 7.15) containing iron (Fe^{2+}) that binds oxygen is linked to the four haemoglobin units by making covalent bonds at the

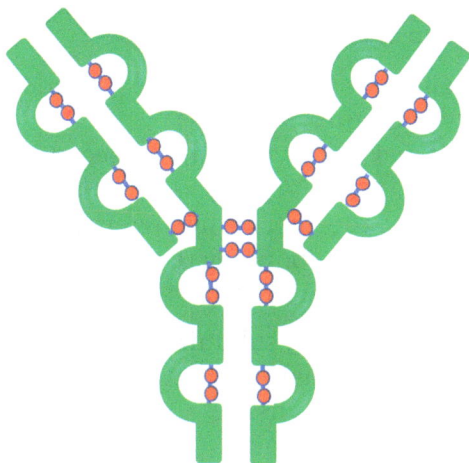

Figure 7.14 General structure of antibodies. The four subunits of a functioning antibody anchored with intra- and inter-chain disulfide bridges are shown.

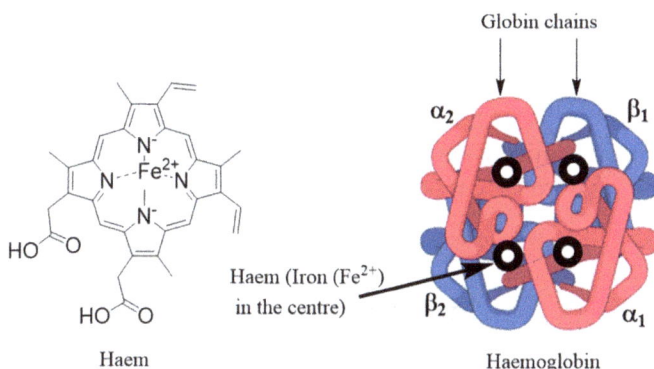

Figure 7.15 Structure of haem. Haemoglobin image: reproduced from https://upload.wikimedia.org/wikipedia/commons/thumb/9/91/1904_Hemoglobin.jpg/1280px-1904_Hemoglobin.jpg, under the terms of the CC BY 3.0 license, https://creativecommons.org/licenses/by/3.0/. Image Credit: OpenStax College.

histidine amino acid residue. Hence the haem group is also bringing the four haemoglobin units together. For haemoglobin to function as an oxygen transporter, the four subunits and their three-dimensional structure must be maintained. Note that the proper function of a protein depends on its amino acid composition and its assembly through primary to quaternary structures. We also have non-polypeptide components in some proteins that we call a prosthetic group – this could be some sort of organic compound (lipids, sugars, or vitamins) or be inorganic in nature, mostly metals.

Quaternary Structure of Proteins – Key Facts

- Several protein chains or subunits are packed together to make a quaternary structure.
- Each subunit has its own primary, secondary, and tertiary structure.
- Subunits are held together by hydrogen bonds, van der Waals forces, and/or covalent bonding (*e.g.* disulfide bridge).
- Examples of quaternary structures in proteins:

  o Haemoglobin has four subunits (two identical α-chains and two identical β-chains).
  o Insulin has two subunits.
  o Aldolase has four subunits.
  o Alcohol dehydrogenase has four subunits.

- A quaternary structure might also incorporate non-amino acid components such as an inorganic group called a prosthetic group. Examples include the haem group:

  o Found in haemoglobin, myoglobin, and cytochromes.
  o Consist of an iron ion coordinated by four nitrogen atoms of porphyrin.

- Biotin (vitamin B_7) is another example of a prosthetic group for many enzymes – carboxyl transferases.

7.5   Amino Acids, Peptides, and Protein Drugs

- There are numerous examples of peptide- and protein-based drugs. If we consider diabetes therapy as an example, insulin as a protein is a prototype drug. Therapy of diabetes using small peptides includes exenatide, liraglutide, and pramlintide. Peptide-based drugs for cancer therapy include degarelix and mifamurtide. Other good examples include enfuvirtide for HIV/AIDS, ziconotide for pain, and ebiratide for heart failure. Whereas proteins serve as hormones (*e.g.* growth hormone, thyroid hormone), peptides serve in a variety of cell signalling, including inflammation (bradykinins) and pain (substance P) mediation. A group of protein mediators in a variety of cell signalling including those in cell growth, differentiation, and death, and also in diseases, are collectively called cytokines. Antibodies and receptors of these signalling molecules are also used in the therapy of numerous diseases. For example, antibodies against pro-inflammatory cytokines and receptors can be used to treat chronic inflammatory conditions such as arthritis. Unfortunately, most of the protein-based drugs must be administered by injection as they are degraded, if taken orally, by digestive enzymes. Overall, we have the following groups of drugs: *Amino acid derived:* Many rare amino acids such as those in plants serve as drugs. Amino acids are also the precursors of many natural and synthetic drugs. Good examples are nitrogen-containing drugs called alkaloids (see Chapter 13).

- *Peptide derived:* Bradykinin as a nine amino acid peptide chain (Arg-Pro-Pro-Gly-Phe-Ser-Pro-Phe-Arg) and kallidin as a ten amino acid chain (Lys-Arg-Pro-Pro-Gly-Phe-Ser-Pro-Phe-Arg) are good examples of bioactive peptides of inflammatory mediators through their potent vasodilatory action. Small peptides of these kinds can be easily synthesised along with several derivatives or modifications to serve as potential antagonists. Small peptides can also be incorporated in a drug molecule. For example, paracetamol is a derivative of Phe-Gly. Several modifications are possible; for instance, peptides with sugar derivatives are called glycopeptides. More examples of peptide-based drugs are discussed in Chapter 13. Of the small peptides, glutathione is a tripeptide that serves the body as a major antioxidant defence. It consists of the amino acids glutamic acid, cysteine, and glycine (Figure 7.16). Upon oxidation, its thiol group undergoes oxidation to form a dimeric structure, hence the molecule exists as a reduced form (monomeric tripeptide form, labelled GSH) or oxidised form (dimeric tripeptide form, labelled GSSG). Many drugs induce their effect by altering this oxidative state of glutathione.

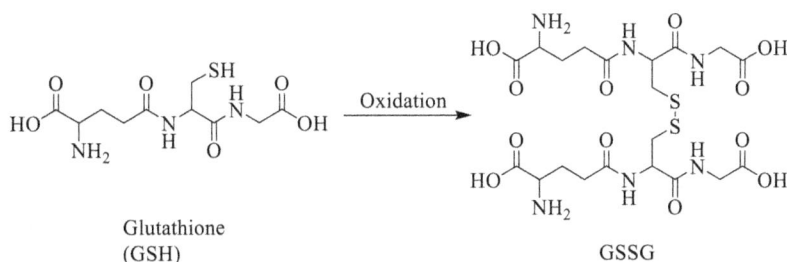

Figure 7.16 Structures of reduced and oxidised forms of glutathione. Note that the oxidised form (GSSG) is a result of disulfide bond formation that brings two glutathione (GSH) molecules together.

- *Protein derived:* The list is impressive and includes hormones, antibodies, and others mimicking protein mediators or their antagonists (see Chapter 13). It should also be noted that proteins with their diverse functions in the body serve as drug targets (Chapter 12). Hence we use drugs either to suppress or to enhance the biological functions of proteins.

Glutathione – Key Facts

- A tripeptide composed of glycine, cysteine, and glutamic acid is referred to as GSH.
- The main non-protein thiol found in cells.
- Potent, naturally occurring endogenous antioxidant found within the intra- and extracellular compartments.
- The conversion between the oxidised and reduced forms is regulated by enzymes – glutathione peroxidase and glutathione reductase.
- Keeping a high level of the reduced form (GSH) is important for maintaining normal body function.

7.6 Summary

In this chapter, we have learned the following:

- Proteins are critical in living organisms with functions as mechanical support, in the catalysis of biological reactions, cellular communications, transport of materials, and cell motility, and as a defence against pathogens.
- Proteins are polymers built from amino acid monomers.
- Structurally, amino acids are based on an amino and a carboxyl group attached mostly at the α-carbon (α-amino acids), or in some cases β-positions (β-amino acids such as β-alanine), or even γ-positions (such as γ-aminobutyric acid).
- Of the several hundred amino acids found in Nature, 20 are α-amino acids that serve as the building blocks of all proteins.
- α-Amino acids are grouped based on the side chains, which could be aliphatic, aromatic, basic, acidic, amide, and imino R groups.
- Non-α-amino acids are represented by β-alanine and γ-aminobutyric acid (GABA).

- Some amino acids are synthesised in the body (non-essential amino acids) whereas others are essential amino acids – must be sourced from the diet.
- A faulty metabolic pathway in the synthesis of a non-essential amino acid could make it essential – a *conditionally essential* amino acid.
- Amino acids could be grouped into proteinogenic and non-proteinogenic. Non-protein amino acids are represented by ornithine, homocysteine, citrulline, DOPA, and 5-hydroxytryptophan.
- Nitric oxide is a local hormone with diverse functions in the body and is formed from arginine.
- Several rare and unique amino acids are found in plants and other living organisms, some of which are toxic or have other pharmacological effects.
- A peptide bond is an amide bond formed through a reaction between two amino acids *via* a dehydration reaction.
- The primary structure of a protein is the linear sequence of amino acids.
- The sequence of amino acids in polypeptides is represented by either a three-letter or a one-letter code.
- A different combination of amino acids is the first source of variations in proteins.
- Hydrogen bonding interaction within the polypeptide chain defines the secondary structure of proteins as α-helices and β-pleated sheets.
- Tertiary structures are ionic, hydrogen bonding, lipophilic interaction, and disulfide bond formation within the polypeptide side chains (R groups).
- Haemoglobin is an example of a globular protein whereas keratin, collagen, and elastin are all fibrous proteins – they are examples of tertiary structures.
- Proteins may be composed of multiples of the same (homo) or variable (hetero) peptides – forming the quaternary structure. Antibodies and haemoglobin are examples of multiple polypeptides in their structure.
- Proteins may also have non-amino acid components that we call prosthetic groups.
- Drugs could be derived from amino acids, peptides, or proteins.
- Protein-based drugs have poor bioavailability and hence are commonly administered *via* injection. The body may develop antibodies against a protein-based drug.

- Synthesis of peptides and proteins is possible while advances in genetic engineering enable their production in high yields.
- Their diverse functions in the body and their alterations under disease conditions make proteins targets for drugs.

7.7 Problems

1. Of the 20 α-amino acids, which one is achiral (or with no chiral centre)?
2. List three basic α-amino acids.
3. A protein undergoes ionic interactions with negatively charged functional groups. Which two amino acids are likely to be involved in this interaction?
4. A basic amino acid with relatively weak ionisation is _____?
5. Which amino acid contains a secondary amine functional group?
6. In what way do the hydroxyl groups in serine, threonine, and tyrosine differ from each other?
7. The structures of serine and cysteine are based on one carbon side chain. In what way do they differ from each other?
8. Homocysteine is a precursor to methionine and is involved in several biochemical pathways. Which amino acid does its chemical reactivity relate to?
9. The linear sequence of amino acids in the protein is called _____?
10. Interactions within a single polypeptide chain (ionic bonds, disulfide bridges, and hydrophobic interactions) are called _____?
11. Name three amino acids that possess an aromatic ring system.
12. Why do amino acids have a higher melting point than compounds of the same molecular weight of other functional groups?
13. The compound shown in Figure 7.17 is a component of fenugreek (*Trigonella foenum-graecum*), which has been shown to display activity in the regulation of glucose and lipid metabolism:
    a. Which amino acid does it relate to?
    b. Name the compound based on the structure of the parent amino acid.

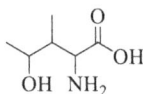

Figure 7.17 Question 13.

14. List the amino acids that are synthesised in the body.
15. Give the structures of the following peptides:
    a. Gly-Cys-Gly.
    b. Ala-Met-Gln.
    c. Phe-His-Ser.
16. You have two amino acids, F and K, in your reaction pot:
    a. How many tripeptides can be formed from them?
    b. Give the different combinations.
17. You have tyrosine (Tyr), glycine (Gly), and valine (Val) in your reaction pot:
    a. How many tripeptides can be formed from them?
    b. Show the number of ways of arranging them with all amino acids present in the tripeptide.
18. Decarboxylation of amino acids is a biosynthetic route for the formation of useful biologically active compounds. For the compounds shown in Figure 7.18, indicate the amino acid origin.
19. The peptide bond represents which functional group?
20. Which two amino acids are amide analogues of aspartic acid and glutamic acid?
21. Explain how the amide groups can serve as both hydrogen bond donors and acceptors.
22. α-Helices and β-sheets are examples of _____?

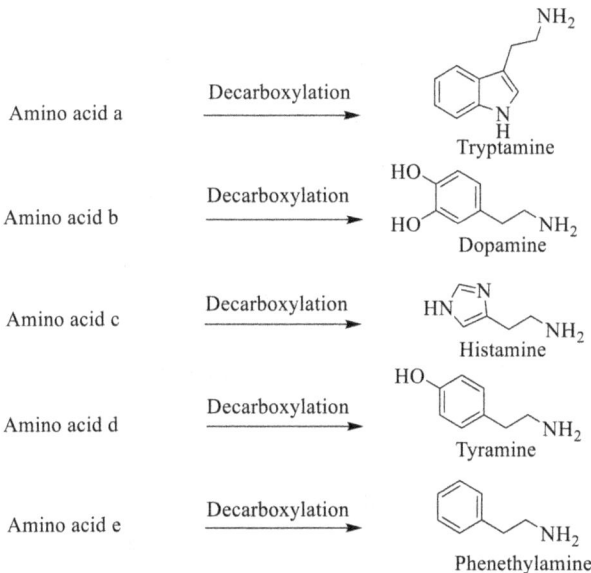

Figure 7.18   Question 18.

Questions 23–25. The proteins from immune cells called cytokines responsible for aggravating (cytokine storm) the disease in COVID patients have been identified. One of the main cytokines travels through the blood and induces inflammation in the body by binding with a specific receptor. Define three strategies for how to design a protein-based drug to tackle this problem:

23. Strategy 1: _____.
24. Strategy 2: _____.
25. Strategy 3: _____.

26. In the formation of a peptide bond by the condensation reaction between amine and carboxyl groups (*i.e.* NH_2 and COOH), what functional group is formed?
27. Hydrogen bonding within a peptide chain between the NH group of one amino acid and the C=O group on another forms _____?
28. Two proteins have exactly the same amino acid composition and sequence order. How do they differ from each other?
29. What is the minimum number of ionisable groups for each amino acid?
30. At pH 7.4, which amino acids become negatively charged.
31. Which amino acids make a positive charge at physiological pH.
32. If we group amino acids into acidic, basic, and neutral, how do we classify alanine, glycine, and leucine?
33. Name three sulfur-containing α-amino acids.
34. Based on water loss and gain, name the following reactions:
    a. A peptide bond formed by losing water.
    b. Breakdown of a peptide bond by adding water.
35. A regular coiled right-hand turn of amino acids formed through hydrogen bonding in proteins is called _____?
36. Interactions between parallel regions of a protein chain form _____?
37. What is the main drawback of protein-based drugs?
38. In proteins, which amino acid residue is most sensitive to oxidation?
39. A single linear unbranched chain formed through multiple peptide bonds is called _____?
40. What kind of interaction between two proteins occurs through the amino acids Arg, Lys, His, and Glu?
41. Consider the amino acids alanine, valine, leucine, and isoleucine. What is common in all of their structures?
42. The side chains of amino acids listed in question 41 undergo what kind of interaction in the tertiary protein structure?
43. Haemoglobin has four polypeptide chains. This is an example of _____?

7.8   Solutions to Problems

1. Glycine.
2. Lysine, arginine, and histidine.
3. Lysine and arginine are positively charged or ionized at physiological pH.
4. Histidine.
5. Proline.
6. Serine (primary alcohol), threonine (secondary alcohol), and tyrosine (phenol).
7. Alcohol (serine) and thiol (cysteine).
8. Cysteine: thiol functional group.
9. The primary structure of a protein.
10. The tertiary structure of a protein.
11. Phenylalanine, tyrosine, and tryptophan.
12. Have polar bonds – amino and carboxyl.
13. Compound:
    a. Typical branched-chain amino acid isoleucine but with an additional alcohol group.
    b. 4-Hydroxyisoleucine.
14. Alanine, arginine, asparagine, aspartate, cysteine, glutamate, glutamine, glycine, proline, serine, and tyrosine.
15. See Figure 7.19.
16. You have two amino acids, F and K, in your reaction pot:
    a. 2^3 possible combinations = 8.
    b. FFF, FFK, FKK, KKK, KKF, KFF, FKF, and KFK.
17. You have tyrosine (Tyr), glycine (Gly) and valine (Val) in your reaction pot:
    a. 3^3 possible combinations = 27.
    b. Tyr-Gly-Val, Gly-Tyr-Val, Val-Tyr-Gly, Ala-Val-Gly, Gly-Val-Tyr, and Val-Gly-Tyr.
18. Indicate the amino acid origin:
    a. Tryptophan → tryptamine.
    b. L-DOPA → dopamine.

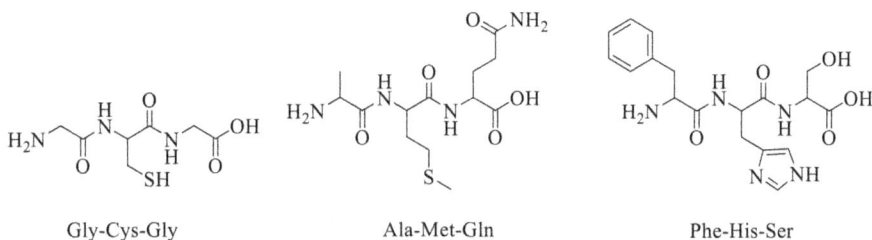

Gly-Cys-Gly   Ala-Met-Gln   Phe-His-Ser

Figure 7.19   Answer to question 15.

c. Histidine → histamine.

d. Tyrosine → tyramine.

e. Phenylalanine → phenethylamine.

19. Amide bond.

20. Asparagine and glutamine, respectively.

21. The carbonyl oxygen of the amides behaves as a hydrogen bond acceptor and the NH group of the amides acts as a hydrogen bond donor.

22. Secondary structure of a protein.

23. Raise antibodies against the cytokine.

24. Raise antibodies against the receptor.

25. Synthesise the receptor itself or a protein that interacts directly with either the cytokine or its receptor.

26. Amide bond.

27. The secondary structure of the protein.

28. Different secondary, tertiary, or quaternary structures.

29. Two: amino and carboxyl groups.

30. Acidic amino acids: aspartic acid and glutamic acid.

31. Basic amino acids: arginine, lysine, and histidine.

32. Neutral.

33. Methionine, cysteine, and homocysteine.

34. Reactions:

a. Dehydration.

b. Hydrolysis.

35. α-Helix.

36. β-Sheets.

37. Poor oral absorption or bioavailability.

38. Cysteine.

39. Polypeptide or primary structure of a protein.

40. Ionic interaction.

41. All contain aliphatic, lipid-soluble, hydrocarbon side chains and have varying steric bulk.

42. Lipophilic.

43. Quaternary structure of a protein.

8 Organic Macromolecules in Cellular Structures, Metabolism, and as Drugs: From Monosaccharides to Complex Carbohydrates

Learning Objectives

After completing this chapter, you are expected to be able to:

- Understand the structural features of acyclic (aldose and ketose forms) and cyclic monosaccharides.
- Identify the common five- and six-carbon monosaccharide sugars.
- Distinguish the various stereoisomers of cyclic monosaccharides by looking into alpha and beta orientations, including that at the anomeric carbon (C-1).
- Describe the various types of glycosidic bonds in disaccharides, oligosaccharides, and polysaccharides.
- Name examples of polysaccharide-based drugs.

Basic Chemistry for Life Science Students and Professionals: Introduction to Organic Compounds and Drug Molecules
By Solomon Habtemariam
© Solomon Habtemariam 2023
Published by the Royal Society of Chemistry, www.rsc.org

8.1 Overview of Carbohydrates – Functional Aspects

Carbohydrates or the saccharides (from the Greek sakharon, meaning 'sugar') are among the most abundant organic molecules in Nature. Constructed from three elements, carbon, hydrogen, and oxygen, their basic monomeric structures, *monosaccharides*, can be represented by the general formula $(CH_2O)_n$, where n represents the number of repeating units of carbon, in most cases from three to six. Like proteins, sugar monomers are assembled to make dimers, trimers, oligomers, and polymers. Hence two monosaccharides make disaccharides, and the chain length can increase to unlimited size to make *polysaccharides*. Carbohydrates are perceived as fuels for cellular metabolism in living organisms and, for this purpose, they are stored in highly polymerised forms such as *starch* in plants and *glycogen* in animals. Carbohydrates also have uses as structural compounds, with the best example being cellulose in plants. In animals, carbohydrates are added to proteins (*glycoproteins*) and have special properties associated with the function of the protein.

8.2 Introduction to Monosaccharides

8.2.1 Acyclic Monosaccharides

Let us consider a monosaccharide with a three-carbon skeleton that we call *triose*, $C_3H_6O_3$. The possible structures of the triose sugars from this molecular formula are shown in Figure 8.1.

Note that monosaccharides can occur in two forms: *aldose* with a carbonyl group occurs as an aldehyde and *ketose* with a carbonyl group occurs as a ketone (Figure 8.1). Hence dihydroxyacetone is a ketose (ketotriose) and glyceraldehyde is an aldose (aldotriose).

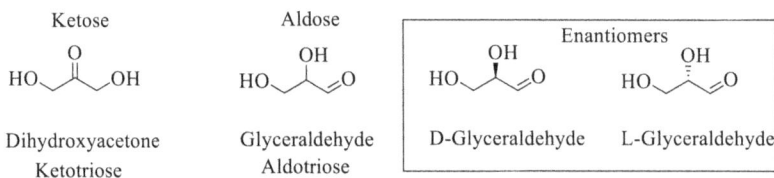

Ketose	Aldose	Enantiomers	
Dihydroxyacetone	Glyceraldehyde	D-Glyceraldehyde	L-Glyceraldehyde
Ketotriose	Aldotriose		

Figure 8.1 Possible structures of a monosaccharide triose. The molecular formula can give two possible structures, one of which is a chiral compound with two enantiomers.

Monosaccharides and sugars in general also possess several *hydroxyl groups*. Another important feature of sugars is their stereochemistry (see Chapter 6). In the simplest monosaccharide, triose, glyceraldehyde has one chiral centre and exists in two enantiomeric forms, D and L. As the number of carbons increases in the monosaccharides, so does the complexity, particularly in their structures resulting from structural isomerism and stereoisomerism (see Chapter 6).

For the four-carbon skeleton sugars, tetroses, we have ketotetrose forms represented by the enantiomeric D and L forms of erythrulose, whereas the aldotetroses are represented by the D and L forms of erythrose and threose. In Nature, however, only the D forms of the enantiomers exist (see Figure 8.2, which presents these isomers in a Fischer projection).

Pentoses (Figure 8.3) are represented by the general molecular formula $C_5H_{10}O_5$. The common aldopentoses are arabinose, ribose, xylose, and lyxose, which exist in either D or L forms. Examples of ketopentoses include ribulose and xylose, which also occur in their enantiomeric (D or L) forms. Whereas ribose (in cyclic form) is a component of RNA, its derivative, deoxyribose, occurs in DNA (see Chapter 10).

Continuing with our presentation of monosaccharides, aldohexoses with four chiral centres have 16 (2^4) possible structures.

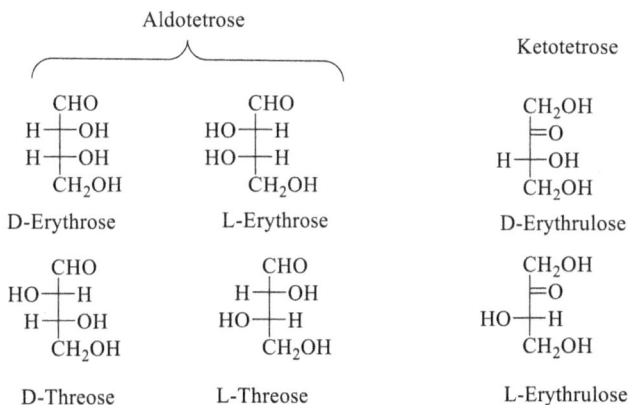

Figure 8.2   Structural features of tetroses. The aldose (aldotetrose) and ketose (ketotetrose) forms are shown using the Fischer projection (from Emil Fischer who, in 1891, devised a two-dimensional representation of organic molecules). The Fischer projection is widely used in the structural drawings of sugars.

D-Arabinose   D-Ribose   D-Xylose   D-Lyxose

L-Arabinose   L-Ribose   L-Xylose   L-Lyxose

Aldopentoses

D-Ribulose   D-Xylulose   D-Deoxyribose

L-Ribulose   L-Xylulose   L-Deoxyribose

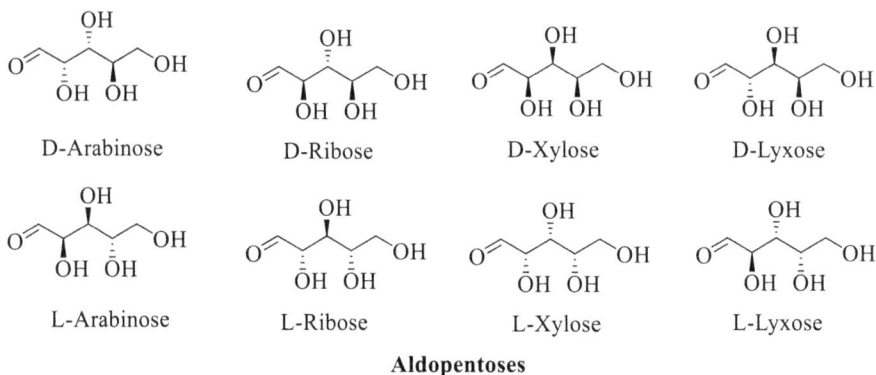

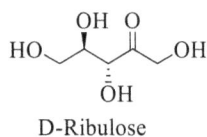

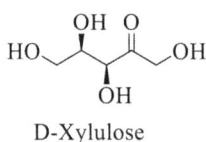

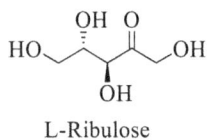

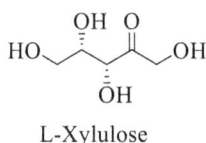

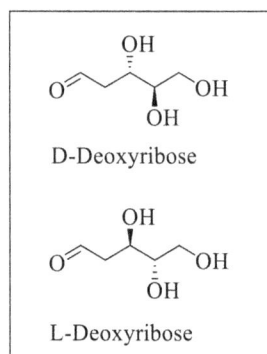

Ketopentoses   **Deoxypentose**

Figure 8.3 Structures of pentoses. The structures of pentoses differ from each other based on whether they are aldoses or ketoses and their stereochemistry. The structure of deoxyribose, which (in its cyclic form) is a component of DNA, is also shown. Note that deoxyribose has one hydroxy group fewer than the general formula for monosaccharides.

The D forms of these aldoses are shown in Figure 8.4, and readers can visualise their mirror images as the L enantiomeric forms. Some of the sugars may differ from each other in the stereochemistry at just one carbon. For example, glucose differs from galactose in the stereochemistry at the C-4 position. Such compounds are called *epimers*.

The common ketohexoses have the carbonyl group position located at C-2 and hence possess three chiral centres. This provides eight (2^3) possible isomers and the four D forms are shown in Figure 8.5.

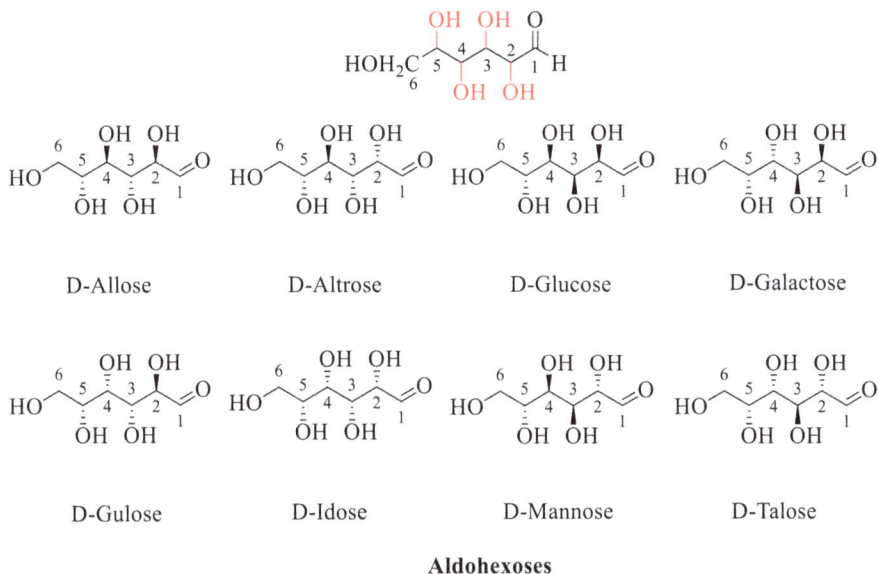

Aldohexoses

Figure 8.4 Structures of the D form of aldohexoses.

Acyclic Monosaccharides – Key Facts

- Monosaccharides are the smallest units of carbohydrates.
- Mostly represented by the general formula $(CH_2O)_n$.
- Named on the basis of the number of carbon atoms: triose, tetrose, pentose, hexose, *etc.*
- Two forms – aldose for the terminal aldehyde group (*e.g.* aldopentose) and ketose for the ketone functional group, usually at the C-2 position (*e.g.* ketohexose).
- Exist in enantiomeric forms: D and L.
- A difference in the stereochemistry of just one carbon atom makes them epimers (glucose *versus* galactose).
- Their structures can be conveniently presented using a Fischer projection.

8.2.2 Cyclic Monosaccharides

Both aldehydes and ketones can react with alcohols to form hemiacetal or hemiketal structures (Figure 8.6). Hence we can expect reactions for the carbonyl groups of aldose or ketose with one of the hydroxyl groups in the chain. The general reaction is summarised in Figure 8.6.

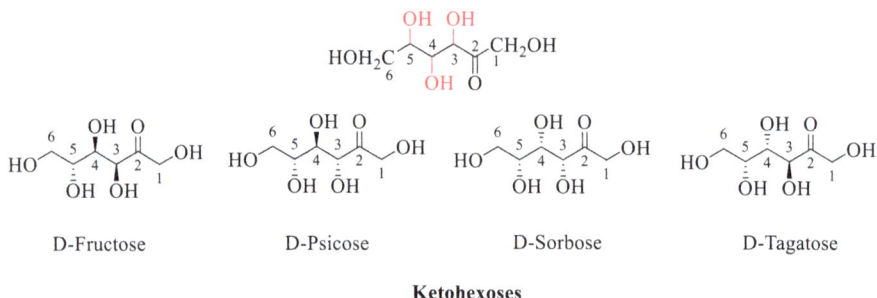

Ketohexoses

Figure 8.5 Structures of 2-ketohexoses. The structures of only the D forms and the carbonyl placed at the C-2 position are shown.

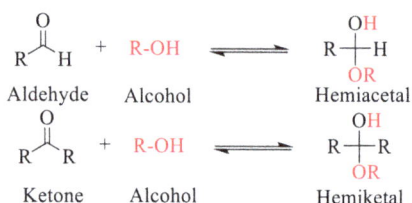

Figure 8.6 Reaction of a ketone or aldehyde with an alcohol to form a hemiacetal or hemiketal structure.

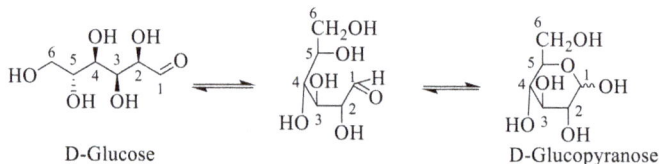

Figure 8.7 Formation of a six-membered ring from acyclic D-glucopyranose. A stable six-membered ring sugar of hemiacetal structure is formed when aldehyde (C-1) interacts with hydroxyl at the C-5 position.

The reaction of the carbonyl group of D-glucose with the hydroxyl group at C-5 gives a six-membered ring structure as shown in Figure 8.7. In theory, reactions with the other hydroxyl groups (C-2, C-3, or C-4) can also occur but the larger ring system (six) is a more stable product and is favoured.

The reaction in Figure 8.7 provides a six-membered cyclic glucose form, *glucopyranose*, with a chiral centre at C-1, which can be presented as beta or alpha forms. The name pyranose is derived

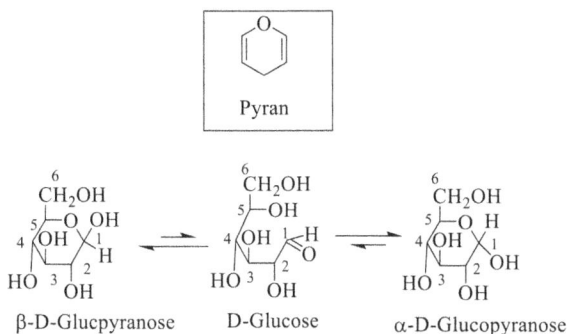

Figure 8.8 Mutarotation of glucose. Glucose exists in an acyclic and two cyclic forms. At equilibrium, nearly all of the glucose molecules exist in the cyclic form with the β-D-glucopyranose form predominating (about 64%) over the α-D-glucopyranose form (about 36%). Hence the conversion between the β- and α-anomers is through the linear (acyclic) aldose form.

from the structural skeleton pyran (Figure 8.8). Position 1 (C-1) of the cyclic glucose structure is called the *anomeric centre* (anomeric carbon – the carbon bonded with two oxygens). Hence C-1 is a hemiacetal group where the carbon is attached to two oxygen atoms. The alpha and beta forms of anomeric glucose (Figure 8.8) have different physical properties, such as optical rotation, and they can be interconvertible in aqueous solution with the beta form appearing to predominate, whereas the aldehyde (acyclic) form occurs in a negligible amount, *i.e.* the aldehyde form serves as an intermediate for the equilibrium between the beta and alpha anomeric forms (Figure 8.8). This interconversion of glucose represented by the three structural forms is called *mutarotation*.

We can show the stereochemistry in sugar structures using different representations. For β-D-glucose, a Haworth projection depicts stereochemistry by placing the substituents up or down in the pyranose skeleton. Since a six-membered ring is used, we indicate this by using pyranose in the naming: glucopyranose (Figure 8.9).

We normally do not show the hydrogen atoms in the structures and the chair conformation is mostly preferred to show the true conformation. It can also be used to reveal the relative positions of substituents positioned either up or down from the skeleton (see Figure 8.10).

For fructose with the carbonyl at position C-2, the most stable ring that can possibly be made is *via* the hydroxyl group at C-5, and this gives a five-membered ring that we call *furanose*. The name furanose is derived from the structural skeleton, furan (Figure 8.11). The alpha

β-D-Glucopyranose   α-D-Glucopyranose

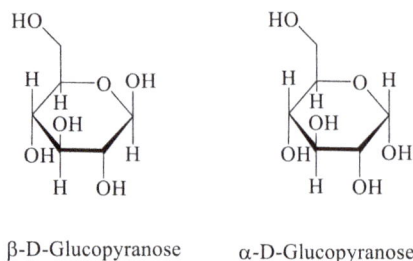

Figure 8.9 Representation of D-glucose using a Haworth projection. This is a common style of presenting cyclic sugars. The bold/thicker lines indicate atoms that are closer to the observer. The projection was the work of the British chemist William Norman Haworth in 1929.

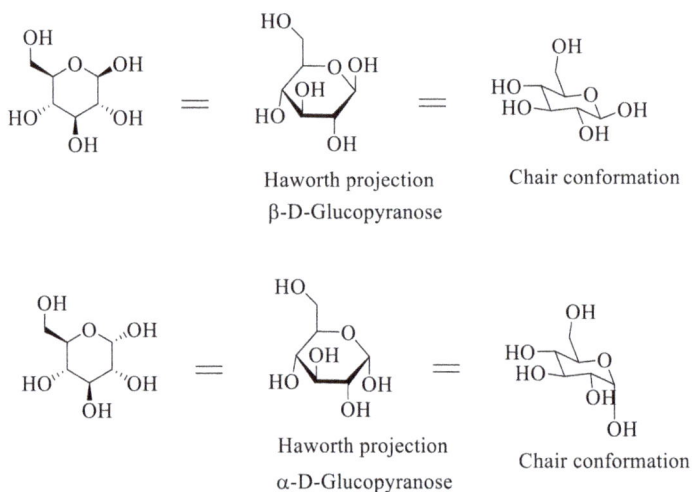

Haworth projection   Chair conformation
β-D-Glucopyranose

Haworth projection   Chair conformation
α-D-Glucopyranose

Figure 8.10 Presentation of D-glucose in the chair conformation.

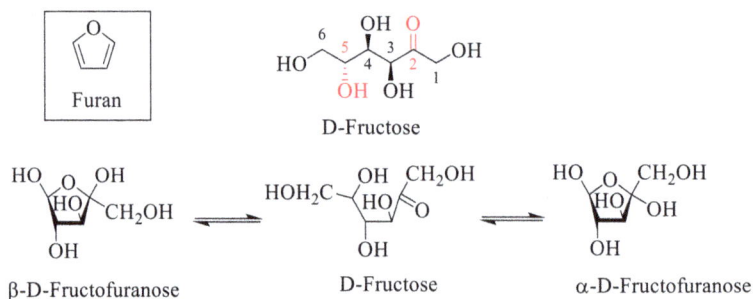

Furan

D-Fructose

β-D-Fructofuranose   D-Fructose   α-D-Fructofuranose

Figure 8.11 Structures of fructose. The five-membered ring, furanose, and acyclic form are shown. Note that the anomeric (C-1) position of fructose is a hemiketal structure, in contrast to glucose, which is hemiacetal.

and beta anomeric forms of fructose are shown in Figure 8.11. Hence ketohexoses (as with fructose) can form a stable cyclic structure in the form of furanose.

A furanose ring system is common for pentoses and some good examples are shown in Figure 8.12. Note that these compounds can also exist in their pyranose form (six-membered ring system), as shown in Figure 8.13 for arabinose.

Based on positional differences for the hydroxyl groups, the eight hexose sugars (see Figure 8.4) that we encounter in biology and chemistry are shown in Figure 8.14.

Cyclic Monosaccharides – Key Facts

- Exist in either hemiacetal (for aldoses) or hemiketal (for ketoses) forms.
- Six-membered ring is pyranose (*e.g.* glucopyranose).
- Five-membered ring is furanose (*e.g.* fructofuranose).
- Stereochemistry at the anomeric centre (C-1) is important (*e.g.* α-D-glucopyranoside or β-D-glucopyranoside).
- In solution, the alpha and beta forms are interconvertible (for glucose the beta form is predominant).
- A difference in stereochemistry of just one carbon makes them epimers (glucose *versus* galactose).
- They can be presented using a Haworth projection or chair conformation.

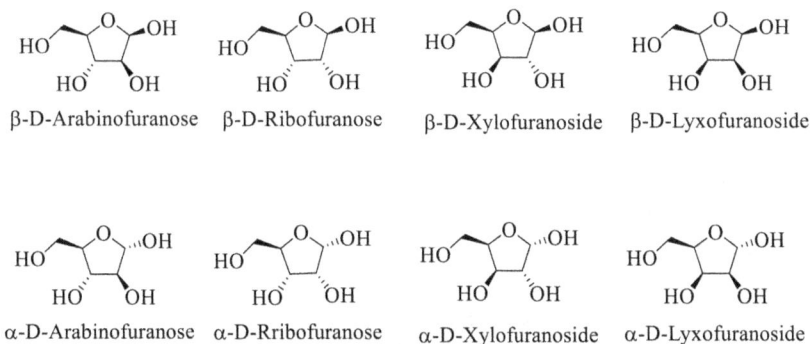

β-D-Arabinofuranose   β-D-Ribofuranose   β-D-Xylofuranoside   β-D-Lyxofuranoside

α-D-Arabinofuranose   α-D-Rribofuranose   α-D-Xylofuranoside   α-D-Lyxofuranoside

Figure 8.12   Examples of pentose sugars in their furanose forms. The alpha and beta anomeric structures are shown.

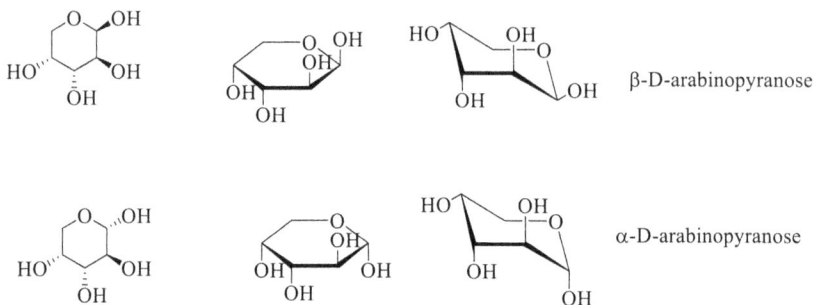

β-D-arabinopyranose

α-D-arabinopyranose

Figure 8.13 Presentation of alpha and beta forms of arabinopyranose.

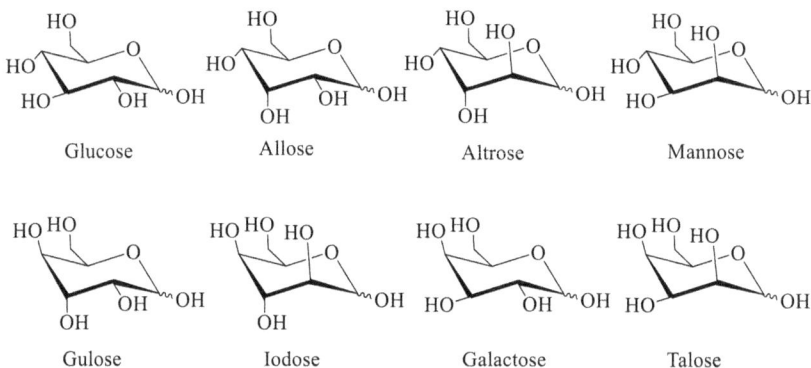

Glucose   Allose   Altrose   Mannose

Gulose   Iodose   Galactose   Talose

Figure 8.14 Common hexoses in pyranose forms. The stereochemistry of the anomeric sugar is not shown and hence could be either beta or alpha. The representation in the chair conformation shows the orientation of the hydroxyl groups in the structures of the D-sugars. You may consider drawing these structures in a Haworth projection.

8.3 Disaccharides

Disaccharides are formed when two monosaccharides condense to form a C–O–C bridge (ether) called a *glycosidic linkage*. This involves a reaction between two hydroxyl groups, one of which is an anomeric hydroxyl group. The resulting disaccharide still has one anomeric position that has either an alpha or beta orientation. Two glucose monomers form a disaccharide, maltose; a disaccharide of glucose and galactose is lactose, and fructose and a glucose disaccharide form sucrose. The position of the linkage between the anomeric hydroxyl of one sugar and another hydroxyl group of the second sugar could vary, hence disaccharides differ in the

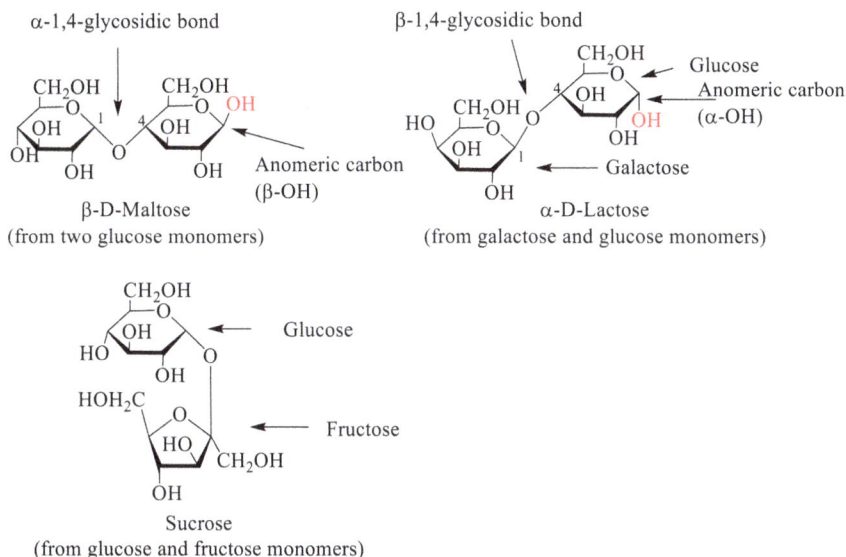

Figure 8.15 Glycosidic bonds in disaccharides. Maltose has a glycosidic bond through the anomeric glucose (C-1) to C-4 position of another glucose. With β-anomeric hydroxyl still available, the sugar is called β-D-maltose. The position of the anomeric hydroxyl group in the glycosidic bond is indicated as an α-1,4-glycosidic bond or α-(1→4). In lactose, the glycosidic bond is from the beta anomeric galactose to the C-4 glucose unit [β-1,4-glycosidic bond or β-(1→4)], but the remaining anomeric hydroxyl group left in glucose is in the alpha position – hence the disaccharide is called α-D-lactose. In sucrose, no anomeric hydroxyl group is left as both anomeric C-1 positions are involved in the bond formation – the sugar is simply called sucrose. The bond is from the C-2 position of fructose to the C-1 position of glucose [β-2,1-glycosidic bond or simply β-(2→1)].

composition of monomers in addition to the glycosidic linkage (Figure 8.15).

The above examples signify the three most common types of disaccharides. Sucrose is obtained commercially from sugarcane and sugar beet; it is a common source of metabolic energy and utilised extensively for its sweet taste. Maltose is common in sprouting grain and is widely used in the brewery industry, where it is released from larger carbohydrates such as starch through the germination process. Barley is a common source of maltose through such a process. Lactose, which is less sweet than sucrose, is a milk sugar. Its commercial source is whey, which is obtained during cheese production.

Glycosidic Linkage – Key Facts

- Two monosaccharides condense to form a C–O–C bridge (ether).
- One of the anomeric hydroxyls reacts with a hydroxyl from another monosaccharide to form the ether bond – glycosidic linkage.
- Disaccharides differ based on sugar composition and linkage (*e.g.* sucrose, maltose, and lactose).
- The anomeric hydroxyl that forms the bond is used to name the linkage (*e.g.* an α-1,4-glycosidic bond for maltose).
- The unreacted anomeric position can be indicated in the name (*e.g.* β-D-maltose).
- In sucrose, both anomeric hydroxyl groups are involved in the glycosidic linkage.

8.4 Oligosaccharides and Polysaccharides

In Nature, carbohydrates mainly occur in the form of polymers of monosaccharides. These polymers with around 10 monosaccharides are called *oligosaccharides* and those with more than 10 monosaccharides as monomers are called *polysaccharides*. Like proteins, oligosaccharides and polysaccharides may differ from each other based on the number and composition of their monomeric units. Since most oligosaccharides are small in molecular size, often up to six monomers, they are water soluble and sweet in taste. They occur in cellular systems such as cell membranes where they serve as a recognition surface for cell–cell and cell–protein binding. In contrast, polysaccharides can be composed of several hundred monomers or monosaccharide residues. In plants they serve for energy storage such as starch in grains, whereas in animals we have glycogen as an energy reserve that is stored in muscles and the liver. In plants, polysaccharides such as cellulose are structural components of cell walls. Polysaccharides are generally not sweet in taste and are insoluble in water.

A polysaccharide may be composed of only one monosaccharide residue (*homopolysaccharide*) and may be called glucan (made of glucose), mannan (a mannose polymer), galactan (a galactose polymer), *etc.* Starch and glycogen are made from only glucose and hence are homopolysaccharides. The glycosidic bond variation in the polysaccharide chain is one major feature of structural diversity. An example is (1→4)-β-D-glucan *versus* (1→6)-β-D-glucan. This indicates anomeric oxygen making a bridge either at a C-4 or a C-6 position, respectively. In addition, polysaccharides vary based on branching patterns, with some monosaccharides in the chain linked to more than two other monosaccharide residues. More than one monosaccharide residue (*heteropolysaccharides*), branching, variation in repeated units of monomers, *etc.*, all lead to the structural diversity of polysaccharides. In the case of starch, it is composed of two units, the *amylose* helical structure composed of α-1,4 linkages [α-(1→4) bond] and the *amylopectin* unit, which has branching of α-1,6 linkages [α-(1→6) bond] that occur about once in 30 monomers. On the other hand, glycogen is composed of α-1,4-glycosidic bonds with branching of α-1,6 bonds that occur once at about every tenth monomer (Figure 8.16). Cellulose, as the most abundant biopolymer or organic molecule on Earth, is also a homopolysaccharide, with unbranched chains of glucose molecules linked *via* β-1,4- glycosidic bonds (Figure 8.16).

In animals and humans, heteropolysaccharides have diverse functions, including *hyaluronic acid* as the synovial fluid of joints; *chondroitin sulfate*, which contributes to the tensile strength and elasticity of cartilage, tendons, and ligaments; *dermatan sulfate*, involved in the coagulation process among many functions; *keratan sulfate* as a structural component of nails and hair; and *heparin* serving as an anticoagulant in the blood.

Polysaccharides are generally considered as the most abundant organic materials on Earth. Chitosan is a natural biodegradable polysaccharide extracted from chitin, which is the exoskeleton component of marine natural organisms such as shrimps and crabs. From these organisms and also others (*e.g.* insects and fungi cell walls), chitosan is released from chitin *via* N-deacetylation.

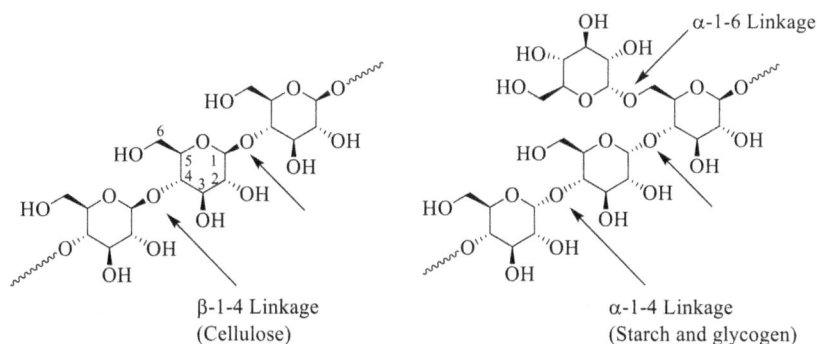

Figure 8.16 Glycosidic bond and branching in polysaccharides. The β-1–4 and α-1–4 linkages are shown.

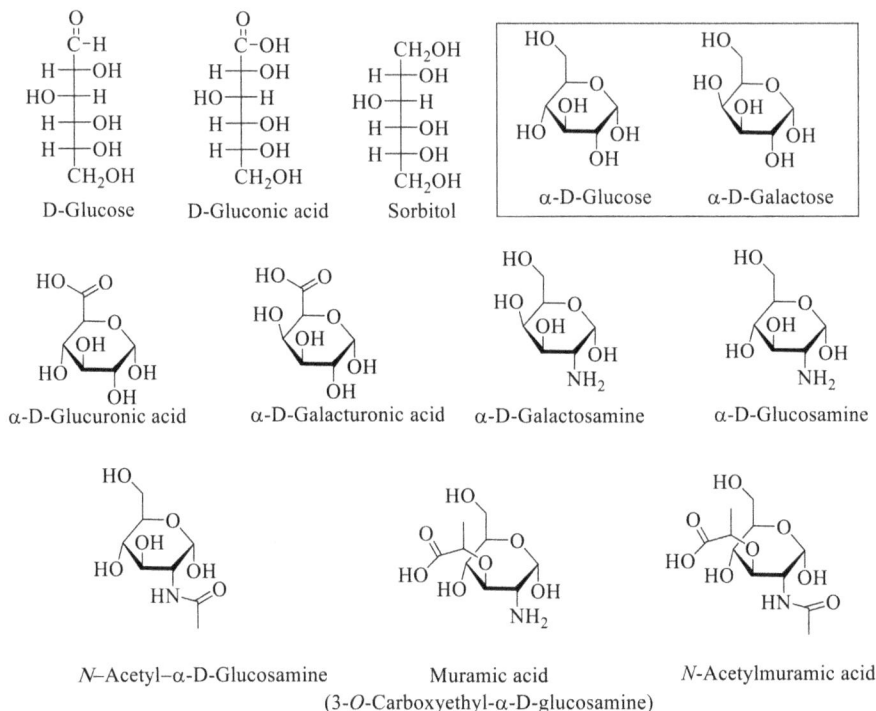

Figure 8.17 Derivatives of monosaccharides that make further structural diversity in polysaccharides. The list is long and only a few examples are shown here.

With respect to the diversity of sugars such as chitosan, there are several derivatives of monosaccharides (see Figure 8.17) that are involved in polymer formation. One such diverse aspect is manifested by amino sugars, which are obtained by replacing a hydroxyl group of a monosaccharide with an amino group. Good examples of amino sugars are 2-aminoaldohexoses such as D-glucosamine and D-galactosamine. Further derivatives of the amino group include *N*-acetyl compounds. Glucosamine incorporating lactic acid as an ether is exemplified by muramic acid, which itself can be *N*-acetylated to form *N*-acetylmuramic acid. In Nature, various derivatives of monosaccharides also occur in polysaccharides. For example, oxidation products of glucose include gluconic acid and glucuronic acids.

8.4.1 Abbreviations of Monosaccharides in Oligo- and Polysaccharides

As with proteins and peptides, showing the structure of carbohydrates, especially polysaccharides, using chemical structures can be cumbersome. Therefore, we use abbreviations to represent the

Table 8.1 Abbreviations used for monosaccharides.

Type	Monosaccharide	Abbreviation
Hexose	Glucose	Glc
	Mannose	Man
	Galactose	Gal
	Gulose	Gul
	Altrose	Alt
	Allose	All
	Talose	Tal
	Idose	Ido
Pentose	Arabinose	Ara
	Lyxose	Lyx
	Xylose	Xyl
	Ribose	Rib

monosaccharides (Table 8.1). Based on these abbreviations and the above-mentioned glycosidic bond representation, we can write the composition of some disaccharide sugars as follows:

Lactose	Galβ1→4Glc
Maltose	Glcα1→4Glc
Sucrose	Fruβ2→1Glc
Cellobiose	Glcβ1→4Glc
Trehalose	Glcα1→1Glc
Melibiose	Galα1→6Glc
Gentiobiose	Glcβ1→6Glcβ

Several legume seeds contain tri- and tetrasaccharides. These include raffinose (Galα1→6Glcα1→2Fruβ) and stachyose (Galα1→-6Galα1→6Glcα1→2Fruβ). Plant tissues also contain other oligosaccharides such as umbelliferose (Galα1→2Glcα1→2Fruβ), planteose (Galα1→6Fruβ2→1Glc), lychnose (Galα1→6Glcα1→2Fruβ1→1Gal), isolychnose (Galα1→6Glcα1→2Fruβ3→1Gal), sesamose (Galα1→-6Galα1→6Fruβ2→1Glc), and verbascose (Galα1→6Galα1→6Galα1→6Glcα1→2Fruβ). Maltotriose (Glcα1→4Glcα1→4Glc) is a hydrolysis product of starch and occurs in glucose syrups.

As indicated earlier, we also have further derivatives of monosaccharides (see Figure 8.18) in biological systems, which include *N*-acetylglucosamine (GlcNAc). This is an amide derivative of glucose and is incorporated as part of the bacterial cell wall, and also chitin, which is a component of the exoskeleton in insects and crustaceans. Other monosaccharides of this nature include *N*-acetylmannosamine (ManNAc), which is a key precursor in the synthesis of sialic acid [*N*-acetylneuraminic acid (Neu5Ac)]. Mammalian cells contain sialic acid, which is negatively charged at physiological pH on the surface of cell membranes. It is also incorporated with lipids and proteins to be involved in several biological processes.

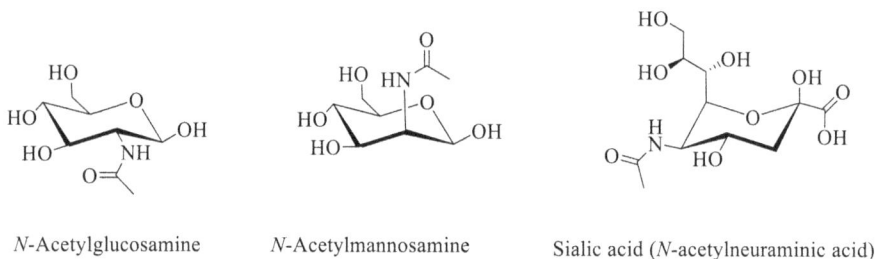

N-Acetylglucosamine   N-Acetylmannosamine   Sialic acid (N-acetylneuraminic acid)

Figure 8.18 Structures of N-acetyl derivatives of monosaccharides in the chair conformation.

8.5 Carbohydrate-based Drugs

Mono-, di-, and polysaccharides may be part of a larger bioactive molecule that contains other functional groups. These are often referred to as *glycosides* in which a sugar unit is attached *via* a glycosidic bond with a non-sugar unit called an *aglycone*. In this section, we only address sugars or carbohydrates as the main components of drugs. Smaller carbohydrate units, normally called sugars, which are mono- and disaccharides, are rarely considered as pharmacological agents. When monosaccharides have other groups attached, however, they show biological effects (see Figure 8.19). For example, the antiepileptic drug topiramate is a sulfamate derivative of a monosaccharide fructose. It also contains a diacetonide structural moiety. Its pharmacological effect is mediated owing to its ability to enhance the level of the excitatory neurotransmitter γ-aminobutyrate (GABA). It also has other effects, including inhibition of the enzyme carbonic anhydrase.

Streptozotocin (Figure 8.19) is a natural antibiotic isolated from the Gram-positive bacterium, *Streptomyces achromogenes*. Owing to its selective toxicity to the beta cells of the pancreatic islets that secrete insulin, it is a classic experimental agent employed to induce diabetes in rodents. Whereas its cytotoxicity is due to the nitroso functional group (nitrosourea), which makes the compound an alkylating agent, its selective toxicity to the pancreas is due to its similarity to glucose and hence is transported *via* glucose transporter-2 (GLUT-2). The high level of GLUT-2 in β-cells means a higher sensitivity to streptozotocin toxicity.

An example of a disaccharide drug is lactulose (Figure 8.19), which is formed from galactose and fructose. As a laxative, it has a clinical use to treat constipation. Based on the structure of sucrose, sucralfate contains sulfuric acid ester and aluminium hydroxide. It has clinical applications with gastric ulcer healing properties.

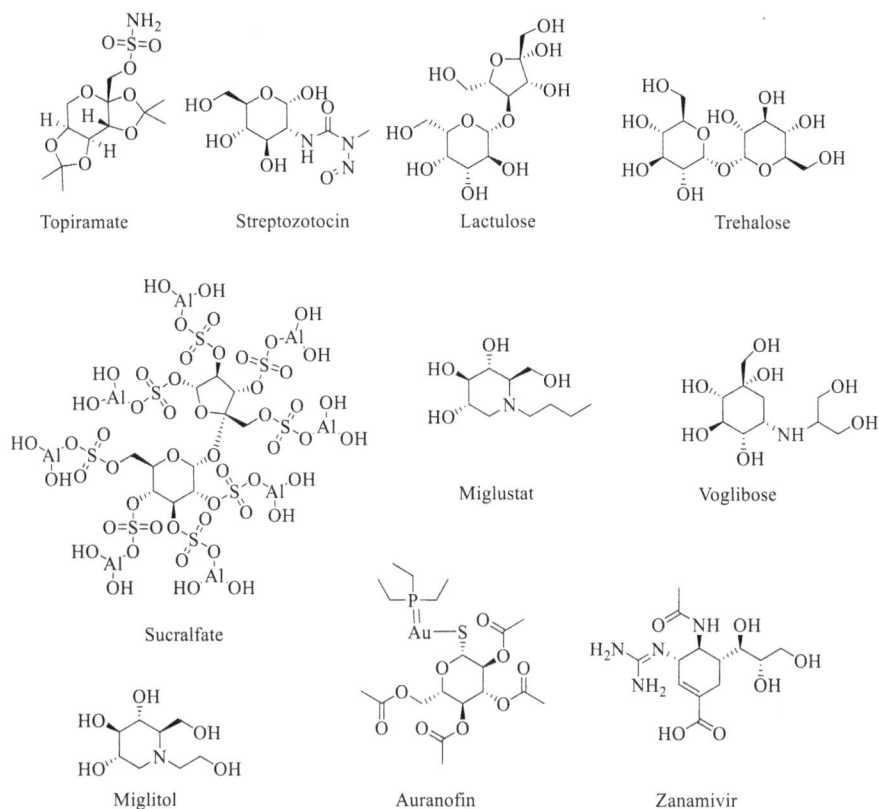

Figure 8.19 Simple sugars and derivatives as drugs.

An intriguing natural disaccharide is trehalose, which is formed by an α-1 glucoside bond between two α-glucose units, *i.e.* α-D-glucopyranosyl-(1→1)-α-D-glucopyranoside. Recently, it was shown to be implicated as a drug for the treatment of a range of conditions from dry eye to neurological disorders such as Huntington's disease and Alzheimer's disease.

On the other hand, sugar derivatives such as volglibose (antidiabetic drug) and miglustat (used in the treatment of Gaucher disease) (Figure 8.19) are drugs with structures containing a nitrogen atom in the heterocyclic ring. Other simple sugar derivatives of medical importance include the antidiabetic drug miglitol, the antirheumatic drug auranofin, which is a gold salt, and the anti-influenza drug zanamivir (Figure 8.19). *N*-Acetylglucosamine (Figure 8.19) is a dietary supplement with claimed benefits for a range of disease conditions.

As the most abundant organic compounds in Nature, polysaccharides commonly occur in plants, animals, bacteria, fungi, algae, arthropods, crustaceans, *etc.* In addition to being used as an energy source and a structural matrix in living organisms, they possess various biological functions by being a component of signalling molecules in cell-to-cell and within-cell communications and also immune functions. With molecular weights that can range from thousands to millions, the structures of polysaccharides contain numerous functional groups such as hydroxyl, amino, and carboxylic acid groups. Hence they also serve as drugs and it is not surprising that scientific reports are regularly published to demonstrate their antibacterial, anti-inflammatory, immunomodulatory, anticancer, antidiabetic and various other effects.

One common application of polysaccharides is as dietary fibres, which are recommended for health benefits both for enabling digestive functions and maintaining a healthy intestinal microflora. Polysaccharides are also used as food additives and in food and medicine preparations as emulsifying, thickening, and/or stabilising agents. Polysaccharides are thus routinely used in prebiotic preparations.

In drug preparations, polysaccharides are extensively used as carriers of drug delivery. Modifications of the various functional groups in polysaccharides allow drug carrier preparations such as the following:

• Drug–polysaccharide conjugates.
• Self-assembling drug-loaded particles.
• Drug molecules encapsulated in hydrogel polysaccharide-based materials.

Polysaccharide-based liposomes, micelles, and hydrogels are routinely used as drug delivery systems to treat various diseases, including cancer. Sustained release of drug materials to target specific disease sites in the body is possible owing to such preparations and nanotechnology.

Overall, polysaccharides as natural products are used extensively in biomedical preparations such as pharmaceutical formulations and clinical applications for the following reasons:

• Abundance in Nature.
• Inexpensive – low cost.
• Can be easily modified chemically.

- Biocompatible.
- Biodegradable.
- Non-toxic.
- Non-reactogenic.

The common natural polysaccharides used in drug delivery systems include chitosan, hyaluronic acid, dextran, arabinogalactan, starch, cyclodextrin, cycloamylose obtained from enzymatic hydrolysis of starch, pullulan, inulin, cellulose, hemicellulose, alginic acid, chondroitin sulfate, heparin, and gums such as pectin and gum arabic.

Polysaccharides extracted from mushrooms, plants, algae, and other sources also have therapeutic applications both in traditional medicines and in modern medicine preparations. Antidiabetic, anticancer, and immunomodulatory effects of these polysaccharide preparations have been routinely reported. Owing to the diversity of polysaccharides and their complex structures, further structural scrutiny is beyond the scope of this book.

Some of the polysaccharide and oligosaccharide drugs are shown in Figure 8.19. Heparin and its low molecular weight derivatives have been used as anticoagulants in a range of cardiovascular conditions such as thrombosis. For its blood-clotting inhibitory properties, heparin is also used in test-tubes while blood samples are collected and kept until use. Structurally, heparin is a glycosaminoglycan with repeating disaccharide units consisting of a uronic sugar and an amino sugar. The structure of heparin can vary greatly, however, and is only defined as a polymer with alternating derivatives of D-glucosamine (*N*-sulfated, *O*-sulfated, or *N*-acetylated) and uronic acid (L-iduronic acid or D-glucuronic acid) joined by glycosidic linkages. The simplified structural form of heparin shows two disaccharide repeating units: L-iduronic acid 2-sulfate linked α-(1→4) to 2-deoxy-2-sulfamido-D-galactose 6-sulfate (structure A, Figure 8.20) and D-glucuronic acid β-(1→4) linked to 2-deoxy-2-sulfamido-D-glucose 6-sulfate (structure B). In animals, the sources of heparin are the liver, lungs, mast cells, and intestinal mucosa. For clinical use, the sodium salt form (heparin sodium) is used with its blood coagulation effect quantified as units. Elmiron, pentosan polysulfate sodium, is a semi-synthetic heparin-like carbohydrate derivative. It has anticoagulant and fibrinolytic properties. Acarbose, which is a pseudo-oligosaccharide, as an antidiabetic agent is specifically used to treat type 2 diabetes. It inhibits the digestion of carbohydrates in the gut, thereby limiting glucose availability, *i.e.* reducing sugar levels in the blood.

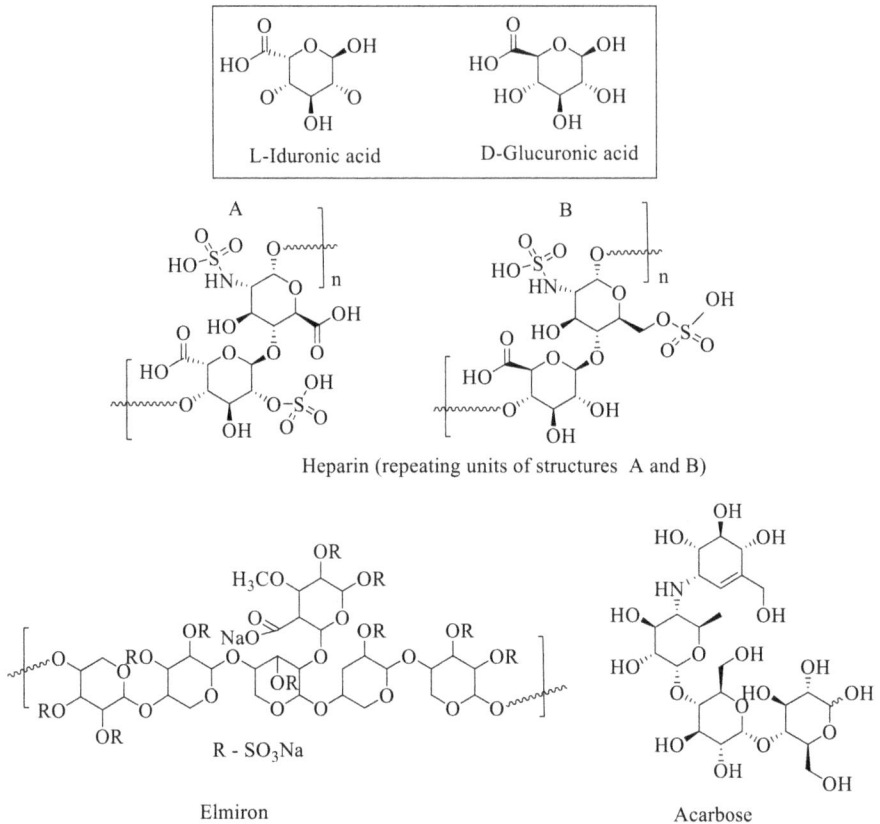

L-Iduronic acid   D-Glucuronic acid

Heparin (repeating units of structures A and B)

Elmiron

R - SO₃Na

Acarbose

Figure 8.20 Structures of heparin, elmiron, and acarbose.

Carbohydrate Digestion – Key Facts

- The digestion of carbohydrates such as oligosaccharides and starches starts in the mouth by salivary amylase.
- The main digestion occurs by α-glucosidase enzymes located in the brush border of the small intestine.
- Drugs such as acarbose and miglitol possess antidiabetic effects by inhibiting these enzymes.
- These drugs reduce the level of glucose available for absorption by the blood.

8.6 Summary

In this chapter, we have learned the following:

- Carbohydrates are constructed from three elements: carbon, hydrogen, and oxygen.

- The smaller units of carbohydrates are monosaccharides, and their polymers are oligo- and polysaccharides.
- Monosaccharides are usually represented by the general formula $(CH_2O)_n$.
- Carbohydrates are largely stored as energy reserves in the form of starch in plants and glycogen in animals.
- Carbohydrates also occur in combination with proteins, as glycoproteins.
- The smallest monosaccharide unit is a three-carbon skeleton, triose.
- Monosaccharides may exist in their acyclic form as aldose (aldehyde) and ketose (ketone) forms.
- The predominant functional group in carbohydrates is the hydroxyl group.
- The aldose form of monosaccharides has more isomers than the ketose form.
- The D and L forms of monosaccharides are enantiomeric forms.
- The reaction between alcohols and a carbonyl (ketone or aldehyde) gives hemiacetal or hemiketal products.
- Aldehyde is the acyclic form of monosaccharides, whereas its cyclic monosaccharides have a hemiacetal structure – the hemiacetal carbon is called the anomeric centre (anomeric carbon). Fructose is a good example that exists in solution in a five-membered cyclic hemiketal form.
- The anomeric hydroxyl can exist as either a beta (*e.g.* β-D-glucose) or an alpha (*e.g.* α-D-glucose) form.
- The interconversion of alpha and beta anomeric forms in solution is called mutarotation.
- A six-membered ring of monosaccharides is called pyranose (*e.g.* β-D-glucopyranose) and a five-membered ring is furanose (*e.g.* β-D-fructofuranose).
- Monosaccharides link together through a glycosidic linkage, which is an ether bridge between two sugars.
- The three most common disaccharides are sucrose, lactose, and maltose. They differ from each other in their glycosidic linkage and monosaccharide components.
- Starch has two major components:

  o Amylose (α-1,4 linkages) has only a linear structure.
  o Amylopectin (α-1,4 linkages + branching of α-1,6 linkages) has a branched structure; a branch point occurs every 25–30 glucose units in the chain.

- Glycogen consists of only glucose molecules that are linked by two types of bonds – the α-1,4-glycosidic bond and the α-1,6-glycosidic

bond, *i.e.* glycogen is composed of α-1,4-glycosidic bonds with branching of α-1,6 bonds.
- Polymers of around 10 monosaccharides are called oligosaccharides whereas those with more than 10 monosaccharides as monomers are called polysaccharides.
- Polysaccharides composed of one monosaccharide residue are called homopolysaccharides.
- Polysaccharides composed of more than one monosaccharide residue are called heteropolysaccharides.
- Cellulose, as the most abundant biopolymer or organic molecule on Earth, is also a homopolysaccharide with unbranched chains of glucose molecules linked *via* β-1,4-glycosidic bonds.
- Examples of heteropolysaccharides are hyaluronic acid, chondroitin sulfate, dermatan sulfate, keratan sulfate, and heparin.
- Monosaccharides, disaccharides, and polysaccharides can serve as drugs:

  o Mostly as derivatives or heteropolysaccharides (*e.g.* heparin).
  o Mostly in combination with organic compounds as glycosides.

- Polysaccharides are also used in drug preparations as carriers, emulsifiers, *etc.*

8.7 Problems

Questions 1–4. The following are classifications of monosaccharides based on functional groups and number of carbons. Name the following:

1. Based on seven carbons, ketone: _____.
2. Based on five carbons, aldehyde: _____.
3. Based on six carbons, aldehyde: _____.
4. Based on three carbons, ketone: _____.

Questions 5–7. Consider glucose, galactose, and fructose:

5. Which are aldoses?
6. Which is a ketose?
7. Which two are epimers to each other?
8. What is the structural difference between D-ribose and D-2-deoxyribose?
9. What is the molecular formula for the seven-carbon monosaccharide heptose?
10. What is the smallest monosaccharide?

Questions 11–13. In the reactions between alcohols and ketones or aldehydes, a hemiketal or hemiacetal form of cyclic monosaccharides is formed. What would be the product (hemiacetal *versus* hemiketal) for the following:

11. Glucose.
12. Fructose.
13. Show structures using a Haworth projection.
14. In the chair conformation of the pyranose ring of glucose, the conformer with the bulky hydroxyl substituents at the equatorial position is more stable. From your knowledge of the cyclohexane conformation, show the two chair conformations.

For questions 15–17, refer to Figure 8.21, which shows the structure of glucose in a Fischer projection.

15. Glucuronic acid is a derivative of glucose where the $-CH_2OH$ group is oxidised to the carboxyl $(-COOH)$ group. Show its structure using a Fischer projection.
16. Gluconic acid is a derivative of glucose where the aldehyde group is oxidised to become a carboxyl functional group. Show its structure using a Fischer projection.
17. Sorbitol is a derivative of glucose where the aldehyde group is replaced with a primary alcohol group. Show its structure using a Fischer projection.
18. In amino sugars, a hydroxyl group is replaced with the amino $(-NH_2)$ group. D-Glucosamine has an amino group at C-2. Show the structure using various presentations as shown in Figure 8.22.
19. The common amide derivative of amino sugar is the *N*-acetyl $[-NH(C=O)CH_3]$ group. Show the structure of *N*-acetyl-D-glucosamine using the structural templates presented in Figure 8.22.

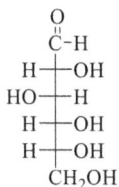

$$
\begin{array}{c}
O \\
\| \\
C\text{-}H \\
H\!-\!\!-\!OH \\
HO\!-\!\!-\!H \\
H\!-\!\!-\!OH \\
H\!-\!\!-\!OH \\
CH_2OH
\end{array}
$$

D-Glucose

Figure 8.21 For questions 15–17.

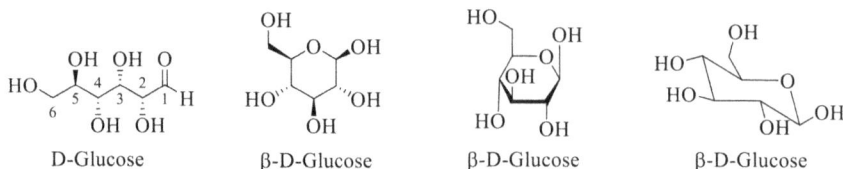

Figure 8.22 For questions 18 and 19.

Questions 20 and 21. Draw the structures of the following:

20. α-D-Galactosamine using a Haworth projection.
21. Galacturonic acid using a Fischer projection.

Questions 22 and 23. Consider D-glucose and L-glucose:

22. What is the structural difference between them?
23. How do you distinguish them experimentally?

Questions 24 and 25. Consider glucose and fructose. How do they differ based on the following:

24. Hemiacetal *versus* hemiketal structural forms.
25. Aldose *versus* ketose forms.

Questions 26–29. When α-D-glucose dissolves in water, the stereochemistry at one of the carbon atoms changes:

26. Which carbon is this?
27. What are the products?
28. If the crystal of α-D-glucose has an optical rotation of +112.2° and that of β-D-glucose +19°, what do you expect to see when α-D-glucose dissolves in water?
29. Which product is predominant or in what ratio?
30. The interconversion of the α- and β-anomers of sugars in aqueous solution is called _____?
31. The hydroxyl group of glucose at the C-1 position is methylated (methyl ether – methyl β-D-glucopyranoside, methyl α-D-glucopyranoside). Show these structures.

Questions 32 and 33. For the structures shown in Figure 8.23, describe the glycosidic bond for:

32. Cellobiose.
33. Gentiobiose.

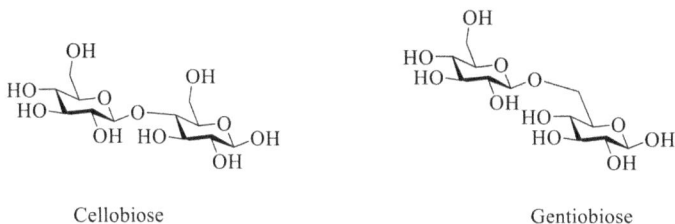

Cellobiose   Gentiobiose

Figure 8.23 For questions 32 and 33.

Questions 34–36. Describe the glycosidic linkage for the following disaccharides:

34. Lactose.
35. Maltose.
36. Sucrose.

Questions 37–42. What would be the monosaccharides obtained by hydrolysis or digestion of the following:

37. Sucrose.
38. Maltose.
39. Lactose.
40. Cellulose.
41. Starch.
42. Glycogen.
43. Disaccharides can be named β-D-maltose, α-D-maltose, α-D-lactose, β-D-lactose, *etc.* Explain why this is not relevant to sucrose.
44. Describe three ways of structural diversity in polysaccharides.

Questions 45–46. Consider starch *versus* glycogen:

45. Name two similarities.
46. Name their difference.
47. What is the similarity between amylose and cellulose?
48. What are the advantages of using polysaccharides in drug preparations?
49. In what forms are polysaccharides used in pharmaceutical formulations?
50. List examples of drugs as:
    a. Simple monosaccharide derived: _____.
    b. Disaccharide derived: _____.
    c. Polysaccharides: _____.

8.8   Solutions to Problems

1. Ketoheptose.
2. Aldopentose.
3. Aldohexose.
4. Ketotriose.
5. Glucose and galactose.
6. Fructose.
7. Galactose and glucose.
8. A hydroxyl group missing at the C-2 position in D-2-deoxyribose.
9. $C_7H_{14}O_7$ from the general formula $(CH_2O)_n$.
10. Glyceraldehyde or other three-carbon derivatives of trioses.
11. Glucose – hemiacetal.
12. Fructose – hemiketal.
13. See Figure 8.24.
14. See Figure 8.25.

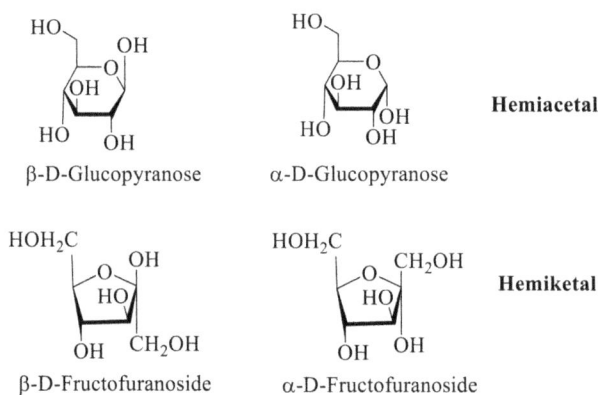

β-D-Glucopyranose   α-D-Glucopyranose

Hemiacetal

β-D-Fructofuranoside   α-D-Fructofuranoside

Hemiketal

Figure 8.24   Answer to question 13.

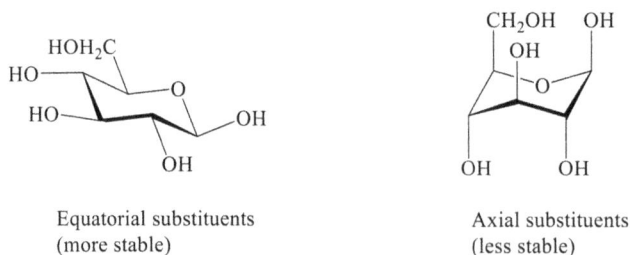

Equatorial substituents
(more stable)

Axial substituents
(less stable)

Figure 8.25   Answer to question 14.

For questions 15–17, see Figure 8.26.
For questions 18 and 19, see Figure 8.27.
For questions 20 and 21, see Figure 8.28.

22. They are enantiomers.
23. Optical rotation measurement.
24. The hemiacetal group for glucose and a hemiketal group for fructose.
25. Aldose in glucose *versus* ketose in fructose.
26. C-1.

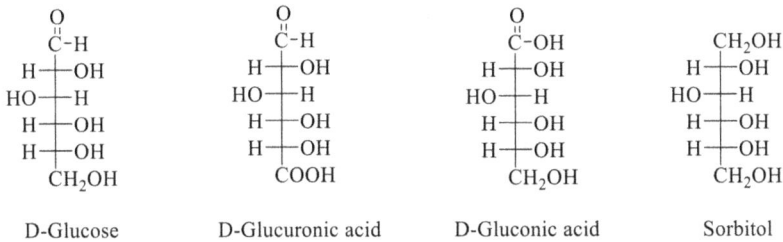

Figure 8.26 Answers to questions 15–17.

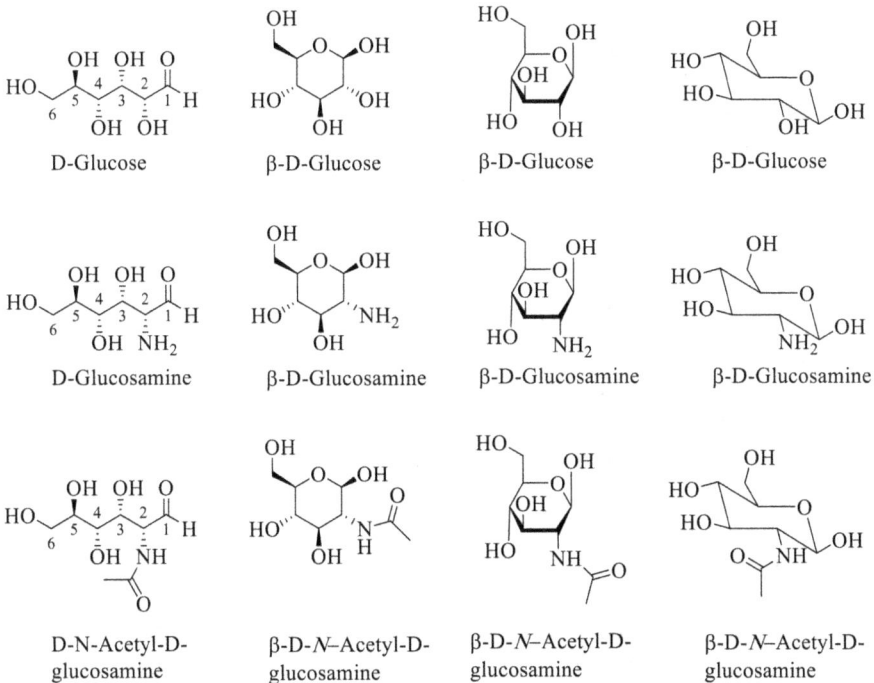

Figure 8.27 Answers to questions 18 and 19.

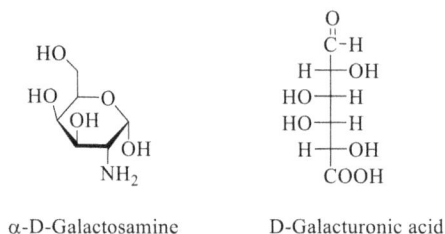

α-D-Galactosamine   D-Galacturonic acid

Figure 8.28   Answers to questions 20 and 21.

27. β-D-Glucopyranoside and α-D-glucopyranoside.
28. The optical rotation would be far less than the rotation for α-D-glucose as some of the molecule changes to β-D-glucose form.
29. The ratio favouring the beta form is 64 : 36, less than that of the equilibrium value of +54° because the beta form dominates.
30. Mutarotation.
31. See Figure 8.29.
32. Cellobiose: β-glycoside bond or β-(1→4) glycosidic bond.
33. Gentiobiose: β-glycoside bond or β-(1→6) glycosidic bond.
34. Lactose: β-1,4-glycosidic bond or β-(1→4) glycosidic bond.
35. Maltose: α-1,4-glycosidic linkage or α-(1→4) glycosidic bond.
36. Sucrose: α-1,β-2-glycosidic (1→2) linkage.
37. Sucrose: glucose and fructose.
38. Maltose: glucose.
39. Lactose: glucose and galactose.
40. Cellulose: glucose.
41. Starch: glucose.
42. Glycogen: glucose.
43. Both anomeric hydroxyl groups are involved in the formation of sucrose.
44. Monosaccharide composition, glycosidic linkage in the chain, and branching pattern.
45. Made from glucose and contain an α-(1→4) bond and an α-(1→6) bond linkage.
46. Starch has two components, amylose and amylopectin units. The patterns of branching in amylopectin and glycogen are different.
47. Glucose molecules linked *via* β-1,4-glycosidic bonds.
48. Widely available, low cost, non-toxic, biodegradable, *etc.*
49. Liposomes, micelles, hydrogels, *etc.*
50. See Figure 8.19.

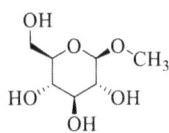

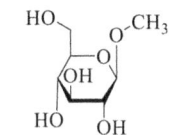

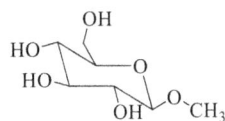

Methyl β-D-Glucopyranoside

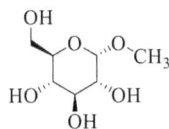

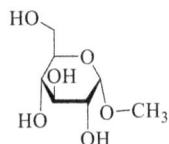

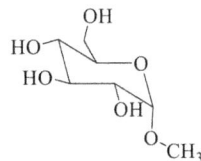

Methyl α-D-Glucopyranoside

Figure 8.29 The methyl ether of glucose at the C-1 position is shown for the two anomeric forms using different models.

9 Organic Macromolecules in Cellular Structures, Metabolism, and as Drugs: From Fatty Acids to Complex Lipids and Fats

Learning Objectives

After completing this chapter, you are expected to be able to:

- Explain the chemical composition of glycerides and their role in biological systems such as structures of cell membranes.
- Explain the chemistry of arachidonic acid as a source of biological mediators and how its metabolism can be targeted by drugs.
- Provide an overview of the lipid chemical composition of animal cell membranes.
- Explain how liposomes can be used in drug delivery.

9.1 Overview of Lipids – Functional Aspects

Traditionally, the term 'lipid' is associated with fats and oil or their fatty acid components. Lipid, however, refers to non-polar biomolecules that are insoluble in water and rather dissolve in non-polar

Basic Chemistry for Life Science Students and Professionals: Introduction to Organic Compounds and Drug Molecules
By Solomon Habtemariam
© Solomon Habtemariam 2023
Published by the Royal Society of Chemistry, www.rsc.org

solvents. Hence membrane components such as sterols and food ingredients such as vitamins (vitamins A, D, E, and K), fatty acids and their glyceride derivatives, and phospholipids are all lipids. Plant carotenoids and plant essential oils (fragrant molecules), which are highly non-polar in nature, can also be classified as lipids. In this chapter, the emphasis is to overview the chemistry of fatty acids and their glycerides or fatty acid esters of glycerol. Membrane lipids also include sterols and are addressed here. In Figure 9.1, the structures of the fatty acid oleic acid in its free form and its glycerol ester are shown. An ester formed from glycerol and fatty acids is called an *acyl-glycerol* or *glyceride*, and for oleic acid, acylation can occur at any site of the three hydroxyl groups of the glycerol structure to yield mono-acylated derivatives (monoglycerides), or it can also be acylated at two sites to make diglycerides, or at three sites to make triglycerides.

Depending on the chemistry of the fatty acid components in glycerides, which may differ in the carbon lengths and the number and

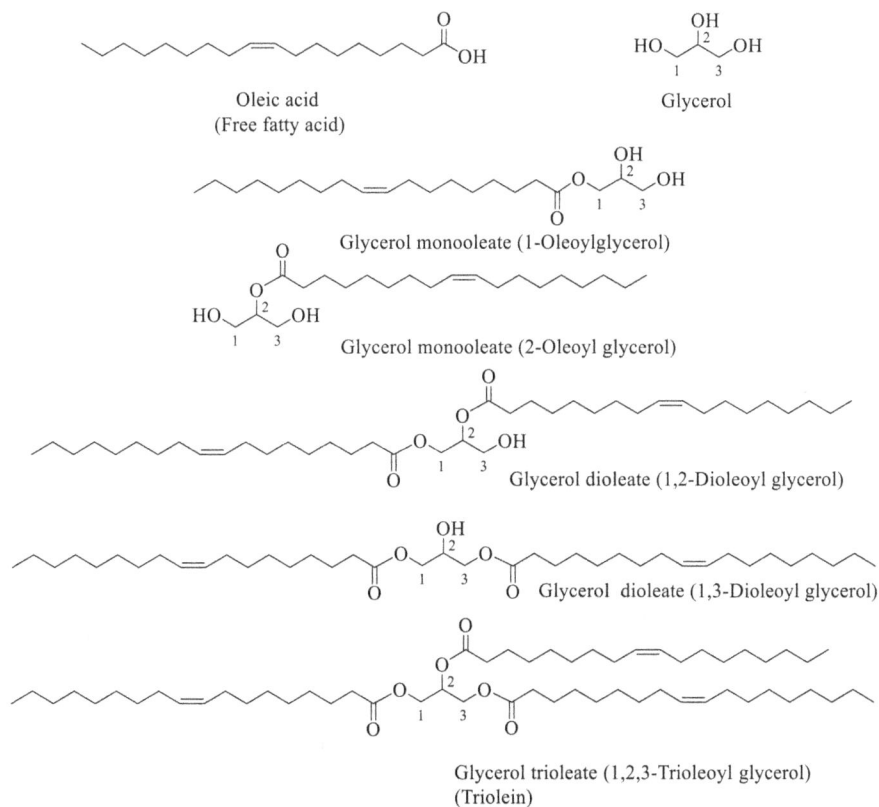

Figure 9.1 Structures of a fatty acid (oleic acid), glycerol, and glycerides.

nature of double bonds (*e.g. cis versus trans* configurations), glycerides can vary including in their physical appearance as fats and oils. In the following sections, we review the various types of fatty acids that contribute to the physical, chemical, and biological properties of fats and oils.

9.2   Introduction to Fatty Acids

Fatty acids consist of a long hydrocarbon chain ($-CH_2-CH_2-$) with a carboxyl group located at the terminal carbon of the molecule. The hydrocarbon chain can be saturated or unsaturated (containing double bonds), depending on the origin of the fatty acid. Organic acids with 1–5 carbon atoms (methanoic acid to pentanoic acid) are sometimes called volatile fatty acids. The short-chain carboxylic acids (fewer than six carbons) are not considered fatty acids because of the lack of a long hydrophobic chain that gives the lipid property of fatty acids, *i.e.* it leaves the polar carboxyl group to dominate in the physical properties of the molecule. For example, methanoic and ethanoic acids are highly soluble in water. As the carbon chain length increases, the non-polar property predominates over the polar influence from the carboxyl group, and they become lipid soluble or lipophilic (see Chapter 5). Fatty acids therefore include carboxylic acids with C_6–C_{24} carbon chains, while C_{25}–C_{40} chains are called long-chain fatty acids. In summary, fatty acids of lipids are acyl chain compounds composed of a carboxylic acid at one end and a methyl group at the other end and they differ from each other in one or more of the following ways:

- the number of carbon atoms in the long hydrophobic chain;
- the number of carbon–carbon double bonds (C=C) that they contain;
- the stereochemistry of the double bond (*cis versus trans*);
- the position of double bonds in the chain.

9.3   Saturated Fatty Acids

A list of some saturated fatty acids is given in Table 9.1. For the sake of convenience, fatty acids with C_3–C_5 carbon chain lengths are also included. Milk contains butyric (butanoic) and caproic (hexanoic) acids. Plant oils (*e.g.* palm kernel oil) are sources of C_8 and C_{10} fatty acids. In Nature, the biosynthetic pathway of fatty acid synthesis dictates an even number of carbon atoms. However, fatty acids with odd

Table 9.1 List of saturated fatty acids.[a]

Common name	Systematic name	Structural formula	Lipid number
Propionic acid	Propanoic acid	CH_3CH_2COOH	C3:0
Butyric acid	Butanoic acid	$CH_3(CH_2)_2COOH$	C4:0
Valeric acid	Pentanoic acid	$CH_3(CH_2)_3COOH$	C5:0
Caproic acid	Hexanoic acid	$CH_3(CH_2)_4COOH$	C6:0
Enanthic acid	Heptanoic acid	$CH_3(CH_2)_5COOH$	C7:0
Caprylic acid	Octanoic acid	$CH_3(CH_2)_6COOH$	C8:0
Pelargonic acid	Nonanoic acid	$CH_3(CH_2)_7COOH$	C9:0
Capric acid	Decanoic acid	$CH_3(CH_2)_8COOH$	C10:0
Undecylic acid	Undecanoic acid	$CH_3(CH_2)_9COOH$	C11:0
Lauric acid	Dodecanoic acid	$CH_3(CH_2)_{10}COOH$	C12:0
Tridecylic acid	Tridecanoic acid	$CH_3(CH_2)_{11}COOH$	C13:0
Myristic acid	Tetradecanoic acid	$CH_3(CH_2)_{12}COOH$	C14:0
Pentadecylic acid	Pentadecanoic acid	$CH_3(CH_2)_{13}COOH$	C15:0
Palmitic acid	Hexadecanoic acid	$CH_3(CH_2)_{14}COOH$	C16:0
Margaric acid	Heptadecanoic acid	$CH_3(CH_2)_{15}COOH$	C17:0
Stearic acid	Octadecanoic acid	$CH_3(CH_2)_{16}COOH$	C18:0
Nonadecylic acid	Nonadecanoic acid	$CH_3(CH_2)_{17}COOH$	C19:0
Arachidic acid	Eicosanoic acid	$CH_3(CH_2)_{18}COOH$	C20:0
Heneicosylic acid	Heneicosanoic acid	$CH_3(CH_2)_{19}COOH$	C21:0
Behenic acid	Docosanoic acid	$CH_3(CH_2)_{20}COOH$	C22:0
Tricosylic acid	Tricosanoic acid	$CH_3(CH_2)_{21}COOH$	C23:0
Lignoceric acid	Tetracosanoic acid	$CH_3(CH_2)_{22}COOH$	C24:0
Pentacosylic acid	Pentacosanoic acid	$CH_3(CH_2)_{23}COOH$	C25:0
Cerotic acid	Hexacosanoic acid	$CH_3(CH_2)_{24}COOH$	C26:0
Carboceric acid	Heptacosanoic acid	$CH_3(CH_2)_{25}COOH$	C27:0
Montanic acid	Octacosanoic acid	$CH_3(CH_2)_{26}COOH$	C28:0
Nonacosylic acid	Nonacosanoic acid	$CH_3(CH_2)_{27}COOH$	C29:0
Melissic acid	Triacontanoic acid	$CH_3(CH_2)_{28}COOH$	C30:0
Hentriacontylic acid	Hentriacontanoic acid	$CH_3(CH_2)_{29}COOH$	C31:0
Lacceroic acid	Dotriacontanoic acid	$CH_3(CH_2)_{30}COOH$	C32:0
Psyllic acid	Tritriacontanoic acid	$CH_3(CH_2)_{31}COOH$	C33:0
Geddic acid	Tetratriacontanoic acid	$CH_3(CH_2)_{32}COOH$	C34:0
Ceroplastic acid	Pentatriacontanoic acid	$CH_3(CH_2)_{33}COOH$	C35:0
Hexatriacontylic acid	Hexatriacontanoic acid	$CH_3(CH_2)_{34}COOH$	C36:0
Heptatriacontylic acid	Heptatriacontanoic acid	$CH_3(CH_2)_{35}COOH$	C37:0
Octatriacontylic acid	Octatriacontanoic acid	$CH_3(CH_2)_{36}COOH$	C38:0
Nonatriacontylic acid	Nonatriacontanoic acid	$CH_3(CH_2)_{37}COOH$	C39:0
Tetracontylic acid	Tetracontanoic acid	$CH_3(CH_2)_{38}COOH$	C40:0

[a]The table includes the first C_3–C_5 carboxylic acids of the homologous series that are not normally included in the list of fatty acids.

carbon number chains are also found in small amounts in animal tissues, and they are common in microorganisms.

In the nomenclature of fatty acids, they are referred to by the carbon number in the chain, for example, C16 for the C_{16} fatty acid palmitic acid. The number of double bonds can also be indicated and, in the case of saturated fatty acids, with no double bonds, a zero entry is used, *e.g.* C16:0 for palmitic acid. As the number of carbon atoms in the chain increases, say above eight, saturated fatty acids occur as solids and an increase in carbon number also means a corresponding increase in their melting points.

Of the saturated fatty acids, C16:0 (palmitic acid) and C18:0 (stearic acid) are the most common fatty acids in Nature or living organisms. The palmitic acid composition of animal fat is known to reach up to 30% whereas in plants its composition varies with its abundance known in palm oil. Vegetable oils contain a significant proportion of stearic acid. Milk fats and animal tissues generally contain C_4–C_{12} fatty acids, whereas medium-chain fatty acids occur in seed oils.

9.4 Unsaturated Fatty Acids

Fatty acids that carry double bonds are called unsaturated, those with one double bond in the molecule are monounsaturated, and those with two or more double bonds are polyunsaturated fatty acids (see Figure 9.2). The presence of a double bond in a molecule means that they occur as liquids and are mostly found in vegetables and fish oils. Some oils, such as olive, peanut, and canola oils, predominantly contain monounsaturated fatty acids, whereas fish oils (*e.g.* salmon) and soybeans contain significant amounts of polyunsaturated fats.

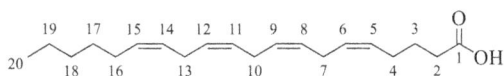

Arachidonic acid

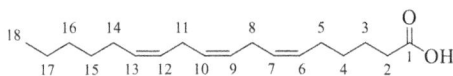

Gamma-Linolenic acid

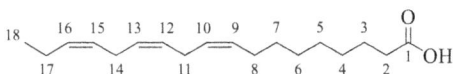

Alpha-Linolenic acid

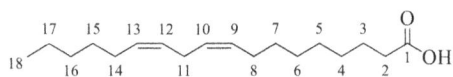

Linoleic acid

Figure 9.2 Examples of polyunsaturated fatty acids. Note their *cis* configuration.

Table 9.2 Examples of unsaturated fatty acids and their nomenclature.

Systematic name	Trivial name	Shorthand designation
cis-9-Hexadecenoic	Palmitoleic	16:1(n-7)
cis-9-Octadecenoic	Oleic	18:1(n-9)
trans-9-Octadecenoic	Elaidic	18:1(n-9)
cis-15-Tetracosenoic	Nervonic acid	24:1(n-9)
11-Octadecenoic	*cis*-Vaccenic	18:1(n-7)
all-*cis*-9,12-Octadecadienoic	Linoleic	18:2(n-6)
all-*cis*-9,12,15-Octadecatrienoic	α-Linolenic	18:3(n-3)
all-*cis*-6,9,12-Octadecatrienoic	γ-Linolenic	18:3(n-6)
all-*cis*-8,11,14-Eicosatrienoic	Dihomo-γ-linolenic	20:3(n-6)
all-*cis*-8,11,14,17-Eicosatetraenoic	ETA	20:4(n-3)
all-*cis*-5,8,11,14-Eicosatetraenoic	Arachidonic	20:4(n-6)
all-*cis*-5,8,11,14,17-Eicosapentaenoic	EPA	20:5(n-3)
all-*cis*-7,10,13,16-Docosatetraenoic	Adrenic	22:4(n-6)
all-*cis*-7,10,13,16,19-Docosapentaenoic		22:5(n-3)
all-*cis*-4,7,10,13,16-Docosapentaenoic	DPA	22:5(n-6)
all-*cis*-4,7,10,13,16,19-Docosahexaenoic	DHA	22:6(n-3)

In their nomenclature (Table 9.2), *cis* or *trans* and the site of double bonds are indicated in addition to the number of double bonds. For example, palmitoleic acid, which is found in marine algae and pine oil, has the systematic name *cis*-9-hexadecenoic acid or a designation of 16:1(n-7). The number of double bonds is indicated following the colon and n- refers to the position of the double bond from the methyl terminal end (omega). Similarly, oleic acid, which is the main component of olive oil and animal tissues, has the systemic name *cis*-9-octadecenoic acid. Natural fatty acids in mammals appear to have a *cis* configuration and, of particular importance in biological systems, are polyunsaturated from the C_{18} carbon chain length. This includes linoleic, γ-linolenic, and arachidonic acid that start their double bond from position 6 from the methyl end of the fatty acid chain (n-6 or omega-6 series), and α-linolenic, eicosapentaenoic, and docosahexaenoic acid with a double bond starting from position 3 from the methyl end (n-3 or omega-3) of the chain (Table 9.2).

In the pathophysiology of inflammation and anti-inflammatory therapeutics, the biology of arachidonic acid [20:4(n-6)] is very important. This fatty acid is an integral part of the cell membrane and is released due to the enzymatic action of phospholipase enzymes. An enzymatic action on arachidonic acid by enzymes such as cyclooxygenases and lipoxygenases leads to a series of biosynthetic pathways that form prostaglandins, leukotrienes, and thromboxanes in addition to other mediators of inflammation. Targeting this biosynthesis pathway by drugs such as aspirin is one way of controlling inflammation.

Arachidonic Acid Metabolism – Key Facts

- Arachidonic acid is a 20-carbon polyunsaturated omega-6 fatty acid that is found abundantly in cell membrane phospholipids.
- It is a precursor of groups of inflammatory mediators collectively called eicosanoids: prostaglandins (PGs), thromboxanes, leukotrienes, *etc.*
- It is released by the enzymatic action of phospholipases (*e.g.* phospholipase A_2), which is a target for steroidal anti-inflammatory drugs.
- Cyclooxygenase, which converts arachidonic acid to prostaglandins (PGs) such as PGE_2 (a potent vasodilator and pain inducer), is a target for aspirin-like anti-inflammatory drugs.
- Lipoxygenases, which convert arachidonic acid to leukotrienes (potent chemotactic factors for leukocytes) are also targets for anti-inflammatory drugs.
- Thromboxane synthase in platelets generates thromboxane, which is a platelet activator and enhances thrombus formation – thrombosis.
- Arachidonic acid metabolism is important in both health and disease.

Some of the fatty acids of biological importance or those serving as precursors for the synthesis of relevant fatty acids must be obtained from a dietary source as they are not produced in the body. These are *essential fatty acids* and include linoleic acid (omega-6) and α-linolenic acid (omega-3). As opposed to the *cis* configuration of fatty acids in mammals, microorganisms including the gut microflora of ruminants (cattle, sheep, and goats) produce *trans*-fatty acids. In the human diet, the main source of *trans*-fatty acids is, however, due to partial hydrogenation of fats in the manufacture of products such as margarine. This is a process of making semi-solid fats by removing double bonds in fatty acids through a hydrogenation reaction. The process, however, also results in the formation of *trans*-fatty acids (the so-called *trans* fats), which are considered unhealthy.

Saturated fatty acids, such as stearic acid (18 carbons) and palmitic acid (16 carbons), are solids at room temperature whereas unsaturated fatty acids, such as linoleic acid (18 carbons with two double bonds at positions 9 and 12) occur as liquids. This is due to the non-straight (often called 'kink') structure of unsaturated fatty acids that is not ideal for the stacking of molecules through good intermolecular attractions, *i.e.* the molecular shapes of double bonds with a *cis* configuration distort the structure of the long chain (see Figure 9.3),

Arachidic acid

Arachidonic acid

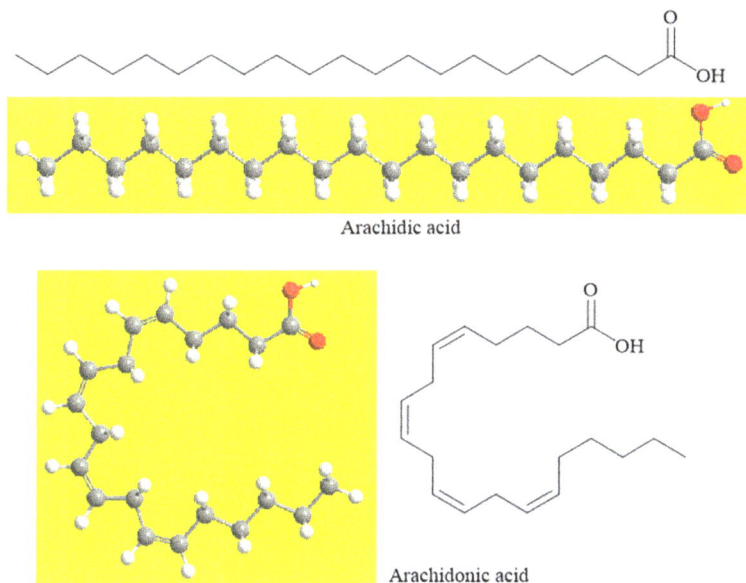

Figure 9.3 Structure of a *cis* configuration leading to a non-straight or kink structure.

resulting in the inability of the molecules to pack closely together. The melting points of unsaturated fatty acids are also lower than those of the saturated analogues for the same reason.

9.5 Physical Properties of Fatty Acids

A common property of fatty acids as with fats and oils is that they are hydrophobic or water-hating molecules. Each fatty acid also has two regions of phases: the carboxylic acid, which is polar and hence a water-loving region, and the hydrocarbon chain, which is a water-hating region. As already described, the hydrophobic nature of fatty acids in general predominates and they appear as lipophilic. When confronted with water, the two regions of fatty acids assemble to form a *micelle* with the carboxyl region facing outside on the water side and the hydrophobic region hidden in a ball-like structure (see Section 9.10).

9.6 Chemical Properties of Fatty Acids

In biochemistry and physiology, we address how fatty acids are absorbed, transported in the body, stored in special sites, and metabolised, including in energy generation reactions. In chemical reactions, we only investigate the two components of the structures: the carboxyl lipophilic and long-chain hydrophobic regions. This can be summarised as follows.

9.6.1 Acidity

The carboxylic acid region gives the fatty acid molecules their weak acid character. They are generally non-polar, however, and this feature increases with increase in the length of the hydrocarbon chain.

9.6.2 Hydrogenation Reaction

As discussed for alkenes (Chapter 4), addition reactions are possible for unsaturated fatty acids. A hydrogenation reaction of fatty acids is applied in practice in order to make liquid lipids (unsaturated) have a hardened physical appearance *via* saturation.

9.6.3 Autoxidation

In the presence of air or oxygen, unsaturated fatty acids can oxidise. This involves free radical chemistry (Chapter 3), leading to the formation of lipid peroxy radicals and lipid hydroperoxides. Cell membranes are particularly liable to oxidation by free radical formation under various physiological and pathological conditions. This is also the reason why we need antioxidants as therapy to remove the deleterious effects of free radicals on cell membranes and other biological molecules such as DNA. The presence of trace heavy metals and light, particularly ultraviolet (UV) light, increases the oxidation process of fatty acids. The three stages (see Chapter 3) of radical generation (initiation), propagation, and termination also apply in this case:

1. *Initiation:*

$$RH \rightarrow R^{\bullet}$$

   A radical ($R^{\bullet}$) is formed from the molecule, say by irradiation with UV light.

2. *Propagation:*

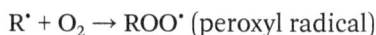

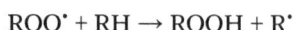

$$R^{\bullet} + O_2 \rightarrow ROO^{\bullet} \text{ (peroxyl radical)}$$

$$ROO^{\bullet} + RH \rightarrow ROOH + R^{\bullet}$$

3. *Termination:*

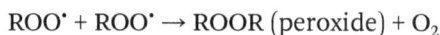

$$ROO^{\bullet} + ROO^{\bullet} \rightarrow ROOR \text{ (peroxide)} + O_2$$

$$R^{\bullet} + R^{\bullet} \rightarrow R\text{-}R \text{ (two fatty acid molecules can dimerise)}$$

$$R^{\bullet} + ROO^{\bullet} \rightarrow ROOR$$

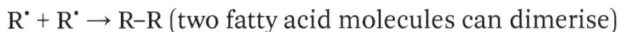

Note that, in biological systems, the regulated oxidation of fatty acids in the mitochondria, called *β-oxidation*, is a key process in the generation of energy and metabolic intermediates. This enzyme-catalysed oxidation is different from a*utoxidation*, or the free radical chemistry described above.

9.7 Glycerides

As indicated in the previous section, glycerides are acylglycerols, which are formed by the esterification of glycerol with fatty acids at any of the three hydroxyl positions. Depending on the degree of esterification, we can have monoacylglycerols, diacylglycerols, or triacylglycerols. Different combinations of these acylated forms and variations in fatty acid composition occur in a given fat or oil of natural origin. For example, plants usually store lipids in the form of triglycerides. Extraction of these lipids from plants such as cereals gives a unique composition specific to that species. Oleic acid (C18:1) and linoleic acid (C18:2) are common fatty acid compositions of glycerides in sunflower, sesame, grapeseed, and soybean oil. Whereas olive oil predominantly contains oleic acid (over 70%), grapeseed and soybean oils have a greater amount of linoleic than oleic acid, sunflower oil has more oleic than linoleic acid, and sesame oils have similar amounts of these two fatty acids. These plant oils have small but different proportions of palmitic, palmitoleic, arachidonic, linolenic, and behenic acid. The actual list of the fatty acid content of glycerides that can be detected in each oil is, however, very long.

9.8 Cell Membrane Lipids

9.8.1 Glycerophospholipids

Being the predominant lipid forms in cell membranes, glycerophospholipids (Figure 9.4) are composed of fatty acid esters of glycerol at positions C-1 and C-2, while the third hydroxyl group of the glycerol is esterified by phosphoric acid (phosphate ester). Hence even more than fatty acids, glycerophospholipids have a well-defined molecular phase in terms of polarity. They are thus truly *amphipathic*, with

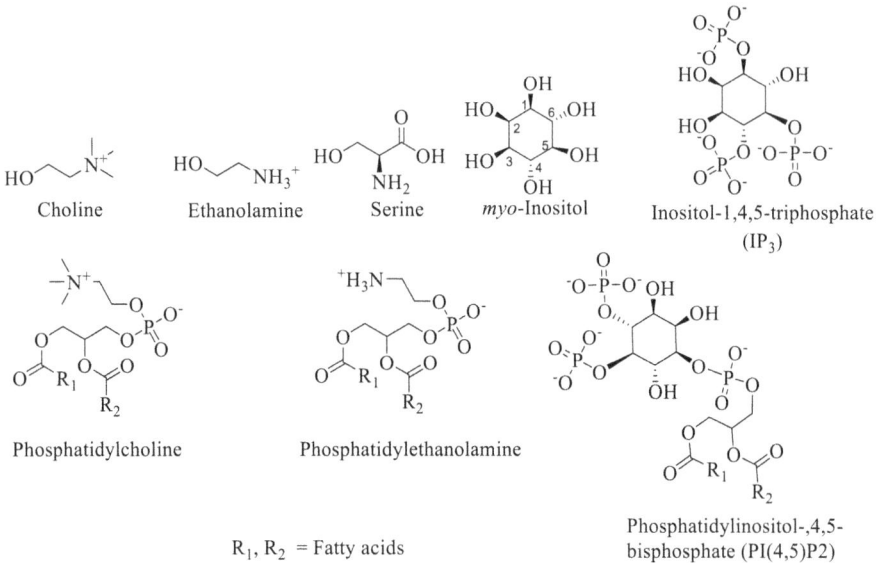

Figure 9.4 Structures of some glycerophospholipids. Common derivatives containing choline, ethanolamine, serine, or inositol are shown. Note that PI(4,5)P$_2$ has a fatty acid component mostly of saturated (*e.g.* stearic acid) at the C-1 and arachidonic acid (unsaturated) at the C-2 position of glycerol. The inositol head of PI(4,5) P$_2$ is further phosphorylated at positions 4 and 5. Enzymes such as phospholipase C act on PI(4,5)P$_2$ to release diacylglycerol and IP$_3$ – second messengers to many signalling molecules.

a polar region or water-loving head of the glycerol and phosphate end, and a non-polar hydrophobic region. The chemical diversity of glycerophospholipids is based on which fatty acid from numerous possibilities is attached to the two fatty acid ester sites of the glycerol. One should therefore assume thousands of possibilities with the C-1-hydroxy ester of glycerol mostly bearing saturated fatty acids and the C-2 position mostly bearing unsaturated fatty acids (*e.g.* arachidonic acid). Although not very common, two fatty acids either saturated or unsaturated at the glycerol (C-1 and C-2) positions also occur as esters. The most common saturated fatty acid esters of phosphatidylcholine, at C-1, are palmitoyl and stearoyl and, at C-2, linolenoyl. In the case of phosphatidylethanolamine, the C-2 fatty acid esters differ but are mostly C$_{20}$ and C$_{22}$ unsaturated acids. Stearic acid is a common fatty acid ester at C-1 and arachidonic acid at C-2 for phosphatidylinositols (Figure 9.4).

Further structural diversity in glycerophospholipids comes from substituents of the phosphate group: one of the OH groups of the phosphate is esterified to make derivatives of glycerophospholipids. Good examples are phosphatidylcholines (the amino alcohol *choline* added to the phosphate group) and phosphatidylethanolamines (amino alcohol ethanolamine derivatives) (Figure 9.4). *Phosphatidylcholine* and *phosphatidylethanolamine* are also called *lecithin* and *cephalin*, respectively. These substituents, just like amino acids, have negative and positive charge sites (dipolar ions, zwitterions) with a net charge of zero. Other derivatives such as phosphatidic acid, phosphatidylserine, and phosphatidylinositol have a net negative charge. The overall charge and amphipathic nature of glycerophospholipids depend on the fatty acid composition and phosphate derivatives. It is worth noting that cell membranes also contain *phosphatidylinositol bisphosphate*, which carries three phosphate groups with additional phosphate groups located at the C-4 and C-5 positions of inositol. This is a precursor to the most diverse cell signalling system molecules, diacylglycerol and inositol 1,4,5-trisphosphate. These are second messenger molecules released to mediate the action of diverse signalling molecules such as hormones and neurotransmitters. The binding of certain hormones/neurotransmitters to their cell surface receptors leads to the release of diacylglycerol and inositol trisphosphate, leading to a physiological response specific to the signalling molecule. By being attached to proteins in cell membranes, glycerophospholipids are also involved in the cell signalling system. In addition to cell membranes, they are also present in very small amounts in fat stores.

Inositol 1,4,5-Trisphosphate (IP_3) – Key Facts

- Serves as a second messenger for many growth factors, hormones, and neurotransmitters.
- Formed from phosphatidylinositol 4,5-bisphosphate.
- Causes a rapid release of calcium ions (Ca^{2+}) from intracellular stores such as endoplasmic reticulum by opening Ca^{2+} channels.
- Ca^{2+} then activates a biological process – in smooth muscles, it causes contraction.

Upon contact with water, glycerophospholipids spontaneously aggregate. This process of micelle formation, however, does not occur in biological membranes as the lipids take more of the lamellar (layered) structures instead of spherical micelles. The water-facing side both inside and outside the cell membrane is where the hydrophilic heads are located whereas the hydrocarbon core is buried inside to create an overall lipid bilayer structure. These molecules arrange in a double layer, with their polar heads facing the aqueous medium (either the cytosol or the external medium bathing the cell) and the non-polar acyl chains are oriented towards the membrane interior (Figure 9.5). The physicochemical properties of glycerophospholipid molecules contribute to the shape and function of cell membranes. This attribute is due to their amphipathic or amphiphilic nature with

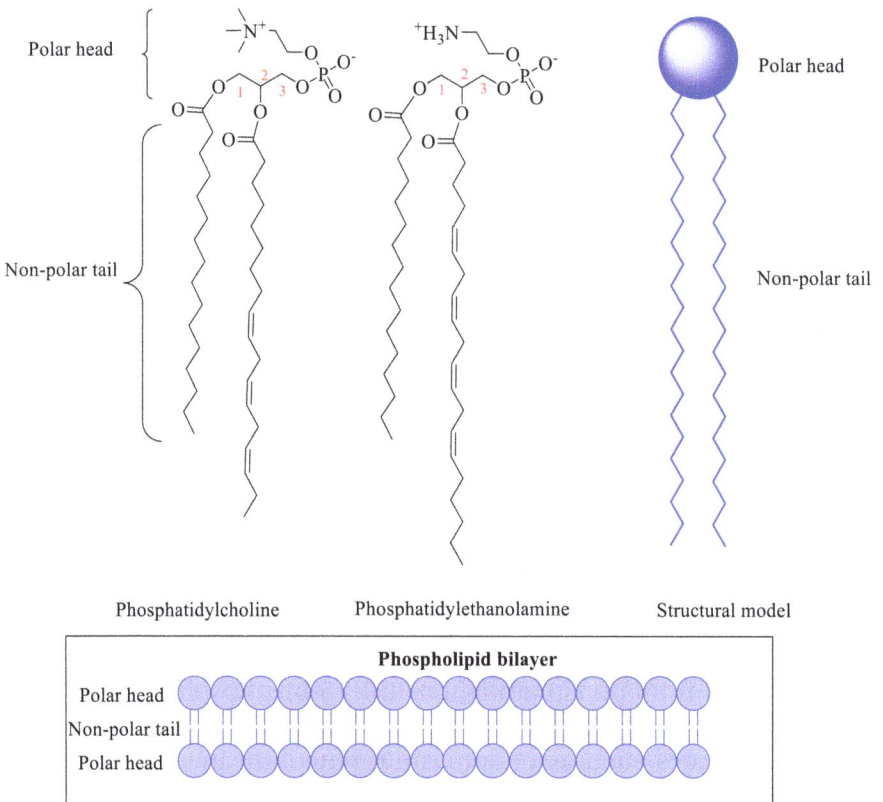

Phosphatidylcholine   Phosphatidylethanolamine   Structural model

Phospholipid bilayer

Figure 9.5 Examples of phospholipids and their physicochemical properties. Phospholipids with a phosphatidylcholine structure containing palmitoyl (C-1) and linolenoyl (C-2) and also phosphatidylethanolamine with a palmitoyl (C-1) and arachidonoyl (C-2) structure are shown. The polar head of hydroxyl and the charged centre and non-polar tail of the hydrocarbon structural model are shown. The image of the phospholipid bilayer (lipid bilayer) as a major component of the cell membrane structure is shown in the box.

a distinct polar head and a non-polar tail. The polar head is associated with the phosphoryl acid moiety that carries free hydroxyl groups that are negatively charged and the basic nitrogen of the amino alcohol. On the other end, a non-polar region is based on the tails of the long hydrocarbon chains of the fatty acids.

9.8.2 Sphingolipids

Another class of lipid components of cell membranes is sphingolipids. Their structure is based on *sphingosine*, which is an 18-carbon amino alcohol with an unsaturated hydrocarbon chain, although (to a lesser extent) a 20-carbon *phytosphingosine* can also occur. To this structural skeleton, a sugar unit or *sphingomyelin* (a phosphorylcholine group) is attached at C-1 (see Figure 9.6). In the latter case, the structure is like that of phosphatidylcholine. Since sphingolipids

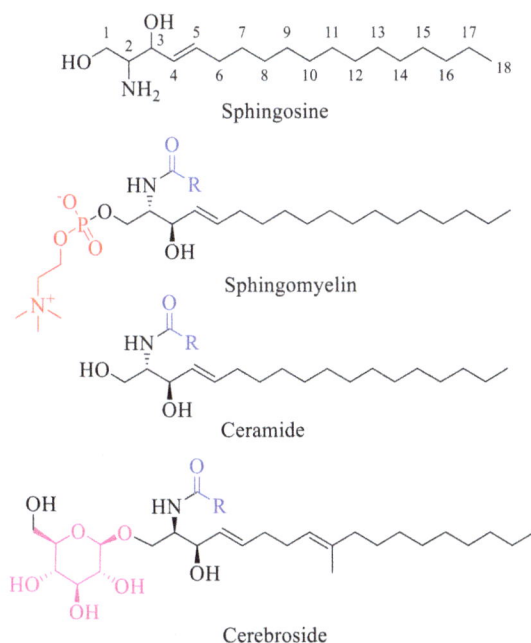

Figure 9.6 Structures of sphingolipids. Note that sphingomyelins differ structurally from phosphatidylcholine by having *N*-acylsphingosine (ceramide) instead of 1,2-diacylglycerol. Cerebrosides are composed of ceramide and a monosaccharide (*e.g.* glucose or galactose) attached *via* a β-glucosidic bond. Although found in small amounts in cell membranes of many tissues, cerebrosides are abundant in the white matter of the brain and myelin sheaths.

have a fatty acid attachment to the amino group of the sphingosine skeleton, they are also amphipathic in nature. A classic example of sphingolipids is sphingomyelin (Figure 9.6), which is a common phospholipid derivative found in cell membranes. Hence the structural difference between phospholipids and sphingolipids is the presence of the lipophilic amino alcohol group in sphingolipids instead of glycerol. Polar sugar units may be attached to sphingosine to make them glycosphingolipids (also called *cerebrosides*), which could be either neutral sugars or with a few sialic acid residues (called *gangliosides*) to make them recognition sites in outer cellular membranes for cell–cell signalling. Hence sphingolipids generally serve as attachment sites for drugs, antigens, and hormones. They play a crucial role in cellular transduction pathways and regulation of cell survival, growth, and differentiation. Derivatives of sphingolipids are ceramides (Figure 9.6), which are metabolic products of the Golgi apparatus and endoplasmic reticulum membranes.

9.8.3 Sterols

Sterols are a class of lipophilic compounds in cell membranes of all living organisms. In plants, they are collectively called *phytosterols* and include three major constituents, β-sitosterol, campesterol, and stigmasterol. In microorganisms (excluding bacterial cell membranes) and fungi, they are called mycosterols, whereas in animals they are sometimes referred as zoosterols with the principal component being cholesterol. All these sterols have a common structural skeleton with a tetracyclic skeleton, a double bond at C-5, and a hydroxyl group at C-3 (Figure 9.7). All steroids in living organisms are synthesised through a terpenoid biosynthesis pathway with five-carbon isoprene units as a building block. In the case of sterols, six isoprene units are assembled to form a triterpene with a tetracyclic structure of the steroid skeleton (see Chapter 13). In animals, steroid hormones and bile acids are also made through a similar biosynthesis pathway. The lipid-soluble vitamins (A, D, E, and K), phytol (a lipid component of the photosynthetic pigment chlorophyll), the insect juvenile hormones, plant hormones (gibberellins), and polyisoprene (the major component of natural rubber) are all examples of the biosynthetic pathway of terpenes. The structures of some common sterols are shown in Figure 9.7.

In terms of polarity, sterols, including cholesterol, are highly lipophilic and the polarity attributes of the hydroxyl group are negligible. As a result, they do not form aggregates in water on their own

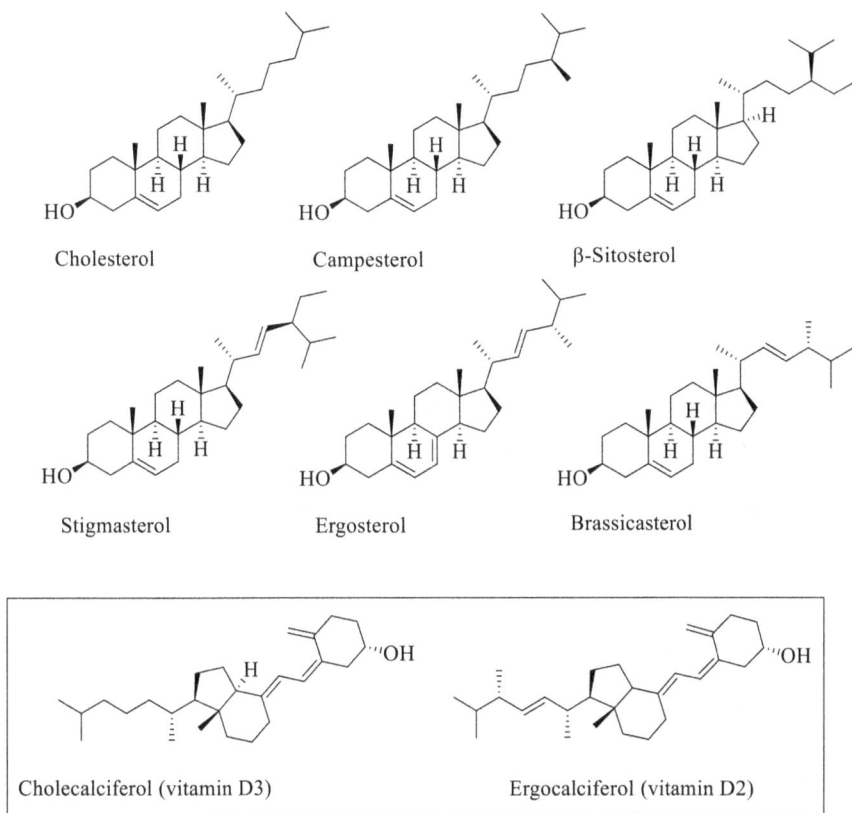

Cholesterol   Campesterol   β-Sitosterol

Stigmasterol   Ergosterol   Brassicasterol

Cholecalciferol (vitamin D3)   Ergocalciferol (vitamin D2)

Figure 9.7 Structures of some common sterols and vitamin D. Vitamin D represents a group of fat-soluble sterol derivatives of mainly vitamin D_2 (ergocalciferol), which is derived from the plant sterol ergosterol, and vitamin D_3 is synthesised in the skin from 7-dehydrocholesterol upon exposure to UV light.

but assemble with the hydrophobic region of the phospholipid membrane bilayer.

9.9 Lipid-based Drugs

Since lipophilicity as a physiochemical characteristic is a general feature that is shared by numerous organic compounds, drug classification such as lipid-based or non-lipid-based drugs is not a useful discussion topic. Many lipophilic drugs such as statins act by interfering with the biosynthetic pathways of lipids such as cholesterol. By inhibiting the key enzyme 3-hydroxy-3-methylglutaryl-coenzyme A (HMG-CoA) reductase (see Section 13.3.1.1) in the synthesis of cholesterol, statins and related drugs have clinical applications in the treatment of a range of cardiovascular diseases. Through inhibition of lipid digestion in the gut, many lipophilic drugs such as orlistat also have antiobesity potential. With respect to the management of obesity with drugs, the digestion of fats in the gut, their absorption, their transportation in the blood, their processing in the liver, and storage sites are all targets for drugs. The level of lipoproteins is also worth mentioning, especially low-density lipoprotein, which mainly transports cholesterol and hence needs to be checked to the lower limit by various therapeutic approaches.

As drug therapy, the lipid components of membranes that are key to cell signalling, cell function, and cell–cell communications serve as targets. These include the second messenger system associated with cell signalling *via* a receptor-mediated action of hormones and neurotransmitters. Interfering with the binding of lipid-based cell surface interaction with antigens can serve as a mechanism for denying entry of intracellular parasites or the infiltration of inflammatory cells to extravascular sites. Hence understanding the biology and chemistry of cell membrane lipids helps in the design of novel drugs for treating human diseases.

In addition to their role as structural components of cell membranes, phosphatidylinositol and other phosphoglycerides function as a reservoir of arachidonic acid, which is the precursor of bioactive lipid-based signalling molecules such as prostaglandins, leukotrienes, and thromboxanes. These compounds are also involved in numerous pathological disorders from chronic inflammation to thrombosis and cardiovascular diseases. The *platelet activating factor* (PAF), or 1-*O*-alkyl-2-acetylglycerylphosphorylcholine, is a kind of glycerophospholipid that triggers platelet aggregation. It is a target for drugs to rectify platelet dysfunction in a range of pathological conditions.

In terms of targeting lipids by drugs (Figure 9.8), we have three main areas, described in the following subsections.

9.9.1   Lipid Digestion

The digestion of dietary fats in the gastrointestinal system is aided by a range of enzymes collectively called lipases. In the process, triacylglycerols or triglycerides are converted to fatty acids and glycerol. As a therapeutic intervention to obesity or hyperlipidaemic conditions, we can use drugs to suppress the digestion of lipids in the gut by inhibiting lipases and hence limiting their availability to the blood. The prototype drug is orlistat.

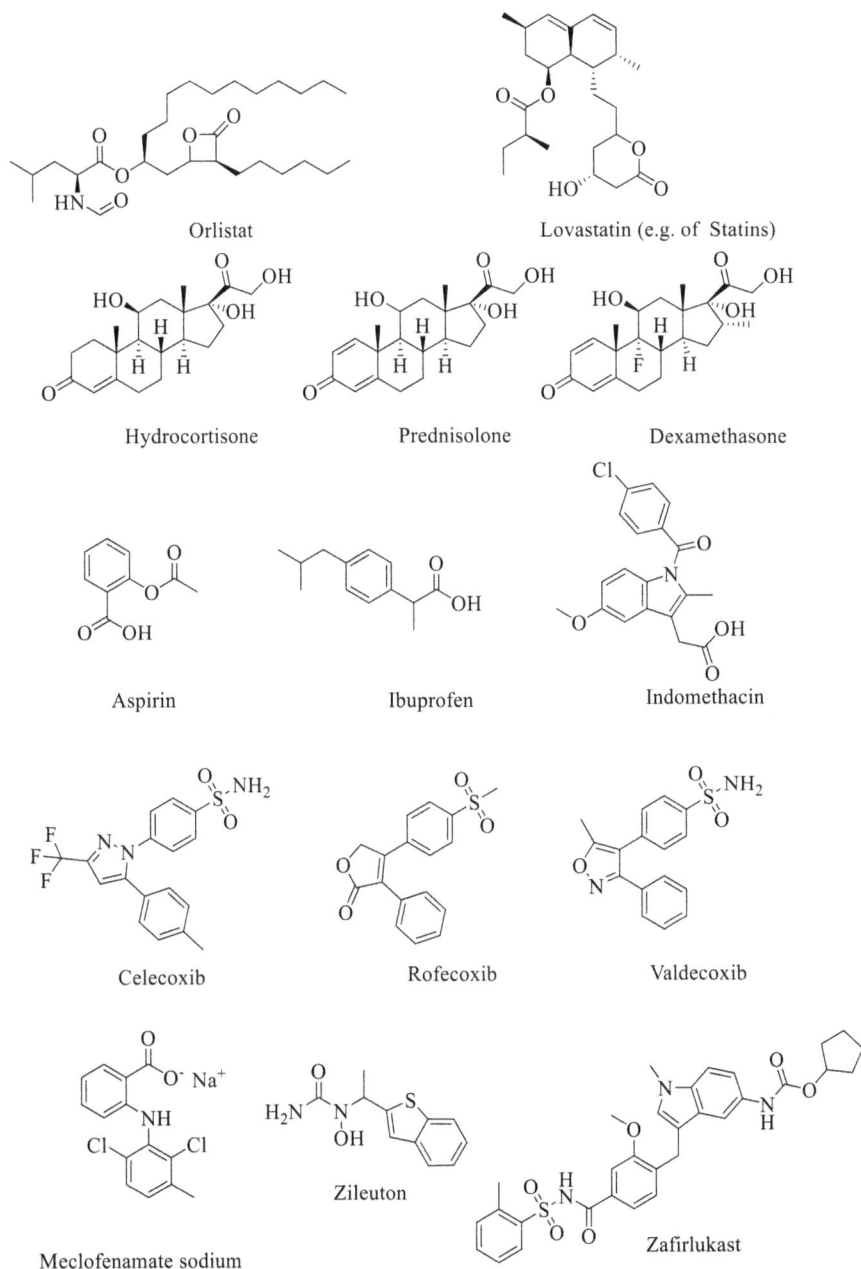

Figure 9.8 Examples of drugs that modulate lipid mediators. Note that statin is a generic name for the group of compounds serving as medicines by targeting cholesterol synthesis. The structure of only one drug, lovastatin, is shown here.

Orlistat is a prototype antiobesity drug that works by inhibiting the activity of pancreatic lipases, thereby inhibiting fat digestion. Cholesterol-lowering agents have a profound effect in the management of cardiovascular diseases and the protype drug, statin, inhibits cholesterol synthesis by targeting a key enzyme (HMG-CoA). The formation of prostaglandin mediators, particularly prostaglandin E, which is also a pain inducer, can be inhibited through inhibition of the key enzyme cyclooxygenase (COX). The enzyme has two isoforms: COX-1, which is present all the time, and COX-2, which is induced during inflammation and must be targeted by drugs. Older drugs such as aspirin, ibuprofen, and indomethacin are non-selective inhibitors, whereas the newer anti-inflammatory drugs such as celecoxib, rofecoxib, and valdecoxib are selective inhibitors of COX-2. Hence selective inhibitors have fewer side effects than aspirin-like drugs. Meclofenamate sodium and zileuton are inhibitors of leukotriene synthesis from arachidonic acid by inhibiting the enzyme 5-lipoxygenase, and zafirlukast is a leukotriene receptor antagonist. The release of arachidonic acid from phospholipids is mediated by phospholipase enzymes and can be inhibited by steroidal drugs such as hydrocortisone, prednisolone, and dexamethasone.

9.9.2 Cholesterol Metabolism

This is discussed in detail in Chapter 13 and the key or rate-limiting step in the synthesis of cholesterol is targeted by drugs such as statins. These drugs have a profound effect on cardiovascular diseases.

9.9.3 Arachidonic Acid Metabolism

The release of arachidonic acid from its cell membrane store by phospholipase A_2 and related enzymes is the first step in the synthesis of inflammatory lipid mediators. This can be targeted by steroidal anti-inflammatory drugs (Figure 9.8) that inhibit phospholipases. Once released, arachidonic acid is acted upon by a variety of enzymes to generate lipid-based inflammatory mediators. Several drugs, including aspirin, act on these enzymes and the overall mechanism can be summarised as follows:

- Arachidonic acid is a 20-carbon polyunsaturated fatty acid that is incorporated in cell membranes (glycerophospholipids).
- Arachidonic acid is released from the plasma membrane by the action of enzymes such as phospholipases A_2, C, and D.

- The two main enzymes that act on arachidonic acid are cyclooxygenases and lipoxygenases.
- Cyclooxygenase converts arachidonic acid to endoperoxides, which are used to synthesise prostaglandins, prostacyclin, and thromboxane (Figure 9.9). These are potent mediators of inflammation.
- Drugs such as aspirin and indomethacin inhibit cyclooxygenase and block the synthesis of prostaglandins (inflammatory mediators) and thromboxane (potent platelet aggregation inducer with implications in thrombosis).
- Inhibiting cyclooxygenase (COX) is the main mechanism of action of the non-steroidal anti-inflammatory drugs (NSAIDs)

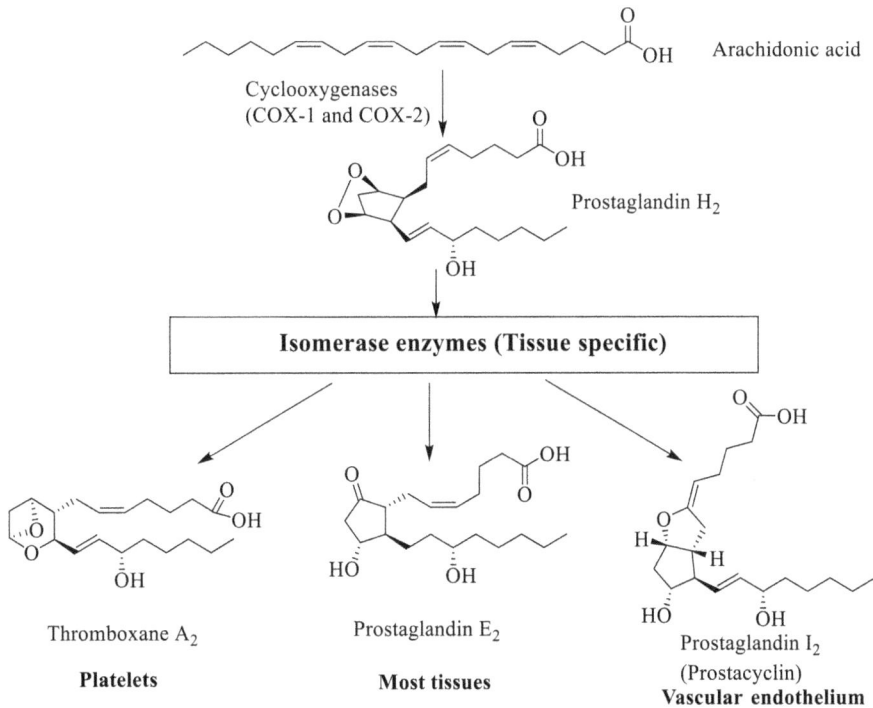

Figure 9.9 Examples of cyclooxygenase (COX) products. Arachidonic acid is processed by COX enzymes to form an intermediate prostaglandin H_2. In the various tissues, isomerase enzymes further act on prostaglandin H_2 to form specific products. For example, thromboxane A_2 is the main product in platelets that is implicated in thrombosis. The vascular endothelium is the main site of prostaglandin I_2 (prostacyclin), which is a vasodilator. Prostaglandin E_2 is produced as an inflammatory mediator in various tissues. Note that there are also other prostaglandin mediators in various tissues.

such as aspirin (see Figure 9.8). Some drugs (celecoxib, rofecoxib, and valdecoxib) are selective to COX-2, which is induced during inflammation and hence is a valid target, whereas others (aspirin, ibuprofen, and indomethacin) are non-selective and inhibit COX-1, which is constitutively expressed or involved in normal body functions (*e.g.* gastrointestinal and kidney functions).

- Lipoxygenase enzymes act on arachidonic acid to form leukotrienes, which are also inflammatory mediators (Figure 9.10). These are a family of lipid-peroxidising enzymes and act on arachidonic acid with their products leukotrienes being implicated in asthma and many other diseases such as inflammation and cancer. There are several isoforms of the enzymes such as the 5-, 12-, and 15-lipoxygenases that facilitate the peroxidation reaction at the indicated site of the arachidonic acid molecule. They are inhibited by lipoxygenase inhibitors (see Figure 9.8) such as meclofenamate sodium and zileuton (both are inhibitors of one type of lipoxygenase, 5-lipoxygenase). The effect of leukotrienes can also be inhibited by using selective inhibitors of their receptors such as zafirlukast (Figure 9.8).

9.10   Lipids in Drug Delivery

Lipids have wide applications in drug delivery systems where drugs are formulated by dissolving or suspending them in lipid excipients. The lipids used for such purposes include glycerides, polyglyceryl/polyalcohol esters, and polyoxyglycerides. These lipids are amphiphilic in nature and can form variable structures in an aqueous medium (Figure 9.11). These include emulsions (>500 nm), microemulsions (10–200 nm), micelles (2–10 nm), or molecular dispersions (<1 nm). By using this technology, drugs that are poorly soluble in water can be formulated using lipid excipients, or intestinal permeability is increased, or the degradation of the drug may be avoided (*e.g.* degradation of peptides by proteases), *etc.* Such formulations may also bypass metabolism by the liver.

Other types of aggregates are also formed in water by certain amphipathic lipids. For example, liposomes are artificial collections of lipids arranged in a bilayer, having an inside and an outside surface (Figure 9.12). The lipid bilayers forming a sphere can trap a molecule inside. The liposome structure can be useful for protecting sensitive molecules that are to be delivered orally.

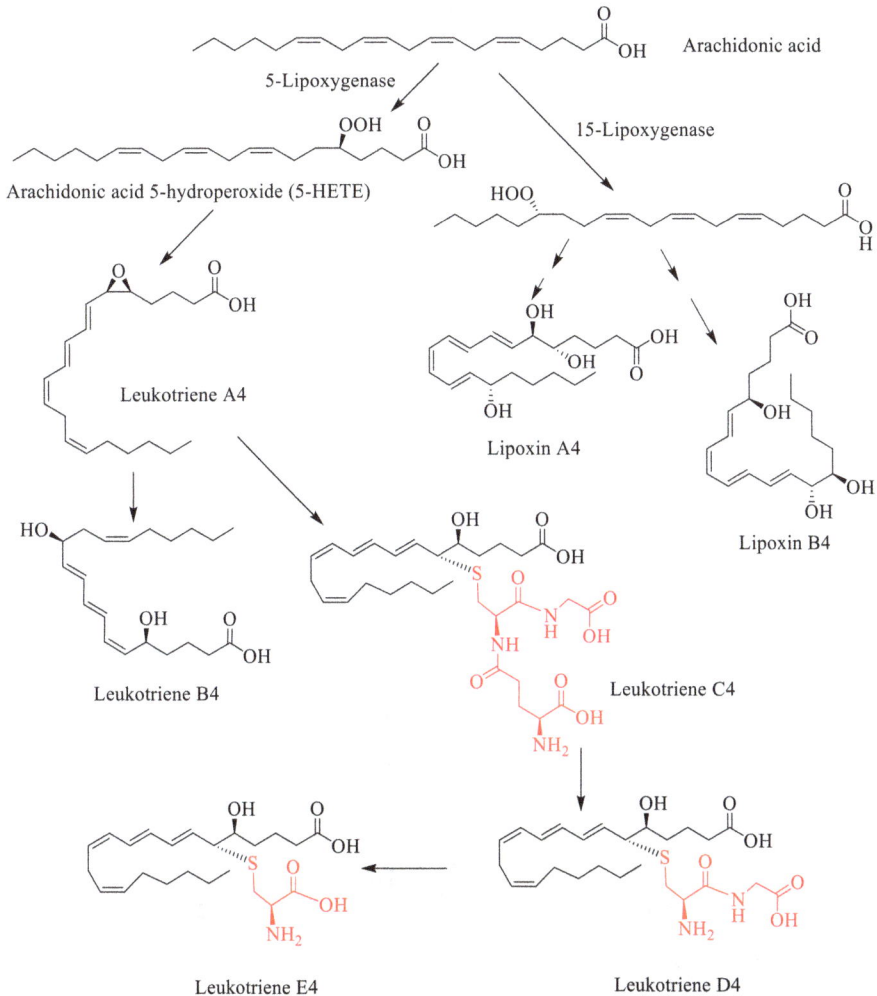

Figure 9.10 Lipoxygenase products. Lipoxygenases are a group of enzymes that incorporate the hydroperoxyl group into a double bond. We have tissue specificity: 5-lipoxygenase common in leukocytes, 12-lipoxygenase common in platelets, and 15-lipoxygenase common in eosinophiles. They make 5-, 12-, and 15-hydroperoxyeicosatetraenoic acid. Lipoxins A_4 and B_4 have anti-inflammatory properties and are made during the end of the inflammatory period after tissue injuries. The 5-lipoxygenase pathway is important in neutrophil-mediated inflammation. Note the structural differences of leukotrienes and the presence of amino acids in leukotrienes C_4, D_4, and E_4.

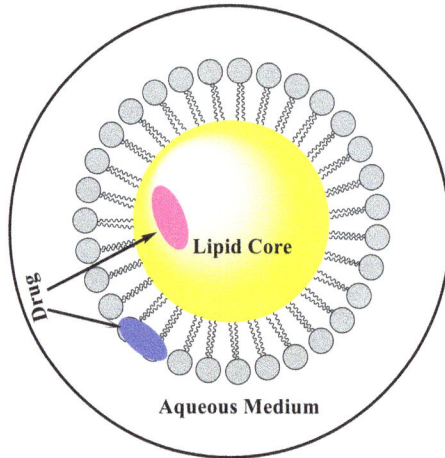

Figure 9.11 Schematic representation of an emulsion. A drug may be loaded in an emulsion by staying in the lipid core or interacting with the hydrophilic components at the outer surface.

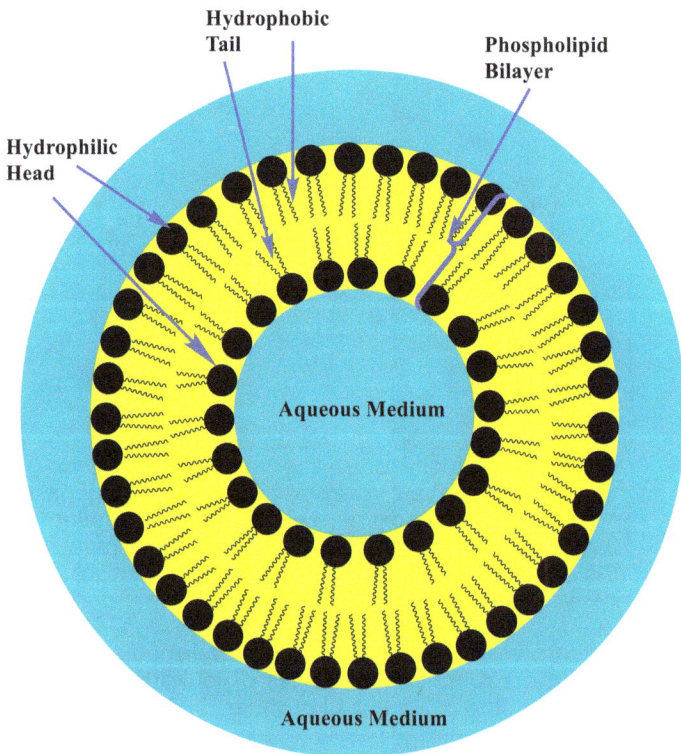

Figure 9.12 Schematic representation of a liposome. Note the lipid bilayer structure that allows hydrophilic drugs to be loaded in the aqueous central core while lipophilic drugs can be trapped in the lipid tail (hydrophobic) region.

9.11 Summary

In this chapter, we have learned the following:

- Acylglycerols or glycerides are structurally fatty acid esters of glycerol.
- Glycerides differ from each other based on the number of fatty acids (mono-, di-, or triglycerides) or the fatty acid composition (which fatty acid is attached to glycerol).
- Fatty acids are grouped into saturated and unsaturated fatty acids.
- Most unsaturated fatty acids occurring in Nature have *cis* double bond configurations.
- The packing of molecules of fatty acids in a *cis* configuration is less tight than that for saturated structures or those with a *trans* configuration.
- Most unsaturated fatty acids occur as liquids whereas saturated fatty acids are mostly in solid or semi-solid forms.
- Unsaturated fatty acids differ from each other not only in the number of double bonds but also in the position of double bonds within the molecules, *e.g. n*-6 and *n*-3 fatty acids.
- Arachidonic acid is a 20-carbon polyunsaturated omega-6 fatty acid stored in cell membranes. It is a precursor to many biologically active metabolites such as inflammatory mediators.
- Unsaturated fatty acids can undergo a hydrogenation reaction to make a saturated or solid (or semi-solid) form of fatty acids. Industrial processing of this kind can lead to some *trans*-fatty acid products which are considered unhealthy.
- Fatty acids have head and tail or lipophilic and hydrophobic ends – called amphipathic in nature.
- Lipids and fats are general terms to refer to non-polar compounds.
- Membrane lipids include fatty acids and their glycerides or fatty acid esters of glycerol and sterols.
- The common sterol in animal cell membrane is cholesterol – it occurs in esterified form.
- Fatty acids are long-chain hydrocarbon compounds with a carboxyl functional group terminus.
- The two common saturated fatty acids are C16:0 (palmitic acid) and C18:0 (stearic acid).
- Polyunsaturated fatty acids of the *n*-6 or omega-6 series include γ-linolenic and arachidonic acids.
- Polyunsaturated fatty acids of the *n*-3 or omega-3 series include α-linolenic, eicosapentaenoic, and docosahexaenoic acids.

- Unsaturated fatty acids are vulnerable to free radical attack – they oxidise.
- Glycerophospholipids are truly amphipathic compounds with well-defined polar and non-polar regions.
- Phosphatidylcholine and phosphatidylethanolamine are examples of glycerophospholipids.
- The hydroxyls of the phosphate group can be esterified to make derivatives of glycerophospholipids, *e.g.* phosphatidylcholines, phosphatidylethanolamines, phosphatidic acid, phosphatidylserine, and phosphatidylinositol.
- Choline, ethanolamine, serine, and inositol are common derivatives incorporated into glycerophospholipids.
- The metabolism of lipids is important in health and disease – it can be targeted by various drugs.
- Targeting lipid digestion by using drugs against lipases is a therapeutic approach in obesity and hyperlipidaemia.
- An anti-cholesterol approach in cardiovascular disease management by statins aims to inhibit cholesterol synthesis.
- Arachidonic acid metabolism is targeted by a range of drugs, including cyclooxygenase and lipoxygenase inhibitors.
- Lipids have a role in transporting drugs – liposomes are common forms that allow the delivery of drugs such as proteins and DNA, which would otherwise not be delivered orally.

9.12   Problems

1. Glycerol belongs to which functional group?
2. In what way do the functional groups in glycerol differ from each other?

Questions 3–7. When glycerol reacts with a carboxylic acid:

3. What kind of bond is formed?
4. What would the product be?
5. If the reaction involves just one fatty acid, how many products can be formed?
6. Name the two groups present in the structures of fatty acids.
7. Why do we say fatty acids are amphipathic?

Questions 8–14. Stearic acid, oleic acid, and linoleic acid are all fatty acids made from 18 carbons:

8. What is the difference between stearic acid and the other two fatty acids?

9. What is the difference between oleic acid and linoleic acid?
10. What is the similarity between oleic acid and linoleic acid?
11. Stearic acid occurs as a solid whereas oleic and linoleic acids are liquids. Why?
12. The melting point of stearic acid is 68.8 °C, oleic acid 29.2 °C, and linoleic acid 8.5 °C. Explain the difference.
13. Which two compounds readily undergo a hydrogenation reaction and what would the product be?
14. In the hydrogenation reaction, what side products could be formed?
15. α-Eleostearic acid [(9Z,11E,13E)-octadecatrienoic acid] and β-eleostearic acid [(9E,11E,13E)-octadecatrienoic acid] are both made from 18-carbon fatty acids and have three conjugated double bonds at positions C-9, C-11, and C-13. The difference is that α-eleostearic acid has one double bond (C-9) *cis* whereas all the others are similar (*trans*). Which one do you expect to have a higher melting point?
16. A 20-carbon fatty acid with four double bonds that are involved in the inflammation pathway is called _____?
17. α-Linolenic and γ-linolenic acids have the same number of carbon atoms and the same number of double bonds. What is the difference between the two?

Questions 18–21. Phosphatidic acid (PA) is a simple phospholipid from which more complex phospholipids can be formed. It is a phospholipid that possesses two acyl chains of fatty acids:

18. In what way do the phospholipids differ from each other?
19. What is the difference between phosphatidic acid and that incorporating choline (phosphatidylcholine) or ethanolamine (phosphatidylethanolamine)?
20. In what way is inositol 1,4,5-trisphosphate incorporated in the cell membrane and what is its relevance?
21. What is the main physicochemical property of glycerophospholipids?
22. Cholesterol is found in all animal cell membranes and is needed for their proper functioning, including membrane permeability and fluidity. Where within the lipid bilayer do you expect to find cholesterol?
23. Define the structural groups or functional groups of a sphingosine.
24. What is the structural similarity and difference between sphingomyelin and phosphatidylcholine?

25. What is the structural difference between ceramide and cerebroside?
26. Name the main sterol present in the cell membrane.

Questions 27–30 are based on the inhibition of the enzyme phospholipase A_2:

27. What is the main class of drugs that target the enzyme phospholipase A_2?
28. To which cell membrane component does the structure of these drugs relate?
29. What is the structural analogue of a hormone in the body to which these drugs relate?
30. What would be the level of free arachidonic acid after taking these drugs?
31. What structural group is formed by cyclooxygenase enzymes?
32. What structural group is formed by lipoxygenase enzymes?
33. What is the main difference in the products catalysed by 5-lipoxygenase and 15-lipoxygenase?
34. Which leukotriene has an epoxide functional group (an oxygen atom joined by single bonds to two adjacent carbon atoms)?
35. Which leukotrienes contain cysteine in their structures?
36. Which leukotrienes contain glycine in their structures?
37. Which leukotriene contains glutamic acid in its structure?
38. What are the two main functional groups in orlistat (Figure 9.8)?

Questions 39–43 are based on phospholipid vesicles used as a means of drug delivery:

39. Phospholipid vesicles consisting of one or more concentric lipid bilayers enclosing discrete aqueous spaces are called _____?
40. Suggest how hydrophobic drugs are transported by these vesicles.
41. Suggest how hydrophilic drugs are transported by these vesicles.
42. Suggest how macromolecules such as DNA and proteins are delivered using this formulation.
43. What is the advantage of this delivery system?

9.13   Solutions to Problems

1. Alcohol.
2. Two primary and one secondary alcohol functional groups.
3. Ester.
4. Glyceride or acylglycerol.

5. Three: mono-, di-, and triglycerides or monoacylglycerols, diacylglycerols, and triacylglycerols.
6. A hydrocarbon tail and carboxy head group.
7. The carboxylic acid can be ionisable and give a negatively charged carboxylate group, which interacts with the polar solvent, whereas the non-polar hydrocarbon chain interacts with the hydrophobic groups.
8. Stearic acid is saturated whereas the others are unsaturated fatty acids.
9. Oleic acid is monounsaturated whereas linoleic acid is polyunsaturated.
10. Both have a *cis* configuration of their double bond.
11. The *cis* double bond in oleic acid makes a kink or bend that prevents the molecules from packing together tightly. Hence many fatty acids with *cis* double bonds occur as liquids at room temperature.
12. The same reason as the answer to question 11. More *cis* double bonds in the molecule mean that there is far less chance of molecular packing and hence they occur as liquids, or have lower melting points.
13. Unsaturated fatty acids (oleic acid and linoleic acid) undergo a hydrogenation reaction – they can be converted to stearic acid.
14. *trans* fatty acids can be formed – partial hydrogenation.
15. The *trans* (*E*) form means a straight chain as in the saturated fats and hence will have good packing of molecules – or a higher melting point with a greater tendency to make a solid form.
16. Arachidonic acid.
17. The difference is the position of the double bond, particularly n-6 (γ-linolenic acid) and n-3 (α-linolenic acid).
18. Difference in the fatty acid components, a further additional group attached to the phosphate group.
19. Phosphatidic acid is negatively charged whereas the other two carry both positive and negative charges (Figure 9.4).
20. Phosphatidylinositol 4,5-bisphosphate and its processing in cell signalling gives IP_3, which is a second messenger.
21. They have a well-defined polar head and non-polar tail – cell membrane structure.
22. It is non-polar, hence it is mostly found within the tail end of the phospholipid.
23. Alcohol, amine, and alkene.
24. The main similarity is the presence of phosphate and choline groups and a hydrocarbon chain; the difference is the presence of the amino group in sphingomyelin.

25. The presence of sugar in cerebroside (Figure 9.6).
26. Cholesterol.
27. Steroidal anti-inflammatory drugs (see Figure 9.8).
28. Cholesterol.
29. Cortisone.
30. Steroids suppress the release of arachidonic acid from the cell membrane store, so the free arachidonic acid level is reduced by the drugs.
31. They make endoperoxides.
32. They make hydroperoxides.
33. Site of addition of the hydroperoxide – 5-lipoxygenase adds at position 5 of the carboxylic acid whereas 15-lipoxygenase adds at the carbon-15 site.
34. Leukotriene A_4.
35. Leukotrienes C_4, D_4, and E_4.
36. Leukotrienes C_4 and D_4.
37. Leukotriene C_4.
38. Ester and amide.
39. Liposomes.
40. Hydrophobic molecules are inserted into the lipid bilayer structure.
41. Hydrophilic molecules can be entrapped in the aqueous centre.
42. The large size of the aqueous centre makes it possible to entrap larger molecules.
43. Liposomes protect compounds from early inactivation in the body or degradation by enzymes (*e.g.* in the gut) or dilution in the circulation. They are also non-toxic.

10 Organic Macromolecules in Cellular Structures, Metabolism, and as Drugs: From Nucleotides to Nucleic Acids

Learning Objectives

After completing this chapter, you are expected to be able to:

- Describe the chemical composition of nucleotides and how nucleotides are assembled to form nucleic acids (RNA and DNA).
- Understand the primary, secondary, and tertiary structures of DNA.
- Explain how drugs affect the structures and functions of nucleic acids.
- List the common drugs that target DNA and RNA.

10.1 Introduction to the Chemistry of Nucleic Acids

Living cells rely on macromolecules called nucleic acids that carry information on inherited characteristics and cellular functions, including protein synthesis. The two forms of nucleic acids are

Basic Chemistry for Life Science Students and Professionals: Introduction to Organic Compounds and Drug Molecules
By Solomon Habtemariam
© Solomon Habtemariam 2023
Published by the Royal Society of Chemistry, www.rsc.org

deoxyribonucleic acid (DNA) and ribonucleic acid (RNA). Except for some viruses that use RNA, all living cells and most viruses use DNA to keep and use their genetic information. On the other hand, RNA is present in all living cells and is primarily involved in the synthesis machinery of proteins. As proteins are polymers of monomeric amino acids, nucleic acids are polymers of *nucleotides*. Nucleotides as monomers or building blocks of nucleic acids are themselves composed of the following structural moieties:

- Carbohydrate residue of either *2-deoxy-*D*-ribose* in DNA or D*-ribose* in RNA. These are sugars of cyclic structures constructed from five-carbon skeletons or aldopentose forms and differ from each other by the presence or absence of a hydroxyl group at the C-2 position (Figure 10.1).
- Heterocyclic bases of purines (adenine and guanine) and pyrimidines (cytosine, thymine, and uracil). They are called bases because of the amine functional groups. The structures of these bases are shown in Figure 10.2. Both adenine and guanine, the purines, are found in both DNA and RNA. There are differences in the occurrence of the pyrimidines in nucleic acids, however. Whereas cytosine occurs in both DNA and RNA, uracil occurs only in RNA and thymine occurs only in DNA.
- Phosphate group – incorporated as phosphoric acid esters of the monosaccharides.

Structurally, a nucleotide (Figure 10.3) has a carbohydrate residue connected to a heterocyclic base by a β-D-glycosidic bond and to a phosphate group at the C-5' or C-3' position. The nucleotide structure without the phosphate group, purine or a pyrimidine base connected to ribose or a deoxyribose sugar *via* a β-glycosidic linkage is called a *nucleoside*.

Composition of DNA and RNA – Key Facts

- Base – DNA is made of two purines (adenine and guanine) and two pyrimidines (cytosine and thymine bases); RNA contains uracil instead of thymine, *i.e.* adenine, guanine, cytosine, and uracil.
- Sugar – DNA is made of 2-deoxy-D-ribose whereas RNA is made of D-ribose.
- Nucleoside – a base attached to a sugar with a β-glycosidic linkage.
- Nucleotide – a phosphate group attached to the 5'-position of a sugar of a nucleoside.

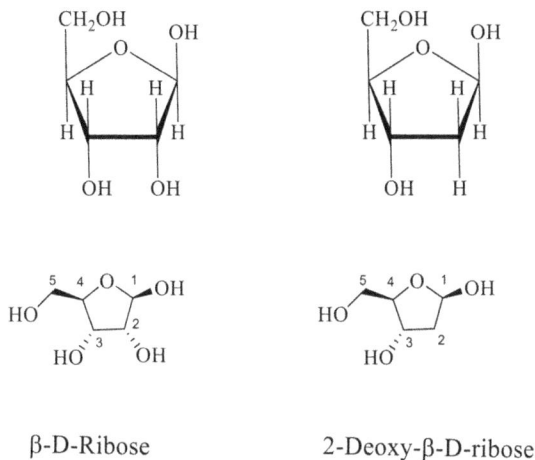

β-D-Ribose   2-Deoxy-β-D-ribose

Figure 10.1   Structures of the two nucleic acid sugars. 2-Deoxy-D-ribose is a component of DNA whereas D-ribose is a sugar in RNA. For the sake of clarity, the conformation of the sugars as Haworth projection formulae (top) is also shown.

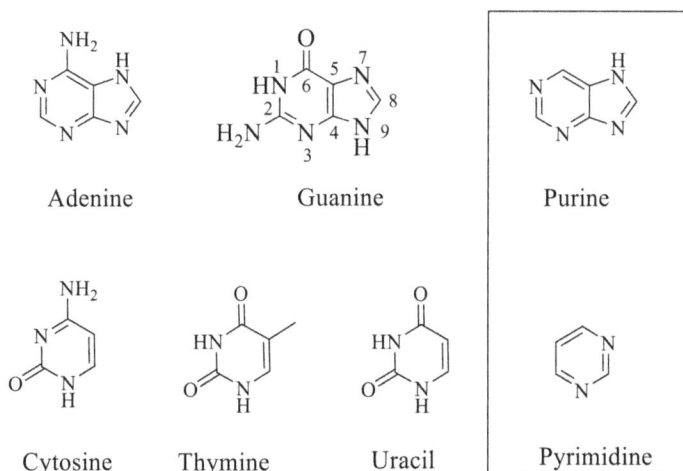

Adenine   Guanine   Purine

Cytosine   Thymine   Uracil   Pyrimidine

Figure 10.2   Structures of nucleic acid bases.

The biological aspects of nucleic acids and their biochemistry are beyond the scope of this book. This chapter is intended to highlight the basic chemistry of how nucleotides are assembled to form DNA or RNA structures. As explained above, uracil (U) is unique to RNA and thymine (T) to DNA, whereas adenine (A), guanine (G), and cytosine (C) occur in both RNA and DNA. In the formation of polymeric nucleotides, *polynucleotides*, the phosphate group at the 5'-hydroxyl group

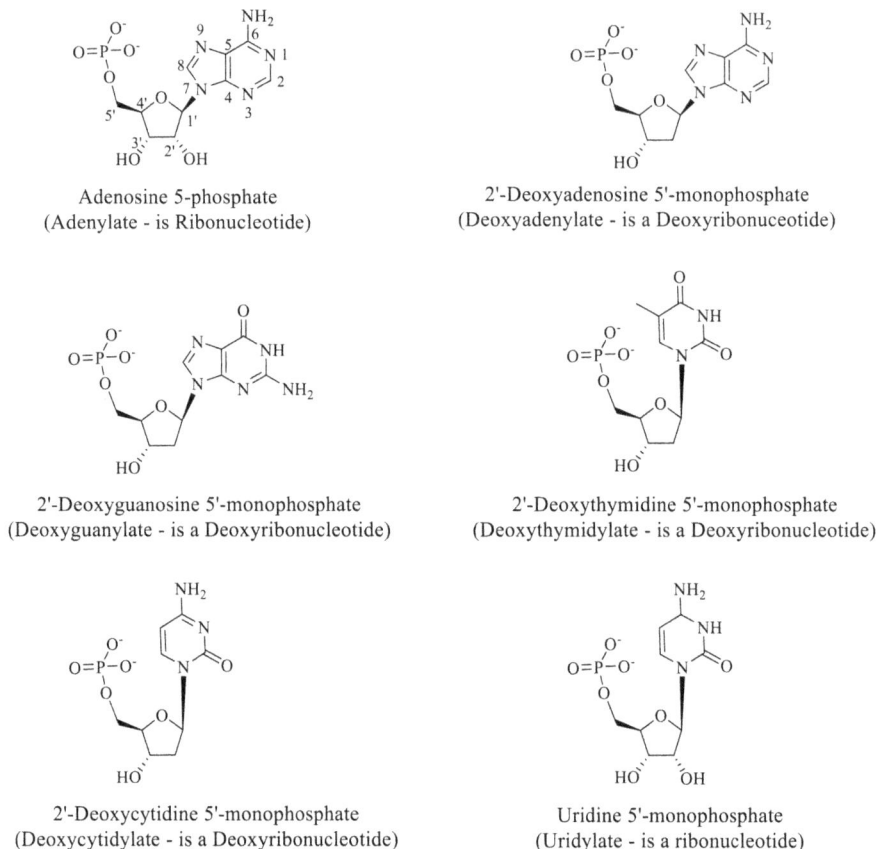

Adenosine 5-phosphate
(Adenylate - is Ribonucleotide)

2'-Deoxyadenosine 5'-monophosphate
(Deoxyadenylate - is a Deoxyribonuceotide)

2'-Deoxyguanosine 5'-monophosphate
(Deoxyguanylate - is a Deoxyribonucleotide)

2'-Deoxythymidine 5'-monophosphate
(Deoxythymidylate - is a Deoxyribonucleotide)

2'-Deoxycytidine 5'-monophosphate
(Deoxycytidylate - is a Deoxyribonucleotide)

Uridine 5'-monophosphate
(Uridylate - is a ribonucleotide)

Figure 10.3 Examples of nucleotides. Note that the heterocyclic base is numbered first, followed by the sugar (as prime numbers). The glycosidic bond in a nucleoside is between the anomeric carbon of the ribose sugar and the nitrogen in the base – also called a β-N-glycosidic bond. The hydroxyl groups of the phosphate group are charged at normal body pH and are shown in their ionised form.

of one sugar makes a bridge *via* the 3'-hydroxyl group of the next nucleotide sugar in the series (Figure 10.4). Whether the nucleic acid is RNA or DNA, the nucleoside linkages arise through *phosphodiester bond formation*. In the biosynthesis of nucleic acids, the phosphate group comes from adenosine triphosphate (ATP) through the enzymatic action of kinases. The nucleotide polymer formed through this process has discrete 5'- and 3'-phosphate attachment ends. In the formation of DNA, a pair of nucleotides are assembled through hydrogen bonding between two complementary bases: A : T and G : C

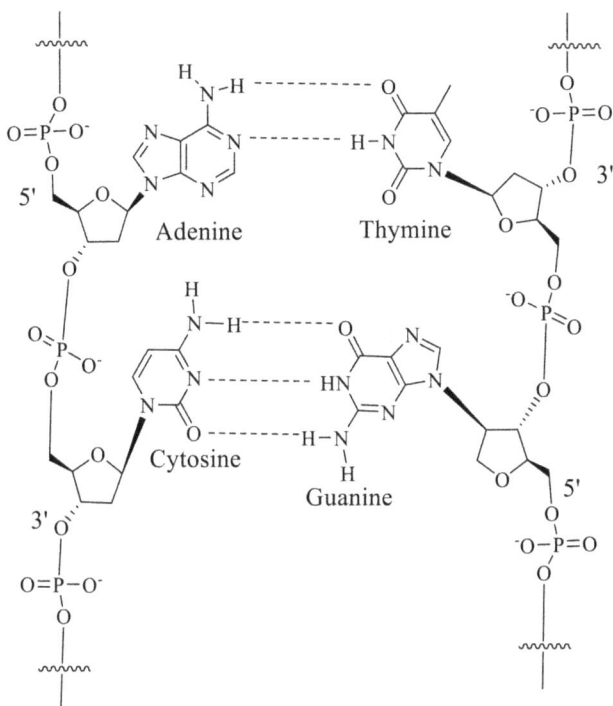

Figure 10.4   Phosphodiester and hydrogen bonding in DNA. Note that one of the hydroxyl groups in the phosphate group of a nucleotide reacts with the sugar of another nucleotide at the C-3 position. The resulting phosphodiester bond is similar in both RNA and DNA and makes a polymer of nucleotides assembled with 5′ and 3′ terminal ends. In the case of DNA, a duplex or double strand is formed due to hydrogen bonding between the complementary base pairs: A=T and G≡C.

pairs (Figure 10.4). These base pairs are what we call complementary pairs: A=T and G≡C.

10.2   DNA – Structural Considerations

The DNA structure as we know it today, both in the double-helical structural model and its function in self-replication and protein synthesis, has been associated with the famous discovery paper by James Watson and Francis Crick in 1953. The study of the chemistry and biology of these biomolecules, however, was begun by scientists at least a century earlier. The contribution of these and more recent studies to our understanding of cellular functions has further helped in designing drugs for numerous pathologies. As shown above, the building block of DNA is a nucleotide that is composed of a sugar deoxyribose attached to a base and phosphate group. A strand of DNA as a polymer is formed through a phosphate bridge between sugar molecules of the nucleotides, while the two strands come together through hydrogen bonding between the complementary base pairs. Hence the polynucleotide of DNA is formed by the phosphodiester bonds linking deoxyribose sugars of the nucleotides. A simplified DNA model is shown in Figure 10.5, including the double-helix structure that resembles a 'twisted ladder'.

In the same way as for proteins, the primary, secondary, and tertiary structures of DNA can be defined. The first source of variation in DNA comes in the form of the repeating units of nucleotides in the sequence that forms the *primary structure*. As with proteins or polypeptides, polynucleotides differ from each other based on the side chains, which are pyrimidine or purine bases. Note that we write polypeptides from left to right in the 5′ to 3′ direction. DNA is made of millions of nucleotides joined in a long chain. The pairing of A with T and

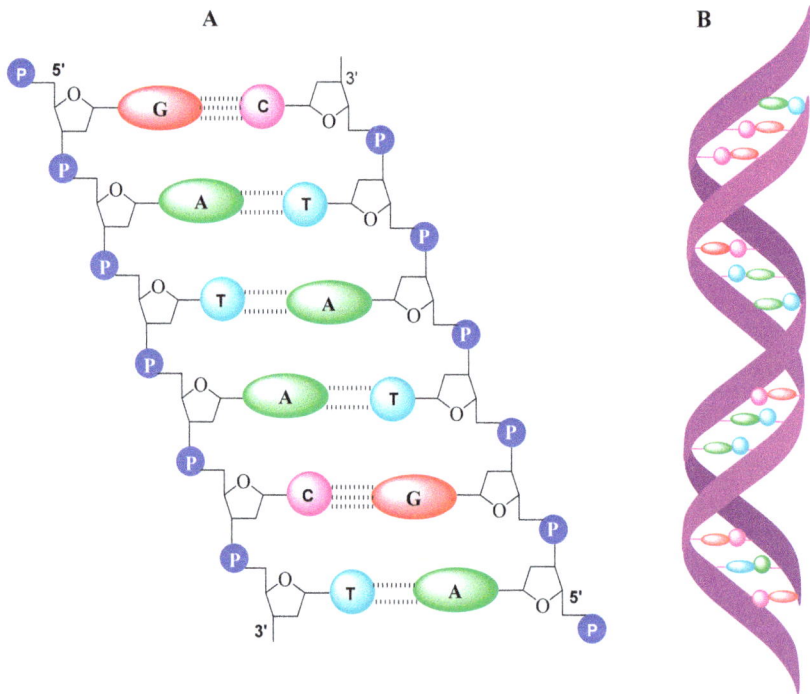

Figure 10.5 The structure of DNA. Variations in the DNA structure come from the nucleotides in the DNA and the order in which they are assembled. The atomic model (A) and the double-helix structure of DNA (ribbon model, B) are shown.

of G with C can form a sequence that is unique to the polynucleotide of DNA. The sugar with the associated phosphate groups is located on the outside of the molecule while the bases are held together through hydrogen bonding in the inside region. The phosphate group, which is ionised at normal body pH (7.4), is negatively charged and hence nucleotides have a net negative charge. It is worth noting that if the DNA is hydrolysed, the A:T ratio is 1:1 and similarly the G:C ratio is 1:1. Knowing the sequence in one strand can also indicate the composition of the complementary strand. Hence the complementary strand for GCTTAC should be CGAATG. The *secondary structure of DNA* is due to the hydrogen bonding between the complementary base pairs. Hence the secondary structure shows two strands of DNA, or two polynucleotides joined together to form the double helix. Visualising this double helix in a three-dimensional shape provides the *tertiary structure of DNA*.

DNA Structure – Key Facts

- Made of repeating units of nucleotides.
- Primary structure – linear sequence of nucleotides.
- Secondary structure – hydrogen bonding: G–C three bonds and A–T two bonds.
- Tertiary structures – 3D shape of the DNA double-helix coils.

From a functional point of view, one major aspect worth mentioning is what we call the *central dogma of molecular biology*: DNA makes RNA and in turn the RNA directs the synthesis of protein. Considering DNA as a massive polymer that does not move out of the nucleus, a chain of communication needs to be established to realise its commanding role in cellular functions, including the decision whether the cell should live or die. The message for protein synthesis in the DNA molecule is stored in a small section, hence activation of the entire genome is not required. To access this information centre of the DNA, the duplex DNA structure must first open (unzip), and the required region copied in the form of RNA in a process called *transcription*. The DNA then zips back to its original form. This RNA formed in the nucleus is a messenger (*messenger RNA*) and moves to the cytoplasm where its information in the ribosomes is read with three base pairs (*codon*) at a time. Each codon directs a specific amino acid that makes a peptide chain in the process of protein synthesis, *i.e.* RNA is translated into polypeptide chains of proteins.

For continued normal cellular functions, including replication, transcription in protein synthesis, and the repair process following chemical/physical damage, the structural integrity of DNA must be maintained. The housekeeping enzymes for this job include the group called DNA topoisomerases. These enzymes correct conformational changes in DNA topology by breaking and rejoining the DNA strands: a transient break in a single strand of DNA by type I DNA topoisomerases and double-strand breaks by type II DNA topoisomerases. Several other enzymes are involved in the DNA replication process and function. For example, *helicase* is involved in unzipping the DNA strands or simply splitting the base pairs. In the DNA synthesis process, two identical DNA duplexes are formed from each unzipped original DNA duplex through the enzymatic action of *DNA polymerase*. Nucleases generally serve as molecular scissors and cleave phosphodiester bonds between the sugars and the phosphate moieties of DNA. They play a role in the DNA repair process – which otherwise the cell would not be able to cope with – such as repairing continuous DNA damage by reactive oxygen species, radiation such as UV light, and other carcinogens. One can see that all these enzymes and biological processes involved in the normal function of DNA regulation can be altered in pathological conditions such as cancer and serve as therapeutic targets. The enzymes that are relevant in both health and disease and also in drug targeting are those involved in DNA replication:

- DNA helicase – unwinds the DNA (transient separation of duplex DNA) to facilitate DNA replication, transcription, or repair. The enzyme breaks down the hydrogen bonds between the complementary bases.
- DNA polymerase – making a covalent bond between nucleotides. Involved both in the synthesis of new DNA and in DNA repair.
- DNA clamp (sliding clamp) – proteins that tether polymerase enzymes to DNA.
- Topoisomerases or DNA gyrase – enzymes that remove positive and negative supercoils formed during the unwinding process of DNA by cutting and resealing one (topoisomerase I) or both (topoisomerase II) strands of the DNA duplex.
- DNA ligase – an enzyme that links matching ends of DNA strands, *i.e.* fragments of strands come together to form a long chain. It adds a phosphate group to the 5' end of one strand to link it to the hydroxyl group of the 3' end to make a phosphodiester linkage.
- Primase – an enzyme that synthesises short RNA sequences or primers.

Transcription is carried out using RNA polymerase, which synthesises RNA molecules from a template of DNA.

10.3 RNA – Functional Considerations

As already explained, RNA is a nucleic acid that is based on the heterocyclic nitrogenous bases A, G, C, and U. The U replaces T of the DNA structure. Unlike DNA, RNA is a single-stranded polymer. The various types of RNAs are considered below.

10.3.1 Messenger RNA (mRNA)

mRNA is formed from the gene segment of the DNA molecule with information specific to the type of protein to be synthesised by the cell. This genetic code information governs the amino acid sequence of protein synthesis within the ribosomes of the cytoplasm. The genetic code reflects the heterocyclic bases in the DNA sequence and hence any fault or change in the gene is reflected in the synthesis of a protein with the wrong amino acid sequence, which in turn affects the function of the protein or the enzyme. The four nucleotides (or bases) with a genetic code in triplicate can give rise to 64 different codes.

10.3.2 Ribosomal RNA (rRNA)

The ribosomes are the site of protein synthesis in the cytoplasm or simply the site of translation of the genetic code that is sent from the DNA (the nucleus) in the form of mRNA. Chemically, ribosomes are composed of rRNA and associated proteins to form the ribosomal structure or nucleoprotein. Composed of two subunits (50S and 30S in bacteria/prokaryotes and 60S and 40S forms in eukaryotes – two density forms), ribosomes carry enzymes and other accessories required for protein synthesis, *i.e.* amino acids complementary to the codon come together to form polypeptide chains. The primary role of rRNA is in protein synthesis, for which it binds with mRNA.

10.3.3 Transfer RNA (tRNA)

This is a relatively small polymer of about 75 nucleotides. In the synthesis of proteins in ribosomes, tRNA brings the amino acid that corresponds to the code (*i.e.* it reads the genetic code) and allows the incorporation of amino acids in the developing peptide chain of the protein. It is interesting to note how the genetic code is read by tRNA. The genetic code in mRNA in triplet bases is read by tRNA using an anticodon that matches the codon through complementary base pairs *via* hydrogen bonding. For example, the tRNA anticodon (GAG) reads the codon (CUC).

Protein Synthesis Inhibitors as Therapeutic Agents – Key Facts

- Many clinically useful antibacterial agents (*e.g.* erythromycin, tetracycline, chloramphenicol, and aminoglycosides) act by inhibiting protein synthesis.
- Selectivity is based on ribosomal difference: bacteria as 70S (two subunits of 50S and 30S) *versus* eukaryotic 80S (larger 60S and smaller 40S subunits) – a division based on sedimentation coefficients.
- Chloramphenicol, macrolides (*e.g.* erythromycin) and lincos-amides (*e.g.* lincomycin and clindamycin) bind to the 50S sub-unit – they prevent peptide bond formation and hence inhibit protein synthesis.
- Aminoglycosides (*e.g.* streptomycin, gentamicin, neomycin, and kanamycin) bind to the 30S subunit – they produce faulty proteins.
- Tetracyclines bind to the 30S subunit – they block the binding of tRNA and inhibit protein synthesis.

10.3.4   Other Structural and Functional Divisions of RNAs

Recent advances in the field have further established the various types of RNAs in addition to the above-mentioned mRNA, tRNA, and rRNA. Our understanding of the chemistry of these various types of RNAs has now opened up avenues to develop a host of therapeutic opportunities to combat human disease. Some of these RNAs are as follows:

- RNAs may be classed as coding (cRNA) or non-coding (ncRNA).
- ncRNAs may function in housekeeping (tRNA and rRNA) or have a regulatory function.
- Regulatory ncRNAs could be long in size (lncRNA) with 200 nucleotides or shorter (small ncRNAs) with fewer than 200 nucleotides.
- Small ncRNAs include micro-RNA (miRNA), small nucleolar RNA (snoRNA), small nuclear RNA (snRNA), small-interfering RNA (siRNA), and PIWI-interacting RNA (piRNA).

- The miRNAs are about 22 nucleotides long and function in gene regulation.
- miRNAs have therapeutic implications owing to their capacity to inhibit (silence) gene expression by binding to target mRNA and inhibiting translation.
- Some miRNAs serve as tumour suppressors whereas others serve as oncogenic (cancer-initiating) miRNAs. Hence some promote tumorigenesis whereas others serve as therapeutics for cancer.
- Circular RNA (circRNA), which has a cyclic structure due to linkage of the 5′ and 3′ ends, may be involved in protein synthesis (as mRNA) or bind with miRNA to neutralise them. They have a role in the transcription of genes.

10.4   Drugs Acting on Nucleic Acids

10.4.1   DNA Intercalating Agents

DNA intercalating agents are chemical compounds that can be inserted between the DNA base pairs of the double-helix structure leading to structural distortion. Such compounds are mostly molecules with a heterocyclic ring system of hydrophobic nature and include *ethidium bromide*, *acridine orange*, and *actinomycin D* (Figure 10.6). Structural changes due to molecular distortion by these agents result in alterations in the normal function of the DNA in the replication, transcription, and repair processes. Actinomycin D serves as a reference standard in research laboratories to study interference of the DNA replication and transcription process. Specifically, in protein synthesis, one can say that the inhibition by actinomycin D occurs not at the translation but at the transcription stage. Ethidium bromide is a DNA intercalating agent with fluorescence characteristics and hence is used in DNA-based studies, *e.g.* in the DNA laddering experiment using electrophoresis. Similarly, acridine orange and fluorescent dyes such as Hoechst 33342 and Hoechst 33258 are used effectively in DNA staining and cell death studies.

Since the process of DNA intercalation leads to mutations, DNA intercalating agents are also regarded as mutagens or carcinogens. A range of DNA intercalating compounds are, however, used in chemotherapy to treat cancer. *Doxorubicin* and *daunorubicin* are anthracycline antibiotics with anticancer activities *via* DNA intercalation, but they also interfere with topoisomerase II activity (see Section 10.4.2).

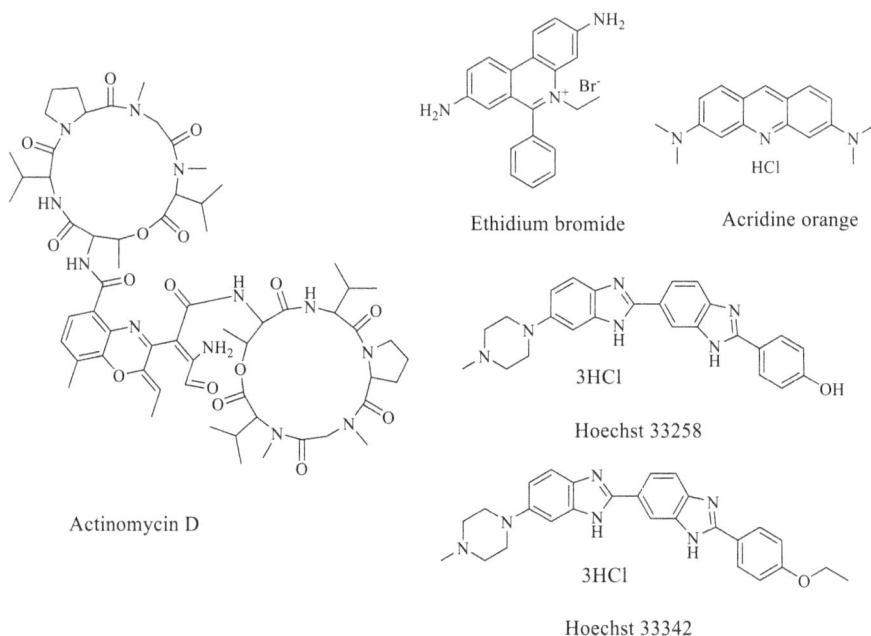

Ethidium bromide   Acridine orange

3HCl

Hoechst 33258

3HCl

Hoechst 33342

Actinomycin D

Figure 10.6 Structures of some DNA intercalating agents. The structure of actinomycin D is composed of a heterocyclic phenoxazine derivative, which is joined with two cyclic pentapeptide lactone rings. Also note that some of the compounds are available in their salt form such as an HCl salt.

DNA Intercalating Agents – Key Facts

- Intercalating agents (e.g. ethidium bromide, acridine orange, and actinomycin D) insert themselves between the stacked base pairs, leading to distortion of the DNA double-helix structure.
- The planar aromatic ring systems in the structures of these compounds help to insert the compounds between the nucleic acid strands.
- Damage to DNA leads to inhibition of replication and transcription, leading to cell death – cancer cells are vulnerable to this damage.
- Some intercalating agents interact not only with DNA but also with DNA-modifying enzymes (*e.g.* topoisomerases).
- Resistance to such drugs can develop, leading to:

  o increased inactivation of the drugs;
  o decreased uptake of the drugs;
  o increased rate of repair of the damaged DNA.

10.4.2   Topoisomerase Inhibitors (Poisons)

Topoisomerases [topoisomerase I (Topo I) and topoisomerase II (Topo II)] are crucial for correcting changes in DNA structure, such as those encountered during DNA replication, chromosome condensation, and chromosome segregation. As therapeutic agents, inhibitors of topoisomerase enzymes are routinely used to treat cancer. As mentioned above, some topoisomerase inhibitors are in fact DNA intercalators.

DNA supercoiling resulting from normal functions such as transcription, replication, and chromatin remodelling is relaxed by Topo I through a transient single-strand break. *Camptothecin* and *irinotecan* (Figure 10.7) are classic examples of inhibitors that induce cytotoxicity in cancer cells. Through hydrogen bonding, camptothecin binds with both the DNA base and Topo I, with the resulting ternary complex formation disrupting normal DNA function or replication. Since the modulation of DNA topology by Topo II involves a transient double-stranded break, inhibitors of these enzymes could have a profound effect when the cleaved DNA is relegated. Good examples are *etoposide*, *daunorubicin*, *doxorubicin*, *epirubicin*, *teniposide*, and *mitoxantrone* (Figure 10.7).

Topoisomerase Inhibitors – Key Facts

- Inhibit the activity of topoisomerase enzymes, which cut and release DNA strands during a critical time such as DNA replication.
- The enzymes remove torsional strain through either transient single-stranded DNA (topoisomerase I) or double-stranded DNA (topoisomerase II) cut.
- Inhibitors of topoisomerase I (*e.g.* irinotecan, topotecan, and camptothecin) and topoisomerase II (etoposide, doxorubicin, and epirubicin) serve as anticancer agents.
- The drugs mostly inhibit the last step (releasing stage) of the enzymes' action, leading to the accumulation of fragmented DNA.
- Inhibiting the ligation step of DNA during either replication or transcription steps leads to single- or double-stranded DNA breaks.
- DNA damage eventually leads to cell death.

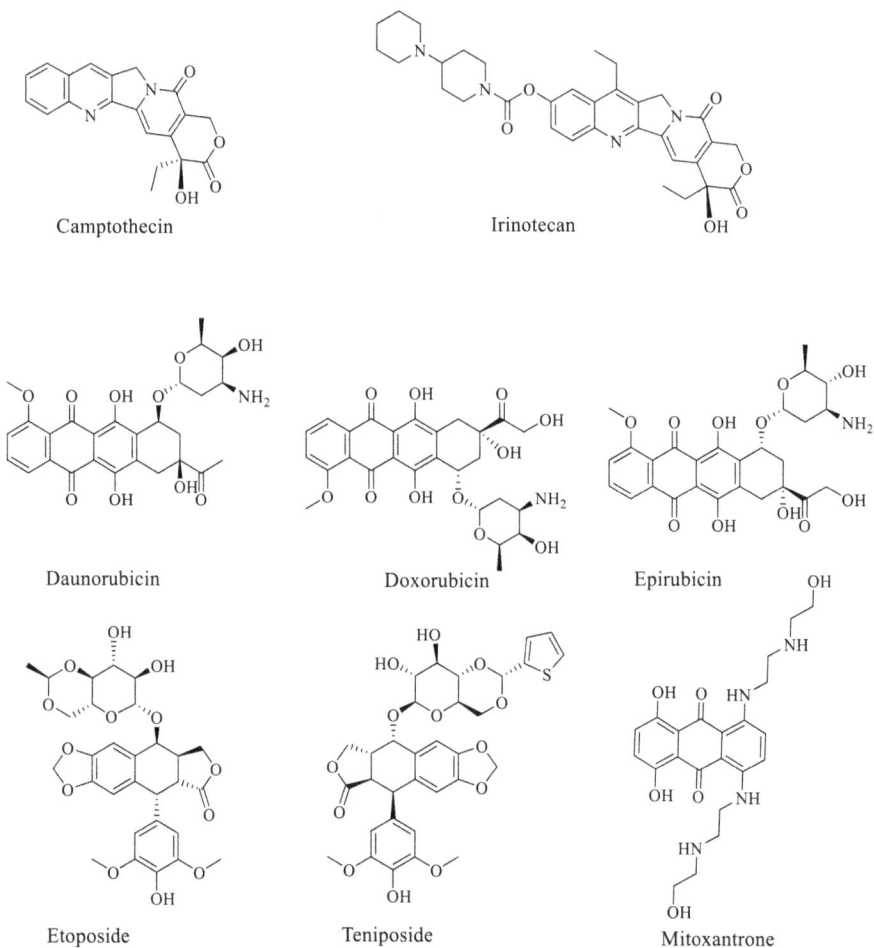

Camptothecin

Irinotecan

Daunorubicin

Doxorubicin

Epirubicin

Etoposide

Teniposide

Mitoxantrone

Figure 10.7 Structures of some topoisomerase inhibitors.

10.4.3 Alkylating Agents

Alkylating agents are highly reactive compounds that make cross-links with DNA strands. They form covalent bonds by reacting with electron-rich atoms, *i.e.* alkylating agents contain electrophilic structural groups. In this reaction, an alkyl group such as a methyl group (from a methylating agent) or, in some cases, a hydrocarbon chain is added to make either cross-links within one strand or a covalent cross-link between two strands. Unless the DNA is repaired, such a reaction leads to DNA malfunction (including the DNA being unable to uncoil and separate) and leads to cell death. Largely non-specific in their action, alkylating agents are anticancer agents with different structural classes including nitrogen mustards, alkyl sulfonates, nitrosoureas, ethylenimines, and triazenes (Figure 10.8). Their non-specific action means that they can also alkylate proteins, and alkylating DNA or RNA bases can also result in miscoding.

Some alkylating agents are not readily electrophilic and need processing in the body to be converted to their active form (Figure 10.9). Thus, they are *prodrugs* that need metabolic activation in the body. For example, *dacarbazine* is processed in the liver and converted to *methyldiazonium* ion, which is an alkylating agent. Mitomycin C is also a prodrug that needs activation before it forms DNA cross-links and toxicity to cancer cells. The activation reaction involves an enzyme-catalysed reduction process of the benzoquinone skeleton to hydroquinone. In this connection, compounds with a quinone structure (*e.g. diaziridinylbenzoquinone* or *diaziquone*) can be activated by cellular reductases to form highly reactive DNA alkylating agents.

Alkylating Agents – Key Facts

- Widely used as anticancer drugs.
- They make cross-links with a DNA strand – prevent DNA transcription and replication.
- They have highly electrophilic groups that form irreversible covalent bonds with nucleophilic sites.
- Guanine (N-7 position, Figure 10.2) is a common site of attack for an alkylating agent.
- In addition to DNA, they also alkylate cellular proteins.
- Most of the alkylating agents have adverse effects such as gastrointestinal effects and toxicity to bone marrow – this limits their dose.
- Beyond their use in cancer therapy, their high reactivity makes them carcinogenic.
- They include nitrogen mustard (cyclophosphamide, chlorambucil, melphalan, busulfan, and ifosfamide), nitrosoureas, the tetrazines (DTIC, or dacarbazine), the aziridines (thiotepa and mitomycin C), and non-classical alkylating agents.

10.4.4 Methylating Agents

Several platinum complexes (Figure 10.10) that cross-link with DNA strands have been used to treat cancer. They bind with DNA, particularly in the guanine-rich area, and in doing so inhibit transcription

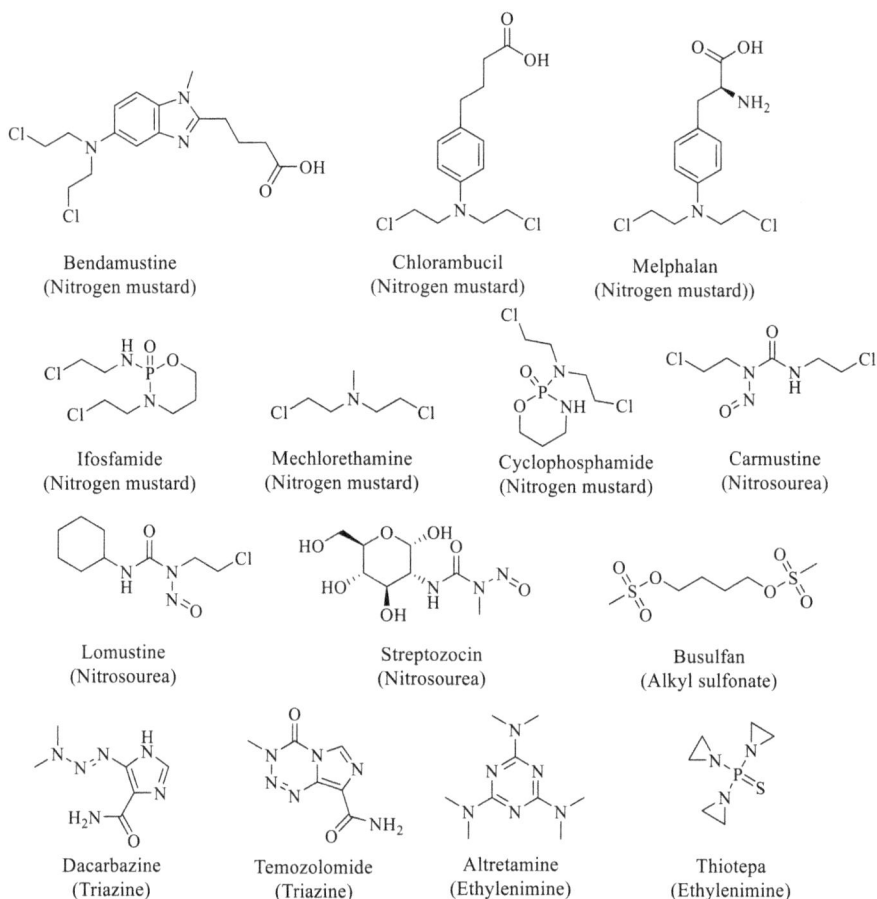

Bendamustine
(Nitrogen mustard)

Chlorambucil
(Nitrogen mustard)

Melphalan
(Nitrogen mustard))

Ifosfamide
(Nitrogen mustard)

Mechlorethamine
(Nitrogen mustard)

Cyclophosphamide
(Nitrogen mustard)

Carmustine
(Nitrosourea)

Lomustine
(Nitrosourea)

Streptozocin
(Nitrosourea)

Busulfan
(Alkyl sulfonate)

Dacarbazine
(Triazine)

Temozolomide
(Triazine)

Altretamine
(Ethylenimine)

Thiotepa
(Ethylenimine)

Figure 10.8 Structures of some common alkylating agents. The structural groups associated with their mechanism of action are given in parentheses. For example, those in the ethylenimine group such as thiotepa are converted in the body into a highly reactive ethylenimine structure that undergoes covalent bonding with nucleophilic molecules (*e.g.* DNA).

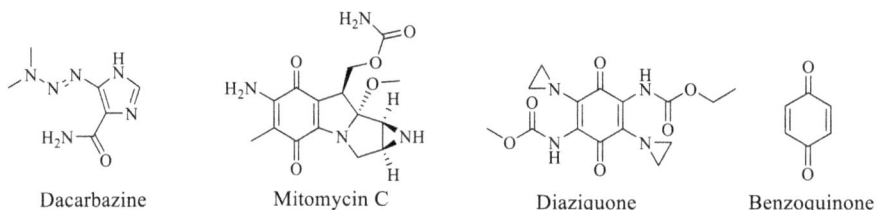

Dacarbazine

Mitomycin C

Diaziquone

Benzoquinone

Figure 10.9 Structures of some prodrugs as alkylating agents and benzoquinone.

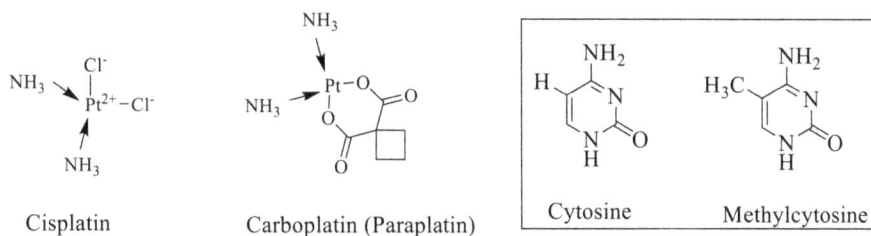

Figure 10.10 Structures of cisplatin and carboplatin. Note that carboplatin differs from cisplatin by replacing the two chlorine atoms with a bidentate cyclopropyl malonato structure. These drugs inhibit DNA methylation or, at the molecular level, methylation of cytosine.

among other DNA functions. *Cisplatin* is a prototype drug, which is also a prodrug as it requires activation for its DNA binding properties. Cisplatin is also an alkylating agent. Other drugs that act as methylating agents include *carboplatin*. They are called methylating agents because they inhibit DNA methylation – a process of incorporation of a methyl group at the C-5 position of cytosine to form 5-methylcytosine. This is catalysed by a group of enzymes called DNA methyltransferases. Since DNA methylation is largely involved in cancer development, methylating agents have therapeutic potential as anticancer agents.

10.4.5 Chain Cutters and Terminators

Several anticancer and chemotherapeutic agents not only interact with DNA or intercalate but also react either by producing radical species or by inhibiting enzymes (*e.g.* repair enzymes), leading to chain cutting. Examples are anticancer antibiotics such as *bleomycin*, *calicheamicin*, and *neocarzinostatin* (Figure 10.11).

Chemical compounds that can be added to the growing DNA during DNA synthesis and inhibit further chain enlargement are called *chain terminators* (Figure 10.12). Inhibition of the human immunodeficiency virus (HIV) enzyme called reverse transcriptase by the anti-AIDS drug *azidothymidine* (*AZT*, also called *zidovudine* or *Retrovir*) is a good example. Such compounds have a heterocyclic structure similar to those of nucleic acid bases. The anti-herpes drug reference compound *acyclovir* (*Zovirax*) and *famciclovir* (*Famvir*) are other good examples of DNA chain terminators. These compounds are prodrugs as they are phosphorylated to triphosphate in the body to serve as drugs.

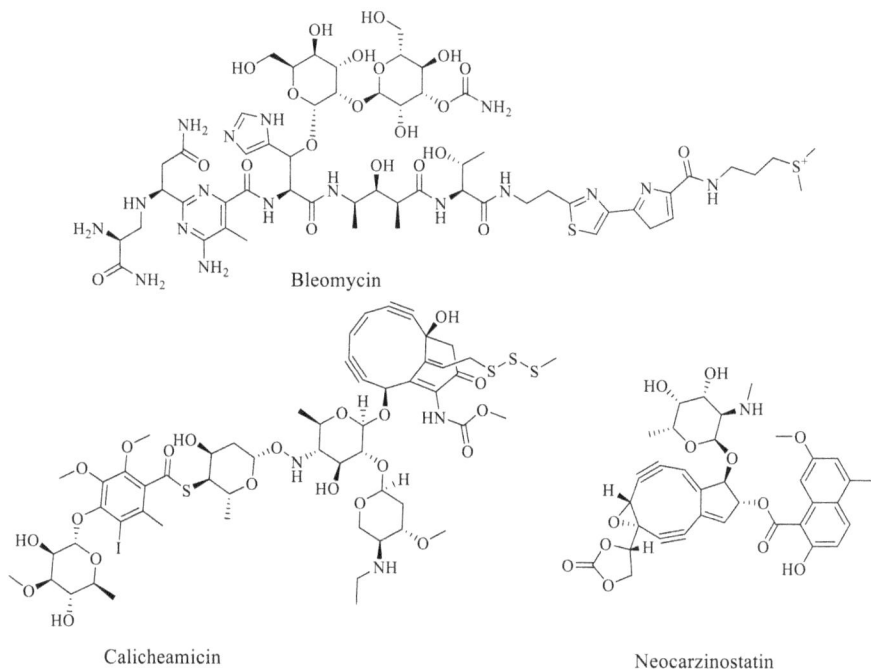

Figure 10.11 Structures of some antibiotics with DNA chain-cutting properties.

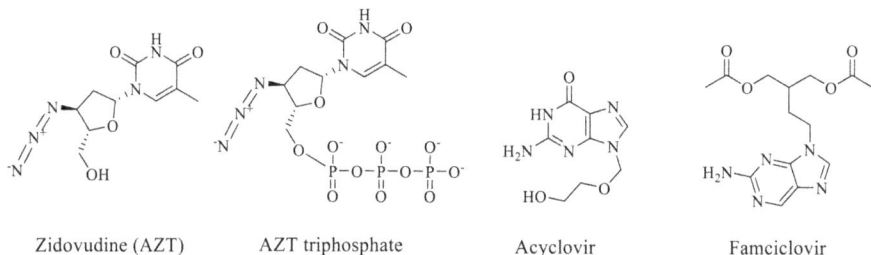

Figure 10.12 Structures of some DNA chain terminators. As shown for AZT, these compounds are phosphorylated in the body.

10.5 Drugs Acting on RNA

10.5.1 Antisense RNA Therapy

Single-stranded oligonucleotides that can make complementary base pairings with certain mRNAs can be prepared synthetically. These compounds can target/inhibit the expression of selected genes and also protein synthesis. This strategy is an example of the knockout of gene expression. Generally, a specific region of the mRNA sequence is selected, complementary sequence engineered, and inserted into cells to stop the translation of certain proteins. A non-coding mRNA, which blocks the translation of a given protein, can also be used.

For the effective therapy of diseases based on the antisense principle, the genetic map or sequence of a particular gene associated with the disease must be known. A synthetic compound including a complementary sequence of nucleic acid can then be used to bind to the mRNA and turn off the gene.

10.5.2 Small Interfering RNA (siRNA) Therapy

Sometimes called short interfering RNAs, these are double-stranded RNAs of about 20–25 base pair (bp) nucleotides. With respect to size and function, they are similar to micro-RNAs. The siRNAs have a specific binding based on the sequence complementarity at a site within a single gene. By knocking down or silencing the expression of a specific gene, siRNAs have therapeutic implications for various diseases, including cancer.

10.5.3 RNA Aptamers

These are single-stranded, highly structured DNA or RNA oligonucleotides that can be designed to bind to a specific target, including proteins/peptides, DNAs, RNAs, small molecules, and ions. They do this through selective and high-affinity binding. Aptamers are often compared in their function with antibodies, but they are generally considered as more thermally and chemically stable and also their syntheses are simpler and cheaper.

10.5.4 mRNAs

As shown by the COVID-19 vaccination programme, mRNAs have great potential to be employed to serve as vaccines to tackle a variety of viral diseases. They can also replace protein- or antibody-based therapies.

10.5.5 Other Drugs Acting on RNA

Several RNA-based technologies, including guide RNAs (gRNAs) and micro-RNAs (miRNAs), are now being extensively developed as therapeutic agents.

Targeting RNA by Drugs – Key Facts

- mRNA – used in vaccination, protein replacement therapy, and antibody therapy.
- rRNA in prokaryotes is targeted by antibiotics (streptomycin, spectinomycin, tetracycline, and puromycin) – inhibition of protein synthesis.
- Antisense oligonucleotides – single-stranded oligonucleotide to selectively inhibit target gene expression *via* complementary base pairings with targeted mRNA.
- Small interfering RNA (siRNA) – small (18–22 bp) double-stranded RNAs used for selective and effective knockdown of target gene expression.
- MicroRNAs – post-transcriptional gene regulation.
- RNA aptamers – single-stranded oligonucleotides of DNA or RNA that bind to molecular targets such as proteins, peptides, DNAs, and RNAs.

10.6 Nucleoside Analogues as Drugs – Drugs Related to Nucleic Acid Building Blocks

Drugs that have structural similarity with the natural nucleoside analogues may have the ability to interfere with DNA replication or cell division. One practical application of this is the development of anti-infectious agents mostly as antiviral drugs. Hence nucleoside analogues are major classes of drugs used in combating infections by hepatitis B virus (HBV), hepatitis C virus (HCV), herpes simplex virus (HSV), the human immunodeficiency virus (HIV), cytomegalovirus (CMV), and varicella-zoster virus (VZV). In the case of HIV, these drugs target key DNA replication enzymes, primarily reverse transcriptase, although they also have an effect on polymerase enzymes of both DNA and RNA. Examples of nucleoside-based anti-HIV drugs (see Figure 10.13) are abacavir, didanosine, emtricitabine, stavudine, tenofovir disoproxil, and zidovudine [azidothymidine (AZT)]. For HBV treatment, the nucleoside analogues used include adefovir, emtricitabine, entecavir, lamivudine, telbivudine, and tenofovir. Sofosbuvir is an anti-HCV agent, cidofovir and ganciclovir (Valganciclovir) are anti-CMV agents, and adefovir, emtricitabine, entecavir, lamivudine, telbivudine, and tenofovir disoproxil serve as anti-HBV drugs. Valacyclovir is a drug used for HSV and VZV, and acyclovir is employed to treat HSV and VZV. Thus, nucleoside analogues appear to be useful in

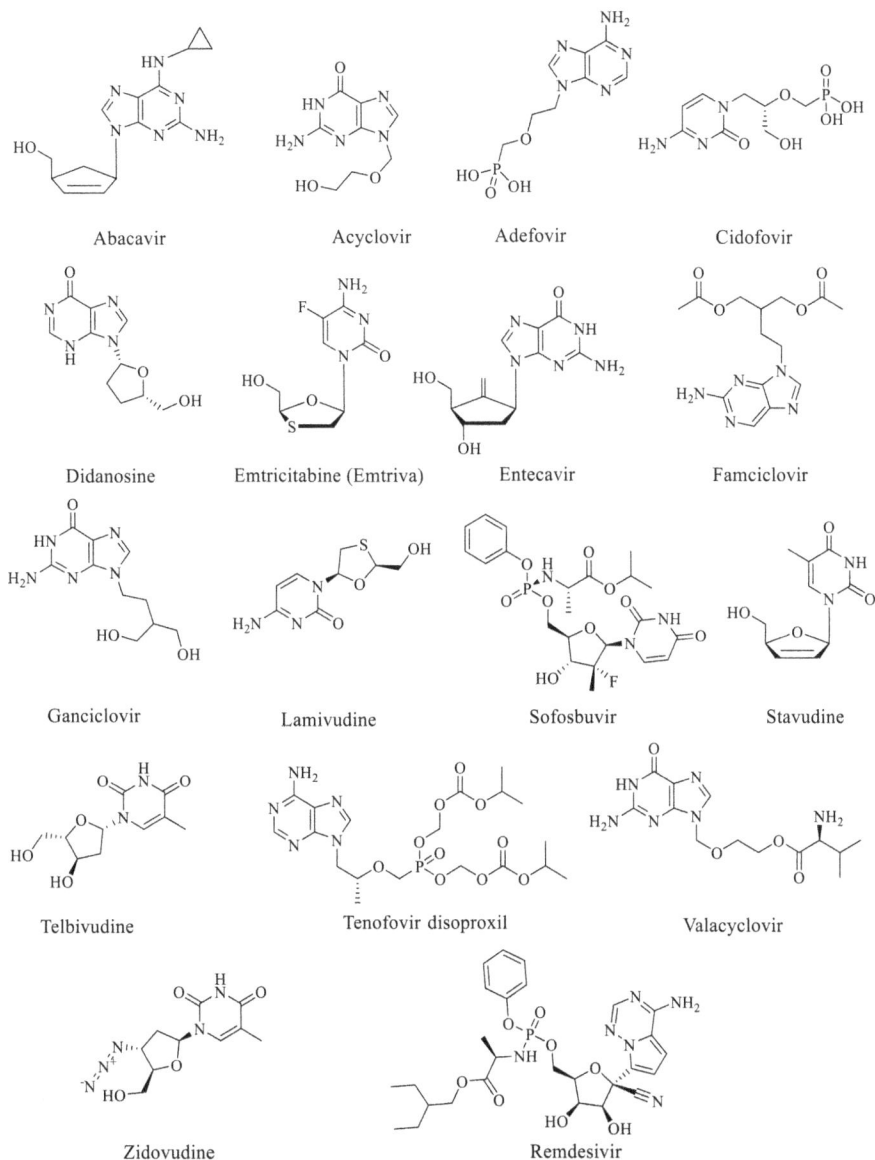

Figure 10.13 Examples of nucleoside analogues as antiviral agents.

treating a broad range of viral infections. One approach in the therapeutic application of these drugs is also to COVID-19, where promising effects of drugs such as remdesivir have been reported.

In addition to viral infections, various nucleoside analogues are also active against bacterial infections (*e.g.* trimethoprim) and many are effectively employed for treating cancer (cytarabine, gemcitabine, mercaptopurine, azacytidine, cladribine, decitabine, fluorouracil, floxuridine, fludarabine, and nelarabine) and inflammatory diseases (azathioprine and allopurinol) (Figure 10.14).

Nucleoside and Nucleotide Analogues as Drugs - Key Facts

- Contain either purine or pyrimidine with a β-N-glycosidic bond of a ribose sugar (nucleoside) that may also have a phosphate ester group (nucleotides).
- Structural modification includes changes in the sugar unit (hydroxyl positions) or replacing oxygen with other atoms, changing the sugar ring size, *etc.*, or changing the base such as by halogenation, *etc.*
- They are largely used in the treatment of cancer and viral infections.
- Nucleoside analogues are altered in the body to the active form (to incorporate the phosphate group) – they are prodrugs.
- The drugs are inserted (more potent to viral enzymes) instead of the normal nucleoside/nucleotide.

10.7 Nucleotide-incorporating Biomolecules Other than Nucleic Acids

The structure of a nucleoside can be incorporated in other structures of biological molecules. This includes the main energy storage biomolecule in living cells, adenosine triphosphate (ATP), and related compounds such as ADP (adenosine diphosphate) and AMP (adenosine monophosphate). Although ATP and related adenine nucleotides are the most common sources of chemical energy in the cell, guanine, cytosine, uracil, and thymine analogues also perform the same function. The metabolic processes in living systems also require coenzymes made from ADP and another base (nicotinamide) to form nicotinamide adenine dinucleotide (NAD) and nicotinamide adenine dinucleotide phosphate (NADP). Both NAD and NADP are dinucleotides containing adenosine and nicotinamide bases and they join together through a diphosphate bridge (Figure 10.15). Reduction and oxidation reactions in biological systems utilise these cofactors: the charged forms (NAD^+ and $NADP^+$) serve as oxidizing agents by accepting electrons and being reduced (to NADH and NADPH). In turn, the reduced forms serve as reducing agents as they lose or donate electrons to oxidise in the form of NAD^+ and $NADP^+$. In addition to the

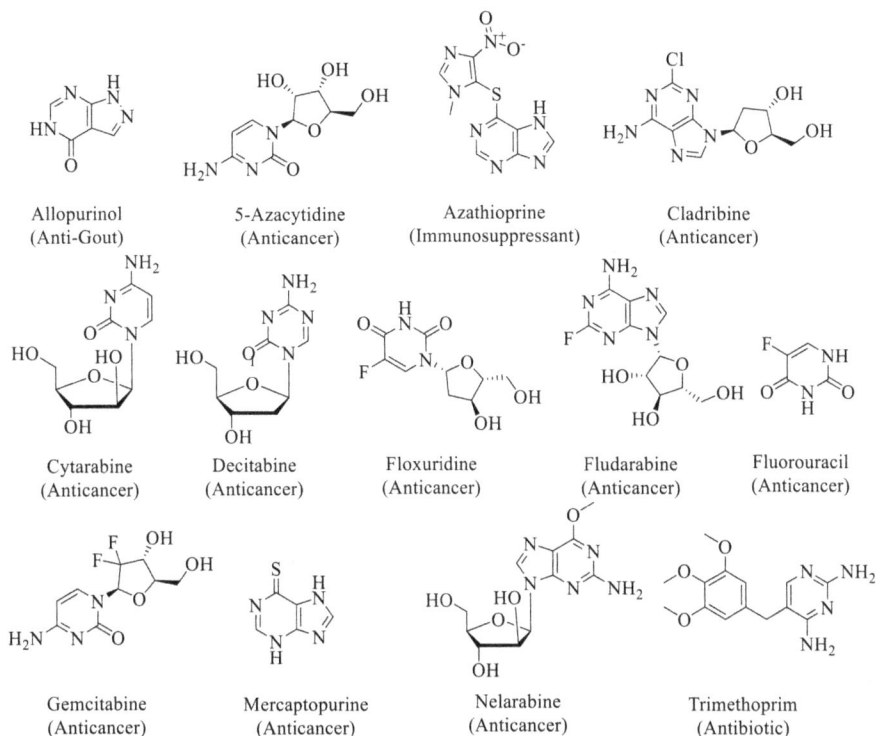

Allopurinol (Anti-Gout)	5-Azacytidine (Anticancer)	Azathioprine (Immunosuppressant)	Cladribine (Anticancer)
Cytarabine (Anticancer)	Decitabine (Anticancer)	Floxuridine (Anticancer)	Fludarabine (Anticancer)	Fluorouracil (Anticancer)
Gemcitabine (Anticancer)	Mercaptopurine (Anticancer)	Nelarabine (Anticancer)	Trimethoprim (Antibiotic)

Figure 10.14 Further examples of nucleosides as therapeutic agents.

NAD and NADP system, other redox coenzymes also occur that facilitate biochemical reactions.

Another redox-sensitive enzyme cofactor is *flavin adenine dinucleotide (FAD)*, which is found in association with some proteins (called flavoproteins). Enzymes that function to keep haemoglobin in a reduced state and the antioxidant enzyme glutathione reductase use FAD as a cofactor. Structurally, FAD has a riboflavin group (vitamin B$_2$) attached to a phosphate group of an ADP molecule (Figure 10.16).

The key feature of FAD in its biological reactions is its ability to donate or accept electrons and interconvert into several intermediate structural forms. As with the NAD and NADPH system, the flavin group can exist simply in two major redox forms, *i.e.* either the oxidised form (FAD) or reduced form (FADH$_2$). A similar redox-sensitive cofactor that incorporates riboflavin (vitamin B$_2$) and adenine is *flavin mononucleotide (FMN)*, or *riboflavin-5'-phosphate*. Note the structural difference between FMN and FAD with respect to the presence of ADP in FAD, whereas only a phosphate group is added to the riboflavin unit in FMN (Figure 10.16). In both cases, the oxidation and reduction processes (see Chapter 11)

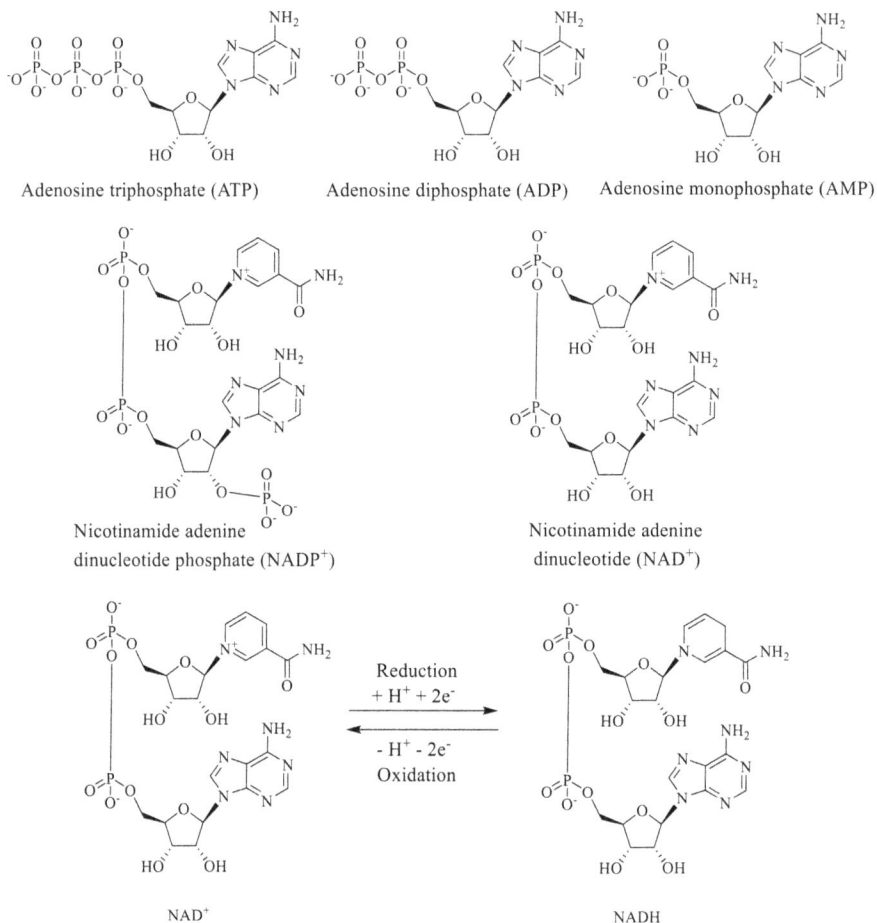

Figure 10.15 Structures of adenosine phosphates and NAD and NADP. The oxidation–reduction reaction using NAD is also shown.

occur in the flavin base skeleton as shown in Figure 10.16. In terms of biosynthesis, FMN is formed by adding a phosphate group from ATP using a riboflavin kinase enzyme. A further addition of the adenosine phosphate group comes from another ATP using the enzyme FAD synthase. FAD can also be converted to FMN and in turn FMN converted to riboflavin using the appropriate enzymes.

Coenzyme A (CoA) is a multifunctional biomolecule involved in both anabolic and catabolic reactions. Structurally, it is based on adenosine, phosphate groups, and organic compound attachment as shown in Figure 10.17. Hence many enzyme cofactors contain nucleotides in their structures. CoA is synthesised from vitamin B_5 (pantothenic acid), the amino acid cysteine, and adenosine triphosphate. In most metabolic reactions in which CoA is involved, it serves as an acyl carrier.

Riboflavin   Flavin mononucleotide (FMN)   Flavin adenine dinucleotide (FAD)

FAD or FMN   FADH$_2$ or FMNH$_2$

Oxidized form   Reduced form

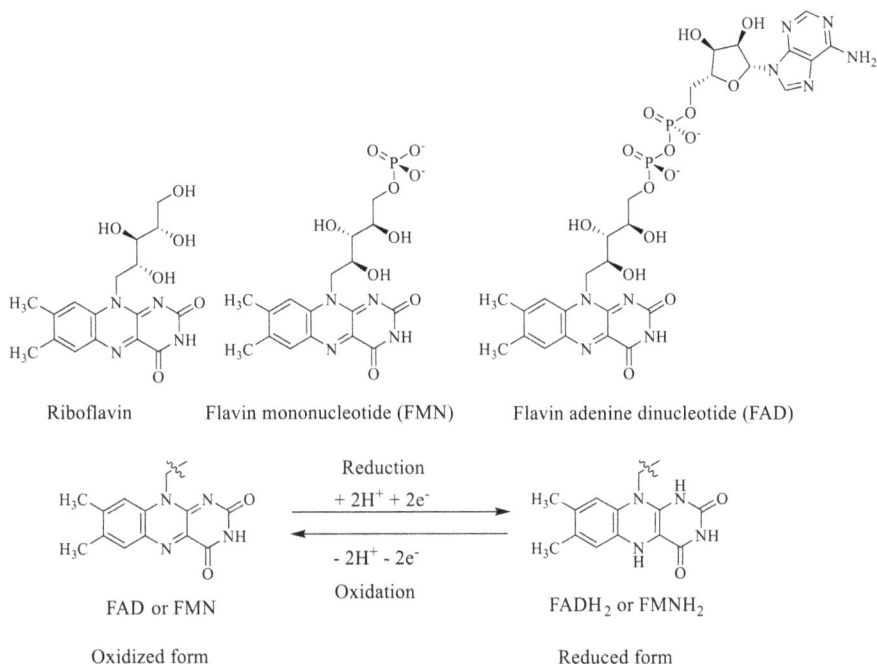

Figure 10.16 Structures of FMN and FAD and their redox states.

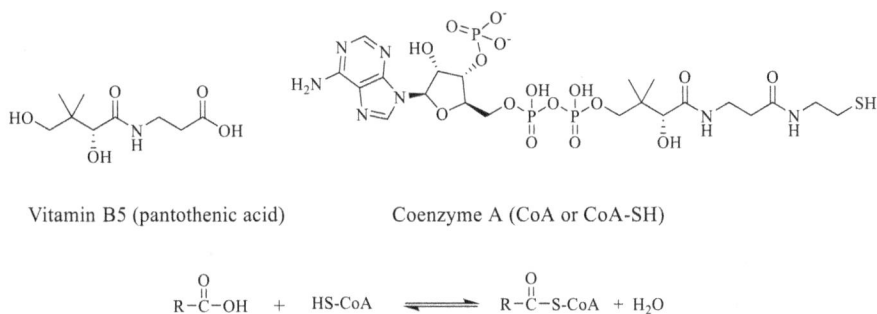

Vitamin B5 (pantothenic acid)   Coenzyme A (CoA or CoA-SH)

Figure 10.17 Structure of coenzyme A (CoA) and its reaction with acids. The reaction of fatty acids with CoA is critical in their oxidation within the mitochondria to generate energy.

Through its critical sulfhydryl group (R–SH), it interacts with carboxylic acids to form thioesters, which are involved in various biological reactions due to the –S–CoA group being displaced by other groups.

Many cell signalling processes mediated through receptors and other systems utilise a second messenger system such as *cyclic AMP (cAMP)* (Figure 10.18). This is crucial in many cellular functions and serves as a target for many drugs. Similarly, *guanosine*

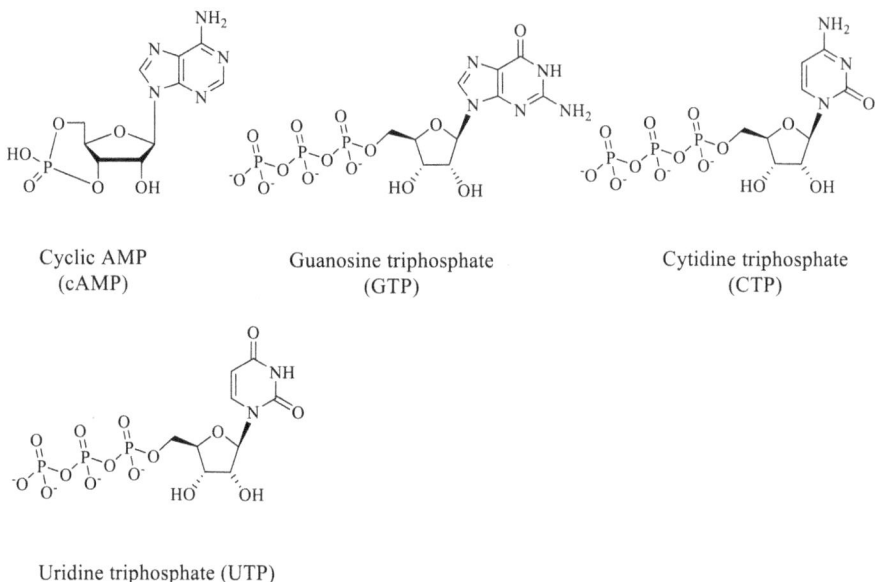

Cyclic AMP
(cAMP)

Guanosine triphosphate
(GTP)

Cytidine triphosphate
(CTP)

Uridine triphosphate (UTP)

Figure 10.18 Structures of cGMP, GTP, CTP, and UTP.

triphosphate (GTP) is a triphosphate based on purine (guanine) nucleoside (Figure 10.18) and serves as a source of energy (just like ATP) in protein synthesis and in the process of glucose formation from a non-carbohydrate source (gluconeogenesis). In G-protein-linked receptors that use a second messenger system such as cAMP or phosphatidylinositol, activation of a receptor leads to modulation of the associated protein (G-protein) and subsequent chain of events by using GTP. Another example of the pyrimidine nucleoside triphosphate is *cytidine triphosphate (CTP)* (Figure 10.18), which differs from ATP in using cytosine as a base instead of adenine. It has various roles in metabolic reactions. On the other hand, *uridine triphosphate (UTP)* (Figure 10.18) uses a heterocyclic amine base, uracil. It is used as a source of energy in biological reactions just like ATP, for example, in the synthesis of glycogen. Note that many drugs interfere with biological processes by modifying the function of these key biological molecules.

Functions of Nucleotides Other than Nucleic Acids – Key Facts

- Source of energy in chemical reactions – ATP, UTP, GTP, and CTP.
- Components of enzyme cofactors – coenzyme A, FAD, FMN, NAD, *etc.*
- Cell signalling – cAMP, cGMP, *etc.*

10.8 Summary

In this chapter, we have learned the following:

- Nucleic acids are of two types – DNA and RNA.
- The two monosaccharides incorporated in nucleic acids are β-D-ribose in RNA and 2-deoxy-β-D-ribose in DNA.
- Nucleic acids are made from purine bases (adenine and guanine) and pyrimidines (cytosine, thymine, and uracil).
- Thymine is unique to DNA whereas uracil is unique to RNA – the other bases are found in both RNA and DNA.
- Nucleic acids are built with monomeric units of nucleotides, which are composed of a base, a pentose sugar, and a phosphate group.
- A base joined with ribose or 2-deoxyribose sugar *via* a β-glycosidic linkage is called a nucleoside.
- The glycosidic bond in a nucleoside is between the anomeric carbon of the sugar (ribose or 2-deoxyribose) and the nitrogen in the base – hence it is called a β-N-glycosidic bond.
- The phosphate group in the nucleotide is attached to the C-5 hydroxyl position of the pentose sugar.
- Two nucleotides join together through a 5'- and 3'-phosphate bridge.
- In DNA, a hydrogen bond between complementary bases forms a double-helical structure.
- Guanine interacts with cytosine through three hydrogen bonding (G≡C).
- Adenine interacts with thymine *via* two hydrogen bonding (A=T).
- The primary structure of DNA is the sequence of nucleotides.
- The base pairing of the two DNA strands through hydrogen bonding between complementary bases is called its secondary structure.
- The three-dimensional shape of nucleic acids is the tertiary structure.
- The copying out of the DNA sequence by using complementary base pairs to form a transcript (RNA) is called transcription. In this case, uracil is used in RNA in place of thymine.
- Several enzymes are involved in the normal function of DNA and RNA. These enzymes also serve as targets for therapeutic agents.
- RNAs are a diverse group of nucleic acids with a basic function in protein synthesis. They also have various other functions depending on their chemical composition.

- Drugs can alter cellular functions by intercalating with DNA. Cancer is targeted by such agents.
- Many anticancer agents act by inhibiting topoisomerase enzymes.
- Alkylating agents interact with DNA by forming covalent bonds. Mostly, they contain electrophilic structural groups and attack electron-rich atoms.
- Methylating agents inhibit the methylation of DNA, which is associated with cancer development. Cytosine is methylated by methyl transferase enzymes to form methylated DNA.
- By using drugs that cut the DNA or prematurely terminate its synthesis, cell division can be targeted by drugs – this is one of the established anticancer mechanisms of drugs.
- Drugs can act on RNA in a variety of ways and we also have small pieces of RNAs as therapeutic agents.
- Nucleoside analogues are drugs with a similar structure to natural nucleosides, hence they interfere with the synthesis of nucleic acids (*e.g.* DNA). Several groups of these drugs are used in antiviral therapy.
- Nucleotides are also incorporated in several biological molecules, such as ATP, NAD, NADP, FAD, FMN, CoA, GTP, UTP, CTP, *etc.* They are also involved in cell signalling.

10.9   Problems

1. Which monosaccharide is present in RNA?
2. Which monosaccharide is present in DNA?
3. Identify nucleic acid bases that contain two keto groups: _____.
4. What is the structural similarity and difference between thymine and uracil?
5. What is the structural difference between cytosine and thymine?
6. A base that is not found in DNA is _____.
7. A base that is not found in RNA is _____.
8. A base and sugar in a nucleotide are attached through which bond?
9. A nucleoside is composed of: _____.
10. A nucleotide is composed of: _____.
11. What is the structural difference between nucleosides and nucleotides?
12. In the formation of a dinucleotide from two nucleotides, what type of bonding is involved and at which site?

13. What are the building blocks of nucleic acids?
14. What intermolecular forces hold together the two DNA strands?
15. Of the base, sugar, and phosphate group, which one is responsible for the formation of a DNA double-helix structure?
16. How many hydrogen bonds are formed between adenine and thymine?
17. How many hydrogen bonds are formed between guanine and cytosine?
18. How are the complementary DNA strands joined together?
19. What is the sequence that complements the strand GCTAGATC?
20. How many hydrogen bonds allow GCTAGATC binding with its complementary pair?
21. If you hydrolyse RNA, what would be the product?
22. If the sequence of DNA helix in one strand is GTCAAA, what would be the sequence on the other strand?
23. Suppose that thymine constitutes 25% of the bases in the DNA. What would be the percentages of adenine, guanine, and cytosine?
24. If the DNA sequence is ATTGGCCA, what would be the sequence of the strand produced by DNA polymerase?
25. If the DNA sequence is ATTGGCCA, what would be the sequence of the strand produced by RNA polymerase?
26. Some antiviral agents are either nucleosides or nucleotides. What is the difference between the two?
27. Actinomycin D can intercalate with DNA. Would it affect DNA replication or transcription?
28. Ethidium bromide is a mutagenic agent (causes mutation) and can kill cells. What is the mechanism of its action?
29. In the analysis of DNA samples by gel electrophoresis, ethidium bromide is sometimes added to the sample mixture before separation. What is the purpose of this?
30. Doxorubicin is an effective anticancer agent. Suggest its main mechanism of action and structural attributes for this action.
31. What is common for the anticancer drugs etoposide, daunorubicin, doxorubicin, epirubicin, teniposide, and mitoxantrone?
32. An anticancer drug molecule is known to make bonds to the N-7 position of the guanine base of DNA. What group of anticancer agents can it be classified under?
33. Etoposide and teniposide belong to a class of drugs called
_____.

34. Bleomycin, calicheamicin and neocarzinostatin can cause DNA fragmentation with predominantly single-stranded breaks. What class of compounds are they classified under?

35. Zidovudine (AZT) is a drug used in the treatment of HIV/AIDS. Its effect is mainly on the HIV reverse transcription. Under what category is this drug classified?
36. Alicaforsen is an anti-inflammatory agent made as a 20 bp single-stranded deoxyribonucleotide, which is complementary to the mRNA target. What kind of therapy is this and how does it work?
37. Give an example of mRNA in vaccine therapies.
38. Gemcitabine is an anticancer agent with the pyrimidine structure attached to a fluorine-containing pentose sugar. What class of compound is this drug?

10.10   Solutions to Problems

1. D-Ribose.
2. 2-Deoxy-D-ribose.
3. Thymine and uracil.
4. Both are pyrimidine bases; a methyl group is present in thymine.
5. An amine group in cytosine is replaced with a keto group in thymine.
6. Uracil.
7. Thymine.
8. *N*-Glycosidic
9. A base and pentose sugar.
10. A base, pentose sugar, and a phosphate group.
11. A phosphate group attached to a nucleoside makes a nucleotide.
12. A phosphodiester bond between the 5′-hydroxyl group on a nucleotide and the 3′-hydroxyl group of another nucleotide.
13. Nucleotides.
14. Hydrogen bonding.
15. Base.
16. Two.
17. Three.
18. By hydrogen bonding.
19. CGATCTAG.
20. $3 + 3 + 2 + 2 + 3 + 2 + 2 + 3 = 20$ hydrogen bonds.
21. A ribose sugar and A, U, G, and C bases and a phosphate group product which is phosphoric acid.
22. CAGTTT.
23. If 25% of the bases in the DNA are thymine, it means that 25% of the complementary pair, adenine, occurs. The other 50% therefore consists of 25% guanine and 25% cytosine.

24. For a 5′ ATTGGCCA 3′ strand, DNA polymerase makes 3′ TAAC-CGGT 5′.
25. For a 5′ ATTGGCCA 3′ strand, RNA polymerase makes 3′ UAAGGU 5′. Note that uracil is used in RNA instead of thymine.
26. Nucleosides lack the 5′-phosphate group on the pentose sugar.
27. Both DNA replication and transcription are inhibited.
28. It affects the secondary structure of DNA through intercalation.
29. Ethidium bromide undergoes strong intercalation with the DNA and the separated DNA can then fluoresce due to ethidium bromide, hence making their detection easier.
30. Doxorubicin intercalates between the bases in double-stranded DNA. Its three aromatic rings in a planar structure help to insert the molecule for this action. It also has other effects such as topoisomerase II inhibition. It is also known to generate free radicals that contribute to the killing of cancer cells.
31. They are topoisomerase inhibitors.
32. Alkylating agent.
33. Topoisomerase poisons.
34. Chain cutters.
35. Chain terminators.
36. This is an example of antisense therapy. A double-stranded structure is formed that is identified as foreign and therefore destroyed by the cell before the unwanted protein is produced.
37. A good example is COVID-19 but other viral vaccines can also be named.
38. A nucleoside analogue.

SECTION III
Physicochemical Properties of Organic Compounds and Drug Molecules

11 Physicochemical Properties of Organic Compounds and Drug Molecules

Learning Objectives

After completing this chapter, you are expected to be able to:

- List the common International System of Units (SI Units) applicable to the analysis of organic compounds and drug molecules.
- Define solution, solvation, and dissociation and their application in the analysis of organic compounds and drug molecules.
- Be familiar with some common physical properties of organic compounds, characteristics of acids and bases, and titration-based quantitative analysis.
- Compare and contrast common reaction types and chemical equilibrium in organic compounds and drug molecules.

11.1 Introduction to Units of Measurements

In biological and chemical experiments or measurements, we use units for volume, mass, density, temperature, *etc.* The use of units may depend on the country; for example, in the UK, a pound may be used as a unit of weight instead of a kilogram (kg), a mile may be used as a unit of distance instead of a kilometre (km), a yard may be used

Basic Chemistry for Life Science Students and Professionals: Introduction to Organic Compounds and Drug Molecules
By Solomon Habtemariam
© Solomon Habtemariam 2023
Published by the Royal Society of Chemistry, www.rsc.org

as a unit of length instead of a metre (m), and a pint or gallon may be used as a unit of volume instead of a litre (L). For area measurements based on centimetre (cm), decimetre (dm), metre (m), and kilometre, we use units of cm², dm², m², and km², respectively. One could also use units in inches, yards, miles, *etc.*, to express length and area. Unfortunately, units such as a hectare or an acre for area may have different meanings in different countries. These could be confusing both for scientists and for the practical application of the units, *e.g.* as doses of drugs to be administered to patients. Luckily, units of measurements have been standardised and the accepted norm in science is to use what we call the *International System of Units* or *SI Units*. The common units of measurement in SI units are given in Table 11.1.

Understanding fractions or multiples of units is also simple using the SI system. For example, the prefix *kilo* means one thousand:

$$\text{One kilometre (1 km)} = 1000 \text{ m} = 10^3 \text{ m}.$$

$$\text{One kilogram (1 kg)} = 1000 \text{ g} = 10^3 \text{ g}.$$

Whatever measurement is used (weight, volume, time, *etc.*), prefixes such as kilo can apply to simplify writing large numbers. Instead of writing one million, for example, we can use the prefix mega, and similarly prefixes for fractions apply, such as micro, referring to 10^{-6}. These common units are listed in Table 11.2.

11.1.1   Length

The SI system is the same as the metric system, which uses metre (m) as a unit:

$$1 \text{ km} = 1000 \text{ m} = 10^3 \text{ m}.$$

$$1 \text{ dm} = 0.1 \text{ m} = 10^{-1} \text{ m}.$$

$$1 \text{ cm} = 0.01 \text{ m} = 10^{-2} \text{ m}.$$

$$1 \text{ mm} = 0.001 \text{ m} = 10^{-3} \text{ m}.$$

Table 11.1   Common units and symbols.

Measurement	Unit	Symbol
Length	Metre	m
Mass	Kilogram	kg
Time	Second	s
Temperature	Kelvin	K
Amount of substance	Mole	mol

Table 11.2 Prefixes used for multiples and submultiples of SI units.

Prefix	Symbol	Factor
Femto	f	10^{-15}
Pico	p	10^{-12}
Nano	n	10^{-9}
Micro	μ	10^{-6}
Milli	m	10^{-3}
Centi	c	10^{-2}
Deci	d	10^{-1}
Kilo	k	10^{3}
Mega	M	10^{6}
Giga	G	10^{9}
Tera	T	10^{12}

11.1.2 Mass

The unit of mass in the SI system is the kilogram (kg), which is equivalent to 1000 grams (1000 g).

11.1.3 Temperature

The kelvin (K) is the main unit of temperature in the SI system. However, degrees Celsius (°C) is commonly used in biology and organic chemistry, and it is also accepted in the SI system. The freezing and boiling points of water are good reference points for the conversion of units:

Water freezes at 0 °C, which is 273.15 K.

Water boils at 100 °C, which is 373.15 K.

The human body temperature of 37 °C is about 310 K. It is also worth noting that degrees Fahrenheit (°F) is commonly used as a unit of temperature in many countries. The conversion between the three units of measurements is shown in Table 11.3.

11.1.4 Time

The base unit of time in the SI system is the second (s):

One microsecond (1 μs) = 0.000001 s = 10^{-6} s.

One megasecond (1 Ms) = 1 000 000 s = 10^{6} s.

We can also use minutes, hours, days, and years as units of measurement of time.

Table 11.3 Temperature conversion formulae.

	To degrees fahrenheit	To degrees celsius	To kelvin
Fahrenheit (°F)	—	$(°F-32)\times\dfrac{5}{9}$	$(°F-32)\times\dfrac{5}{9}+273.15$
Celsius (°C)	$\left(°C\times\dfrac{9}{5}\right)+32$	—	°C + 273.15
Kelvin (K)	$(K-273.15)\times\dfrac{9}{5}+32$	K – 273.15	—

The number of periods or cycles per second is called *frequency*. In electromagnetic radiation and spectroscopic measurements, we use hertz (Hz) as the SI unit for cycles per second:

One hertz (1 Hz) = one cycle per second.

One megahertz (1 MHz) = 1 000 000 Hz = 10^6 Hz.

11.1.5 Volume

The cubic metre (m^3) is used as the standard SI unit of volume from the base unit of length the metre (m). The common unit of volume in science laboratories is, however, the cubic decimetre (dm^3), which is based on a length in decimetres (dm):

One decimetre (1 dm) = 0.1 m = 10 cm.

One litre (1 L) = one cubic decimetre (1 dm^3).

One cubic centimetre (1 cm^3) = one millilitre (1 mL) = 10^{-3} L.

One cubic micrometre (1 μm^3) = one microlitre (1 μL) = 10^{-6} L.

One cubic nanometre (1 nm^3) = one nanolitre (1 nL) = 10^{-9} L.

11.1.6 Density

The *density* of a substance is the ratio of the mass to its volume:

$$\text{Density} = \frac{mass}{volume}.$$

Kilograms per cubic metre ($kg\ m^{-3}$) is used as a unit in the SI system, although we commonly use the following:

- Densities of solids and liquids can be expressed as grams per cubic centimetre ($g\ cm^{-3}$). Liquid drugs and oily substances have their characteristic density cited at a given temperature. Their mass can therefore be calculated from the volume of the liquid samples taken for the measurement.
- Densities of gases are expressed as grams per litre ($g\ L^{-1}$).

11.1.7   Mole

In the SI system, one mole (1 mol) of substances such as atoms, molecules, ions, or electrons is defined as the exact numerical value of Avogadro's number of $6.02214076 \times 10^{23}$ particles. Thus, 1 mol of ethanoic acid (CH_3COOH) contains $6.02214076 \times 10^{23}$ molecules, *i.e.*

$$1\ mol = 6.02214076 \times 10^{23}\ particles.$$

The common element used as a reference for the definition of mole is carbon (C), where one mole refers to the number of atoms in exactly 12 g of pure carbon-12:

$$1\ mol\ of\ C\ atoms = 12\ g\ of\ C = 6.02214076 \times 10^{23}\ C\ atoms.$$

For calculation of the moles of chemical compounds, Avogadro's number of $6.02214076 \times 10^{23}$ is used, whereby the mass of one mole in grams is taken as equal to the average mass of one molecule of the compound in daltons (atomic mass units, symbol Da). Ethanoic acid (CH_3COOH) has a molecular mass of 60.052 g:

$$1\ mol\ of\ CH_3COOH = 60.052\ g = 6.02214076 \times 10^{23}\ molecules.$$

Hence the molecular mass of CH_3COOH is simply given as 60.052 g mol^{-1}. If we consider ethanol (CH_3CH_2OH) and water (H_2O):

CH_3CH_2OH with a molecular mass of 46.07 is taken as 46.07 g mol^{-1}.
H_2O with a molecular mass of 18.0153 is taken as 18.0153 g mol^{-1}.

11.1.8   Mole Fraction

From the above information, we can calculate the *mole fraction* of chemical compounds in solution as follows:

$$Mole\ fraction = \frac{moles\ of\ component}{total\ moles\ in\ solution}$$

Let us consider 23 g of ethanol dissolved in 54 g of water:

1 mol of ethanol = 46.07 g; 23 g of ethanol = 0.49924 mol.

1 mol of water = 18.0153 g; 54 g of water = 2.99745 mol.

Total moles of the solution given above = 0.49924 + 2.99745 = 3.49669 mol.

$$\text{Mole fraction of ethanol} = \frac{0.49924}{3.49669} = 0.142775.$$

Note that mole fraction is dimensionless, and it simply tells us about the proportions in moles of the components in a mixture or a solution.

11.1.9   Mole Percent

Once we know the mole fraction of a component, then multiplying it by 100 gives the mole percentage of that component. In the above example, the mole percentage of ethanol in water is 11.764706%.

Mole fractions are often used in mixtures, solutions, and multiple components of mixtures. If the percentage of mass of the mixture components is known, the mole fraction can also be calculated.

Let us consider a solution of caffeine in ethanol. What is the mole fraction of caffeine that has a mass percentage of 10% in ethanol?

The molecular mass of ethanol is 46 g mol^{-1}.
The molecular mass of caffeine is 194.19 g mol^{-1}.
Of a total mass of 100.0 g:

10% caffeine = 10 g = 0.05149596 mol.

90% ethanol = 90 g = 1.95652175 mol.

Total moles = 0.05149596 + 1.95652175 = 2.00801771.

$$\text{Mole fraction of caffeine} = \frac{0.05149596}{2.00801771} = 0.02564517.$$

Mole percentage of caffeine = 2.564517%.

11.1.10   Molality, Molarity, and Normality

In solutions, molality (m) is a measure of the amount of a dissolved substance per unit mass of the solvent, whereas molarity (M) measures the amount of a dissolved substance per unit volume of the solvent.

Molality (m) = moles of solute divided by kilograms of solvent:

$$m = \frac{\text{moles of solute}}{\text{kilograms of solvent}}$$

The SI unit of molality is mol kg^{-1}.

Molarity (M) = moles of a solute per litre of solution:

$$M = \frac{\text{moles of solute}}{\text{litres of solution}}$$

Molarity is a measure of the molar concentration of a solution. The units of molarity are M or mol L^{-1}. A 1 M solution is said to be 'one molar'.

In many biological and chemical experiments, you are required to prepare concentrations of drug solutions or other chemicals in molar concentrations. Your reference will be a solution with a concentration of solute of 1 mol L^{-1} (1 mole of solute per litre of solution), *i.e.* one molar (1 M). This can be expressed as

$$1 \text{ mol L}^{-1} = 1 \text{ mol dm}^{-3}.$$

Let us consider that you prepared 100 mg of aspirin (solute) in 2 mL of ethanol (solvent). This is equivalent to 50 000 mg (50 g) of aspirin in 1000 mL (1 L) of ethanol.

The molecular mass of aspirin is 180.158 g mol^{-1}.

$$50 \text{ g of aspirin} = 0.27753416 \text{ mol.}$$

$$0.27753416 \text{ mol L}^{-1} = 0.27753416 \text{ M.}$$

In both biological and chemical experiments, we often prepare a stock solution from which several dilutions are prepared. The relationship of these dilutions can be established by using the equation

$$C_1 V_1 = C_2 V_2$$

where C_1 and V_1 are the concentration and volume of the starting solution, respectively, and C_2 and V_2 are the concentration and volume of the final solution, respectively.

Let us consider that you prepared a 5.0 M solution of aspirin in ethanol, and you need to use in your experiment 200 mL of 2.0 M aspirin solution. The question would be how much ethanol and how much 5.0 M aspirin solution from the stock should be used to make up the required 200 mL of 2.0 M aspirin solution? As

$$C_1 V_1 = C_2 V_2$$

then

$$5.0 \text{ M aspirin} \times V_1 = 2.0 \text{ M aspirin} \times 200 \text{ mL},$$

and from this

$$V_1 = \frac{2 \text{M} \times 200 \text{mL}}{5 \text{M}} = 80 \text{ mL of 5 M aspirin solution.}$$

To prepare 200 mL of 2 M aspirin solution, we need to take 80 mL of 5 M aspirin solution and dilute it with 120 mL of ethanol, *i.e.*

$$200 \text{ mL} - 80 \text{ mL} = 120 \text{ mL}.$$

You will encounter various problem-solving exercises in laboratories based on molar calculations and dilutions. For example, if you transfer 50 mL of the 5 M aspirin solution into a flask and dilute it to a total volume of 250 mL, the new molarity of the solution would be

$$C_1 V_1 = C_2 V_2$$

$$5.0 \text{ M aspirin} \times 50 \text{ mL} = C_2 \times 250 \text{ mL}.$$

$$C_2 = \frac{5 \text{M} \times 50 \text{mL}}{250 \text{mL}} = 1 \text{M}.$$

Another unit of measurement used in assessing drug solutions is normality (N), which is the moles of reactive species of a solute (number of gram equivalents, Eq) per litre of solution. Its units are Eq L^{-1}. Let us consider the following reactions:

$$HCl \rightarrow H^+ + Cl^-$$

$$NaCl \rightarrow Na^+ + Cl^-$$

In these examples, the concentration of the hydrogen ion $[H^+]$ is the same as that of HCl, [HCl], or they are the same equivalent. If we have 1 M [HCl] we also have 1 M $[H^+]$; NaCl also gives $[Na^+]$ with the same equivalence. Hence the molarity and normality of these compounds are the same: 1 M HCl is the same as 1 N HCl.

On the bases of the ionisation in solution and mole equivalence:

1 mol of HCl gives 1 mol of H^+; 1 M HCl = 1 N HCl.
1 mol of $CaCl_2$ gives 2 mol of Cl^-; 1 M $CaCl_2$ = 2 N $CaCl_2$.
1 mol of H_2SO_4 gives 2 mol of H^+; 1 M H_2SO_4 = 2 N H_2SO_4.

We can now apply the same principle to organic compounds. In the following examples, the ionisation of the organic acid salts gives the same equivalent ions as the starting salts. Hence normality is the same as molarity for these compounds:

sodium acetate (CH_3CO_2Na);
ammonium butyrate $(CH_3CH_2CH_2CO_2NH_4)$;
sodium benzoate $(C_6H_5CO_2Na)$.

In the following examples, however, 1 mol of the salt gives 2 mol of ionised species, hence 1 M = 2 N:

magnesium propanoate $[(CH_3CH_2COO)_2Mg]$;
calcium oxalate $[(O_2C-CO_2)_2Ca]$.

11.2 Solubility of Organic Compounds and Drug Molecules

11.2.1 Solutes, Solvents, and Solubility

In this topic, we have two concepts: the *solute*, which may be in any physical state such as solid, liquid, or gas, and the *solvent*, which dissolves the solute. Most often solvents are liquids, but in principle they can also be a gas or a solid. The resulting mixture, which has a uniform distribution of the solute in the chosen solvent, is called a solution. Solubility is a measure of the ability of a chemical substance (solute) to dissolve in a solvent to make a solution. Salts and ionic compounds are polar and dissolve in polar solvents such as water, whereas organic compounds may preferentially dissolve in organic solvents. We often express this as *'like dissolves like'*. It should be noted that this is a physical process and does not include solutes that disappear as solids in solvents because of a chemical reaction. Hence the first criterion of solubility is that it depends on the nature of the solute and the solvent. Let us consider water dissolving a solute to make an aqueous solution. When sodium chloride (NaCl) dissolves in water it becomes fully charged as Na^+ and Cl^- ions because of the water molecules breaking the bonds and aligning between the two ions (Figure 11.1). Hence the two ions are represented in the solution as Na^+ (aq) + Cl^- (aq). An aqueous solution of NaCl is thus highly charged and conducts electricity. As a result, the solution is also called an *electrolyte*.

In organic compounds, unlike the ionic interaction shown for the above-mentioned NaCl, the molecules are held together through intermolecular forces such as hydrogen bonding, dipole–dipole interactions, *etc.* (see Chapter 2). These kinds of intermolecular interactions are also relevant in solvent–solvent, solute–solute, and solvent–solute interactions. Hence solubility depends on the nature of both the solute and the solvent. If we add hexane or petrol to water, its solubility is negligible as the components differ from each other in their chemical properties. Thus hexane is *hydrophobic* (*water hating*) or *lipophilic* (*lipid*

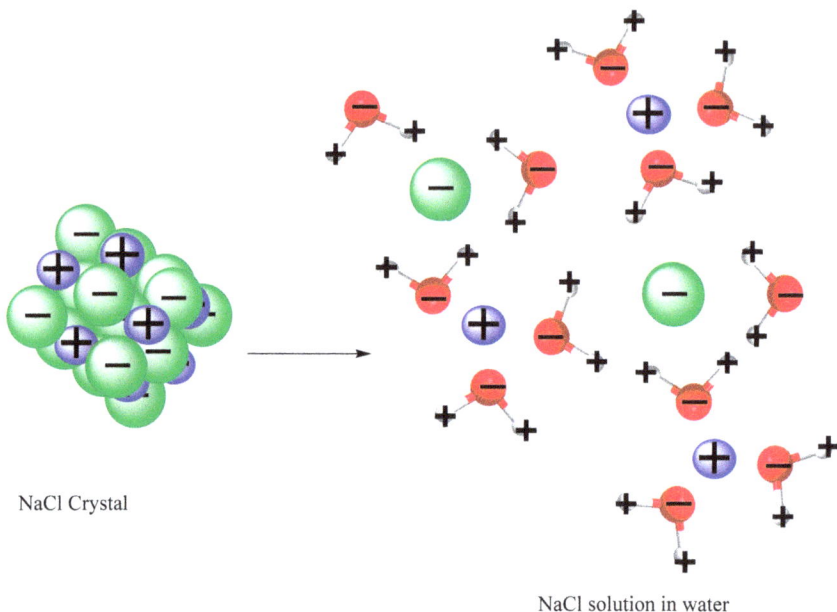

NaCl Crystal

NaCl solution in water

Figure 11.1 Arrangement of sodium and chloride ions in an NaCl crystal and upon dissolution in water. In the solution, the chloride and sodium ions are surrounded by water molecules in line with the dipole water molecular structure. The resulting Na$^+$ (aq) + Cl$^-$ (aq) ions are shown.

loving) and is insoluble in water, whereas NaCl and other water-soluble compounds are called *hydrophilic* (also *lipophobic*). In alcohols (Chapter 5), we have seen that those with shorter hydrocarbon chains such as methanol and ethanol are completely miscible (soluble) in water. Butanol is slightly soluble in water but as the size of the hydrocarbon chain increases (*e.g.* decanol), the alcohols become insoluble in water.

Organic compounds with polyhydroxy functional groups such as sugars are soluble in water. Amino acids which normally exist as zwitterions (Chapter 7) generally interact with water like ionic compounds and are therefore soluble in water. We have also seen that the carboxyl functional group makes molecules more hydrophilic provided that the hydrocarbon chain is not too long. For example, methanoic, ethanoic, and propanoic acids are soluble in water. Removing the hydroxyl group in alcohols by making them ethers or converting carboxylic acids into esters makes them non-polar or hydrophobic. As a result, their solubility in water diminishes and they rather dissolve in organic solvents. For organic compounds and drug molecules, one good way to make them water soluble is to convert them, when possible, into salt forms. For example, benzoic acid, which is highly soluble in alcohols (*e.g.* ethanol), is poorly soluble in water. At 20 °C, only about 0.3 g of benzoic acid can dissolve in 100 g of water. On the other hand, sodium benzoate is the salt form of benzoic acid and is widely used as a preservative and can be found in many foods and drinks and medicinal products. According to the PubChem database (https://pubchem.ncbi.nlm.nih.gov), 1 g of sodium benzoate can dissolve in only 1.8 mL of water or 1.4 mL of boiling water. Generally, we can increase the solubility of benzoic acid in water by about 185-fold by converting it to its salt form, sodium benzoate (Figure 11.2). Another good example is phenol, which is moderately soluble in water, with a solubility of about 84.2 g L^{-1} (8.42 g per 100 g). The sodium salt of phenol, sodium phenoxide, however, is very soluble in water just like salts. Amines behave like alcohols, those with shorter hydrocarbon chains being soluble in water whereas those with longer carbon chains are insoluble in water but soluble in organic solvents. For decylamine, which is miscible in ethanol, its water solubility is negligible at about 0.078 g L^{-1} at 25 °C (PubChem database; https://pubchem.ncbi.nlm.nih.gov). Decylamine can be made completely soluble by converting it into a salt form, *e.g.* decylamine acetate (Figure 11.2).

On the other hand, converting acids to esters or alcohols to ethers makes them non-polar and reduces their solubility in water (Figure 11.3). Whereas ethanol is completely miscible with water, diethyl

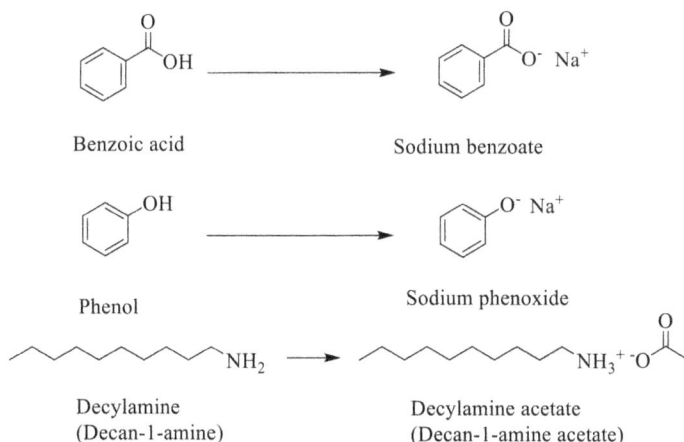

Benzoic acid   Sodium benzoate

Phenol   Sodium phenoxide

Decylamine   Decylamine acetate
(Decan-1-amine)   (Decan-1-amine acetate)

Figure 11.2 Increasing the solubility of alcohols, phenols, organic acids, and amines in water by salt formation. Through this approach, organic compounds which are not water compatible can be made into or formulated as water-soluble form for use as medicines.

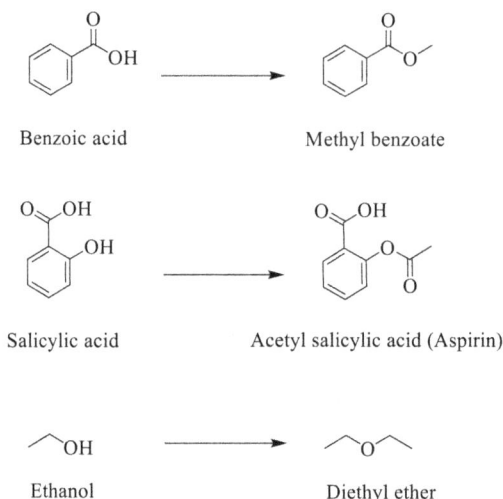

Figure 11.3 Acylation and esterification of compounds make them non-polar or less soluble in water.

ether is extremely lipophilic, *i.e.* it is a non-polar compound. As a highly volatile organic compound, it is used in anaesthesia and as an organic solvent for highly lipophilic compounds. The water solubility of aspirin as an ester is far lower than that of salicylic acid and, similarly, esterification of benzoic acid makes it even more non-polar (more hydrophobic).

As we continue to add more solute to a solvent to make a solution, we will reach a point of *saturation*, beyond which adding further solute will not dissolve more of it or increase the solution concentration. Based on how much solute can be added to a given solvent before we reach saturation, the extent of solubility can be quantified. Some solutes, such as ethanol, when dissolved in water do not reach the saturation level and are called *completely miscible* or *infinitely soluble*. At the other end of the scale, a solute is considered insoluble when it hardly dissolves to make a solution. Solubility can be quantified as molarity, molality, mole fraction, mole ratio, mass (solute) per unit volume (solvent), and other units.

The solubility of a solute in a solvent depends on temperature and pressure. For solutes such as sugars dissolving in liquid solvents, an increase in temperature generally increases the solubility. A practical application of this is to crystallise compounds out of solution, and for this an excess amount of solute is dissolved using heat. Upon cooling, the compound crystallises out of the solution. Pressure may not have a significant effect for solids and liquids but affects gases. Hence in many drug preparations, as solids dissolve in liquids, pressure has little practical effect on solubility.

A term associated with solubility is *solvation* (or its kinetic process, *dissolution*), which refers to the process of forming a solution. In the process of dissolving NaCl in water, the interaction of the solid particles of NaCl with water is called solvation, and this leads to the formation of solvated ions surrounded by water molecules. On this basis, we can now summarise the distinction between solubility, solvation, and even dissolution.

11.2.2 Solvation

Solvation refers to the process of attraction between a solute and a solvent or the process of association of solvent molecules with solute molecules or ions. When ions dissolve in a solvent (often polar solvents such as water), they are evenly dispersed and become surrounded by solvent molecules. Hence solvation is a measure of the interaction of a solvent with the dissolved solute in the solution. When water is used as a solvent, solvation is also called *hydration*. This interaction makes a stable environment for the solute to remain in the solvent environment or solution.

11.2.3 Dissolution

Dissolution is a kinetic process of solvation and is quantified by its rate, *i.e.* it is the speed at which the solute dissolves in the solvent and is measured in moles per second (mol s^{-1}).

11.2.4 Solubility

Solubility is a measure of the state of dynamic equilibrium reached when the rate of dissolution equals the rate of precipitation. It indicates the maximum amount of a solute that can dissolve in a particular solvent at a given temperature. Hence solubility is the outcome of dissolution and is measured as the amount of solute (moles) per unit amount of solvent (kilograms), *i.e.* mol kg^{-1}.

With the concept of '*like dissolves like*', we need to know which solvent is appropriate to dissolve a particular drug molecule or an organic compound. These solvents can be arranged based on the *polarity index*, which is a relative measure of the degree of solvent interaction with polar solutes. Starting from the most lipophilic (hydrophobic) solvent such as pentane at the top, the list can go down to water at the bottom (Table 11.4).

Table 11.4 Order of polarity of common organic solvents.

Solvent	Polarity
Pentane	**Least polar**
Cyclopentane, heptane, hexane, isooctane, petroleum ether	
Cyclohexane	
n-Butyl chloride	
Toluene	
Methyl *tert*-butyl ether, *o*-xylene	
Chlorobenzene, *o*-dichlorobenzene	
Diethyl ether	
Dichloromethane	
Ethylene dichloride	
n-Butyl alcohol, isopropyl alcohol	
n-Butyl acetate, isobutyl alcohol, methyl isoamyl ketone, *n*-propyl alcohol, tetrahydrofuran	
Chloroform	
Methyl isobutyl ketone	
Ethyl acetate	
Methyl *n*-propyl ketone	
Methyl ethyl ketone	
1,4-Dioxane	
Acetone	
Methanol	
Pyridine	
2-Methoxyethanol	
Acetonitrile	
Propylene carbonate	
N,N-Dimethylformamide	
Dimethyl acetamide	
N-Methylpyrrolidone	
Dimethyl sulfoxide	
Water	**Most polar**

In much of the literature, the polarity index is given as a relative value of polarity with water at the highest end mostly at 10 or 10.2 and pentane as the lowest with a value of zero. What is important here is the order of polarity that helps you choose the right solvent for the analysis of your drug/organic compound's molecules.

An organic compound or a drug molecule may form an adduct with water to form a *hydrate.* Hence a drug molecule may exist in either an anhydrous form (no water) or a hydrate form. Hydration appears to be a common phenomenon since about one-third of active pharmaceutical substances are known to make a hydrate form. Note that the presence of water in the crystalline lattice of drug molecules can change their physical properties, including their solubility and even their chemical stability.

11.3   Boiling Point, Density, and Melting Point

Another physical property of organic compounds and drug molecules that are in liquid form is the boiling point. This normally refers to the temperature at which the vapour pressure is equal to the pressure of the gas above it. It is simply a temperature point at which a liquid changes into a gas. The measurement of boiling point is given at an atmospheric pressure of one (1 atm = 760 torr). Hence the boiling point of a liquid is lower if the atmospheric pressure is reduced. This explains why the boiling point of water, which is defined as 100 °C at sea level, is lower at higher altitudes. The boiling point of water at the top of Mount Everest is said to be as low as about 70 °C.

The boiling and melting points of organic compounds depend on the intermolecular forces, which are discussed in Chapter 2 for various groups of compounds.

The density of liquids is a measure of mass per unit volume:

$$\text{Density} = \frac{\text{mass}}{\text{volume}}$$

The density of water is taken as 1 g mL^{-1} or one *gram per cubic centimetre* (1 g cm^{-3}). It could be lower for many organic compounds that appear as liquids. Both boiling point and density for liquids are a function of intermolecular forces that bring molecules together. Once again, the relative strength of the four intermolecular forces is

ionic > hydrogen bonding > dipole–dipole > van der Waals dispersion forces.

There are two other factors that affect the boiling point in organic compounds:

- Molecular size – the boiling point increases with an increase in carbon chain length.
- Branching disturbs or reduces the packing of molecules and reduces the boiling point.

The overall density and boiling point of an organic compound are thus governed by the intermolecular forces involved, depending on the atomic composition, the way in which the atoms are arranged (*e.g.* functional groups), the molecular size, and branching. We have seen these also for gaseous compounds in alkanes (Chapter 3). Ionic compounds such as NaCl and organic salts appear as solids. Whereas methanol (CH_3OH), which forms hydrogen bonds between its molecules, occurs as a liquid, butane ($CH_3CH_2CH_2CH_3$) occurs as a gas.

More hydrogen bonds mean a stronger attractive force in organic compounds, which also means a higher density and a higher boiling point compared with compounds that have little effect from hydrogen bonding. The physical characteristics of organic compounds within the same series of functional groups are described in Chapter 5.

Any organic compound also has a *melting point*, but we normally use this term for solids. When heat is applied to solids, the temperature at which the solid state changes to liquid is its melting point. For organic compounds, the melting point is measured from crystallised samples, and for a very pure compound, the melting point lies within a very narrow temperature range of about 1 °C. At this point of transition between two states, we normally have a range of temperature where the two forms exist side-by-side. The melting point of aspirin, which is commonly reported as 135 °C, actually lies in the range 134–136 °C.

11.4   Acid–Base Properties

11.4.1   Introduction and Definitions

In Chapter 5, we studied the functional groups of organic compounds called carboxylic acids (carboxyl groups) and amines, which are acids and bases, respectively. Both acids and bases of organic and inorganic compounds are common in Nature and in living systems, so we need to see their distinction in order to understand their physical and chemical properties. There are two ways of defining acids and bases, outlined below.

11.4.1.1   Brønsted Definition

In a chemical reaction, an acid is a hydrogen ion (H^+) or proton donor while a base is a species that accepts a proton. This is called the Brønsted–Lowry theory of acids and bases, as two chemists (Johannes Nicolaus Brønsted and Thomas Martin Lowry) independently developed this definition simply based on the donation or acceptance of H^+. The definition has since been expanded, however, to include both hydrogen (H^+) and hydroxide (OH^-) ions. Let us consider an aqueous (aq) solution of an acid and a base as follows:

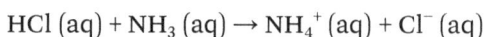

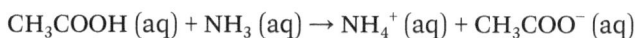

$$HCl\,(aq) + NH_3\,(aq) \rightarrow NH_4^+\,(aq) + Cl^-\,(aq)$$

$$CH_3COOH\,(aq) + NH_3\,(aq) \rightarrow NH_4^+\,(aq) + CH_3COO^-\,(aq)$$

In these examples, the hydrochloric acid (HCl) and acetic acid (CH_3COOH) in aqueous medium (aq) donate a proton (H^+) to be negatively charged, while ammonia (NH_3) accepts a proton (H^+) to form a positively charged ammonium ion (NH_4^+).

Extending the definition to the hydroxide (OH^-) ions, a metallic salt of halides can generate OH^- ions in aqueous solution:

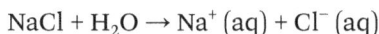

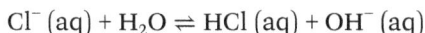

$$NaCl + H_2O \rightarrow Na^+ (aq) + Cl^- (aq)$$

$$Cl^- (aq) + H_2O \rightleftharpoons HCl (aq) + OH^- (aq)$$

In this example, a basic salt takes proton from water to generate OH^-. The symbol $\rightleftharpoons$ indicates a reversible reaction.

Bringing the above two examples of Brønsted's acid–base definition together, acids release hydrogen ions (H^+) in the solution whereas bases take up protons from the solvent (water) to generate OH^-.

The Brønsted theory of acids and bases shows that water acts both as a base and as an acid – note that water has a neutral pH of 7. The aqueous hydrogen ion (H^+) is called the oxonium ion, which is represented as H_3O^+ (aq). Water can then be represented as H_3O^+ and OH^- ions at equilibrium:

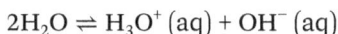

$$2H_2O \rightleftharpoons H_3O^+ (aq) + OH^- (aq)$$

An acidic substance in water that lowers the pH increases the H^+ concentration, whereas a base substance forming OH^- ions makes an alkaline solution, which increases the pH. Hence water reacting as both a proton acceptor and a proton donor can act as a base or an acid in a reaction:

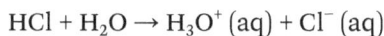

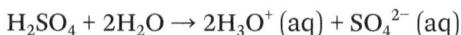

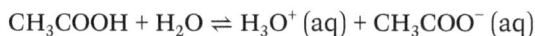

$$HCl + H_2O \rightarrow H_3O^+ (aq) + Cl^- (aq)$$

$$H_2SO_4 + 2H_2O \rightarrow 2H_3O^+ (aq) + SO_4^{2-} (aq)$$

$$CH_3COOH + H_2O \rightleftharpoons H_3O^+ (aq) + CH_3COO^- (aq)$$

In the above examples, water acts as a base. As proton donors, HCl, H_2SO_4, and CH_3COOH are acids. The products are also acids and bases called conjugate acids and conjugate bases. Cl^-, SO_4^{2-} and CH_3COO^- are conjugate bases; H_3O^+ is the conjugate acid.

Let us consider a base reacting with water:

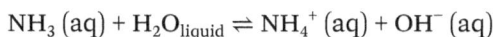

$$NH_3 (aq) + H_2O_{liquid} \rightleftharpoons NH_4^+ (aq) + OH^- (aq)$$

with water acting as an acid to form aqueous ammonia. In this case, ammonia as a base reacts with water, which acts as an acid to form a conjugate acid (ammonium ion, NH_4^+) and a conjugate base (OH^-).

In the physiology topic that covers the buffering effect of hydrogen carbonate (HCO_3^-) and reactions in the CO_2 exchange mechanism in the lung and tissues, you may address reactions of this species acting in an amphoteric manner – just like water. By accepting a proton from an acid, HCO_3^- may act as a base, or donate a proton like an acid to the hydroxide ion (base):

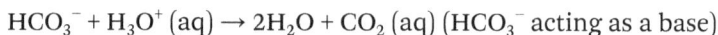

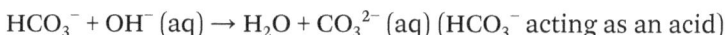

$$HCO_3^- + H_3O^+ \text{ (aq)} \rightarrow 2H_2O + CO_2 \text{ (aq) } (HCO_3^- \text{ acting as a base})$$

$$HCO_3^- + OH^- \text{ (aq)} \rightarrow H_2O + CO_3^{2-} \text{ (aq) } (HCO_3^- \text{ acting as an acid})$$

11.4.1.2   Lewis's Acid–Base Definition

An acid or Lewis acid is like H^+ that can accept a pair of non-bonding electrons whereas a base is like OH^- that can donate a pair of non-bonding electrons. Hence a Lewis acid is an acceptor and a Lewis base is a donor of an electron pair, *i.e.* acids react with bases to share a pair of electrons, with no change in the oxidation numbers of any atoms.

Other concepts relevant to chemical reactions based on Lewis's definition of acids and bases are nucleophilic and electrophilic groups (see below).

11.4.2   Nucleophile

A nucleophile is usually a reactive species (molecule, ion, or atom) with excess electrons that can be shared. They are examples of a Lewis base and are of two types: those containing a negatively charged atom (*e.g.* HO^-) or neutral with a lone pair of electrons (*e.g.* O in H_2O) that can be donated to other species. A nucleophile is a source of a pair of electrons to form a covalent bond.

11.4.3   Electrophile

An electrophile is a molecule, ion, or atom that is deficient in electrons. In a chemical reaction, an electrophile accepts a pair of electrons to form a covalent bond. Hence Lewis acids are electrophilic.

11.4.4   Lewis Acids and Bases – Some Examples

Lewis bases can be an ion, or a molecule with a lone pair of electrons that are nucleophilic and hence attack a positively charged species with their lone pair (Figure 11.4). Other species of Lewis base include

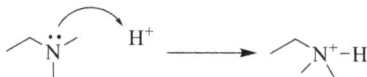

Figure 11.4 Reaction of Lewis bases with a proton.

OH^-, CN^-, CH_3COO^-, NH_3, H_2O, and CO. Amines such as $C_6H_5CH_2NH_2$ that donate a pair of electrons from the nitrogen atom are bases. On the other hand, Lewis acids accepting an electron pair are electrophilic or an electron-attracting group such as charged metal ions (*e.g.* Cu^{2+}, Fe^{2+}, and Fe^{3+}). Hence, according to Lewis's definition, every cation is an acid. There are also other groups that are Lewis acids such as CO_2 and SO_2 with multiple bonds between two atoms of different electronegativities.

Let us consider a neutralisation reaction where acids and bases react to make salt and water:

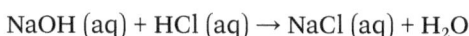

$$NaOH\ (aq) + HCl\ (aq) \rightarrow NaCl\ (aq) + H_2O$$

This reaction can be considered as a sum of Brønsted's type of reaction of the acid (HCl) and the base (NaOH) in aqueous medium:

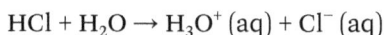

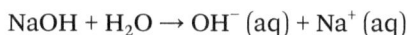

$$HCl + H_2O \rightarrow H_3O^+\ (aq) + Cl^-\ (aq)$$

$$NaOH + H_2O \rightarrow OH^-\ (aq) + Na^+\ (aq)$$

The net neutralisation reaction that obeys the Lewis acid–base definition is therefore the hydroxide acting as a base to donate its electron pair to H^+:

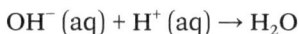

$$OH^-\ (aq) + H^+\ (aq) \rightarrow H_2O$$

11.4.5 Strong Acids and Bases

As shown in the preceding section on acid–base definition, both acids and bases react with water to produce ionised species. Strong acids that are 100% ionised in an aqueous solution include sulfuric acid (H_2SO_4), nitric acid (HNO_3), hydrochloric acid (HCl), hydrobromic acid (HBr), and hydroiodic acid (HI). Strong bases include sodium hydroxide (NaOH), potassium hydroxide (KOH), and calcium hydroxide $[Ca(OH)_2]$.

For strong acids and bases, their ionisation is complete, hence the reaction is shown by using a forward arrow:

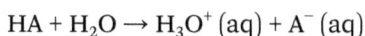

$$H_2O \rightleftharpoons H^+ + OH^-$$

$$HA + H_2O \rightarrow H_3O^+\ (aq) + A^-\ (aq)$$

Water reacts with a strong acid (HA) to give the conjugate base (A⁻). For a base:

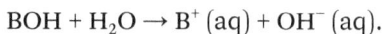

$$BOH + H_2O \rightarrow B^+ (aq) + OH^- (aq).$$

Water reacts with a strong base (BOH) to give the conjugate acid (B⁺). This means that for strong acids, the concentration of acid is equal to that of the conjugate base:

$$[H_3O]^+ = [H^+] = [A^-].$$

Species in square brackets indicate molar concentration.

From this relationship, calculation of the acidity and basicity of strong acids as a measure of pH is straightforward. The pH values of acids and bases are calculated using the expression

$$pH = -\log[H_3O^+]$$

which is the same as

$$pH = -\log[H^+]$$

As an example, calculate the pH of an HCl solution in water at a concentration of 0.5×10^{-3} M:

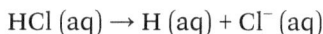

$$HCl (aq) \rightarrow H (aq) + Cl^- (aq)$$

$$[HCl] = [H^+] = 0.5 \times 10^{-3}$$

$$pH = -\log(0.5 \times 10^{-3}) = 3.30103$$

Instead of pH, we can also express pOH for bases. The calculation of pOH in this case is similar to the acid example:

$$pOH = -\log[OH^-]$$

Calculate the pOH of a KOH solution in water at a concentration of 0.5×10^{-3} M:

$$KOH \rightarrow K^+ + OH^-$$

In the above case for a strong base:

$$[KOH] = [OH^-] = 0.5 \times 10^{-3}.$$

$$pOH = -\log(2.5 \times 10^{-3}) = 3.30103$$

What if we have 0.5×10^{-3} M $Ca(OH)_2$, which liberates two OH⁻ ions in the following reaction:

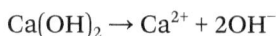

$$Ca(OH)_2 \rightarrow Ca^{2+} + 2OH^-$$

$$[OH^-] = 2[Ca^{2+}]$$

i.e. the molar concentration of OH^- is double that of $Ca(OH)_2$:

$$[OH^-] = 2 \times 0.5 \times 10^{-3} \, M$$
$$= 1 \times 10^{-3} \, M$$

$$pOH = -\log[1 \times 10^{-3}]$$
$$pOH = 3.0$$

11.4.6 Weak Acids and Weak Bases

As opposed to strong acids and strong bases, weak acids and weak bases only partially ionise in water. These groups of chemicals are highly relevant to organic compounds and drug molecules and include many organic acids and amines. The ionisation is best expressed as an equilibrium with the reactants and products as follows:

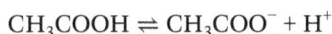

$$CH_3COOH \rightleftharpoons CH_3COO^- + H^+$$

You should note two points from this equation:

- The reaction is at equilibrium and only a small proportion of the acid is ionised to form the conjugate acid and conjugate base.
- The concentration of conjugate acid is equal to the conjugate base, thus

$$[H^+] = [CH_3COO^-]$$

By measuring the pH of the solution, the degree of ionisation and the concentration of the acid can be determined. If the pH is recorded as 1.4, we can work out the concentration of the CH_3COO^- or H^+:

$$pH = -\log[H] = 1.4$$

$$[H^+] = [CH_3COO^-] = 0.0398107 \, M = 3.98107 \times 10^{-2} \, M$$

In the above example, we have seen the pH as a measure of the concentration of hydrogen ions in an aqueous solution. We can also use another related concept, pK_a, which is calculated using the *Henderson–Hasselbalch equation*. Let us consider again the general equation for weak acids in aqueous solution:

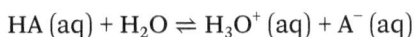

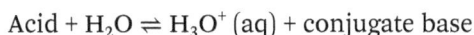

$$HA \, (aq) + H_2O \rightleftharpoons H_3O^+ \, (aq) + A^- \, (aq)$$

$$Acid + H_2O \rightleftharpoons H_3O^+ \, (aq) + \text{conjugate base}$$

$$K_a = \text{dissociation constant} = \frac{\left[H_3O^+\right]\left[A^-\right]}{\left[HA\right]}$$

$$pK_a = -\log K_a$$

We can now see the relationship between pK_a and pH as follows:

$$pH = pK_a + \log\left(\frac{\left[A^-\right]}{\left[HA\right]}\right)$$

This equation allows us to determine the proportions of the conjugate base $[A^-]$ and unionised acid $[HA]$ in the aqueous solution at a particular pH of the solution. We can also make the following generalisation:

- where the pH = pK_a, the concentration ratio of $[A^-]$ to $[HA]$ is 1;
- where the pH is higher than pK_a, it means that $[A^-]$ must be greater than $[HA]$;
- where the pH is lower than pK_a, it means that $[HA]$ must be greater than $[A^-]$.

The relative acidity of compounds can be compared by using their pK_a values. A lower pK_a value indicates a higher ionisation potential which, in turn, means a lower pH in aqueous solution. The traditional pK_a value of 14 at the top end in aqueous solution does not apply in reactions using organic solvents. Both pH and pK_a values exceeding 14 are therefore quite common. Accordingly, the pK_a value of a drug molecule could vary depending on which solvent is used to make the solution. pK_a tables are available for a vast array of organic compounds.

Several drugs contain carboxylic acid as part of their molecules (Figure 11.5). These include non-steroidal anti-inflammatory drugs (NSAIDs) such as aspirin, ibuprofen, naproxen, indomethacin, diclofenac, and mefenamic acid. The overall acidity of the molecule may depend on the structural feature of the other part of the molecule (non-polar *versus* polar), but the carboxylic acid group of such drugs behaves like an acid. With the pK_a value for these indicated drugs between 3 and 5, they are ionised at the body or physiological pH of 7.4. Benzylpenicillin is another example of an acidic drug (pK_a, $\approx$2.87).

Basic drugs include adrenaline, atropine, amphetamine, cocaine, codeine, lignocaine, and procaine with pK_a values between 8 and 11 (Figure 11.6).

The Henderson–Hasselbalch equation can also be applied to estimate the degree of ionisation of a given drug by comparing the pK_a

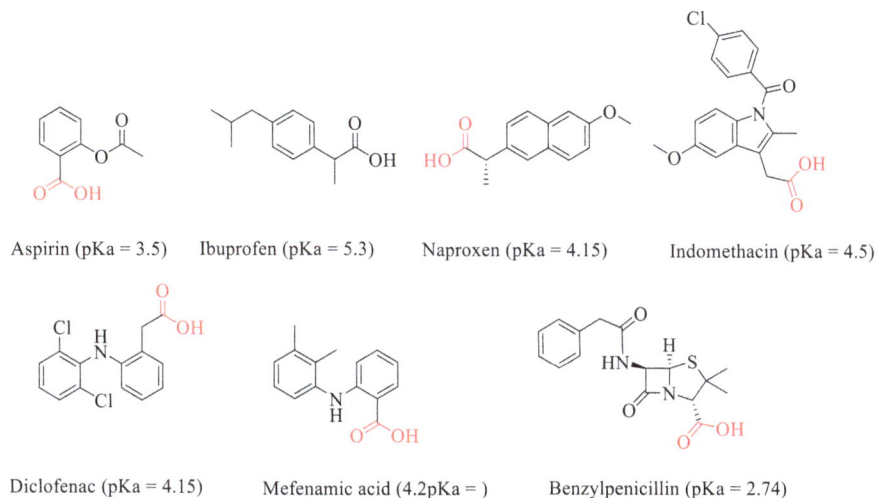

Figure 11.5 Acidic drugs that contain a carboxylic acid functional group. Data on pK_a were sourced from PubChem (https://pubchem. ncbi.nlm.nih.gov).

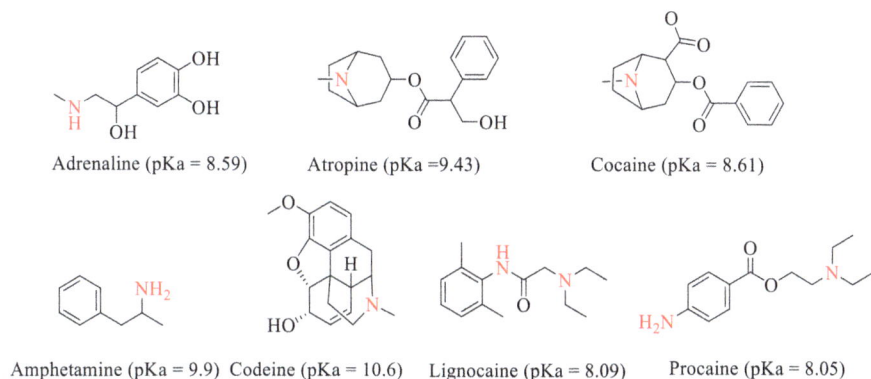

Figure 11.6 Examples of basic drugs or amines with pK_a values higher than 8. The stereochemistry of the compounds is not shown. Data on pK_a were sourced from PubChem (https://pubchem.ncbi.nlm. nih.gov).

value and the pH of the medium. For example, one can estimate the degree of ionisation of a drug in the stomach where the pH is acidic, in the blood where the pH is close to neutral, *etc.*

For acidic drugs:

$$HA \rightleftharpoons H^+ + A^-$$

where A⁻ is the ionised and HA is the unionised group:

$$\log\left(\frac{[\text{ionised}]}{[\text{unionised}]}\right) = \text{pH} - \text{p}K_a$$

$$\log\left(\frac{[\text{A}^-]}{[\text{HA}]}\right) = \text{pH} - \text{p}K_a$$

$$\frac{[\text{ionised}]}{[\text{unionised}]} = 10^{(\text{pH}-\text{p}K_a)}$$

Considering that pK_a is the pH at which the drug is 50% ionised, we can now estimate the degree of ionisation of drugs at various pH values. Let us now consider the absorption of an orally administered drug with a pK_a of 5.5 in the stomach where the pH is 3.5:

$$\log\left(\frac{[\text{ionised}]}{[\text{unionised}]}\right) = \text{pH} - \text{p}K_a$$

$$\log\left(\frac{[\text{ionised}]}{[\text{unionised}]}\right) = 3.5 - 5.5 = -2$$

$$\log\left(\frac{10^{-2}}{1}\right) = -2$$

$$\log\left(\frac{1}{100}\right) = -2$$

Only 1% of the drug (one out of 100 molecules) is ionised at the indicated stomach pH. The drug is thus highly fat soluble or easily absorbed from the stomach (ionised groups are not easily absorbed from tissues unless there is a special transport system for them).

11.5 Overview of Common Reactions

11.5.1 Addition Reaction

In an addition reaction, an atom or group of atoms or a functional group is added to a molecule. In Chapter 4, we described alkenes as being more reactive than alkanes because they have at least one double bond in their molecules. We have seen that several species such as bromine, iodine, and other halogens or hydrogen halides, when added to alkenes, change the bonding of carbons from a double bond to a single bond. Hence addition reactions are typical of unsaturated organic compounds such as alkenes and alkynes. A classic example using ethene is shown in Figure 11.7.

In Figure 11.7, X–Y represents any group including hydrogen (hydrogenation reaction), halide (bromination, iodination, chlorination, *etc.*, reaction), and water (hydration reaction). Ethene and related derivatives such as vinyl chloride can also polymerise (polymerisation reaction) in a continuous addition reaction to form polymeric macromolecules such as plastics and rubbers (Figure 11.8). Asymmetric addition reactions in alkenes and possible products are discussed in Chapter 4.

Alkynes also undergo addition reactions just like alkenes. For example, hydrogen iodide can be added to ethyne to form iodoethene (Figure 11.9).

As discussed in Chapter 2, the bonding between carbonyl carbon and oxygen in aldehydes and ketones is polarised (electron-withdrawing oxygen partially charged as δ−), leaving the carbon to be an electron-deficient centre (δ+). An electron-rich group (nucleophile) can be added to this centre, and such a reaction is called nucleophilic addition. A good example used in the literature is the addition of cyanide

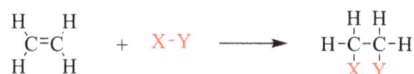

Figure 11.7   General mechanism of the addition reaction of alkenes.

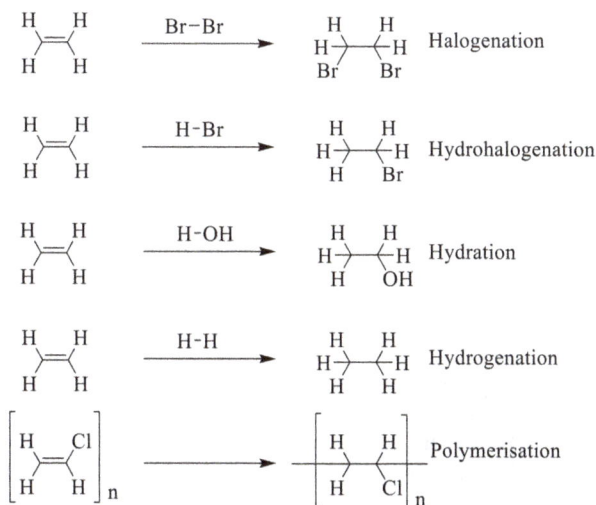

Figure 11.8   Examples of the addition reactions of alkenes.

H≡≡H + H–I ⟶ Iodoethene (H₂C=CHI structure)

Ethyne   Hydrogen   Iodoethene
              iodide

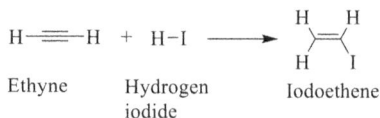

Figure 11.9 Addition reaction in alkynes. Hydrogen iodide can be added to ethyne to form an alkene (iodoethene). Note that an alkene further reacts with hydrogen iodide to form an alkyl halide.

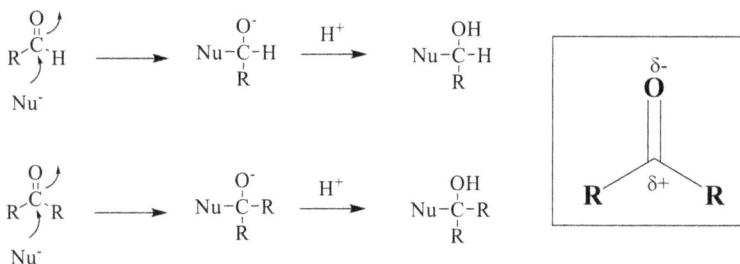

Figure 11.10 General mechanism of the nucleophilic addition reaction. In organic reactions, several reagents acting as nucleophiles are available. These include HCN, alcohols, $NaHSO_3$, and RMgX. A nucleophile is added to a molecule *via* reaction with the carbonyl carbon. Aldehydes without the stabilising effect of an alkyl group are more unstable and hence are expected to react faster.

to aldehydes and ketones (Figure 11.10). Once again, electrophiles and nucleophiles can be defined based on Lewis acids and Lewis bases as follows:

- Electrophile (electron loving): an electron-deficient species that accepts electrons from nucleophiles in a chemical reaction. Electrophiles are also *Lewis acids.*
- Nucleophile (nucleus loving): a species with electron availability that donates electrons to electrophiles in a chemical reaction. Nucleophiles are *Lewis bases.*

11.5.2   Substitution Reaction

In a substitution reaction, an atom, ion, or group of atoms, or even a functional group in a molecule, is replaced with another atom, ion, or group, *e.g.* an alkyl halide reacting with OH⁻ to form an alcohol:

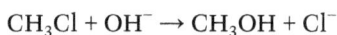

$$CH_3Cl + OH^- \rightarrow CH_3OH + Cl^-$$

A substitution reaction may involve an electron-pair donor (the *nucleophile*, Nu) and an electron-pair acceptor (the *electrophile*, E). In a fully saturated system (sp³-hybridised carbons), a nucleophilic substitution takes place when a leaving group (X) is replaced with a nucleophile. Note that a nucleophile has an electron excess such as a lone pair of electrons usually on negatively charged species (anionic) such as CN^- and OH^-, or a neutral species, partially charged ($\delta-$), or those with lone pair electrons (*e.g.* NH_3). As a nucleophile, the order of reactivity is as follows:

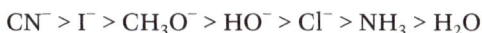

$$CN^- > I^- > CH_3O^- > HO^- > Cl^- > NH_3 > H_2O$$

Hence negatively charged nucleophiles are expected to be more reactive than neutral nucleophiles. Depending on the stages involved in the substitution process, the reaction could be termed either S_N2 or S_N1. In the S_N2 substitution (Figure 11.11), the attack by the nucleophile occurs simultaneously with removal of the leaving group from the molecule. Since the attack occurs on the opposite side of the molecule, the product formed, where chiral carbon is involved, is the mirror image of the original molecule, *i.e.* a reversal of the stereochemistry or configuration is expected at the chiral centre. Can you think why the attack occurs at the opposite side of leaving group? (See Figure 11.11.)

As explained in Figure 11.11, a nucleophilic substitution reaction of S_N2 type leads to one product by inversion of the stereochemistry

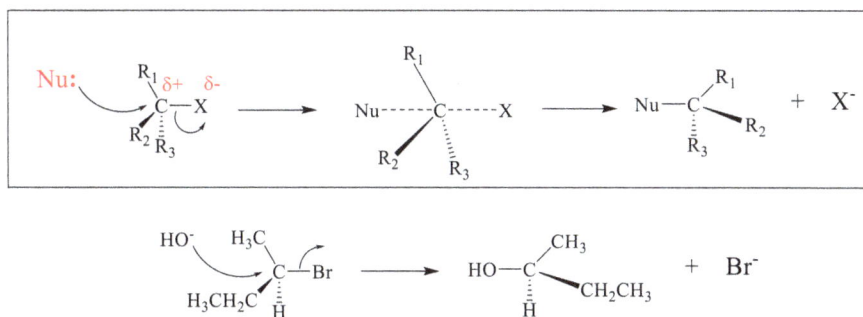

Figure 11.11 The S_N2 substitution reaction leading to the stereochemistry of the product as a mirror image of the reactant. The mechanism of an S_N2 reaction is shown in the box. The leaving group (*e.g.* halogen) has a partial negative charge ($\delta-$), which repels the electron-rich nucleophile (Nu:). Hence the nucleophile attacks at the opposite side to form a transition state (partially formed and partially broken bonds at 180° to each other) showing both nucleophile and the leaving group opposite to each other. As the leaving group is pushed out from the molecule, the tetrahedral arrangement of the carbon is restored. leading to the new stereochemistry as a mirror image of the original molecule.

of the carbon carrying the leaving group. Therefore, provided that the carbon involved in the reaction is chiral, one can expect the stereochemistry of the product to be the mirror image of the reactant. We can also make some generalisations regarding the rate of reactions of the S_N2 type. Under given experimental conditions such as a known temperature, the rate of the reaction is dependent on the concentration of both reactants: the attacking nucleophile (Nu:) and the molecule with the leaving group being attacked (R_3C–X). Increasing the concentration of either of the reactants increases the rate of reaction. On this basis, the S_N2 type of reaction can be defined as follows:

- S – substitution;
- N – nucleophilic;
- 2 – bimolecular reaction: the rate of the reaction depends on both reactants.

In the S_N2 reaction, polar solvents with a high dipole moment (*e.g.* water and alcohols) that form hydrogen bonds with the nucleophile create shielding (make a shell around the nucleophile). This stabilisation effect reduces the reaction rate. Hence the S_N2 reaction is favoured in solvents that do not participate in hydrogen bonding. Polar aprotic (no hydrogen bonding) solvents such as acetone, dimethyl sulfoxide (DMSO), acetonitrile, and dimethylformamide (DMF) are favoured. These are solvents that are polar enough to dissolve samples but are not involved in hydrogen bonding.

The S_N1 reaction proceeds through a carbenium ion intermediate (Figure 11.12), which further reacts with the nucleophile to form a racemic mixture. In this reaction, the departure of the leaving group forms a carbenium ion (carbocation), which is then attacked by the nucleophile from either side of the molecule to form the two stereoisomeric products.

As shown in Figure 11.12, the S_N1 reaction is a two-step reaction, *i.e.* the bond formation with the nucleophile and bond breakage with the leaving group do not occur simultaneously. The departure of the leaving group creates an electron-deficient group, a carbocation, with a positive charge. The nucleophile then attacks from either side of the trigonal carbocation centre to form a racemic mixture (50:50 ratio of enantiomers). The formation of the carbocation is a slow process (rate-limiting step) and the overall reaction is dependent on the concentration of the carbocation. On this basis, we can now define the S_N1 reaction as follows:

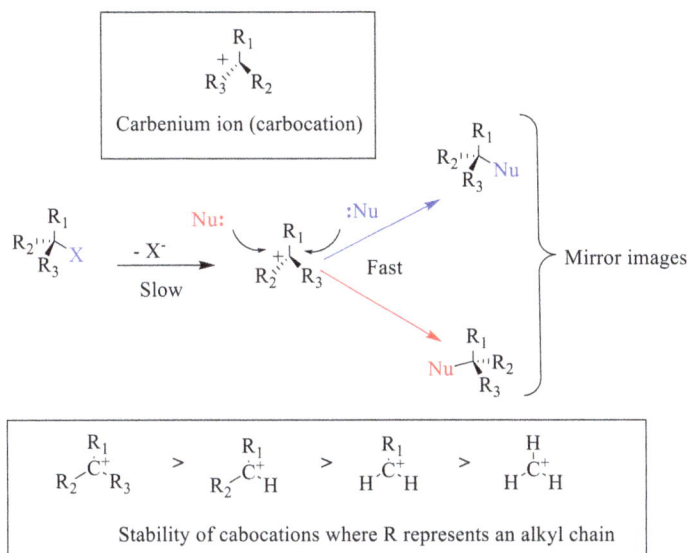

Figure 11.12 S$_N$1 substitution reaction leading to the formation of an enantiomeric mixture. Note the two-step reaction with a slow rate of carbocation formation followed by a fast rate of reaction of the nucleophilic attack. Where chirality is involved, the product is a racemic mixture. A compound that forms a stable carbocation is likely to give a better yield or faster reaction than a compound with an unstable carbocation intermediate (see the box at the bottom).

- S – substitution;
- N – nucleophilic;
- 1 – unimolecular – the rate of the reaction is dependent on only one of the reactants (the electrophile, not the nucleophile).

When considering carbocations as electrophiles, assess the stability of the charged species based on the number of substituents on the charged carbon. This is like the stability of double bonds discussed for alkenes (Chapter 4). The more substituents there are on the carbon carrying the positive charge, the more stable is the carbocation. Hence tertiary carbocations are more stable than secondary carbocations and, in turn, secondary carbocations are more stable than primary carbocations. For example, tertiary alkyl halides are expected to be more reactive than either secondary or primary alkyl halides.

Since the S$_N$1 reaction is dependent on the formation of carbocations, any reaction environment or polar solvents that stabilise the carbocations increase the rate of reaction. In this case, polar protic solvents such as water, alcohols, and carboxylic acids are favoured.

Protic solvents are those with hydrogen bonds to either oxygen, nitrogen, or fluorine (where hydrogen bonding is possible).

In a nucleophilic substitution reaction, there is competition between the leaving group and the nucleophile to be part of the molecule. If the leaving group can form a stable ion on its own, it is regarded as a good leaving group. From the electronegativity characteristics of elements of the Periodic Table that we discussed in Chapter 2, on going down the column from fluorine to iodine in group 17 the elements increase in size. For iodine, the valence electrons are far away from the nucleus and hence the tendency to gain electrons in covalent bonding is higher for fluorine than iodine. As a leaving group in alkyl halides, fluoroalkanes do not undergo nucleophilic substitution, and iodine (in iodoalkanes) leaves more readily than chlorine in chloroalkanes. On this basis, we expect the reactivity of haloalkanes in nucleophilic substitution to increase as we move down the column of the given group in the Periodic Table. Examples of good leaving groups are halide ions (I^-, Br^-, and Cl^-) and water (H_2O). Weaker bases are generally considered to be strong leaving groups. Because of this, knowing the properties of a leaving group or what constitutes a good nucleophile is important in understanding substitution reactions.

11.5.3   Elimination Reaction

In an elimination reaction, a pair of atoms or groups of atoms are removed from a molecule. Such a reaction could be a result of that facilitated by treatment with acids, bases, or metals or heating. When discussing alkanes in Chapter 3, we observed an elimination reaction leading to the formation of alkenes from alkyl halides. Alkenes can also be formed from alcohols through a dehydration reaction or elimination of water. When both leaving atoms are hydrogen atoms, the reaction is known as dehydrogenation.

An example of elimination reactions is homolytic and heterolytic cleavage reactions. These involve cleavage of the covalent bond such that each bonded atom retains one electron of the shared pair. Homolytic bond fission is also called symmetrical fission as it leads to the formation of two identical products with unpaired electrons. This creates two products consisting of free radicals. In heterolytic fission, which is unsymmetrical, the two products are not identical in that one of the products takes both shared electrons forming the bond and the other has none. This creates a net charge of positive (electron loser) and negative (electron excess) products. The general reaction is shown in Figure 11.13.

$$A\!-\!B \xrightarrow{\text{Heterolysis}} A^{\oplus} + B^{\ominus} \quad \text{Ions}$$

$$A\!-\!B \xrightarrow{\text{Homolysis}} A^{\bullet} + B^{\bullet} \quad \text{Radicals}$$

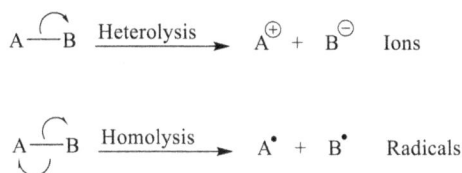

Figure 11.13 General features of homolytic and heterolytic bond fission. The pair of electrons making bonds between A and B are shown. The curved arrows indicate the movement of electrons: a single-barbed arrow indicates the movement of a single electron and a double-barbed arrow depicts the movement of a pair of electrons. Note that a single bond represents a pair of shared electrons.

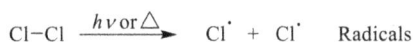

$$Cl\!-\!Cl \xrightarrow{h\nu \, or \, \triangle} Cl^{\bullet} + Cl^{\bullet} \quad \text{Radicals}$$

Figure 11.14 Homolytic bond cleavage or fission in the formation of a chlorine free radical. Light or UV irradiation and also heat ($\triangle$) can induce covalent bond cleavage.

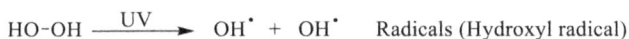

$$HO\!-\!OH \xrightarrow{UV} OH^{\bullet} + OH^{\bullet} \quad \text{Radicals (Hydroxyl radical)}$$

Figure 11.15 Homolytic bond fission in hydrogen peroxide induced by UV irradiation.

Let us consider cleavage of the chlorine gas molecule in the presence of high energy such as ultraviolet (UV) radiation. Generally, light (abbreviated as $h\nu$) or heat [delta (Δ) as a symbol of heat] energy is required to initiate the homolytic fission, which creates unpaired electrons or free radicals (Figure 11.14).

Similarly, hydrogen peroxide (H_2O_2) can give rise to hydroxyl radicals under UV irradiation (see Chapter 3). This is one of the most important chemical reactions relevant to medicine and is an example of homolytic bond fission, *i.e.* once generated, the highly reactive hydroxyl radicals (Figure 11.15) interact with biological molecules to alter their function. The chlorination of alkanes and cycloalkanes as examples of free-radical chemistry through the three stages of chain reactions (initiation, propagation, and termination) is discussed in Chapter 3.

In biology topics, you will learn about the role of oxygen-derived species collectively called reactive oxygen species (ROS). The most deleterious one is a free radical, the hydroxyl radical (HO$^{\bullet}$), and others include superoxide anion ($O_2^{-\bullet}$), peroxyl (ROO$^{\bullet}$), and alkoxyl (RO$^{\bullet}$) radicals. We also have non-radical species such as hydrogen peroxide

Carbocation   Carbanion   Radical

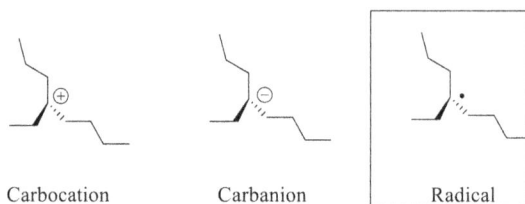

Figure 11.16 Heterolytic bond fission in organic compounds leading to the formation of carbocations or carbanions. Compare this with the free radical shown in the box.

(H_2O_2) and hypochlorous acid (HOCl), which are sources of free radicals. Although ROS at low concentrations have useful roles in normal physiological processes such as cell signalling, a higher level of their production or a weakened antioxidant defence in the body leads to a range of pathological conditions including cancer, inflammatory diseases, diabetes, and age-related diseases. You can therefore apply your knowledge of free radical chemistry in understanding disease pathology and therapies.

In organic reactions, heterolytic fission can give rise to carbocations or carbanions. This is in addition to the possibility of the free radicals generated, discussed in the previous sections (Figure 11.16).

11.5.4 Oxidation and Reduction Reactions

Oxidation and reduction reactions can be defined in three ways, as a gain or loss of oxygen, hydrogen, or electrons. The transfer of any of these three can be considered as either reduction or oxidation.

11.5.4.1 Oxygen Transfer

- Gain of oxygen – oxidation.
- Loss of oxygen – reduction.

In the example shown in Figure 11.17, copper lost oxygen (reduction) whereas magnesium gained oxygen (oxidation). In this kind of reaction with oxygen transfer, reduction and oxidation take place simultaneously and the reaction is called a *redox reaction*.

Other examples are as follows:

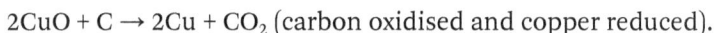

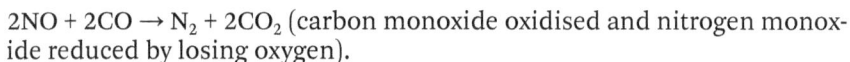

$2CuO + C \rightarrow 2Cu + CO_2$ (carbon oxidised and copper reduced).

$2NO + 2CO \rightarrow N_2 + 2CO_2$ (carbon monoxide oxidised and nitrogen monoxide reduced by losing oxygen).

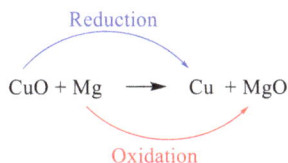

Figure 11.17   Oxidation–reduction reaction as a gain or loss of oxygen.

On the bases of oxygen gain and loss, we can also define oxidising and reducing agents as follows:

- Oxidising agent: oxidises something else.
- Reducing agent: reduces something else.

Based on oxygen gain and loss:

- Oxidising agents: give oxygen to another substance or it is a substance that loses oxygen in a reaction.
- Reducing agents: remove oxygen from another substance or it is a substance that gains oxygen in a reaction.

Now reconsider the reaction between nitrogen monoxide and carbon monoxide:

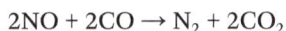

$$2NO + 2CO \rightarrow N_2 + 2CO_2$$

- Nitric oxide loses or donates oxygen and is an oxidising agent.
- Carbon monoxide gains or accepts oxygen and is a reducing agent.

Further examples are as follows:

$H_2O + Mg \rightarrow MgO + H_2$ [water reduced (loss of oxygen) and magnesium oxidised (gain of oxygen)].

You can now apply this concept of oxidation and reduction reactions in organic compounds based on the simple gain or loss of oxygen. Consider the interconversion of alkenes and alcohols discussed in Chapter 4: alkenes oxidise to make alcohols and alcohols reduce to make alkenes.

11.5.4.2   Hydrogen Transfer

- Gain of hydrogen – reduction.
- Loss of hydrogen – oxidation.

Let us consider the reaction between ammonia and bromine to form hydrogen bromide and nitrogen gas (g). The reaction shown in Figure 11.18 exemplifies oxidation or reduction based on loss and gain of hydrogen, respectively. Ammonia is oxidised by losing hydrogen, hence it is a reducing agent. Bromine is reduced by gaining hydrogen, hence it is an oxidising agent.

Another example is hydrogen sulfide, serving as a hydrogen donor when reacting with chlorine to make hydrogen chloride and sulfur (Figure 11.19).

In some reactions, both oxygen and hydrogen are involved in the loss and gain process. Consider the reaction of copper oxide with ammonia (Figure 11.20).

Copper oxide can also react with hydrogen as shown in Figure 11.21. This reaction involves a transfer of oxygen from copper oxide to hydrogen, where copper oxide is reduced to copper and hydrogen is oxidised to water.

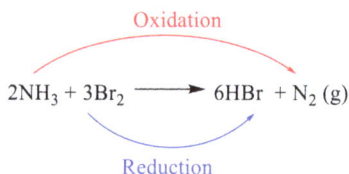

Oxidation

$$2NH_3 + 3Br_2 \longrightarrow 6HBr + N_2 \text{ (g)}$$

Reduction

Figure 11.18 Oxidation–reduction reaction as a gain or loss of hydrogen.

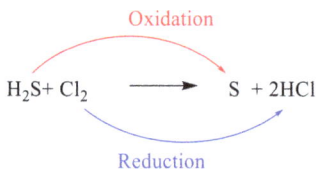

Oxidation

$$H_2S + Cl_2 \longrightarrow S + 2HCl$$

Reduction

Figure 11.19 Reaction of hydrogen sulfide with chlorine as an oxidation-reduction reaction. Hydrogen sulfide oxidises and is a reducing agent whereas chlorine reduces and is an oxidising agent.

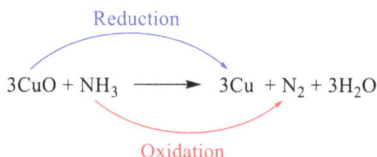

Reduction

$$3CuO + NH_3 \longrightarrow 3Cu + N_2 + 3H_2O$$

Oxidation

Figure 11.20 Reaction of copper oxide with ammonia. Copper oxide is reduced to copper by losing oxygen, *i.e.* reduction, and ammonia loses hydrogen to become nitrogen gas, *i.e.* oxidation.

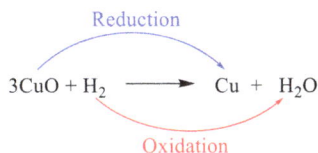

Figure 11.21 Reduction of copper oxide by hydrogen.

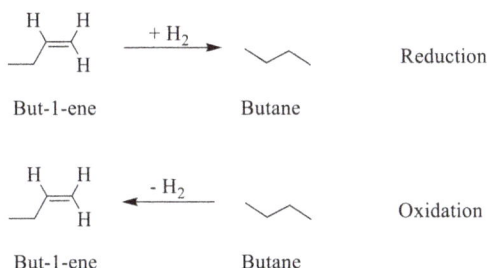

Figure 11.22 Interconversion of alkanes and alkenes through an oxidation-reduction reaction based on gain or loss of hydrogen.

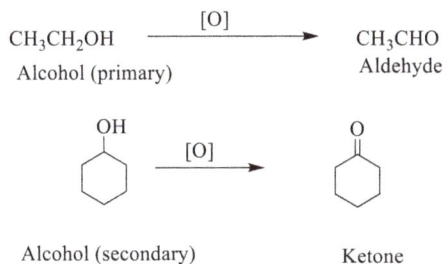

Figure 11.23 Oxidation of alcohols using oxidising agents. [O] indicates oxidation.

Now we can apply this principle of oxidation–reduction reactions to organic chemistry. Consider the interconversion of alkanes and alkenes (Figure 11.22).

Let us consider reactions of other functional groups, such as the conversion of an alcohol to an aldehyde:

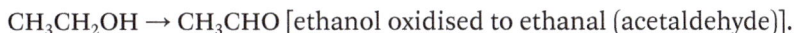

$CH_3CH_2OH \rightarrow CH_3CHO$ [ethanol oxidised to ethanal (acetaldehyde)].

By using oxidising agents such as an acidic solution of potassium permanganate, alcohols can sequentially oxidise ([O]) through removal of hydrogen to form aldehydes or ketones (Figure 11.23).

Note that the reaction in Figure 11.23 can proceed to form carboxylic acids but that process also involves a gain of oxygen and is not discussed here. Generally, a weak oxidising agent leads to the conversion of primary alcohols to aldehydes whereas strong oxidising agents convert them to carboxylic acids. Secondary alcohols can also be converted to ketones.

The two fundamental processes of life, photosynthesis and respiration, also involve oxidation and reduction reactions, as shown in Figure 11.24.

The antioxidant activity of ascorbic acid (vitamin C) is related to its conversion to dehydroascorbic acid by losing hydrogen in an oxidation process and, in turn, dehydroascorbic acid can gain hydrogen to form ascorbic acid. The loss of hydrogen from ascorbic acid can be captured using a colour reagent, 2,6-dichloroindophenol, which changes from red to colourless upon reduction as shown in Figure 11.25.

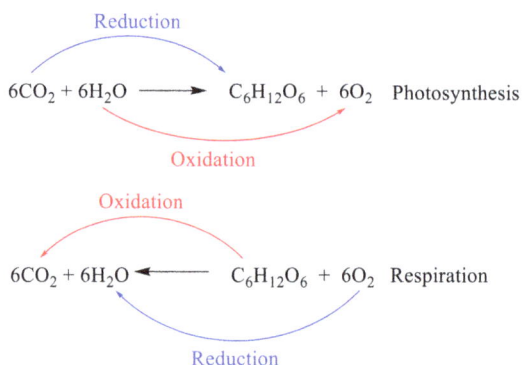

Figure 11.24   The net reactions of photosynthesis and respiration are fundamentally oxidation–reduction reactions. Note the direction of the arrows in the two reactions, *i.e.* respiration is the reverse reaction of photosynthesis.

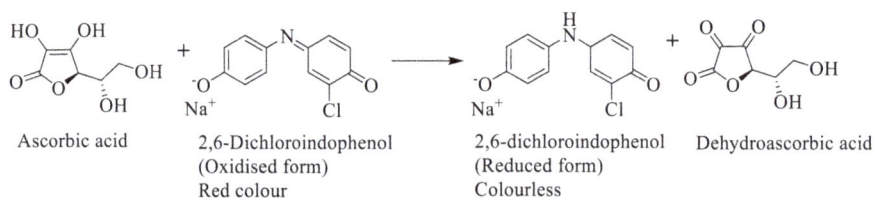

Figure 11.25   Monitoring the oxidation state of ascorbic acid using a colour reagent, 2,6-dichloroindophenol. Note that the two hydroxyl groups of ascorbic acids are oxidised to a ketone form in dehydroascorbic acid.

11.5.4.3 Electron Transfer

Consider the following reaction between magnesium and iron ions (Fe^{2+}):

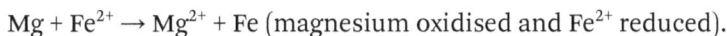

$$Mg + Fe^{2+} \rightarrow Mg^{2+} + Fe \text{ (magnesium oxidised and Fe}^{2+} \text{ reduced)}.$$

Magnesium loses electrons whereas Fe^{2+} gains electrons. This is an electron transfer reaction involving metal ions whereby a more reactive metal (magnesium) displaces a less reactive metal (copper). Based on the reactivity order of metal ions or the ability to lose electrons, a displacement reaction *via* electron gain and loss can occur in solutions. Now, consider first the reactivity order based on the ability to lose electrons or metallic characteristics (Table 11.5).

In chemical reactions, the addition of a reactive metal displaces a less reactive one from its solution. For example, the addition of solid iron to a copper sulfate solution forms iron sulfate solution by displacing copper, which precipitates as a solid:

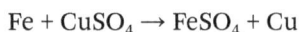

$$Fe + CuSO_4 \rightarrow FeSO_4 + Cu$$

In this case, the reaction is either a gain or loss of two electrons as follows:

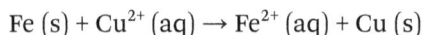

$$Fe\,(s) + Cu^{2+}\,(aq) \rightarrow Fe^{2+}\,(aq) + Cu\,(s)$$

[note the solid (s) and aqueous (aq) states].

Silver nitrate can react with copper in a displacement reaction as follows:

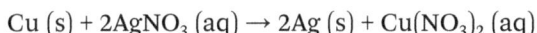

$$Cu\,(s) + 2AgNO_3\,(aq) \rightarrow 2Ag\,(s) + Cu(NO_3)_2\,(aq)$$

Table 11.5 Order of reactivity of some metals and hydrogen.

Element	Symbol	Reactivity
Potassium	K	**Most reactive**
Sodium	Na	
Calcium	Ca	
Magnesium	Mg	
Aluminium	Al	
Carbon	C	
Zinc	Zn	
Iron	Fe	
Tin	Sn	
Lead	Pb	
Hydrogen	H	
Copper	Cu	
Silver	Ag	
Gold	Au	
Platinum	Pt	**Least reactive**

This can also be expressed as

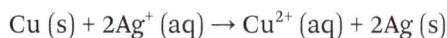

$$Cu\,(s) + 2Ag^+\,(aq) \rightarrow Cu^{2+}\,(aq) + 2Ag\,(s)$$

In the displacement of iron from its salt by a more reactive metal, consider a reaction with zinc and iron sulfate as follows:

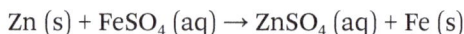

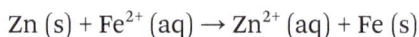

$$Zn\,(s) + FeSO_4\,(aq) \rightarrow ZnSO_4\,(aq) + Fe\,(s)$$

$$Zn\,(s) + Fe^{2+}\,(aq) \rightarrow Zn^{2+}\,(aq) + Fe\,(s)$$

The addition of solid magnesium to aqueous hydrogen bromide results in the formation of magnesium chloride solution and hydrogen gas (g). This oxidation–reduction reaction can be seen as a metal–acid reaction:

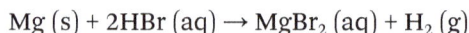

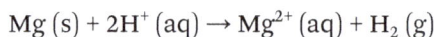

$$Mg\,(s) + 2HBr\,(aq) \rightarrow MgBr_2\,(aq) + H_2\,(g)$$

$$Mg\,(s) + 2H^+\,(aq) \rightarrow Mg^{2+}\,(aq) + H_2\,(g)$$

11.5.5   Energy Requirement of Chemical Reactions

Reactions of organic compounds and drug molecules can be broadly divided into two: exothermic and endothermic. This can be expressed as a *potential energy diagram* as an energy difference between reactants and products. The change in energy, called enthalpy change (ΔH), for these two types of reactions is shown in Figure 11.26.

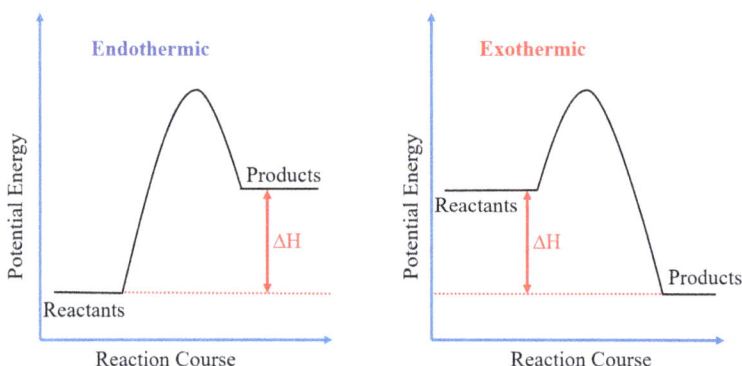

Figure 11.26   Potential energy diagram for endothermic and exothermic reactions. Note that the energy level of the products is higher than the energy of the reactants in exothermic reactions. With positive ΔH values, endothermic reactions absorb energy from the reaction environment. On the other hand, the energy level of the products is lower than the energy of the reactants in exothermic reactions. With negative ΔH values, exothermic reactions release energy to the environment.

For a chemical reaction to occur, there must be an energy input, which is called an *activation energy* (E_a) or *energy of activation*. This is the minimum energy required to cause a reaction to start. For a reaction with a low activation energy requirement, the reaction is fast, whereas a high activation energy means a requirement of high energy to bring the reactant particles in motion or to collide with each other. The activation energy can be seen as a barrier that must be overcome for the reactants to form the products. Hence exothermic reactions have low activation energy and endothermic reactions have high activation energy (Figure 11.27).

In chemical reactions, somewhere in the energy levels the molecular structure exists in a transitory form between the reactant and the product – a *transition state*. This is the highest energy level in the potential energy diagram (Figure 11.28).

The *heat of reaction* refers to the amount of heat that must be added for the reaction to proceed or that is released during the reaction.

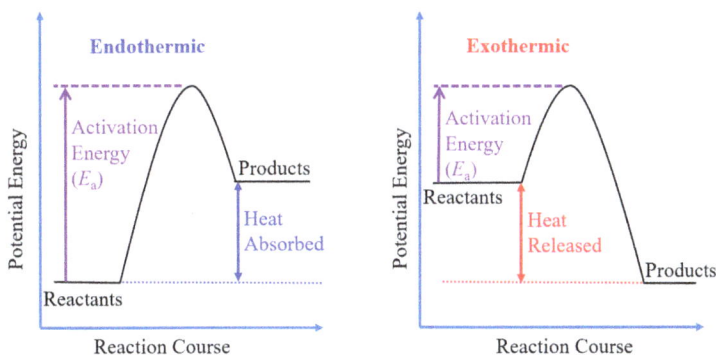

Figure 11.27   Illustration of activation energy in potential energy diagrams.

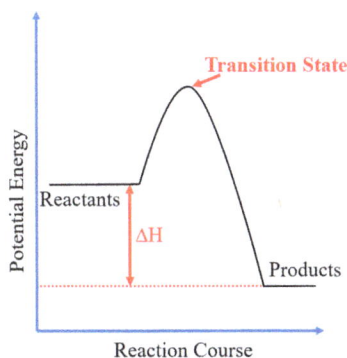

Figure 11.28   Transition state in a potential energy diagram.

Keeping the pressure of the reaction environment constant, the heat of reaction is the enthalpy of reaction (ΔH). Experimentally, the heat of reaction or ΔH can be measured using a calorimeter; a calorimeter is a device that allows one to measure the transfer of heat into or out of a system during a chemical *reaction*.

11.5.6   Catalyst

Chemical reactions may be slow to proceed and sometimes require heating, which may not be possible in biological systems. The use of substances to make a chemical reaction faster is a process of catalysis. A catalyst is therefore a substance that increases the rate of reaction without itself being changed at the end of the reaction. In biological reactions we have enzymes as catalysts, whereas in laboratories and industry several substances of organic and inorganic materials are used as catalysts.

11.5.7   Chemical Equilibrium

Equilibria in chemical reactions relate to a reversible reaction in which reactants produce a product(s) while at the same time a product(s) also breaks down to form the reactants. Reaction depends on temperature, pressure, and the concentration of the reactants, and if these variables are kept constant, the state of the forward and backward reaction rates being constant is the equilibrium of the reaction. In organic chemistry, many reactions are reversible, hence the conversion of the reactants to products is less than 100%. Note that the rates of forward and backward reactions are the same at equilibrium, but the reaction yield of the product could vary between 0 and 100%.

Let us consider a strong acid, such as HCl, which ionises almost completely in aqueous solution:

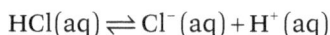

$$HCl(aq) \rightleftharpoons Cl^-(aq) + H^+(aq)$$

At equilibrium, the concentrations of the ionised products and the acid in the aqueous solution are not the same as we have a very high concentration of ionised products. Hence the reaction yield is very high and is close to 100%. This means that the equilibrium of the reaction is towards the *right-hand side*. If we start with 1 mol dm^{-3}, we may end up with 0.99 mol dm^{-3} of the products:

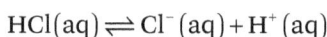

$$HCl(aq) \rightleftharpoons Cl^-(aq) + H^+(aq)$$

$$0.01 \, \text{mol dm}^{-3} \rightleftharpoons 0.99 \, \text{mol dm}^{-3} + 0.99 \, \text{mol dm}^{-3}$$

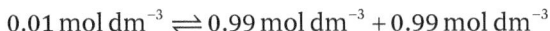

(Starting from 1 mol dm^{-3} HCl, this could be the yield at equilibrium.)

The ionisation of organic acids in aqueous solution is weak and the yield is very low. This means that the position of the equilibrium is towards the *left-hand side*. Let us consider ethanoic acid:

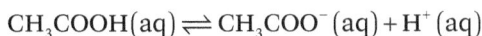

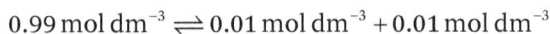

$$CH_3COOH(aq) \rightleftharpoons CH_3COO^-(aq) + H^+(aq)$$

$$0.99 \, \text{mol dm}^{-3} \rightleftharpoons 0.01 \, \text{mol dm}^{-3} + 0.01 \, \text{mol dm}^{-3}$$

(These values are for illustration only.)

The yield of the product also varies depending on the reaction environment and concentration. For example, an increase in temperature in endothermic reactions pushes the equilibrium position forwards, whereas the reverse is true for exothermic reactions, *i.e.* lowering the temperature favours the forward reaction in an exothermic reaction. The use of a catalyst increases the rate of reaction to reach the equilibrium, but there would be no change in the equilibrium position.

The equilibrium rate constant (K_c) can be defined as the concentration of products divided by the concentration of the reactants:

$$K_c = \frac{\left[Cl^- \right]\left[H^+ \right]}{[HCl]}$$

for the ionisation of HCl, and

$$K_c = \frac{\left[CH_3COO^- \right]\left[H^+ \right]}{[CH_3COOH]}$$

for the ionisation of CH_3COOH.

As a rule, consider the K_c of reactions as

$$A + B \rightleftharpoons C + D$$

$$K_c = \frac{[C][D]}{[A][B]} = \frac{[\text{Products}]}{[\text{Reactants}]}$$

11.6   Titration

In organic chemistry and biological measurements, we often need to determine the concentration of compounds in an unknown solution such as drug substances dissolved in a solvent (*i.e.* in a solution).

This could be a pure drug substance in solution or in a mixture. A simple and rather old method of quantitative analysis of organic compounds and drug molecules is titration. It involves the addition of a titrant, which is a known concentration of a solution, to a known volume of another solution of unknown concentration. We continue to add the titrant until we reach an equilibrium or neutralisation, which we measure by a colour change or other means (Figure 11.29). Since titration primarily involves the measurement of volume, it is also called *volumetric analysis*.

The most common example of titration is acid–base titration with an experimental setup as shown in Figure 11.29. By using an acid–base

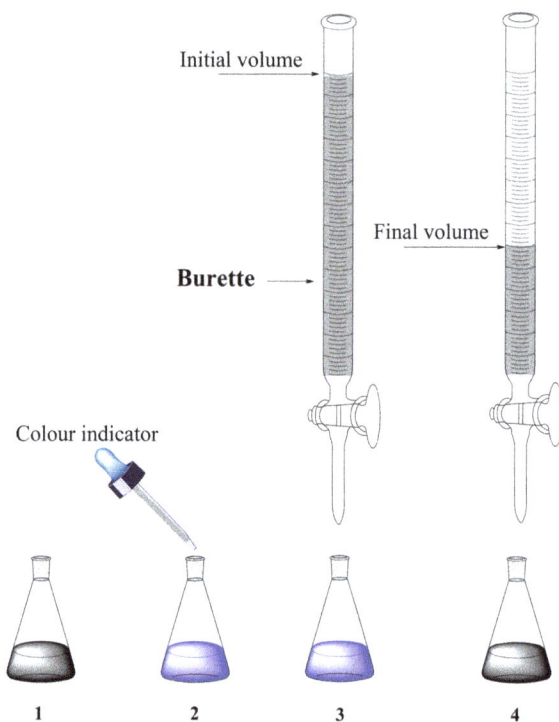

Figure 11.29   Pictorial representation of titration. (1) Prepare the acid or base of the unknown concentration to be measured. Place a known volume of this sample in a conical flask. (2) Add a few drops of the neutralisation or endpoint indicator (*e.g.* phenolphthalein for strong acid–base reactions) used for a neutralisation reaction. (3) Place the known concentration of the acid or base titrant in a burette (*e.g.* an acid if what you are measuring in the conical flask is a base). (4) Add the burette contents in small increments or drop by drop until the colour disappears – endpoint reached. Record the volume of the titrant solution dispensed from the burette.

reaction, we can determine the concentration of an unknown acid or base through titration. We use a small volume of an indicator that quickly changes colour near its pK_a value. If the sample to be analysed is a weak base, we use an indicator with a pK_a of less than 7. Readers should note the following regarding acid–base titration:

- The method is based on a neutralisation reaction between an acid and a base when they are mixed in solution.
- The acid–base indicator shows the endpoint of the titration by changing colour.

Let us consider that we want to determine an unknown concentration of an acid. For this, we need to prepare a standard solution of a base and place it in a burette or similar glassware apparatus. We place a known volume of the acid (unknown concentration) in a flask and add to it a few drops of a universal indicator. We then add the standard base from the burette drop by drop to the acid in the flask while gently mixing the flask contents until the colour change indicating neutralisation is seen. The volume of the standard base dispensed from the burette is used to calculate the concentration of the unknown acid.

For example, an unknown concentration (molar) of HCl needs to be determined by titration with a known concentration of NaOH. The neutralisation endpoint being pH 7, we can use litmus with a pK_a of 6.5 as the indicator, *i.e.* we choose an indicator with a pK_a value close to the endpoint measurement. If we place 50 mL of HCl in a flask together with a few drops of the indicator, and use 10 mL of a 0.1 M solution of NaOH from the burette to record the colour change, then:

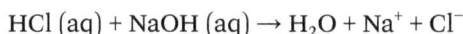

$$HCl\,(aq) + NaOH\,(aq) \rightarrow H_2O + Na^+ + Cl^-$$

$$H^+ + OH^- \rightarrow H_2O$$

The concentration (molarity, C) multiplied by the volume (mL, V) of the acid and base must be balanced at equilibrium:

$$(C \times V)_{NaOH} = (C \times V)_{HCl}$$

$$(0.1\,M \times 10\,mL)_{NaOH} = (C \times 50\,mL)_{HCl}$$

$$C_{HCl} = \frac{0.1\,M \times 10\,mL}{50\,mL} = 0.02\,M$$

Other forms of titrations are also commonly used in chemistry and biology and include precipitation titration, complexation titration, redox titration, *etc.*

11.7 Summary

In this chapter, we have learned the following:

- Using the International System of Units (SI Units) makes scientific measurements and recorded data easier to understand by the reader.
- Common SI units are metre (length), kilogram (mass), second (time), kelvin (temperature), mole (amount of substance), *etc.*
- The use of prefixes for larger multiple units (kilo, mega, giga, tera, *etc.*) and smaller submultiple units (deci, centi, milli, micro, nano, pico, femto, *etc.*) help when writing large digit values or decimals.
- Density (measure of mass divided by volume) can be used in the quantitative analysis of liquids and oily drug molecules.
- Mole, mole fraction, and mole percentage analysis are common measurements for organic compounds and analysis of drugs.
- Molar mass is the mass of one mole (1 mol) of a substance.
- For drug components in a solution, the mole fraction of one compound is its number of moles divided by the total number of moles of all components in the solution.
- Molality (m) is the number of moles of a solute divided by the amount of the solvent in kilograms.
- Molarity (M) is the number of moles of a solute per litre of solution.
- Normality (N) is the number of moles of a reactive species of the solute per litre of solution.
- Dilutions from stock solutions can be calculated using the equation $C_1 V_1 = C_2 V_2$.
- Solvation is a measure of the interaction of a solvent with the dissolved solute in the solution.
- Dissolution is a measure of the speed at which the solute dissolves in the solvent – measured as moles per second (mol s^{-1}).
- Solubility is a measure of the maximum amount of a solute that can dissolve in each solvent at a given temperature.
- Physical property analysis of organic compounds and drug molecules includes measurements of boiling point, density, and melting point.
- Acids and bases can be defined based on two definitions: the Brønsted–Lowry and Lewis's acid–base definitions.
- Acids and bases can be grouped into strong or weak based on the rate of ionisation.

- Rate of ionisation can be determined using dissociation constant, pH, and pK_a measurements.
- Common reactions in organic compounds include addition, substitution, elimination, and oxidation–reduction reactions.
- In reactions, an electron pair donor is a nucleophile whereas an electron pair acceptor is an electrophile.
- Potential energy diagrams are used to show the energy differences between reactants and products.
- Reactions may be classed as endothermic or exothermic based on the energy requirement and release from the reactions.
- Acid–base titration is used in quantitative measurements to determine the concentration of the components of unknown samples based on an acid–base neutralisation reaction.

11.8 Problems

1. In your pharmacology experiment, you are asked to inject an experimental drug at a dose of 10 mg kg^{-1}. If the drug is prepared as a 50 mg mL^{-1} solution, what volume do you need to inject into a rat that weighs 200 g?
2. Convert the following:

   a. 0.012 litre (L) to mL.
   b. 157 87 nanograms (ng) to mg.
   c. 1.476 micrograms (µg) to mg.

3. With 25 µg vitamin D tablets, you are required to take a dose of 0.05 mg per day. How many tablets do you take?
4. You have prepared a 5% solution of ibuprofen. How many milligrams (mg) do you have in 2 mL of this solution?
5. You are monitoring an enzyme reaction that converts a substrate at the rate of 10 000 units of substrate per second.

   a. How many units are converted in 0.5 s at the optimum conditions for the enzyme?
   b. If 1 mg of the enzyme contains 100 000 units, what would the required weight of the enzyme for the reaction?

6. 0.02 mol of aspirin is dissolved in 100 g of boiling water. Calculate the mole fraction and mole percentage of aspirin in the solution.
7. A stock solution of a drug is prepared at 5×10^{-4} mol L^{-1} in methanol. For your experiments, you will require 50 mL each of 20.0×10^{-6}, 40.0×10^{-6}, 60.0×10^{-6}, and 80.0×10^{-6} mol L^{-1} in methanol.

Calculate how many mL are required to make up the required concentrations.

8. Two acidic drugs A and B have pK_a values of 1.7 and 4, respectively. Show if they can be charged in the stomach at a pH of 1.7.

9. Sodium benzoate is a weak acid with poor solubility in water. You prepared its salt form (sodium benzoate), which gives an aqueous alkaline (base) solution. If you were given an unknown concentration of sodium benzoate solution, you can determine it by titrating it with an acid such as HCl.

   a. Show the chemical reaction in the titration.
   b. In the titration assay, you may be given a known volume of sodium benzoate (unknown concentration) to be placed in a conical flask with the addition of a known amount of water–diethyl ether mixture (*e.g.* to 5 mL of sodium benzoate, add 50 mL of water and 30 mL of diethyl ether). The amount of HCl needed for the titration using a colour indicator is to be measured. Why do you use diethyl ether in this experiment?

10. A drug molecule that contains an acidic (carboxylic acid) group has a pK_a value of 2.9. Comment on its ionisation in blood plasma (pH = 7.4), at urinary pH (6.0), and at stomach pH (1.8).

11. The drug atenolol has a pK_a value of 9.58. Comment on its ionisation in the stomach.

12. For acidic (HA) and basic (B) drugs, show their dissociation equations in an aqueous medium.

13. For the following questions, choose the right terminology from the choice of endothermic and exothermic:

   a. Reaction that transfers heat energy to the surroundings.
   b. The temperature of the reaction mixture decreases.
   c. The energy level diagram shows a negative energy change.
   d. Methane reacts with oxygen in a combustion reaction.
   e. An organic compound decomposes when heat is applied.

14. The molecular mass of cocaine is 303.35 g mol^{-1}. Calculate its molarity in the following solution prepared using diethyl ether:

   a. 2.139 mol in 2.3 L of solution.
   b. 0.89 g in 1.5 L of solution.
   c. 11.6 g in 1945 mL of solution.
   d. 20 g in 100 mL of solution.

15. A 1.6 L volume of a 2.5 M solution of a protein drug is diluted to a final volume of 2.5 L. What would be the molarity?
16. List the factors that affect the solubility of an organic compound.
17. While undergoing a nucleophilic substitution reaction to convert alkyl halides to alcohol, you have obtained a product with an optical rotation of −33°, while the reading for the starting material was +33°. Comment on the type of substitution reaction and reaction mechanism. What would be the type of the nucleophilic substitution reaction if the observed optical rotation for the product was zero (0°)?
18. In a nucleophilic substitution reaction, which type (S_N2 *versus* S_N1) is favoured under the following solvent conditions?

    a. Methanol.
    b. Acetonitrile.
    c. Chloroform.
    d. Ethanoic acid.

19. When a DNA molecule was incubated with hydrogen peroxide and irradiated with UV light, a substantial amount of damage was recorded. Comment on the type and mechanism of reaction.

11.9 Solutions to Problems

1. For a rat of 200 g, the required dose of 10 mg kg^{-1} means 10 mg per 1000 g or 2 mg per rat. In a 50 mg mL^{-1} drug solution, you have 50 mg in 1 mL – which means that the required dose of 2 mg is achieved by taking 0.04 mL = 40 µL.
2. Conversion:
    a. 0.012 L is 12 mL.
    b. 157 87 ng is 15.787 µg = 0.015787 mg.
    c. 1.476 µg is 0.001476 mg = 1.476×10^{-3} mg.
3. 0.05 mg per day means 50 µg per day – hence two 25 µg vitamin D tablets need to be taken.
4. A 5% solution is 5 g in 100 mL, which is 5000 mg in 100 mL or 50 mg mL^{-1}, *i.e.* 100 mg per 2 mL.
5. Enzyme reaction:
    a. 10 000 units per s = 5000 units per 0.5 s.
    b. 100 000 units per mg means 5000 units per 0.05 mg, *i.e.* 0.05 mg of the enzyme is needed.

6. 0.02 mol of aspirin is dissolved in 100 g of boiling water.

$$\text{Water} = 18.0153 \text{ g mol}^{-1}.$$

$$\text{No. of moles of water} = \frac{100}{18.0153} = 5.55 \text{ mol.}$$

$$\text{No. of moles of aspirin} = 0.02 \text{ mol.}$$

$$\text{Total no. of moles} = 5.55 + 0.02 = 5.57.$$

$$\text{Mole fraction of aspirin} = \frac{0.02}{5.57} = 0.0035907.$$

$$\text{Mole percentage of aspirin} = 0.35907\%.$$

7. You can use the equation $C_1V_1 = C_2V_2$:

$$5 \times 10^{-4} \text{ mol L}^{-1} \times V_1 = 20 \times 10^{-6} \text{ mol L}^{-1} \times 50 \text{ mL}$$

$$V_1 = \frac{20 \times 10^{-6} \text{ mol L}^{-1} \times 50 \text{ mL}}{5 \times 10^{-4} \text{ mol L}^{-1}} = 2 \text{ mL.}$$

- We take 2 mL of the stock solution and dilute it using 48 mL of methanol to make up 50 mL of 20×10^{-6} mol L^{-1} solution.

Using the same calculation:

- We take 4 mL of the stock solution and dilute it using 46 mL of methanol to make up 50 mL of 40×10^{-6} mol L^{-1} solution.
- We take 6 mL of the stock solution and dilute it using 44 mL of methanol to make up 50 mL of 60×10^{-6} mol L^{-1} solution.
- We take 8 mL of the stock solution and dilute it using 42 mL of methanol to make up 50 mL of 80×10^{-6} mol L^{-1} solution.

8. Drugs A and B have pK_a values of 1.7 and 4, respectively. To show if they can be charged in the stomach at a pH of 1.7:

Let us use the equation $\dfrac{\text{ionised}}{\text{unionised}} = 10^{(\text{pH}-\text{p}K_a)}$.

For drug A, $\dfrac{\text{ionised}}{\text{unionised}} = 10^{(1.7-1.7)} = 1$. The ratio of ionised to unionised drug is 1, meaning that 50% of the drug is ionised at the indicated stomach pH.

For drug B, $\dfrac{\text{ionised}}{\text{unionised}} = 10^{(1.7-4)} = 10^{-2.3} = \dfrac{1}{10^{2.3}}$. The drug is almost unionised at the indicated stomach pH.

Since unionised drugs readily pass through the cell membrane, drug B is more likely to be absorbed from the stomach than drug A.

9a. $C_6H_5COONa + HCl \rightarrow NaCl + C_6H_5COOH$.

9b. The product of the titration is benzoic acid with poor water solubility. It would precipitate out in the aqueous solution and may interfere with the endpoint colour measurement. Hence we add diethyl ether to the benzoic acid, with the ether layer as the top organic layer, while sodium benzoate is in the aqueous layer. Continuous shaking/stirring is necessary.

10. For an acidic drug, the plasma pH (7.4) is more basic than the functional group: $pH > pK_a$. The drug is thus ionised – an acid functional group would ionise in a basic environment. The urinary pH (~6) is also more basic than the functional group, hence the drug would be primarily ionised. In the stomach, with $pH < pK_a$, the environment is more acidic than the drug, hence the acidic functional group is not ionised.

11. $pH < pK_a$. A basic drug is ionised in an acidic environment.

12. The equations are

$$HA + H_2O \rightleftharpoons A^- + H_3O^+$$

$$B + H_2O \rightleftharpoons BH^+ + OH^-.$$

13. The terminology is as follows:
    a. Exothermic.
    b. Endothermic.
    c. Exothermic.
    d. Exothermic.
    e. Endothermic.

14. The concentrations are as follows:

    a. $mol\,L^{-1} = \dfrac{2.139}{2.3} = 0.93\,M.$

    b. $moles = \dfrac{0.89}{303.35} = 0.0029339; moles\,per\,1.5\,L = 0.00195594\,M.$

    c. $moles = \dfrac{11.6}{303.35} = 0.0382397; 1945\,mL = 1.945\,L; mol\,L^{-1} = 0.0196605\,M.$

    d. $moles = \dfrac{20}{303.35} = 0.0659304; 100\,mL = 0.1\,L; mol\,L^{-1} = 0.6593044\,M.$

15. $C_1V_1 = C_2V_2$; $2.5\,M \times 1.6\,L = C_2 \times 2.5\,L$; $C_2 = 1.6\,M.$

16. Temperature, pH, solute characteristics, solvent type, and volume of solvent. You can also add a decrease in particle size as greater access to the solvent increases solubility.

17. S_N2 reaction gives a product (optical rotation of −33°) that is a mirror image of the reactant (+33°). S_N1-type reaction yielding an enantiomeric mixture [optical rotation of zero (0°)].

18. The reactions are as follows:
    a. Methanol S_N1.
    b. Acetonitrile S_N2.
    c. Chloroform S_N2.
    d. Ethanoic acid S_N1.
19. This is an example of a homolytic fission reaction, and it generates a free radical (hydroxyl radical). The hydroxyl radical is highly unstable and reacts with DNA – it oxidises DNA.

SECTION IV
Drug–Target Interactions and Common Sources of Drugs and their Structural Classes: Inspiration from Nature, Synthesis and Recombinant Technology

12 Drug–Target Interactions

Learning Objectives

After completing this chapter, you are expected to be able to:

- Describe the types of interactions between drugs and their biological targets.
- Explain why covalent drug–target interactions are useful in treating bacterial infections.
- Explain how amino acids are involved in electrostatic interactions between drugs and their targets.
- Identify functional groups in drugs and their targets that are attributed to hydrogen bonding interactions.
- Identify all functional groups in a drug molecule that contribute to binding with their targets.

12.1 Introduction to Drug–Target Interactions

For a drug molecule to act in the body, it must be administered through a convenient route such as an oral, parenteral (injection), sublingual, rectal, optic, ocular, nasal, or vaginal route. While being transported from its site of administration to its target, a drug molecule is subjected to numerous challenges, such as destruction by the host enzymes (*e.g.* the digestive systems) and unfavourable environments (*e.g.* low gastric acidity), detoxification and elimination by the liver and the kidney, and transportation by binding to proteins and

Basic Chemistry for Life Science Students and Professionals: Introduction to Organic Compounds and Drug Molecules
By Solomon Habtemariam
© Solomon Habtemariam 2023
Published by the Royal Society of Chemistry, www.rsc.org

other components (*e.g.* in the blood). Having reached the target site, a drug may stimulate or inhibit receptors, activate or inhibit enzymes, modulate the function of ion channels or transporter proteins, *etc.* The action of a drug molecule in the body is called *pharmacodynamics* (*PD*), while the movement of a drug molecule into, through, and out of the body is called *pharmacokinetics* (*PK*). Both PD and PK involve the interaction of a drug with biological molecules through specific and/ or non-specific binding. A good drug is one that selectively binds to its target molecule, induces the desired pharmacological effect with little or no side effects, and readily metabolises and is eliminated from the body. For the subject of drug–target interactions in this chapter, we focus on specific interactions between a drug molecule and its biological targets such as receptors and enzymes. A drug interacts with its target molecules through one or more of the following mechanisms: covalent bonding, hydrogen bonding, electrostatic, and lipophilic interactions.

The Movement and Action of a Drug in the Body – Key Facts

- Pharmacodynamics (PD) – the action of a drug molecule in the body.
- Pharmacokinetics (PK) – the movement of a drug molecule into, through, and out of the body.
- Both PK and PD involve interactions of drugs with various targets of cellular or acellular components.
- Drugs interact with targets through one or more of the following: electrostatic, covalent bonding, hydrogen bonding, and lipophilic interactions.

12.2   Covalent Interactions

Chapter 2 presented examples of *covalent bonding* between two non-metal elements, and we studied covalent bonding further in Chapters 3–5 by reviewing the various structural groups of organic molecules. Drugs based on organic compounds all involve bonding between atoms through the sharing of a pair of electrons. This interaction is very strong and cannot be broken unless high energy is applied. A drug molecule binding through covalent bonding with its target molecule such as enzymes or receptors is thus considered as a permanent or an irreversible binding. An irreversible binding also means that the effect is long-lasting. If this happens to a key biological molecule (*e.g.* a protein) in the body, some degree of toxicity is expected at least until the body removes and replaces the targeted (or dysfunctional) biomolecule. This kind of interaction works well if the targeted enzymes or receptors belong to a foreign body such as bacteria, fungi, or pathogens or parasites invading the body. Let us consider that a drug binds covalently to either the cell surface or metabolic targets of a particular pathogen. As it is unable to disassociate from the targeted biomolecule(s), it permanently inactivates the pathogen until such time that a drug resistance mechanism is developed by the pathogen. Hence covalent interaction of an anti-infective agent with less toxicity to the host can be designed.

β-Lactam Antibiotics – Key Facts

- Contain a β-lactam ring system in their molecular structure.
- Include penicillins and cephalosporins.
- They are the most widely used antibacterial agents in the world.
- Interact with penicillin-binding proteins and disrupt peptidoglycan synthesis.
- β-Lactamase enzymes produced by antibiotic-resistant bacteria also interact with these drugs through covalent interactions.

The binding of the β-lactam class of antibiotics with pathogenic bacterial targets represents the best example of covalent interactions of drugs. These include penicillins and cyclosporines with a structural moiety of a four-membered ring containing an amide bond. Covalent bonding between a β-lactam antibiotic at a specific amino acid site of proteins, called the penicillin-binding protein, inhibits bacterial cell wall synthesis. Since the biological target is unique to bacteria, the process of covalent interaction does not show toxicity towards the host or human body. Bacteria also have the capacity to overcome this damage by β-lactam antibiotics as they develop resistance through the synthesis of an enzyme called *β-lactamase*. By breaking the β-lactam ring of these antibiotics, those bacteria that produce the enzyme and secrete it, upon exposure to β-lactam antibiotics show multi-resistance to many groups of antibiotics, including penicillins, cephalosporins, and cephamycins. Overall, both the action of β-lactam antibiotics and their inactivation by β-lactamase involve covalent bond formation between the drugs and target proteins/enzymes (Figure 12.1).

Platelet aggregation is a normal physiological process that is required in blood clotting processes to limit the shedding of blood from damaged blood vessels. Unfortunately, it is also a major pathological

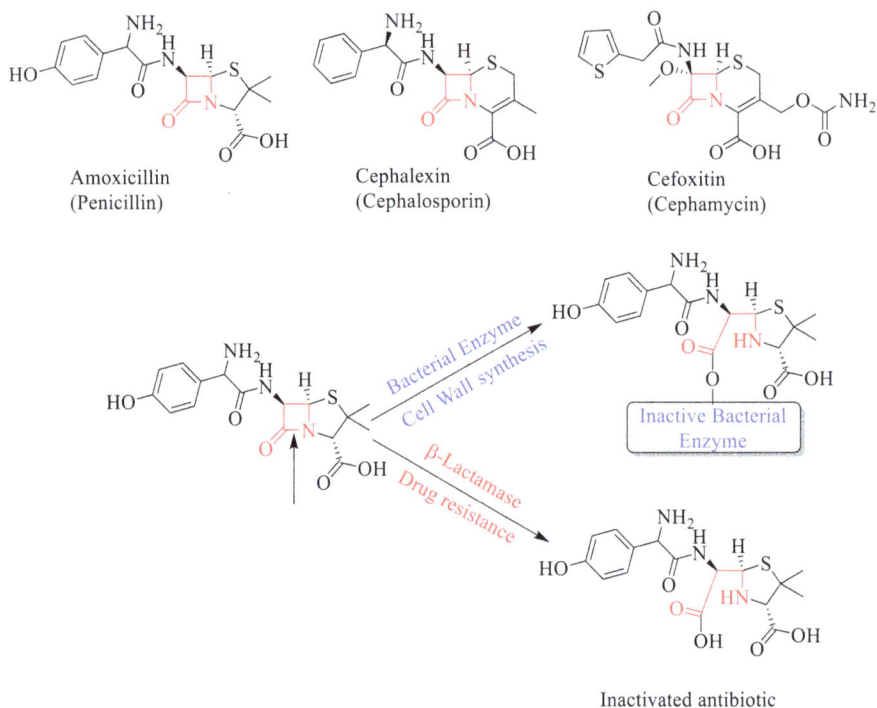

Figure 12.1 Structures of common β-lactam antibiotics and their covalent interaction with bacterial cell wall synthesis target and enzyme (β-lactamase). Note the covalent bonding formation by opening of the β-lactam ring indicated by an arrow.

occurrence in diseases such as thrombosis and leads to occlusion of blood vessels. Hence antiplatelet drugs such as aspirin are prescribed for a range of cardiovascular conditions to avoid thrombosis formation and/or enable normal blood flow through blood vessels. The maintenance of normal homeostasis control means that platelets are subjected to a balanced act of stimuli for aggregation and disaggregation. Thromboxane production in platelets is one of the major stimuli for platelet aggregation. Its synthesis is dependent on the activity of the cyclooxygenase (COX) enzymes that produce prostaglandins followed by the formation of thromboxane by the action of thromboxane synthase. In previous chapters, we have already considered the aspirin structure as a class of compound with an ester functional group. The covalent interaction of aspirin with COX enzyme of platelets leads to *permanent acetylation* at the enzyme's active site (Figure 12.2). As a result, platelets are unable to synthesise a key biological molecule (thromboxane) and are inhibited from aggregation for their whole

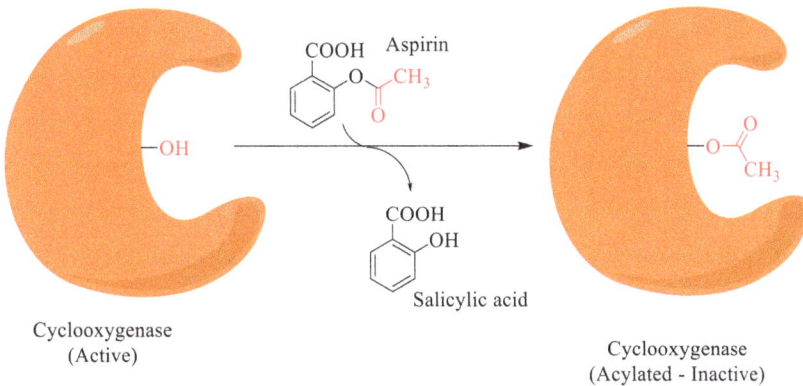

Figure 12.2 Covalent interaction of aspirin with cyclooxygenase (COX) enzyme. Aspirin acetylates the active site of COX, leading to inactivation of the platelet enzyme. This leads to inhibition of platelet aggregation. Many anti-inflammatory drugs work through this mechanism.

life span. Since platelets do not have a nucleus and cannot form new proteins/enzymes, the effect of aspirin is more pronounced in platelets than other cells. Given that COX enzymes are available in various tissues and organs, the effect of aspirin is widespread, although a small dose is enough to switch off the COX enzyme isoform found in platelets.

Aspirin – Key Facts

- It is one of the oldest pharmaceutical agents and still in use today.
- It is an anti-inflammatory and antiplatelet agent.
- It interacts with and inactivates a target enzyme, cyclooxygenase, through covalent interaction.
- Acetylation of the active site of the enzyme deprives platelets of a key mediator that promotes platelet aggregation.
- Many anti-inflammatory agents work through this mechanism of action.

Note that covalent interaction between drugs and targets is a kind of irreversible binding that leads to a long-lasting biological effect. As indicated above, it has some advantages, especially in targeting foreign bodies such as microorganisms, *i.e.* targeting a unique biological process in the parasite/pathogen that is not shared by the host.

Starting from the synthesis of aspirin by the pharmaceutical company Bayer during the 1890s and the discovery of penicillin V in 1928, numerous drugs that act through covalent interactions with their targets have been developed. Good examples of such drugs in use today are discussed below.

12.2.1 Anti-infective Drugs that Act Through Covalent Interactions With Targets

As explained above, several antibiotics of the β-lactam series bind to penicillin-binding proteins (PBPs) and inhibit cell wall synthesis in bacteria. Antibiotics of this group with effective therapeutic value against bacterial infection include amoxicillin, cefaclor (Ceclor), ceftriaxone (Rocephin), cefuroxime axetil (Ceftin), cephalexin (Keflex), meropenem, omnicef, and penicillin V.

The first committed step of peptidoglycan synthesis as part of bacterial cell wall synthesis is catalysed by the MurA enzyme. A prototype drug that acts as an antibacterial agent by covalently binding to this enzyme at the active site residue (Cys115) is fosfomycin.

12.2.2 Antidiabetic Drugs that Act Through Covalent Interactions With Targets

Vildagliptin (Galvus) and saxagliptin (Onglyza) are drugs used for treating type-2 diabetes. Their main target is dipeptidyl peptidase-4 (DPP-4), a serine protease enzyme that degrades the glucagon-like peptide 1 (GLP-1) and other incretin hormones. The incretins promote the production of insulin when it is needed, and they also reduce the amount of glucose being produced by the liver (gluconeogenesis). The levels of these hormones are particularly high at meal times. By stopping the breakdown of these hormones (incretins) by DPP-4, we can reduce the amount of glucose in the blood in diabetic patients. Many DPP-4 inhibitors have an electrophile nitrile (R–CN or R–C≡N) structure (some of them have boronic acid, diphenyl phosphonate, or other structures instead) that form a covalent bond with an active site (amino acid serine) of the enzyme. Examples of DPP-4 inhibitors are shown Figure 12.3. Note that even though covalent adduct formation is involved in the activity of these drugs, their binding with the active site of the enzyme requires other forms of interaction, including extensive hydrophobic, van der Waals, and hydrogen bonding interactions.

Targeting Dipeptidyl Peptidase-4 (DPP-4) to Treat Diabetes – Key Facts

- Glucagon-like peptide 1 (GLP-1) and other similar peptides enhance the secretion of insulin and suppress the release of glucagon (a physiological insulin antagonist) by the pancreas.
- The life span of these peptides is short, however, owing to the activity of degrading enzymes, primarily DPP-4.
- Increasing the life span of these useful peptides is an important therapeutic strategy in diabetes.
- Several DPP-4 inhibitors that act through covalent interaction are now available for clinical use.

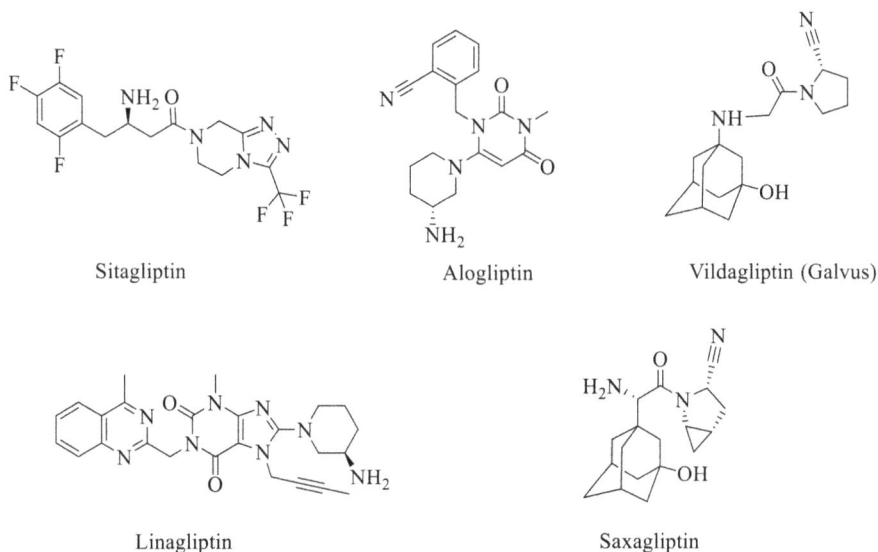

Sitagliptin   Alogliptin   Vildagliptin (Galvus)

Linagliptin   Saxagliptin

Figure 12.3 Structures of some clinically useful DPP-4 inhibitors.

12.2.3 Drugs for Parkinson's Disease that Act Through Covalent Interactions With Targets

Parkinson's disease results from excessive death of neuronal cells that use dopamine as a neurotransmitter. These neuronal cells are located in the substantia nigra region of the brain. One therapeutic strategy for treating Parkinson's disease is to increase the level of dopamine to compensate for the loss of these neurons and this can be achieved by inhibiting the enzymes, monoamine oxidase (MAO) type A and B, that destroy dopamine. Rasagiline and selegiline are such drugs that bind irreversibly to MAO-B through covalent interactions. The structures of these compounds along with their covalent interactions with the enzyme are shown in Figure 12.4.

Parkinson's Disease Therapy: MAO-B Inhibition Through Covalent Inter-actions – Key Facts

- Rasagiline is a drug used to treat Parkinson's disease – it reduces motor fluctuations.
- The *R*-isomer is a selective, potent, and irreversible inhibitor of the enzyme MAO-B that destroys the neurotransmitter dopamine.
- The *S*-isomer has a neuroprotective effect, but it acts through a different mechanism as it is less potent in inhibiting MAO-B.
- The inhibition of MAO-B by rasagiline and its analogues such as selegiline is through their reactive propargylamine moiety.
- The interaction of this drug is through covalent linkage with the enzyme cofactor (FAD), leading to the formation a flavocyanine adduct.

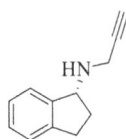
Rasagiline

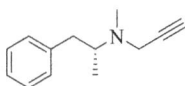
Selegiline

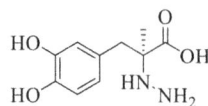
Carbidopa

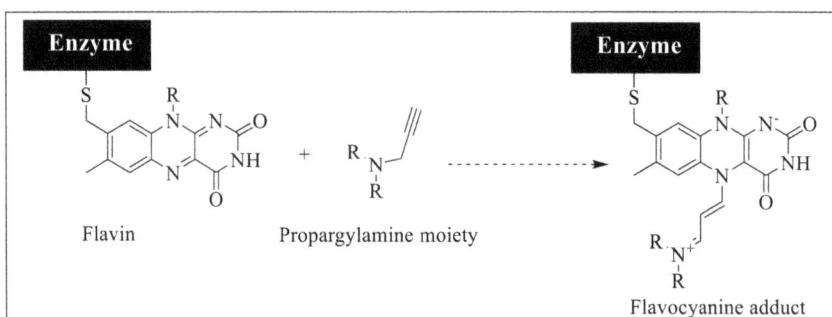

Figure 12.4 Anti-Parkinson's disease drugs that act through irreversible inhibition of enzymes. The interaction of rasagiline and selegiline with MAO-B is shown in the box. Although multiple steps are involved in the reaction, the indicated propargylamine moiety of these compounds interacts with the cofactor of the enzyme, flavin adenine dinucleotide (FAD). The flavin nucleus in the FAD is altered through the reaction to form a flavocyanine adduct, which makes the enzyme permanently inhibited.

Another therapeutic approach for Parkinson's disease is to increase the rate of synthesis of dopamine in neuronal cells. Since dopamine is synthesised from its precursor L-DOPA, making the precursor available to the brain while inhibiting its unnecessary synthesis (through the enzymatic action of DOPA decarboxylase) in the peripheral system has a therapeutic advantage in Parkinson's disease. Carbidopa (Figure 12.4) is administered together with L-DOPA and its effect through covalent interaction on DOPA decarboxylase is to inhibit the utilisation of L-DOPA outside the central nervous system (CNS) (in the peripheral tissues). For the benefit of clarifying this mechanism of action, the following notes are also added here:

- Dopamine cannot cross the blood–brain barrier and hence cannot be peripherally administered as a drug to treat Parkinson's disease.
- We use instead the precursor of dopamine, L-DOPA, that crosses the blood–brain barrier and hence reaches the substantia nigra region of the CNS where dopamine synthesis is needed.
- A substantial amount of L-DOPA administered orally or through the peripheral system is lost by the enzymatic action of DOPA decarboxylase, which converts L-DOPA to dopamine outside the CNS (unnecessary outcome).
- By inhibiting the activity of DOPA decarboxylase outside the CNS using carbidopa, a therapeutic benefit in Parkinson's disease is achieved.
- Carbidopa cannot cross the blood–brain barrier and its effects are limited to the peripheral system, leaving the effect of the enzyme (DOPA decarboxylase) in dopamine biosynthesis in the CNS unaffected.

12.2.4 Drugs for Alzheimer's Disease that Act Through Covalent Interactions With Targets

Alzheimer's disease (AD) is characterised by a significant loss of neurones involved in learning and memory. The pathological hallmark of the disease is primarily linked to the loss of neurones with acetylcholine (ACh) as a neurotransmitter. Since acetylcholinesterase (AChE) is the main neuronal enzyme that breaks down ACh, inhibiting this enzyme to prolong the life span of ACh is a therapeutic strategy in AD. Rivastigmine is an approved therapy that inhibits AChE through covalent interactions. Its phenolic carbamate structure acylates the amino acid serine at the active site of the enzyme (Figure 12.5). Other drugs such as physostigmine and neostigmine are reversible AChE inhibitors, which are prototype drugs for treating AD.

Acetylcholinesterase (AChE) Targeted by Drugs Through Covalent Interactions – Key Facts

- Acetylcholine (ACh) is a neurotransmitter for cholinergic neurons.
- In the CNS, cholinergic neurons in the cortex are involved in learning and memory processes.
- Loss of cholinergic neurons in the brain is a pathological feature of Alzheimer's disease (AD).
- Increasing the life span of ACh by inhibiting the degrading enzyme (AChE) is a therapeutic strategy in AD.
- Reversible inhibitors of drugs that acetylate the enzyme are therapeutically relevant for treating AD.
- Irreversible inhibitors of the enzyme such as nerve poisons have limited therapeutic application – they have applications instead in chemical warfare.

While reversible inhibitors of AChE have therapeutic implications for AD and other peripheral diseases (*e.g.* myasthenia gravis), irreversible inhibition of the enzyme through covalent interactions is also a mechanism of action of various toxins/poisons. The long-lasting inhibition of AChE by these agents leads to excessive accumulation of ACh with severe central and peripheral consequences. Nerve gases such as VX, tabun, soman, sarin, and cyclosarin interact through their phosphorus group with the active site of the enzyme to make strong irreversible covalent bonds (Figure 12.6). They are what we call the organophosphate class of nerve gases and are used in chemical warfare. Many insecticides also act by targeting AChE through irreversible covalent interactions.

12.2.5 Inhibitors of Gastric H⁺/K⁺-ATPase Through Covalent Interactions With Targets

In the process of acid secretion in the stomach, the final step is mediated by the proton pump called gastric H^+/K^+-ATPase. Located within the gastric membrane vesicles, it is responsible for the exchange of intracellular H^+ and extracellular K^+ by using the hydrolysis of cytoplasmic ATP. Acid-related diseases such as peptic ulcers can be targeted by

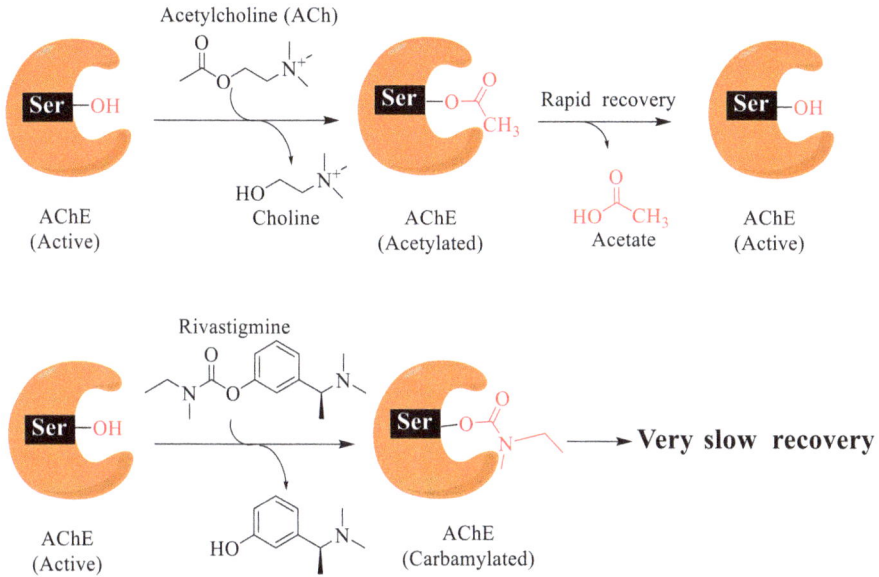

Figure 12.5 Covalent interaction of rivastigmine with acetylcholinesterase (AChE). In the hydrolysis of the neurotransmitter acetylcholine (ACh), the active site of the enzyme with serine (Ser) amino acid residue is transiently acylated followed by rapid recovery. Rivastigmine is similarly hydrolysed by the enzyme but the acetylated enzyme (with a carbamyl group – carbamylated) is far too slow to recover. Hence the activity of AChE is inhibited, leading to the accumulation of vital ACh in the brain of Alzheimer's disease patients where the neurotransmitter is deficient.

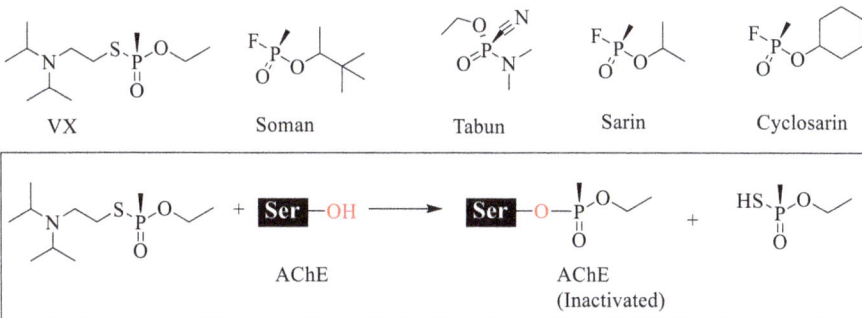

Figure 12.6 Irreversible inhibitors of acetylcholinesterase. Through strong covalent interactions, nerve gases have a very long-lasting inhibition effect on AChE. Whereas reversible AChE inhibitors serve as drugs, primarily for treating AD, irreversible inhibitors such as nerve gases and insecticides are regarded as poisons.

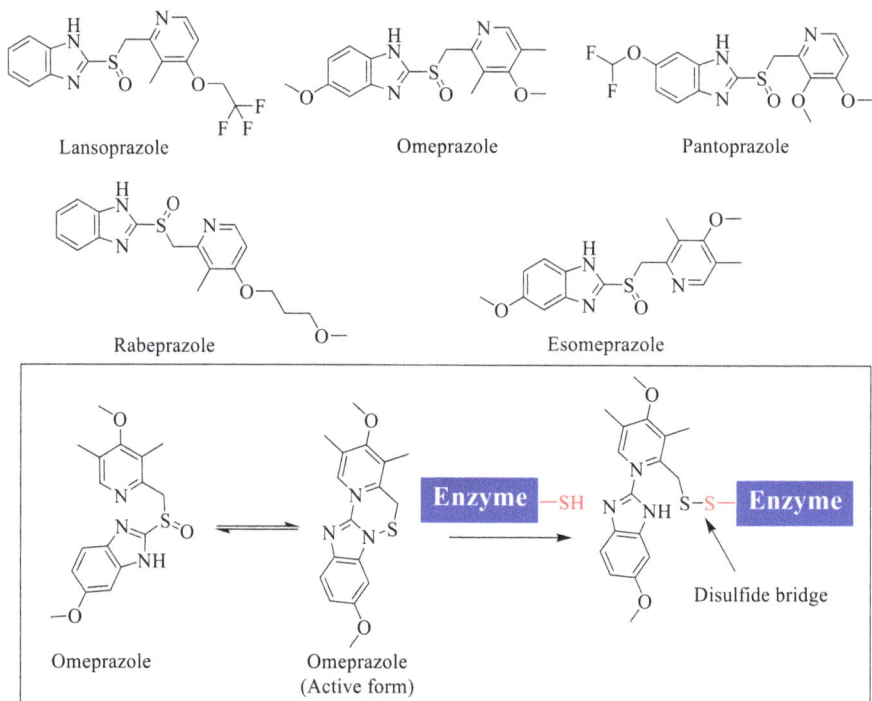

Figure 12.7 Inhibition of gastric secretion through covalent interaction with gastric H⁺/K⁺-ATPase. Omeprazole is converted in the body to a cyclic sulfenamide structure, its active form, which interacts with the enzyme to form a disulfide bridge. This process being favoured in acidic environments, the effect of omeprazole is specific to the gastric H⁺/K⁺-ATPase.

drugs that act on this pump and include (see Figure 12.7) Prevacid (lansoprazole), Prilosec (omeprazole), Protonix (pantoprazole), Aciphex (rabeprazole), and Nexium (esomeprazole). These compounds inhibit H⁺/K⁺-ATPase by forming a disulfide bond with the sulfhydryl (thiol or R–SH) group. Although they have an adverse effect with long-term use, these drugs have been effectively used in the clinical management of stomach ulcers.

12.2.6 Drugs Used to Treat Cardiovascular Diseases Through Covalent Interactions With Targets

Several enzymes that play key roles in cardiovascular biology can be targeted by drugs that bind covalently with crucial enzymes (Figure 12.8). These include inhibition of aromatase by exemestane

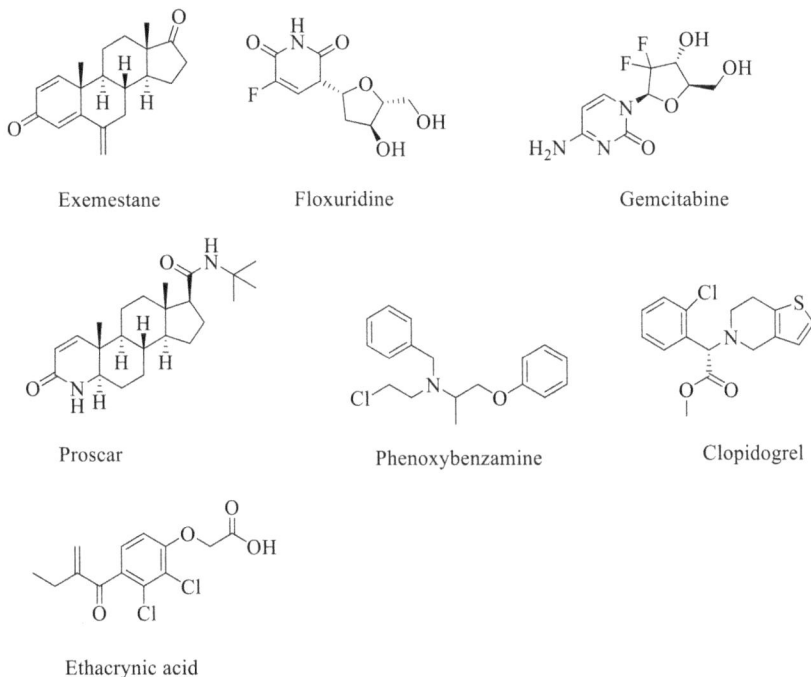

Figure 12.8 Examples of drugs used to treat cardiovascular diseases *via* covalent interactions with targets.

(Aromasin), thymidylate synthase by floxuridine, ribonucleoside reductase by gemcitabine (Gemzar), and 5-α-reductase by finasteride (Proscar). Receptors of neurotransmitters and hormones such as noradrenaline (norepinephrine) and adrenaline (epinephrine) can also be targeted by drugs through covalent bond interactions. For example, the α-adrenoceptor is targeted by phenoxybenzamine hydrochloride. Through long-lasting irreversible inhibition of these receptors, the drug has the potential to treat cardiovascular diseases such as hypertension.

The antiplatelet drug clopidogrel must undergo metabolic reactions to generate the active form in the body. Hence it is called a prodrug. The two-step conversion of the drug in the body leads to the production of the metabolite with the thiol–carboxylic acid group that binds irreversibly with the –SH group of its target. Ethacrynic acid is a diuretic drug that inhibits the Na^+–K^+–$2Cl^-$ cotransport system in the kidneys. By inhibiting glutathione *S*-transferase, it is used to treat several cardiovascular conditions, including hypertension.

12.2.7 Anticancer Drugs that Act Through Covalent Interactions With Targets

Several anticancer drugs that we call the electrophile class are used to treat cancer through molecular mechanisms of covalent interaction with their targets. Although the interaction of these compounds with cancer targets is not highly specific and they have general toxicity, their use in cancer therapy is justified given the severity of the disease. Their structures include epoxides, a vinylogous amide, a boronic acid, a β-lactone, and a variety of acrylamides. Given their diverse structures and that some of them have already been addressed in other chapters (*e.g.* DNA interactive agents in Chapter 10), they are not listed here.

The epidermal growth factor receptor (EGFR) is a receptor tyrosine kinase and is one of the established targets for cancer. Electrophile drugs such as afatinib (Figure 12.9) that bond covalently to the cysteine residue in the epidermal growth factor receptor have been developed. Dacomitinib is another anticancer agent acting as an irreversible inhibitor of EGFR. Zanubrutinib (Brukinsa) (Figure 12.9) is an anticancer agent with a similar action on Bruton's tyrosine kinase (BTK). Other key cancer-associated enzymes as drug targets through covalent interactions include methyltransferase by azacytidine (Vidaza) and decitabine or deoxyazacytidine (Dacogen), proteasome by bortezomib (Velcade), and 5-α-reductase by dutasteride (Avodart) and finasteride (Propecia or Proscar) (Figure 12.9). The identification of BTK as a target for cancer and autoimmune disorders led to the discovery of anticancer drugs such as ibrutinib (Figure 12.9). Another enzyme with a critical role in cancer development is the mitogen-activated protein kinase kinases 1 and 2 (MEK1 and MEK2), which is targeted by a covalent drug interaction with trametinib (Figure 12.9). The purine nucleotide synthesis can also be targeted by drugs such as mercaptopurine (Purinethol) (Figure 12.9). Hence cancer therapy appears to be a good example of the covalent interaction of drugs with their targets.

12.2.8 Other Diseases Targeted by Covalent Drug Interactions

Readers should bear in mind that there are numerous drugs and toxins that act through interactions with their target (biological molecules) *via* covalent bonding. For example, the antiobesity drug orlistat (see Chapter 9) targets an enzyme that processes fats in the digestive tract. By inhibiting the activity of pancreatic and gastric lipases, the

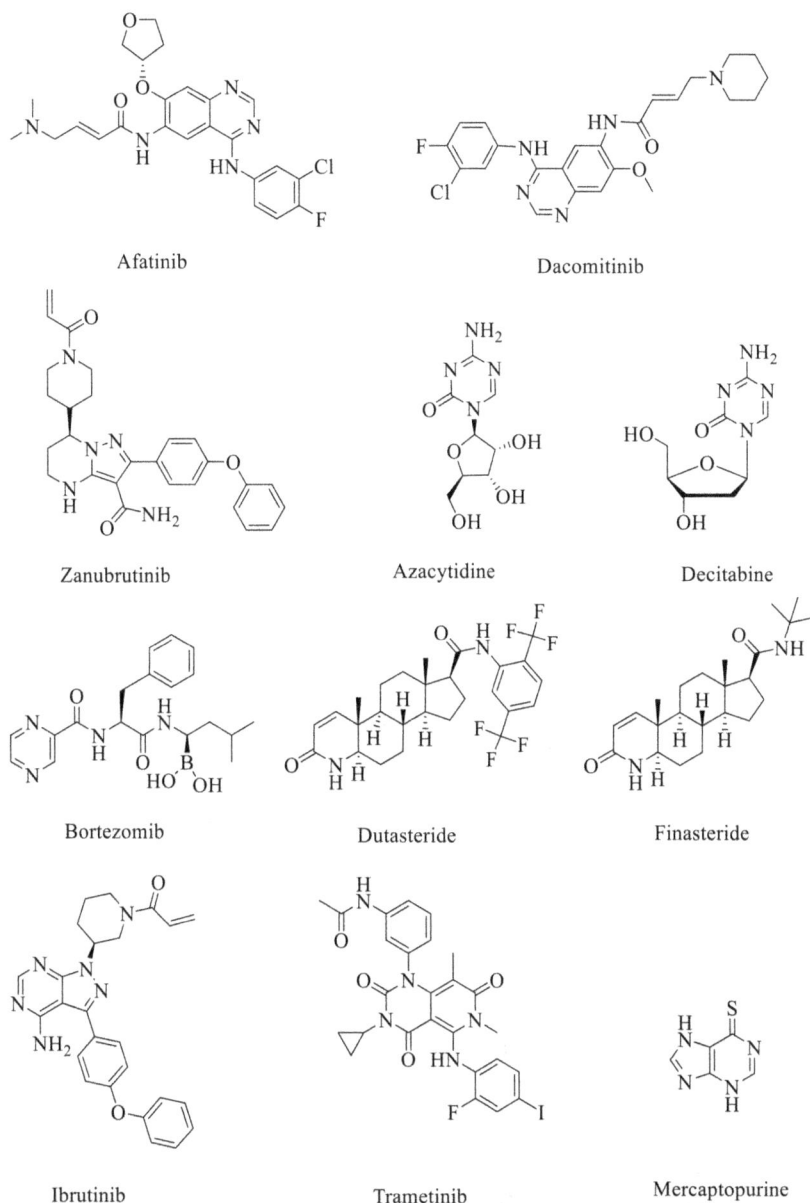

Figure 12.9 Examples of anticancer drugs that target key enzymes through covalent interactions.

availability of fat to the body is restricted by orlistat. As already discussed in the preceding section, aspirin is an anti-inflammatory and antithrombic agent that inhibits the cyclooxygenase enzyme through covalent interactions. Further examples of covalent drug interactions are shown in Figure 12.10: GABA aminotransferase as a target for the

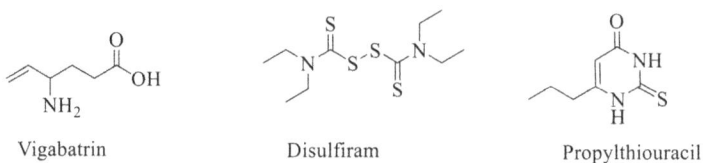

Figure 12.10 Structures of vigabatrin, disulfiram, and propylthiouracil.

antiepileptic drug vigabatrin (Sabril), aldehyde dehydrogenase as a target for drug therapy of chronic alcoholism by disulfiram (Antabuse), and thyroxine-5-deiodinase as a target for the hyperthyroidism drug propylthiouracil (Procasil), *etc.*

12.3   Non-covalent Interactions

Unlike the covalent interactions discussed above, the non-covalent interactions between drugs and their targets do not involve the sharing of electrons between molecules. Instead, intermolecular interaction forces such as electrostatic, hydrogen bonding, aromatic structures (π-effects), van der Waals forces, and hydrophobic effects are involved. These interactions are also crucial to the structural integrity of large molecular weight biomolecules such as proteins and nucleic acids that we discussed in Chapters 7 and 10, respectively. It is important to note that the interaction between drugs and their targets often involves a combination of different intermolecular forces of attractions. The major non-covalent interactions relevant to the action of drugs in the body are discussed below.

12.3.1   Electrostatic Interactions

In ionic interactions, two oppositely charged atoms come together, such as Cl^- and Na^+ making NaCl. Molecules that carry opposite charges also come together whereas those with the same charge repulse each other. It is therefore easy to envisage a charged drug molecule being attracted, pulled towards, and binding to an oppositely charged target biomolecule. Since proteins have sites of charged areas, one of the common attractions between drugs and their binding site is electrostatic attractions. Many drug targets, largely being proteins such as receptors, enzymes, and ion channels, charge–charge interactions are possible owing to the presence of amino acids with charged branches. Those with acid side-chains are readily negatively charged, while an amine group in the side-chain tends to be positively charged at physiological pH or neutral pH environment. Such interactions are illustrated in Figure 12.11.

In Chapter 7, we have seen acidic amino acids such as aspartic acid and glutamic acids creating sites in proteins as negatively charged areas, whereas basic amino acids such as lysine, arginine, and histidine create cationic centres. This is one way of interaction between two proteins, one of which could also be a drug (see Figure 12.12).

In addition to the common negatively charged acidic functional groups of organic matter such as RCOO⁻, many biomolecules, including DNA, RNA, and ATP, have phosphate groups. Where they occur,

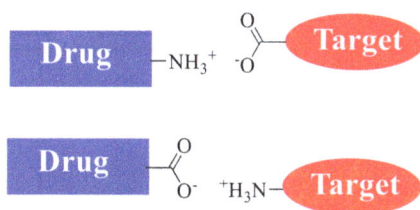

Figure 12.11 Example of electrostatic interactions between a drug molecule and its target. At physiological pH, many drug molecules contain ionisable functional groups such as carboxylic acids or amines (bases). The resulting ionic group can interact with target molecules to bind the drug with its targets. Note that the charge on both the drug and target may come from other ionisable functional groups. The degree of ionisation of a drug molecule at a given pH depends on its pK_a value (see Chapter 11).

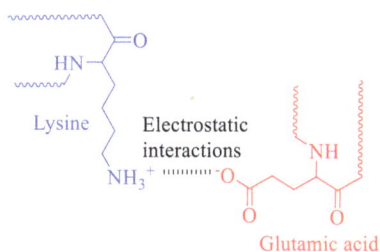

Figure 12.12 Electrostatic interactions between proteins. Amino acid residues with a positively charged side chain (*e.g.* lysine) interact with residues with a negatively charged side chain (*e.g.* glutamic acid). The electrostatic interaction brings these proteins together. The same principle applies to the interaction of a drug with its target. Note also that some drugs are proteins in nature.

the phosphate and sulfate groups in organic compounds provide additional anionic or negatively charged areas. As discussed above, the neurotransmitter acetylcholine is broken down by the action of the enzyme AChE. In this process, the quaternary nitrogen (N^+) of acetylcholine interacts with the anionic site of AChE. Once anchored to the enzyme, the esteratic site is removed to liberate acetic acid and choline (Figure 12.13).

The interaction of tetrodotoxin and saxitoxin with neuronal ion channels involves the quaternary N^+ guanidinium group(s) on the drug molecules (Figure 12.14). Ionic interaction at the outer surface of the Na^+ channels guarantees their binding to initiate the inhibitory effect on the activity of the Na^+ channels. Local anaesthetics in cationic form also bind to the inner surface of Na^+ channels and block nerve conduction.

Ionic Interactions in Protein–Protein Binding – Key Facts

- The most common source of a negatively charged or anionic site in an organic molecule is the acidic functional group – COOH $(-COO^-)$.
- The amino functional group is a common source of positively charged sites (ammonium cation) in organic compounds.
- Basic amino acids such as lysine, arginine, and histidine create cationic sites in proteins.
- Acidic amino acids such as aspartic and glutamic acids create negatively charged sites in proteins.
- Whether or not a drug molecule is charged at a given pH depends on the pK_a value of the drug.

Whereas charged drugs that readily form ionic groups in an aqueous medium readily interact with their biological targets through electrostatic attractions, the ionisation of weakly acidic and weakly basic drugs depends on the pH of the medium and their pK_a values (see Chapter 11).

As outlined above, there are also phosphate groups in biological systems as part of the DNA or nucleic acid structures and in proteins. In addition, there are phospholipids as part of the cell membrane structure (see Chapter 9). Energy-rich molecules such as ATP (adenosine triphosphate) and ADP (adenosine diphosphate) and also AMP (adenosine monophosphate) contain phosphate group(s). Other less common energy sources in the body with a phosphate

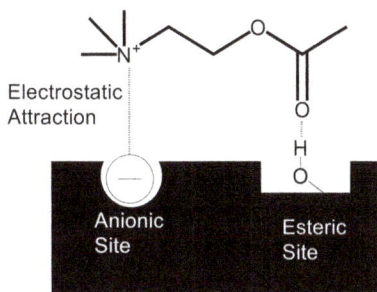

Figure 12.13 Model of acetylcholine (ACh) binding with the active site of acetylcholinesterase (AChE). The structural feature of the active site of AChE is shown. The enzyme has a site for ionic interaction with the substrate, acetylcholine. The electrostatic attraction firmly anchors the substrate while the other site interacts for the removal of the acetate group from the molecule. This leads to the breakdown of acetylcholine to choline and acetic acid. Note that other types of interactions (hydrogen bonding at the esteric site) also help to anchor the substrate with the enzyme.

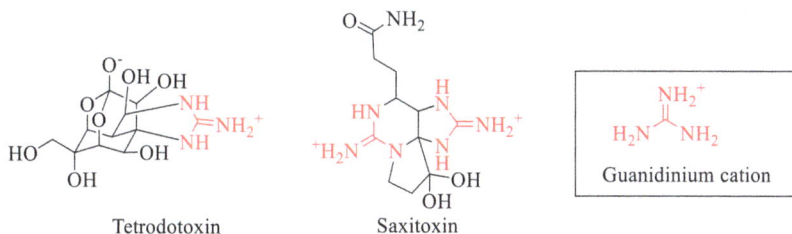

Figure 12.14 Structures of tetrodotoxin and saxitoxin. These compounds contain the structural group guanidine that has a positively charged unit. It undergoes interaction with sodium ion channels (targets) through electrostatic interaction.

group as an integral component include guanosine triphosphate (GTP), cytidine triphosphate (CTP), and uridine triphosphate (UTP). Signalling molecules such as cyclic AMP and cyclic GMP are other examples of phosphate groups in biological molecules. The bacterial cell wall component called a *lipopolysaccharide* has an active component, *lipid A* (see Chapter 13, Figure 13.67), that contains two phosphate groups. Phosphate groups in such biological molecules are negatively charged and often serve as targets through electrostatic interactions with cationic drugs. Hence electrostatic interactions are quite common both in normal physiological processes and in drug therapies.

12.3.2 Hydrogen Bonding

Hydrogen bonding occurs when hydrogen is covalently bonded to strongly negatively charged elements such as N, O, or F (see Chapter 2). The intermolecular force of attraction based on hydrogen bonding involves interaction between this hydrogen (bonded to an electronegative atom that we call a hydrogen donor) and an electronegative atom (which is a hydrogen acceptor). Weaker than the electrostatic attraction, hydrogen bonding plays a crucial role in the structural integrity of macromolecules such as proteins and nucleic acids. In the case of nucleic acids, the helical structure of DNA is based on hydrogen bonding between complementary base pairs (Chapter 10). For optimal binding in drug–target interactions through hydrogen bonding, the *donor-H* must be placed directly at the lone pair of electrons (*e.g.* N or O) at 180°. The relative strength of hydrogen bonding for various functional groups as hydrogen acceptors is shown in Figure 12.15.

In organic molecules, acids, alcohols or phenols, and amines serve as H-donors. Electron-deficient groups such as quaternary ammonium compounds are strong hydrogen donors compared with primary and secondary amines (Figure 12.16).

Once again, hydrogen atoms attached to oxygen, nitrogen, and fluorine are involved in hydrogen bonding. Hence these groups also serve as *H-donors*. In water molecules, hydrogen atoms serve as H-donors whereas oxygen atoms serve as H-acceptors (Chapter 2). Through this interaction, water interacts with organic compounds by serving as both an H-bond donor and an H-bond acceptor (Figure 12.17).

In hydrogen bonding interactions, molecules often have several regions of H-acceptors and H-donors. Consider adenine in Figure 12.18,

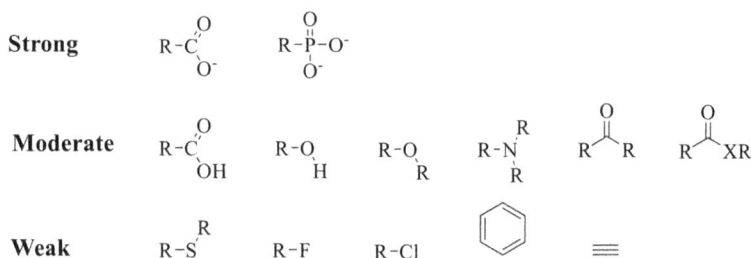

Figure 12.15 Relative strength of hydrogen bond acceptors. Increased electron density increases the capacity to accept hydrogen in hydrogen bonding interactions. Anions such as carboxylate and phosphate groups are strong hydrogen acceptors. Moderate hydrogen acceptors in molecules include carboxyl, hydroxyl, ether, and ketone groups.

which has five nitrogen atoms in its molecule that serve either as an H-acceptor or an H-donor.

Drug–Target Interactions Through Hydrogen Bonding – Key Facts

- Hydrogen bonding occurs where hydrogen is covalently bonded to strongly negatively charged elements such as N, O, and F.
- The interaction between an H-donor and an H-acceptor occurs at 180°.
- Anions such as carboxylate and phosphate groups are strong hydrogen acceptors.
- Increasing electron density increases the capacity to accept hydrogen.
- Electron-deficient groups such as quaternary ammonium compounds are strong hydrogen donors.
- Water serves as both a hydrogen donor and acceptor.

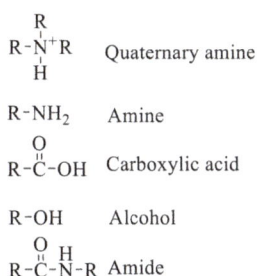

$R-\overset{R}{\underset{H}{N^+}}-R$	Quaternary amine
$R-NH_2$	Amine
$R-\overset{O}{\underset{}{C}}-OH$	Carboxylic acid
$R-OH$	Alcohol
$R-\overset{O}{\underset{}{C}}-\overset{H}{N}-R$	Amide

Figure 12.16 Examples of hydrogen bond donors. Species with hydrogen attached to oxygen or nitrogen in organic compounds serve as H-donors.

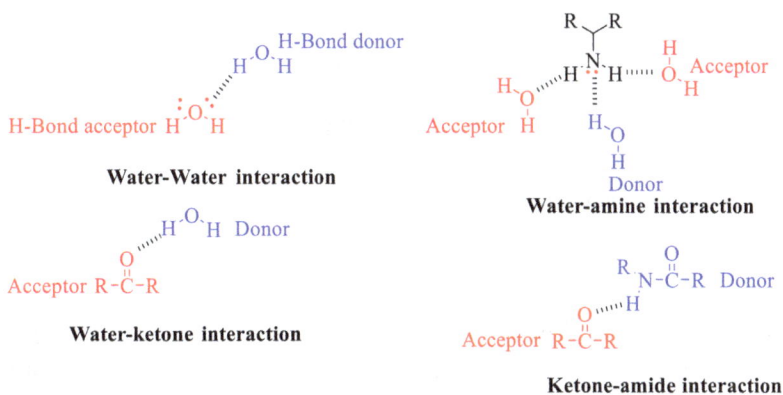

Water-Water interaction

Water-amine interaction

Water-ketone interaction

Ketone-amide interaction

Figure 12.17 Examples of hydrogen bonding interactions.

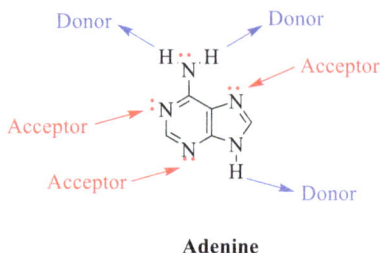

Adenine

Figure 12.18 Hydrogen acceptor and donor sites of the adenine molecule.

12.3.3 Lipophilic Interactions

Lipophilic hydrophobic interactions occur between non-polar hydro-carbon groups on a drug molecule and those in the receptor site, enzymes, ion channels, or other drug targets. Interactions between aromatic rings are also common and are important in biological systems where they influence the structure of both proteins and protein–ligand complexes.

12.3.3.1 The van der Waals or London Dispersion Force

This is an example of a hydrophobic interaction with very small and rather weak energy interactions. Through this interaction, which is based on temporary dipole–dipole attractions (see Chapter 2), hydrophobic regions of different molecules such as aliphatic substituents can interact with each other. This plays an important role in the interaction of drugs with their targets and drug–drug interactions.

12.3.3.2 Pi–Pi (π-π) Stacking

Aromatic compounds and alkenes interact with targets through pi (π) stacking. Even though molecules of aromatic compounds come close to each other, benzene rings do not sit directly on top of one another owing to variable electron densities. The face of the benzene ring or the π orbitals have more electron density than the edge, leading to a staggered stacking orientation of molecules, as shown in Figure 12.19.

12.3.4 Other Interactions

Dipole–dipole and ion–dipole interactions can also occur in the interactions of drugs with their targets. In this sense, a permanent dipole instead of temporary dipole of van der Waals interactions may be involved. Note that hydrogen bonding is a special form of

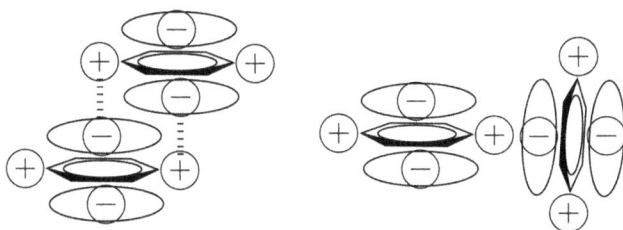

Figure 12.19 Model of pi (π) stacking to illustrate the interaction between two aromatic structures. Anticancer drugs such as doxorubicin interact with DNA through a π–π stacking mechanism.

dipole–dipole interaction (Chapter 2). We also have repulsive interactions that push or stop molecules from coming together. Molecules of similar charges repulse each other. When various charges occur in one molecule, they may align to have the best fit with the receptor or target molecule.

Although water molecules can surround an ionic group, they also repel hydrophobic compounds. Remember that most drug targets such as proteins and DNA exist in aqueous environments. Similarly, drugs in a biological system are also surrounded by water. Hence drug–target interactions require desolvation.

The interaction of low molecular weight drugs with proteins and other macromolecules often involves a combination of different kinds of intermolecular interactions. This is because drugs often contain various functional groups that are involved in different forms of interaction with the target. Observe the various functional groups in the structures of the antibiotic penicillin G and siponimod (a drug for multiple sclerosis therapy) (Figure 12.20).

12.4 Making Sense of Drug–Target Interactions

The interactions of drug molecules with biological targets could occur at the level of cell surfaces such as the bacterial cell wall, or at a macromolecular level such as proteins in the form of enzymes, receptors, ion channels, transporters, or DNA and RNA. Hence drug targets may be located inside or outside cells, at the cell surface (*e.g.* cell membrane), or within cell membranes. The interaction of drug molecules with their target through one or a combination of attractions listed in the previous section is called *binding*.

Drug affinity refers to how tightly a drug binds with its target. The binding of drugs with receptors, enzymes, ion channels, or other

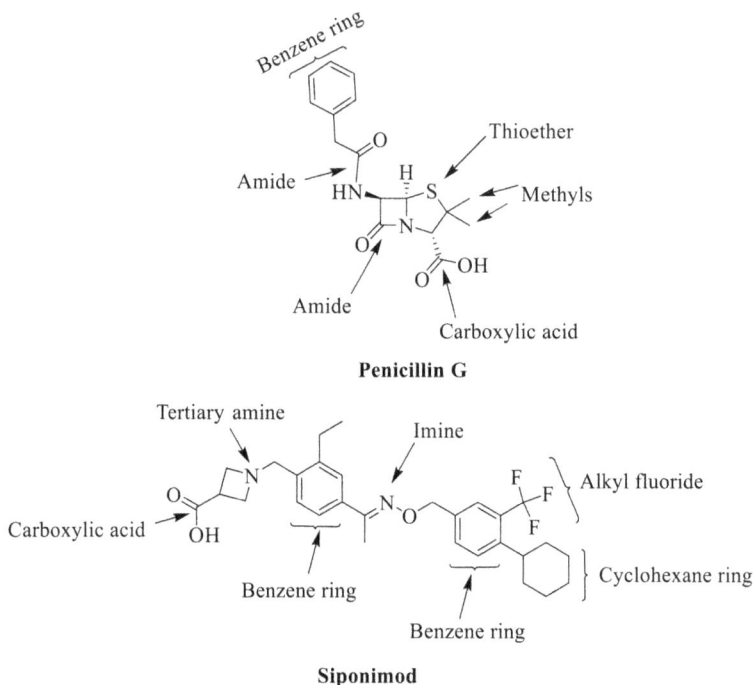

Figure 12.20 Functional groups in drug molecules attributed to different interactions with targets. Note the structural groups in penicillin G and siponimod.

biological targets is the initial step in the induction of their therapeutic effects. As pharmacology involves the study of a drug's effect on the body, those pursuing studies in this area of science deal with the affinity of drugs in detail.

In terms of drugs binding with their targets, we should also consider chemistry topics other than functional groups. In Chapter 6, stereochemistry as the basis for the specific interaction of drugs with their targets and the distinction between drugs being more effective, better selective, or less toxic as a function of stereochemistry are discussed.

12.5 Summary

In this chapter, we have reviewed the different kinds of intermolecular forces of attraction, and also covalent bonding, which are involved in drug–target interactions. In many cases, drug targets are proteins that are composed of amino acids. Depending on the type of amino acids involved, we could have a hydrophobic area or a highly ionis-able region that promotes electrostatic interactions. The overall inter-action would be, however, the sum of several types of interactions. In covalent interactions, a firm bond formation with a foreign agent such as a bacterial structure/metabolism that is not shared by the host organism is favoured. However, we have seen in this chapter several applications of covalent interactions for drugs such as anti-inflammatory and anticancer agents, among others. The binding of drug molecules or biologically active agents such as hormones and neurotransmitters with their receptors also involves the various types of interactions described in this chapter. Their binding affinity is one of the parameters that we need to study when assessing their intrinsic biological activity.

12.6 Problems

1. What are the chemical bases of drug–target interactions?
2. Why is a covalent drug–target interaction considered safe to neu-tralise foreign bodies such as pathogens?
3. How are antibiotics of the β-lactam series activated and inacti-vated through covalent interactions?
4. Explain how acetylation at the active site of enzymes serves as a mechanism of covalent interaction-based therapy.
5. Using rasagiline and selegiline as examples, explain how enzyme cofactors could be targeted by drugs through covalent interactions.
6. Using carbidopa as an example, explain how the effect of a drug is limited to the peripheral nervous system.
7. What are the reversible and non-reversible inhibitors of AChE?
8. How can disulfide bridge formation with the sulfhydryl group (or thiol, R–SH) of an enzyme lead to inhibition of gastric enzymes by drugs?
9. Identify drugs relevant to treat cardiovascular diseases and can-cer through covalent interactions.
10. What is the most common functional group in organic com-pounds that offers an anionic site, and which one offers a cat-ionic site for electrostatic interactions?
11. Explain how ACh (acetylcholine) binds to AChE (acetylcholines-terase) through both ionic and hydrogen bonding interactions?
12. How do the sodium channel toxins act through electrostatic interactions?

13. Which amino acids have side chains for cationic interactions and which have side chains for anionic interactions, and how do these apply for the interaction of protein-based drugs with protein targets?
14. When does a hydrogen bond occur?
15. What are hydrogen bond acceptors and in what order is their strength?
16. What are the common hydrogen bond donors?
17. How does water serve as both a hydrogen bond donor and an acceptor?
18. Identify a hydrogen donor and acceptor in a molecule (*e.g.* adenine).
19. Explain lipophilic interactions by using van der Waals and π–π stacking models.
20. Explain how pharmacodynamics and pharmacokinetics are possible through the interaction of drugs with various cellular and acellular components.

12.7 Solutions to Problems

1. You can answer this question by defining the five major types of interactions between a drug molecule and a receptor. These are further explained in the following answers:
   a. Covalent interaction.
   b. Hydrogen bonding interaction.
   c. Dipole interaction.
   d. Electrostatic interaction.
   e. Lipophilic interaction.

2. When a drug molecule interacts with its target, the order of forces of interaction is covalent bonding > electrostatic > hydrogen bonding > other dipole interactions > lipophilic interactions. When a covalent bond occurs, the effect could be long lasting; sometimes it is a permanent inhibition. When the biological process is not shared with the host system, such inhibition guarantees the permanent inactivation of an unwanted foreign body such as pathogens. The permanent inhibition of vital enzymes and other targets may have unwanted side effects, although we have many drugs in use through this mechanism.
3. See Figure 12.1.
4. See Figures 12.2 and 12.5. The active sites of many enzymes have amino acids such as serine with a hydroxyl group that is prone to

attack by drugs. The acetylation reaction is often a mechanism of inactivation whereas other similar mechanisms of covalent bond formation could also inactivate the enzyme.

5. See Figure 12.4.

6. Carbidopa is a DOPA decarboxylase inhibitor, but its effect is seen only in the peripheral nervous system as it cannot pass the blood–brain barrier. We can increase the life span of L-DOPA if we administer it together with carbidopa, as the degrading effect of DOPA decarboxylase on L-DOPA in the peripheral system is suppressed. Thus, much of the administered L-DOPA is available to enter the brain where it is needed.

7. Reversible AChE (acetylcholinesterase) inhibitors have a similar mechanism of binding as ACh (acetylcholine) and include physostigmine and neostigmine. The effect of rivastigmine is long lasting and all of these drugs have therapeutic implications for Alzheimer's disease. On the other hand, nerve gases such VX, tabun, soman, sarin, and cyclosarin bind irreversibly to AChE.

8. See Figure 12.7.

9. Antihypertensive drugs include aromatase inhibitors or the non-selective irreversible α-adrenoceptor antagonist phenoxybenzamine, the antiplatelet drug clopidogrel, and the diuretic drug ethacrynic acid. There are many anticancer agents that act through covalent interactions, a good example being the electrophile drug afatinib.

10. Ionisable functional groups include carboxylic acids, phenols, sulfates, and phosphates that liberate hydrogen ion (H^+) to become negatively charged (anion) and nitrogen-containing compounds that quaternise to become positively charged (cation).

11. See Figure 12.13.

12. See Figure 12.14. They contain a charged (cation) guanidinium structure.

13. Aspartic and glutamic acids have side chains for the extra anionic group, whereas lysine, arginine, and histidine have side chains for cationic groups. Proteins can interact with their target through these ionic sites – interacting with opposite charges in their target.

14. In compounds where hydrogen is bonded to N, O, or F.

15. See Figure 12.15.

16. See Figure 12.16.

17. See Figure 12.17.

18. See Figure 12.18.

19. Lipophilic interactions are the weakest interactions but play a significant role by allowing non-polar regions of a drug to stack together with non-polar parts of the target – like interacting with like. π–π stacking involves aromatic ring systems (see Figure 12.19).

20. A general question to highlight that both the movement of a drug and its biological action in the body involve interaction with several biological matrices, *i.e.* the diverse covalent and/or non-covalent interactions.

13 Structural Diversity and Sources of Drugs: From Nature to Synthetic and Recombinant DNA Technology

Learning Objectives

After completing this chapter, you are expected to be able to:

- Describe how large molecules in Nature are built from small building blocks.
- Identify the biosynthetic origin of natural compounds.
- Explain how natural compounds serve as drugs, are altered to make semi-synthetic derivatives, or serve as a skeleton for the synthesis of novel drugs.
- Explain why drug discovery is an expensive and multi-year process.
- Identify the common animal sources of drugs and the potential of recombinant technology in drug discovery.

Basic Chemistry for Life Science Students and Professionals: Introduction to Organic Compounds and Drug Molecules
By Solomon Habtemariam
© Solomon Habtemariam 2023
Published by the Royal Society of Chemistry, www.rsc.org

13.1   Introduction

In pharmacology and related sciences, the term 'drug' refers to a chemical substance administered to a living organism to produce a biological effect of either physiological or psychological nature. As a pharmaceutical product, drug refers mainly to medicines that improve wellbeing, treat or cure illness, prevent an illness, or help diagnose a disease. Although these definitions account for many therapeutic agents used by humans, the general population often associate the term 'drugs' with legal or illegal drugs of abuse, which are often addictive, such as marijuana, Ecstasy, cocaine, LSD, crystal meth and heroin. In recent years, many nutraceuticals and medicinal foods and their ingredients have further been marketed for their claimed potential to treat an illness or improve wellbeing. There are also some mineral or inorganic components that have the same composition as that within the body but are still claimed to have therapeutic benefits. Hence the distinction between drugs, foods, medicinal foods, and nutraceuticals is becoming narrower. In this book, the term 'drug' refers to a medicine or any substance, legal or illegal, of good or toxic outcome, that has a physiological/psychological effect when administered to a living system. Drugs have toxic effects also, hence toxins in this sense can also be referred to as drugs.

Thousands of years ago, our ancestors were heavily reliant on Nature to source potential therapies for human diseases. These natural sources, collectively called *natural products*, could be crude extracts of plants, animals, or mineral sources. Perhaps identified through serendipity, the medicinal value of selected natural products is often unique to certain local traditions and regions where they are used. The knowledge and skill of the prescription were in most cases kept secret by a few wise men or wise women healers who passed the information to the next generation of healers. Now, however, drug discovery is a multibillion pound/dollar business and refers to the multidisciplinary process of identifying and developing new medicines. The business model of drug discovery includes a comprehensive study of the biology, chemistry, and pharmaceutical preparations of potential drugs. The clinical validity of potential drugs also needs to be established through phases of clinical trials. This chapter is designed to give an overview of drugs sourced through different approaches. Special attention is given to natural products, both primary and secondary metabolites, as they give readers the best foundation of the structural diversity of organic compounds and also drugs and their targets.

13.2 Natural Compounds and Their Role in Modern Drug Discovery

The traditional systems of medicines still practiced today, including Chinese and Ayurvedic traditional medicines, are good examples of natural products utilised effectively by humans as drugs. Crude drugs of dried herbal powders and their extracts in some form are employed by millions of people throughout the world. About 80% of the world's population today use plant medicines as a primary means of health-care, which also means, by and large, crude plant extracts. The active ingredients of some of these plants have been characterised and, in some cases, developed as modern medicines. While morphine preparations have been developed as modern pharmaceutical products, the opium plant is still used in crude form as it has been for thousands of years. In addition to the significant proportion of therapeutic drugs today that trace their origin to natural sources, we still have untapped resources of plants, animals, and microorganisms from marine and land environments yet to be studied. Some of the iconic active drug ingredients discovered from natural sources are listed here under the source categories, plants, animals, microorganisms, *etc.*

13.3 Plants and Microorganisms as Sources of Drugs – Natural Products and Their Synthetic Analogues

The best way to understand drugs of microbial and plant origin is to assess the metabolic pathways in these organisms. The growth and survival of living organisms depend on the function of macromolecules such as DNA, proteins, carbohydrates, and lipids and also their metabolism. The metabolic activities required for the immediate survival of the organism are called the *primary metabolism*, and the metabolites are called *primary metabolites*. These include the metabolic process of photosynthesis in plants, anabolic reactions to build macromolecules, and catabolic reactions in living systems used to generate metabolic energy. There are also metabolic reactions, which may play a crucial role for the long-term but not for the immediate survival of the organism. You may wonder why caffeine is produced in coffee and tea plants, morphine in opium plants, cocaine in coca leaves, *etc.* Such chemicals are claimed to give the plants an ecological advantage, say by reducing competitors or avoiding herbivores or attracting favourable animals such as insect pollinators or microorganisms (mycorrhizae), *etc.*

These chemicals are called *secondary metabolites* and the metabolism is called *secondary metabolism*. In many textbooks, secondary metabolites are mainly considered as defensive chemicals produced by plants or other organisms and serve as signalling molecules in interspecies interactions within their ecosystem. Even without knowing the type of chemicals or chemical structures, humans have been exploiting secondary metabolites in their crude forms by extracting them as medicines, foods, flavours, fragrances, and colourings/dyes, and for various other purposes. Several thousand secondary metabolites have been isolated from natural sources and one should bear in mind also that there are still more many plants, fungi, and microorganisms yet to be studied. Secondary metabolites are also often complex in their structures, with several stereoisomers or chiral centres to be considered in their molecules. They are all derived through a handful of biosynthetic pathways, however, and understanding them is easier by looking into how they are produced in a living system. Recent advances in the identification of enzymes involved in the biosynthesis of these chemicals also allow genetic engineering and manipulation of the production of secondary metabolites. Starting from simple primary metabolites of photosynthetic and respiratory chemical intermediates, complex secondary metabolites are formed owing to the unique enzymes expressed in these organisms. An overview of the synthesis of major secondary metabolites such as terpenoids, alkaloids, and flavonoids is depicted in Figure 13.1.

Primary *versus* Secondary Metabolism – Key Facts

- Primary – anabolic and catabolic metabolic reactions.
- Primary – required for the immediate existence of the organism.
- Primary – includes DNA, proteins, lipids, and carbohydrate metabolism.
- Secondary – chemical compounds not involved in primary metabolism.
- Secondary – important for long-term survival of the species.
- Secondary – used as defence against pathogens and interaction with other living organisms.

13.3.1 Terpenoids

13.3.1.1 General Structure and Classification

Also called isoprenoids, terpenoids, or terpenes, these compounds are formed through the *mevalonic acid pathway*. Their basic building

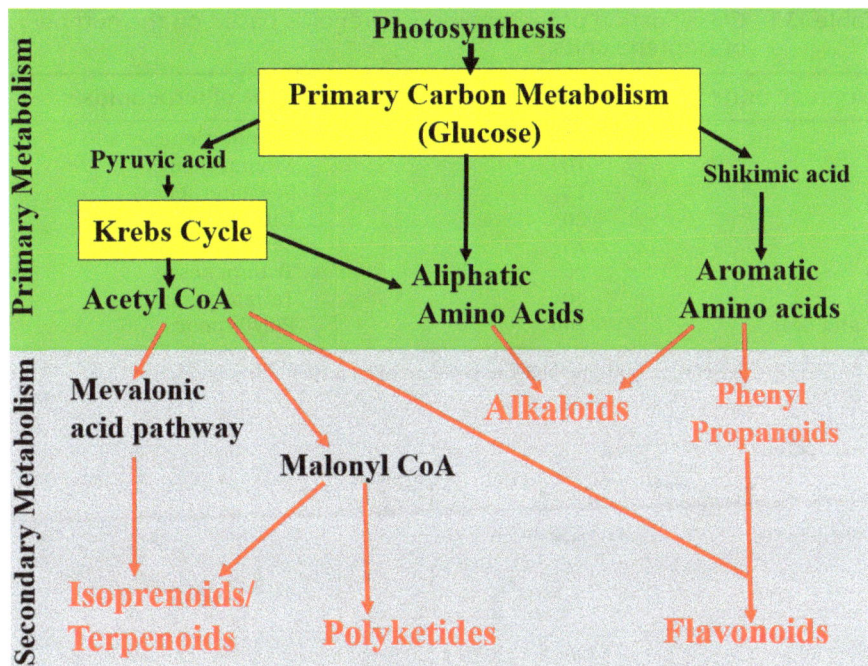

Figure 13.1 Overview of the production of secondary metabolites in living organisms. The synthesis of secondary metabolites starts from photosynthetic products and metabolites from mitochondrial respiratory metabolism (Krebs cycle) such as acetyl-coenzyme A (CoA). The mevalonic acid pathway is a classic example of the synthesis of terpenoids and malonyl-CoA products are the so-called polyketides. Alkaloids are mostly formed from amino acid precursors whereas phenolic compounds are derived from aromatic amino acids, which may further combine with acetyl-CoA products to give polyphenolic compounds such as flavonoids. Further structural modifications of these secondary metabolites also occur to yield complex compounds and polymers such as tannins.

blocks are five-carbon isoprene units called isopentenyl pyrophosphate (IPP) and dimethylallyl pyrophosphate (DMAPP). The numerous terpenoids reported from natural sources are simply formed through further condensation of these two-isoprene building blocks. Two isoprene units form a 10-carbon building precursor, geranylgeranyl pyrophosphate (GGPP), to generate monoterpenes, three isoprene units form farnesyl pyrophosphate (FPP) that produces sesquiterpenes, four isoprene units condense to form geranylgeranyl pyrophosphate that gives diterpenes, and six isoprene units form a triterpenoid precursor, squalene (Table 13.1). Representing the largest and most diverse

Table 13.1 Classification of terpenoids/isoprenoids based on the number of isoprene units.[a]

Isoprene units	Carbon atoms	Type of terpenoids
1	5	Hemiterpenes
2	10	Monoterpenes
3	15	Sesquiterpenes
4	20	Diterpenes
5	25	Sesterterpenes
6	30	Triterpenes
8	40	Tetraterpenes
9 and over	>40	Polyterpenes

[a]Isoprene is a five-carbon building block or skeleton of all terpenoids – see Figure 13.2.

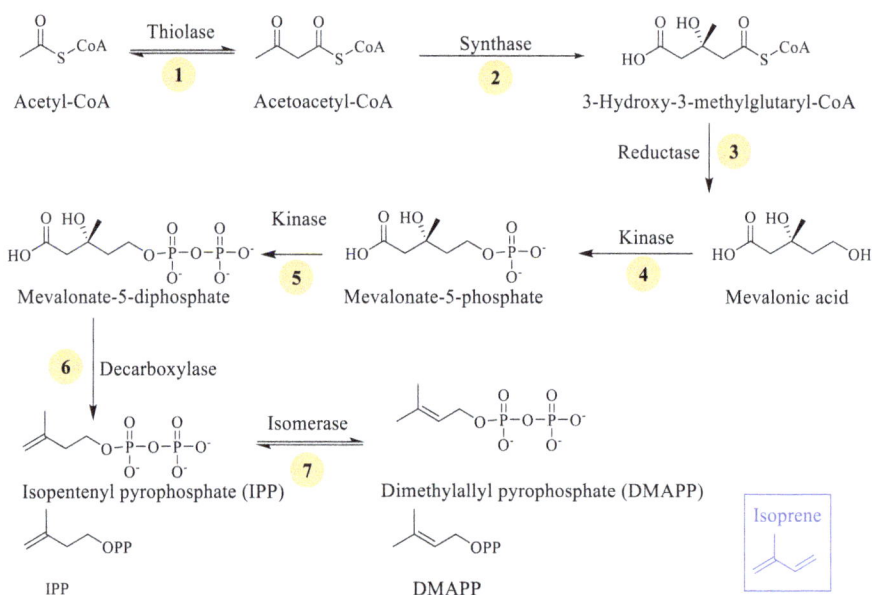

Figure 13.2 The common mevalonic acid pathway for the formation of the five-carbon isoprene building blocks of terpenoids. The metabolic process is catalysed by enzymes: 1, acetoacetyl-CoA thiolase; 2, HMG-CoA synthase; 3, HMG-CoA reductase; 4, mevalonate kinase; 5, phosphomevalonate kinase; 6, mevalonate pyrophosphate decarboxylase; 7, isopentenyl pyrophosphate:dimethylallyl pyrophosphate isomerase. Note that the biosynthesis of terpenoids starts from the primary metabolite acetyl-CoA and three molecules of acetyl-CoA condense to form a six-carbon intermediate, mevalonic acid. The five-carbon building blocks of terpenoids are isopentenyl diphosphate (IPP) and dimethylallyl pyrophosphate (DMAPP), which is also called dimethylallyl diphosphate. There is also an alternative mevalonate pathway of IPP formation that is not discussed here.

group of secondary metabolites, the terpenoid structural skeleton is quite common in many drugs.

From the biosynthesis point of view, the mevalonate pathway is a common metabolic process that occurs in living organisms as diverse as eukaryotes and some bacteria. Hence it also occurs in humans although the production of many terpenoids is unique to a selective group of organisms (species, genera, or families) which activate the relevant genes to produce the required enzymes. The process starts from acetyl-coenzyme A (CoA), which is the mitochondrial metabolic product. As the name of the pathway (mevalonic acid pathway) implies, mevalonic acid is an intermediate in the biosynthesis of terpenoids. Figure 13.2 shows mevalonic acid (mevalonate) formation through the first committed step of terpenoid synthesis: the conversion of 3-hydroxy-3-methylglutaryl-CoA (HMG-CoA) to mevaloate, which is catalysed by the enzyme HMG-CoA reductase (HMGCR). This pathway being important in the synthesis of cholesterol, HMGCR is a key drug target for therapeutic intervention of cardiovascular diseases where cholesterol is implicated in the pathology.

A brief overview of the biosynthesis of terpenoids is outlined in Figure 13.3. Note the head-to-tail and head-to-head fashion of addition reactions in the biosynthesis pathway. The five-carbon skeleton terpenoids are called hemiterpenes, which are the smallest units, but they are not diverse in Nature. The smallest and most diverse units of terpenoids are thus considered as monoterpenes, which are based on a 10-carbon skeleton.

13.3.1.2 Monoterpenes

The key feature of the synthesis of terpenoids is the presence of the good leaving group diphosphate from the immediate precursor. In the case of GPP, the possibility of double bond formation, hydroxyl group addition, and possible cyclic structures is enormous. Most monoterpenes are small in structure and therefore are volatile in nature. They are components of the fragrances in plants and essential oils that are widely utilised in the cosmetics (perfumery) and food (flavouring) industries. Further classification of monoterpenes could be based on functional groups such as alcohols (*e.g.* geraniol, nerol, citranellol, linalool), aldehydes (*e.g.* geranial, neral), acids (*e.g.* geranic acid), esters (*e.g.* linalyl acetate), phenols (*e.g.* carvacrol, thymol), ketones (*e.g.* carvone, thujone), hydrocarbons (*e.g.* myrcene, citronellene, ocimene), or acyclic, monocyclic, bicyclic, *etc.* (Figure 13.4).

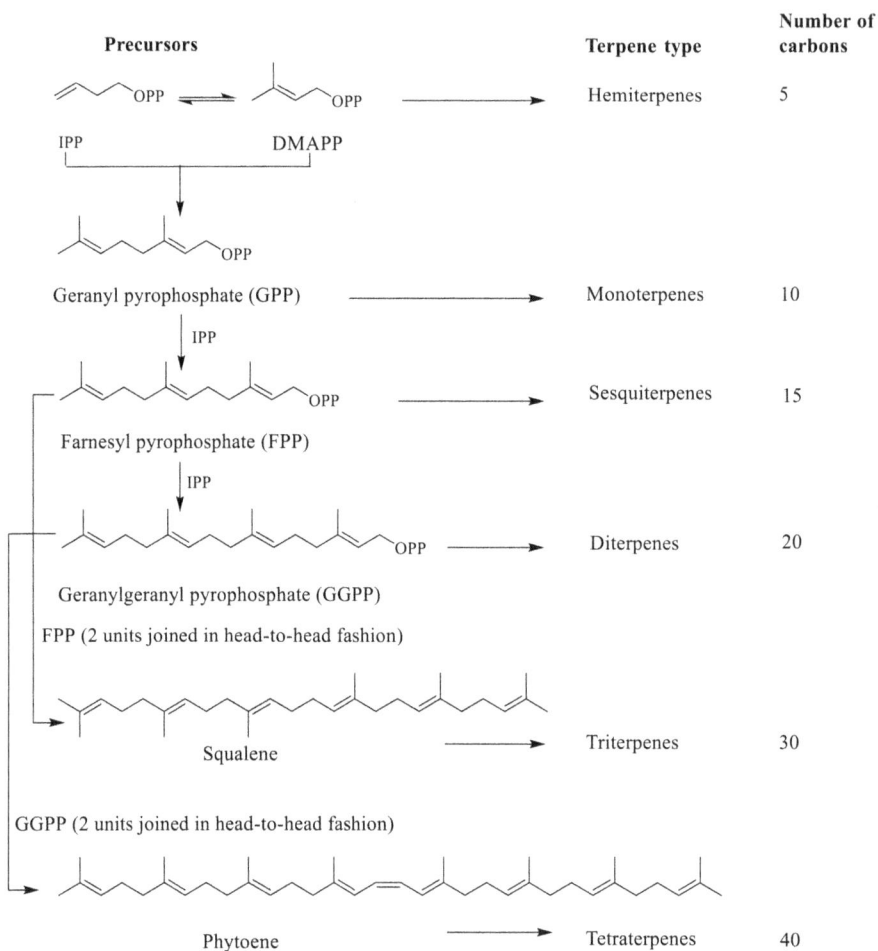

Figure 13.3 Overview of the synthesis of terpenoids. DMAPP and IPP condense in head-to-tail fashion to form geranyl pyrophosphate (GPP), a 10-carbon skeleton precursor of monoterpenoids. Addition of another five-carbon unit (IPP) to GPP forms farnesyl pyrophosphate (FPP) as an immediate precursor of the 15-carbon skeleton terpenoids, sesquiterpenes. A further addition of IPP to FPP leads to the formation of geranylgeranyl pyrophosphate (GGPP) as an immediate precursor of the 20-carbon terpenoids, diterpenes. Two FPP units dimerise in head-to-head fashion to form triterpenes (30-carbon skeleton) and head-to-head dimerisation of two GGPP units forms tetraterpenes (40-carbon skeleton).

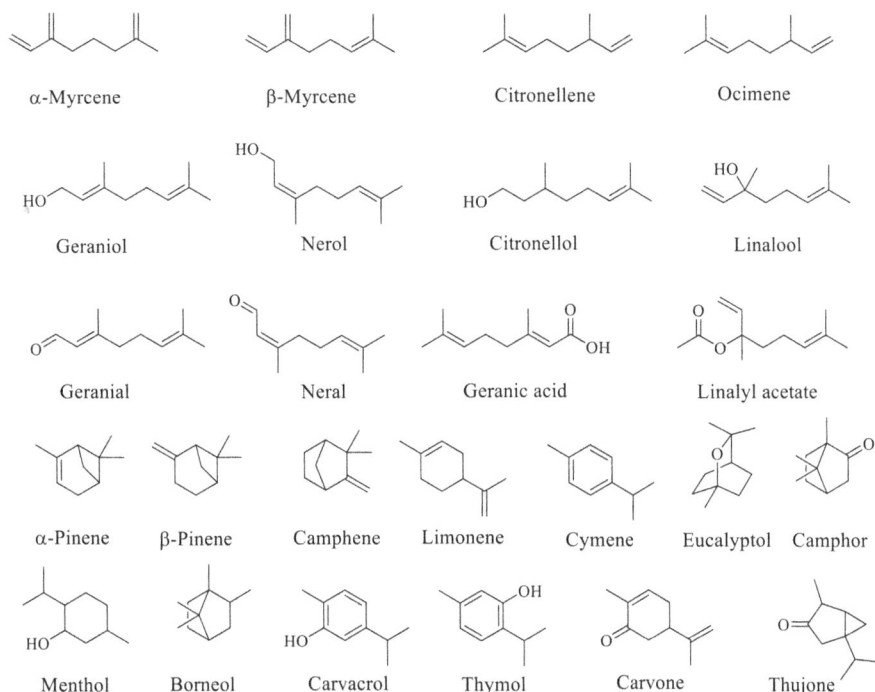

Figure 13.4 shows structures with the following labels:

α-Myrcene, β-Myrcene, Citronellene, Ocimene

Geraniol, Nerol, Citronellol, Linalool

Geranial, Neral, Geranic acid, Linalyl acetate

α-Pinene, β-Pinene, Camphene, Limonene, Cymene, Eucalyptol, Camphor

Menthol, Borneol, Carvacrol, Thymol, Carvone, Thujone

Figure 13.4 Structures of some cyclic and acyclic monoterpenes.

Terpenes – Key facts

- All terpenes trace their biosynthetic origin to isoprenoids – DMAPP and IPP.
- They polymerise to form the basic skeleton of monoterpenes, sesquiterpenes, diterpenes, *etc.*
- From the same skeleton, structural diversity comes through oxidation, reduction, cyclisation, hydroxylation, glycosylation, *etc.*
- Smaller units of terpenoids are volatile and are generally non-polar.
- The glycoside form of terpenoids is water soluble.
- Several thousand terpenoids are known to occur in Nature and more are to be identified from natural sources.

Monoterpenes are the main components of many essential oils. Although one or a few compounds predominate in their content, many essential oils are mixtures of several dozen components comprising monoterpenes and other classes of compounds. Some herbs are particularly sourced in the aroma and fragrance industries for their high-yielding essential oils.

Monoterpenes also have medicinal properties, as shown by the antidiabetic potential of many derivatives (Figure 13.5). They also

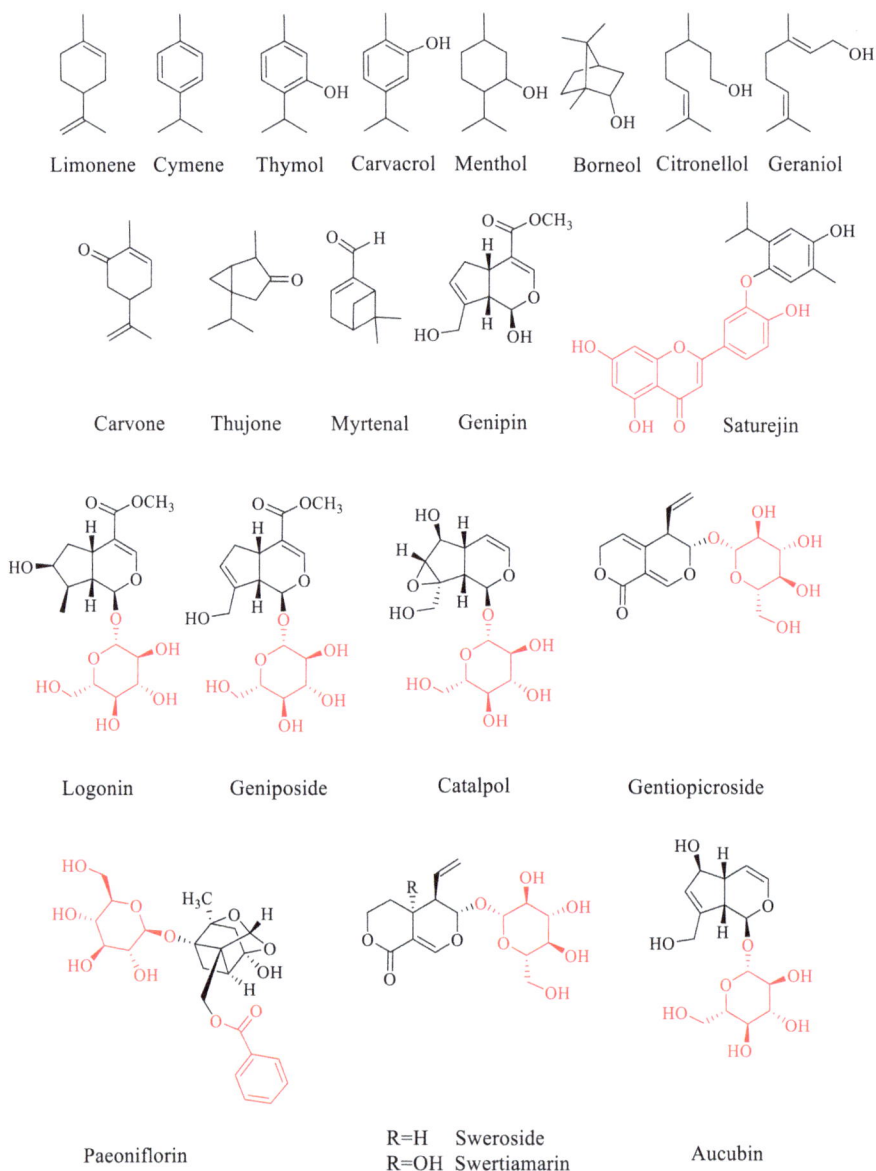

Figure 13.5 Monoterpenes that have been shown to display antidiabetic effects. Reproduced from ref. 1, https://doi.org/10.3390/ijms19010004, under the terms of the CC BY 4.0 license, https://creativecommons.org/licenses/by/4.0/.

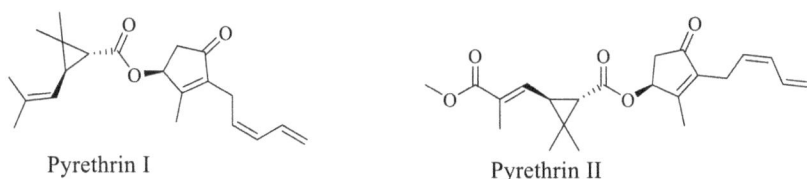

Figure 13.6 Structures of pyrethrin I and II.

Figure 13.6 Structures of pyrethrin I and II.

combine with other structures such as phenolic compounds and sugars to form complex structures (Figure 13.5). The main pharmacological properties of monoterpenes include antibacterial, antioxidant, and anti-inflammatory effects. They are also used as nasal decongestants (*e.g.* eucalyptol, Figure 13.4). Other pharmacological effects include a central nervous system (CNS) effect such as potential therapy for Alzheimer's disease that has attracted attention in recent years.[2]

Monoterpenes play a crucial role in insect–plant interactions. For instance, monoterpenes with an insecticidal effect are utilised in the agroindustry. Pyrethrins (Figure 13.6) are natural insecticidal and insect-repellent compounds extracted from the flowers of *Chrysanthemum cinerariifolium*. Since natural pyrethrins can easily decompose when exposed to air, light, and heat, synthetic derivatives have also been developed.

13.3.1.3 Sesquiterpenes

Based on a 15-carbon skeleton and originating from three isoprene units, sesquiterpenes have greater structural complexity than monoterpenes. Their acyclic and cyclic structural diversities are shown in Figure 13.7.

Acyclic sesquiterpenes are not as diverse as the cyclic counterparts. A few examples that occur in essential oils are shown in Figure 13.8.

Monocyclic sesquiterpenes are represented by α-, β- and γ-bisabolanes, which differ from each other in the position of the double bond within the aliphatic side chain (Figure 13.9). The rhizomes of *Curcuma longa* (turmeric) and related curcuma species are well known spices and medicines, particularly in Asia. *Zingiber* is another genus with similar usage and is best represented by ginger (*Z. officinale*). The fragrances of these rhizomes and extracted essential oils are rich in bisabolene-type sesquiterpenes. Representative compounds of these sesquiterpenes known for their medicinal, flavouring, and cosmetic uses are shown in Figure 13.9. Phenolic structures of the sesquiterpene class have also been isolated from both plants and marine organisms such as sponges.

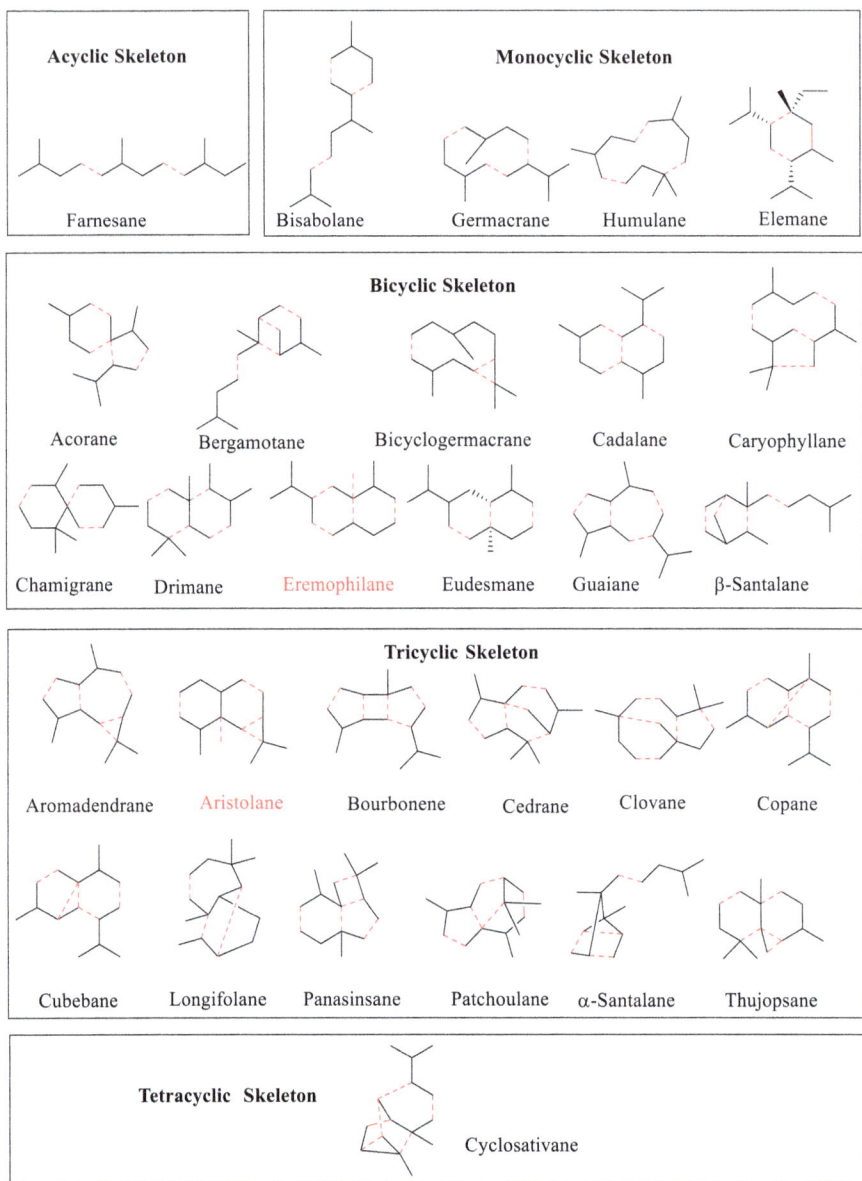

Acyclic Skeleton

Farnesane

Monocyclic Skeleton

Bisabolane   Germacrane   Humulane   Elemane

Bicyclic Skeleton

Acorane   Bergamotane   Bicyclogermacrane   Cadalane   Caryophyllane

Chamigrane   Drimane   Eremophilane   Eudesmane   Guaiane   β-Santalane

Tricyclic Skeleton

Aromadendrane   Aristolane   Bourbonene   Cedrane   Clovane   Copane

Cubebane   Longifolane   Panasinsane   Patchoulane   α-Santalane   Thujopsane

Tetracyclic Skeleton

Cyclosativane

Figure 13.7   Structural skeletons of sesquiterpenes. The five-carbon isoprene units are shown in black and the bonding between these
units to form the skeleton is shown as dashed red lines. In some
cases, migration of methyl groups occurs, as shown for the
structures of eremophilane and aristolane.

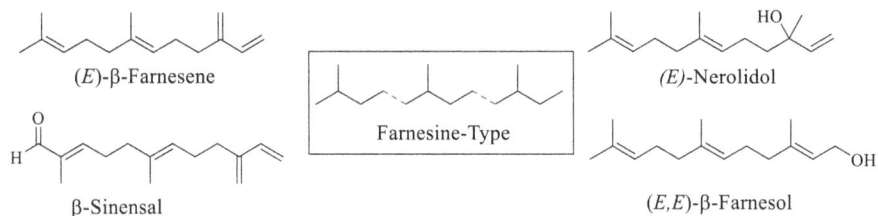

(E)-β-Farnesene

Farnesine-Type

(E)-Nerolidol

β-Sinensal

(E,E)-β-Farnesol

Figure 13.8 Examples of acyclic sesquiterpenes.

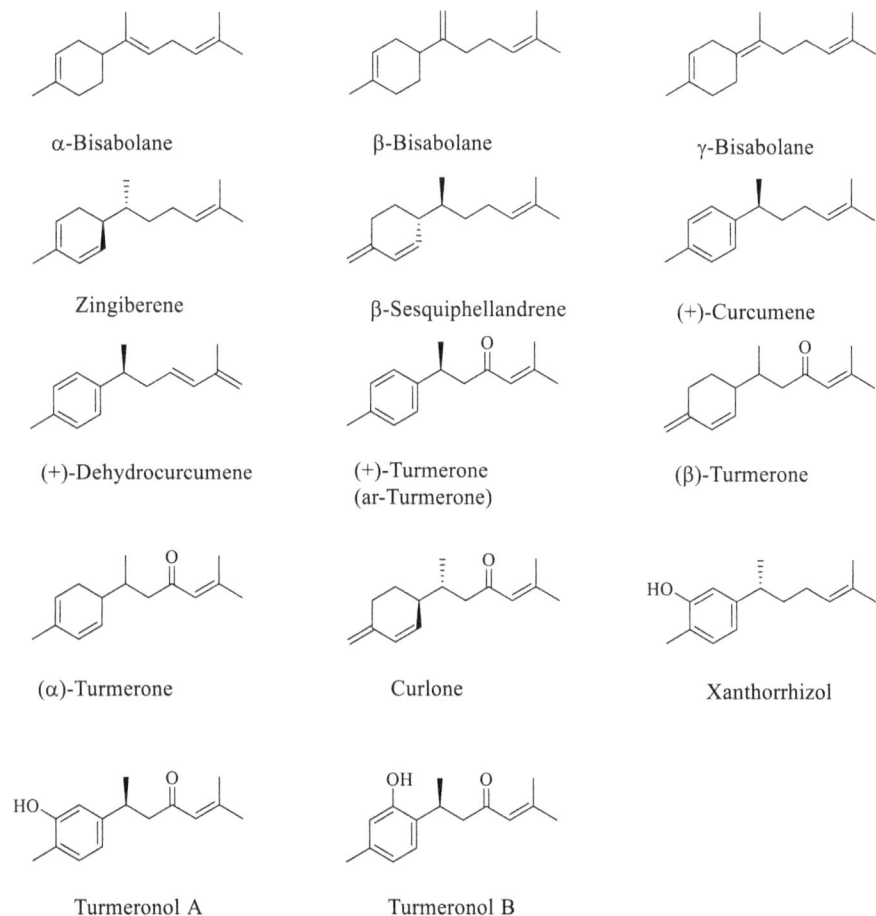

α-Bisabolane

β-Bisabolane

γ-Bisabolane

Zingiberene

β-Sesquiphellandrene

(+)-Curcumene

(+)-Dehydrocurcumene

(+)-Turmerone
(ar-Turmerone)

(β)-Turmerone

(α)-Turmerone

Curlone

Xanthorrhizol

Turmeronol A

Turmeronol B

Figure 13.9 Examples of monocyclic sesquiterpenes.

Germacranes (Figure 13.10) are a class of sesquiterpenes based on the cyclodecane ring system. The simple germacrenes with variations in the positions of double bonds include germacrene A–D. Represented by parthenolide, sesquiterpene lactones based on the

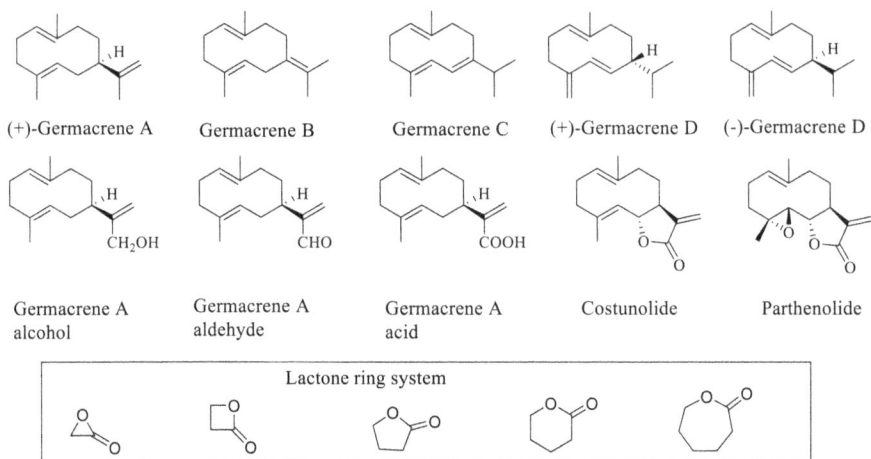

(+)-Germacrene A   Germacrene B   Germacrene C   (+)-Germacrene D   (-)-Germacrene D

Germacrene A   Germacrene A   Germacrene A   Costunolide   Parthenolide
alcohol   aldehyde   acid

Lactone ring system

Figure 13.10   Examples of natural germacrene-type sesquiterpenes. Those with a lactone ring (*e.g.* costunolide and parthenolide) are called germacranolides.

germacrene skeleton are called germacranolides. Parthenolide is the main active ingredient in feverfew (*Tanacetum parthenium*) and has long been known for its diverse pharmacological activities. In addition to the numerous therapeutic claims in traditional medicine, feverfew is used as an antimigraine agent. Parthenolide also occurs in tansy (*T. vulgarum*) and many other members of the plant family Asteraceae. Biosynthetically, sequential oxidation of germacrene A through alcohol, aldehyde, and acid derivatives leads to the first germacranolide skeleton, costunolide, that serves as the precursor to the biosynthesis of parthenolide (Figure 13.10). The anti-inflammatory and potential anticancer activities of parthenolide and costunolide derivatives and plant sources have been extensively studied.

Good examples of sesquiterpene skeletons without oxygenation are shown in Figure 13.11. These are hydrocarbons that are volatile owing to their low molecular weight and non-polar nature. In Nature, however, they are found mostly in oxygenated forms (see below).

Most of the biologically active sesquiterpenes have a lactone structural moiety that plays a significant role in their therapeutic efficacy. As with their structural subclass/skeleton shown in Figure 13.11, their lactones are also called eudesmanolide, guaianolide, pseudo-guaianolide, germacranolide, and xanthanolide (Figure 13.12). The xanthanolide-type sesquiterpenes, for example, have been isolated from *Xanthium strumarium* and other species of the Asteraceae family.

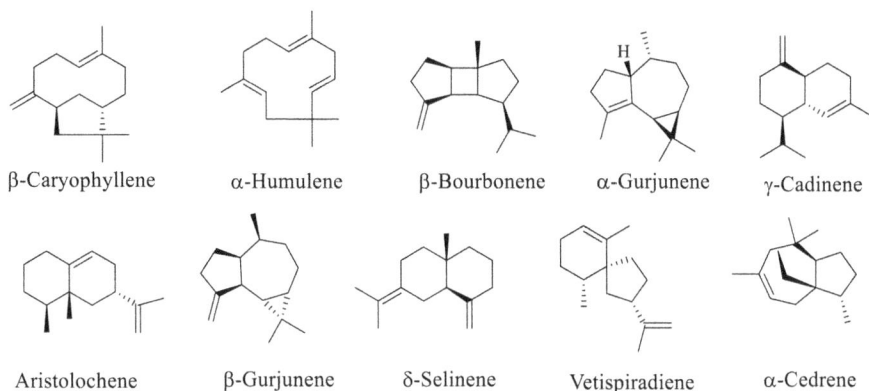

β-Caryophyllene   α-Humulene   β-Bourbonene   α-Gurjunene   γ-Cadinene

Aristolochene   β-Gurjunene   δ-Selinene   Vetispiradiene   α-Cedrene

Figure 13.11   Sesquiterpene skeletons without oxygenation.

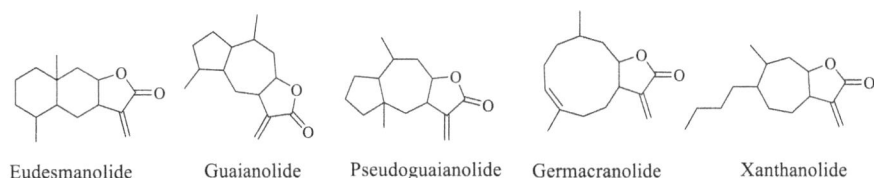

Eudesmanolide   Guaianolide   Pseudoguaianolide   Germacranolide   Xanthanolide

Figure 13.12   Structural classes of sesquiterpene lactones.

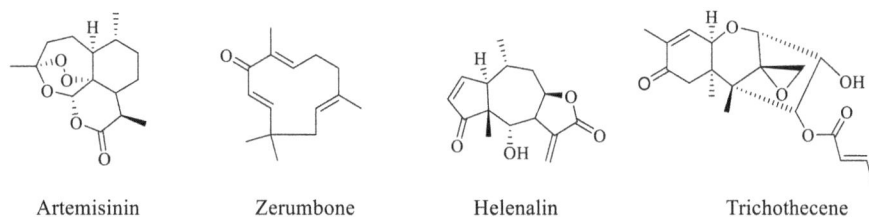

Artemisinin   Zerumbone   Helenalin   Trichothecene

Figure 13.13   Examples of biologically active sesquiterpenes. Numerous trichothecenes based on the skeletal structure illustrated exist (see Section 13.4.1.2).

These sesquiterpene lactones are generally known for their cytotoxic effect and anticancer properties.

An exemplary sesquiterpene of pharmacological importance is artemisinin (Figure 13.13), isolated from the Chinese medicinal plant *Artemisia annua*, which is one of the best therapies for malaria. Its derivatives have also been shown to display potent anticancer effects. Overall, many natural cyclic sesquiterpenes are known for their therapeutic potential. The sesquiterpene zerumbone is one of the active compounds found in the rhizome of the ginger relative *Zingiber zerumbet*. It has shown anti-inflammatory, anticancer, and chemopreventive potential in experimental studies. Helenalin, isolated from several plants of the family Asteraceae, has anti-inflammatory properties. Readers should bear in mind that describing the vast number of pharmacologically active sesquiterpenes is beyond the scope of this book. From simple structures to complex trichothecenes (*e.g.* mycotoxins) of the tetracyclic ring system (Figure 13.13), they have been shown to display numerous pharmacological effects.

13.3.1.4 Diterpenes

With a 20-carbon building block, diterpenes are common in both terrestrial and marine organisms. The immediate precursor of diterpenes is geranylgeranyl pyrophosphate (GGPP), which undergoes several rearrangement reactions to form different structural types, most of which are shown in Figure 13.14.

   In Nature, diterpenes play many physiological roles in the plants or animals that produce them. Some biologically active compounds of the diterpenes class are shown in Figure 13.15. For example, gibberellins serve as hormones and stimulate plant growth, whereas other diterpenoids called prodolactones have the opposite effect (inhibit plant growth). Some diterpenes are poisonous or promote cancer growth. Good examples are phorbol and phorbol esters that activate protein kinase C, thereby promoting tumour growth. They are based on the tigliane structural type of diterpenes. Phorbol (Figure 13.15) was originally isolated from croton oil obtained from the seeds of the purging croton (*Croton tiglium*). The plant families Euphorbiaceae and Thymelaeaceae are particularly known for the synthesis of phorbol esters. Many pharmacological experiments on tumour initiation and activation of white blood cells are based on the use of phorbol esters. A good example of a diterpene-based drug is that obtained from the Indian medicinal plant (Hindu and Ayurvedic traditional medicine) *Coleus forskohlii* (Lamiaceae). The compound forskolin (Figure 13.15) activates cyclic adenosine monophosphate (cAMP) and has numerous therapeutic indications including an antihypertensive effect. Ginkgolides are a group of diterpenoids isolated from *Ginkgo biloba* (Ginkgoaceae). The plant is extensively used in both traditional and modern medicine, particularly in Europe, to treat circulatory diseases. Based on lactone structures (also called diterpene lactones), they also inhibit platelet aggregation by inhibiting the platelet-activating factor.

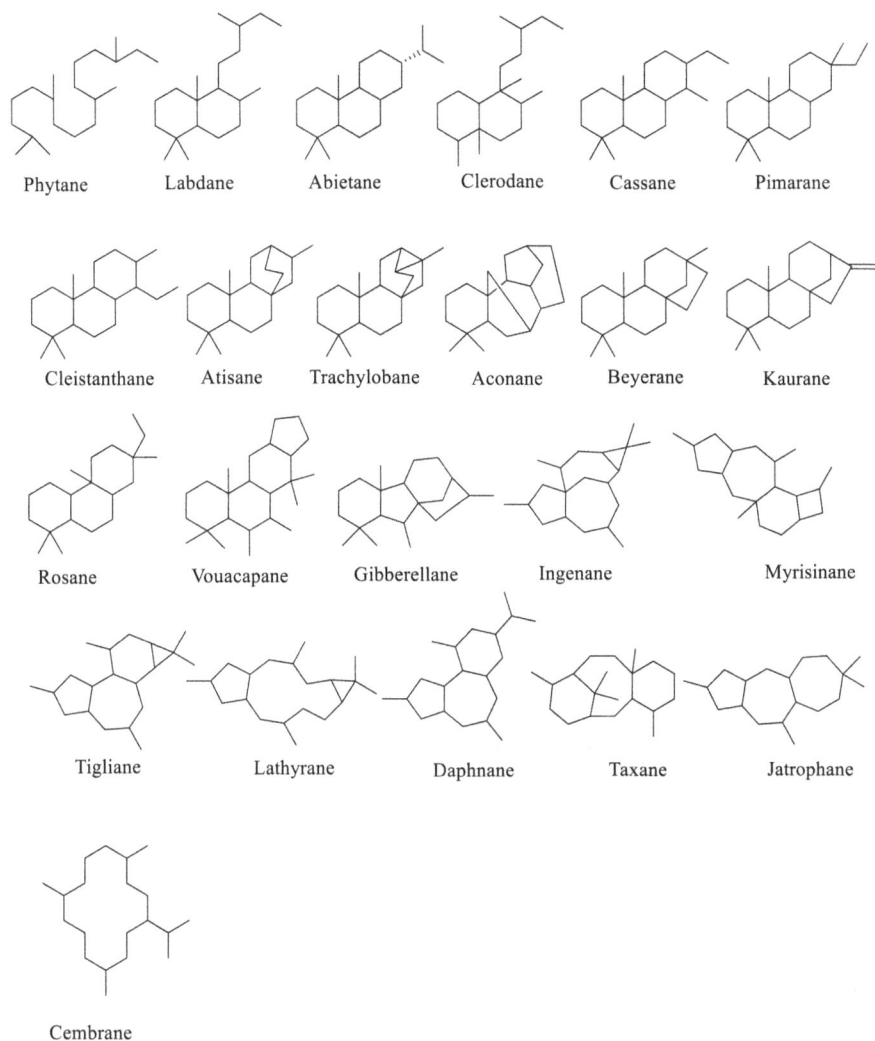

Phytane Labdane Abietane Clerodane Cassane Pimarane

Cleistanthane Atisane Trachylobane Aconane Beyerane Kaurane

Rosane Vouacapane Gibberellane Ingenane Myrisinane

Tigliane Lathyrane Daphnane Taxane Jatrophane

Cembrane

Figure 13.14 Structural skeletons of diterpenes.

The anticancer drug taxol (or paclitaxel) (Figure 13.15) is a classic example of natural products as drugs obtained through random screening for biological effects. By stabilising microtubules, it inhibits cancer cell multiplication. Readers should note that the biological effects of diterpenes are diverse and far beyond the scope of this book. In our laboratories, we have identified several novel diterpenes of various structural classes with potent antibacterial and anticancer properties.

Ginkgolide A

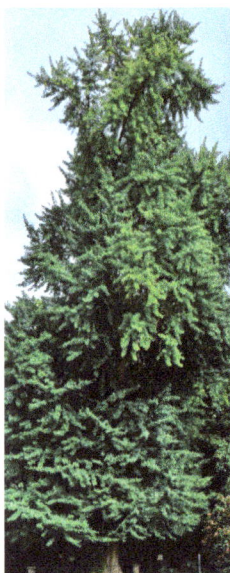

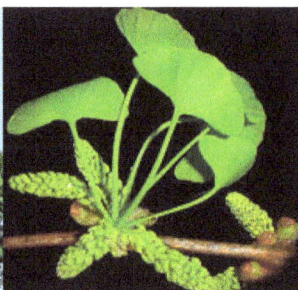

Ginkgo (*Ginkgo biloba*)

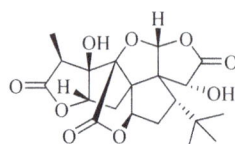

Phorbol

Gibberellic acid

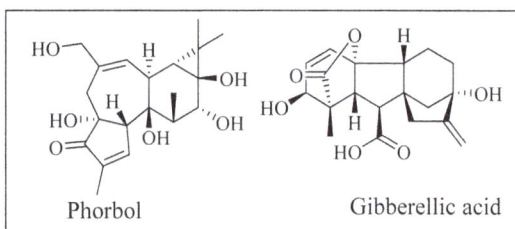

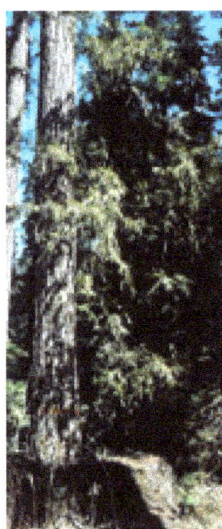

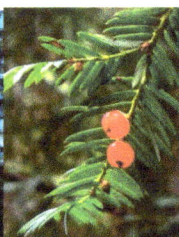

Pacific yew tree
(*Taxus brevifolia*)

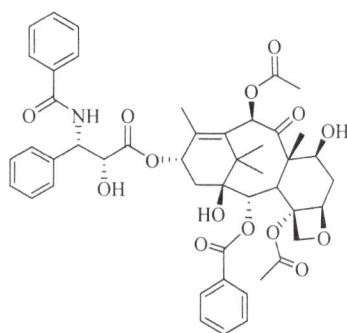

Taxol

Figure 13.15   Examples of biologically active diterpenes. One of the best examples of drug discovery from natural sources is taxol, an anticancer drug extracted from the Pacific yew tree (*Taxus brevifolia*). The diterpene skeleton in taxol is modified through addition of various other structural groups. Another good example of diterpenes is ginkgolides from ginkgo (*Ginkgo biloba*). This tree (also called a maidenhair tree) is one of the oldest trees on Earth (known to exist 290 million years ago) and has been cultivated and used for medicinal purposes to the present day. Gibberellic acid is a plant hormone whereas phorbol and its other diterpene derivatives are from other plants, most of which are poisonous.

Taxol – Key Facts

- Humans have made use of the yew tree for thousands of years, but the discovery of taxol was not based on traditional medicine information.
- Taxol is a potent microtubule-stabilising agent.
- It induces cytotoxicity in cancer cells through inhibition of microtubule formation.
- It has broad activity in several cancers, including breast cancer, endometrial cancer, non-small cell lung cancer, bladder cancer, and cervical carcinoma.
- Unfortunately, thousands of trees need to be killed to obtain a few kilograms of the drug.

13.3.1.5 Triterpenes

The chemical diversity of triterpenes is even more complex than that of mono-, sesqi- and diterpenes. They can be broadly divided into acyclic or linear, monocyclic, bicyclic, tricyclic, tetracyclic, and pentacyclic compounds. They also commonly occur in Nature as glycosides (with sugar units attached) called saponins. The precursor of triterpenes, squalene (Figure 13.3), is found in plants and in oils such as olive oil and the liver oil of sharks. The common triterpenes are phytosterols or simply sterols and include compounds such as α-amyrin, β-amyrin, ursolic acid, oleanolic acid, betulinic acid, sitosterol, stigmasterol, campesterol, and α-spinasterol (Figure 13.16). They display numerous pharmacological effects, including anti-inflammatory properties. Sterols are also common in animals, fungi, and yeasts. For example, ergosterol (Figure 13.16) is the cholesterol equivalent and is found in the cell membranes of fungi and protozoa.

Triterpenoids are also commonly found in animals in various forms. Cholesterol as an integral part of a cell membrane is synthesised through the mevalonic acid (terpenoids) pathway in the liver. Bile acids in the liver are also synthesised from cholesterol. Hence the synthesis of cholesterol is a key target in the regulation of a variety of diseases. For example, statins as lipid-lowering drugs target the key enzyme in the mevalonic acid pathway, 3-hydroxy-3-methylglutaryl-CoA (HMG-CoA) reductase. The most common bile acids in the body are shown in Figure 13.17. They exist either as free acids or conjugated with glycine or taurine.

Steroidal hormones (Figure 13.18) such as the glucocorticoids (cortisol) and mineralocorticoids (aldosterone) are also products of the

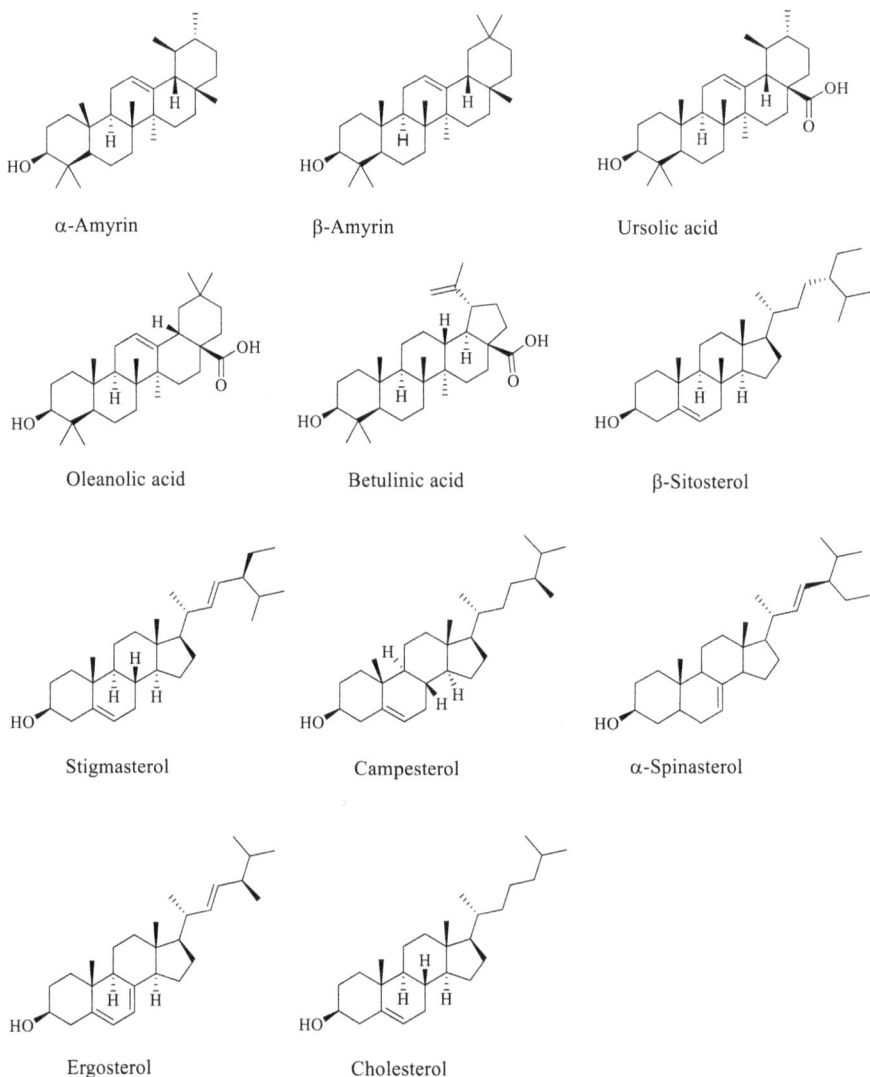

Figure 13.16   Structures of common sterols.

terpenoid biosynthesis pathway *via* cholesterol as a precursor. They are critical in the regulation of various body functions, and drug mimics such as dexamethasone are effectively used to treat inflammation and various diseases including COVID-19.

Oestrogens (estradiol and progesterone, see Figure 13.19) in females and androgens (testosterone and androstenedione) in the testes of males are the principal steroidal sex hormones in mammals. They are formed from cholesterol as a precursor. One of the most effectively

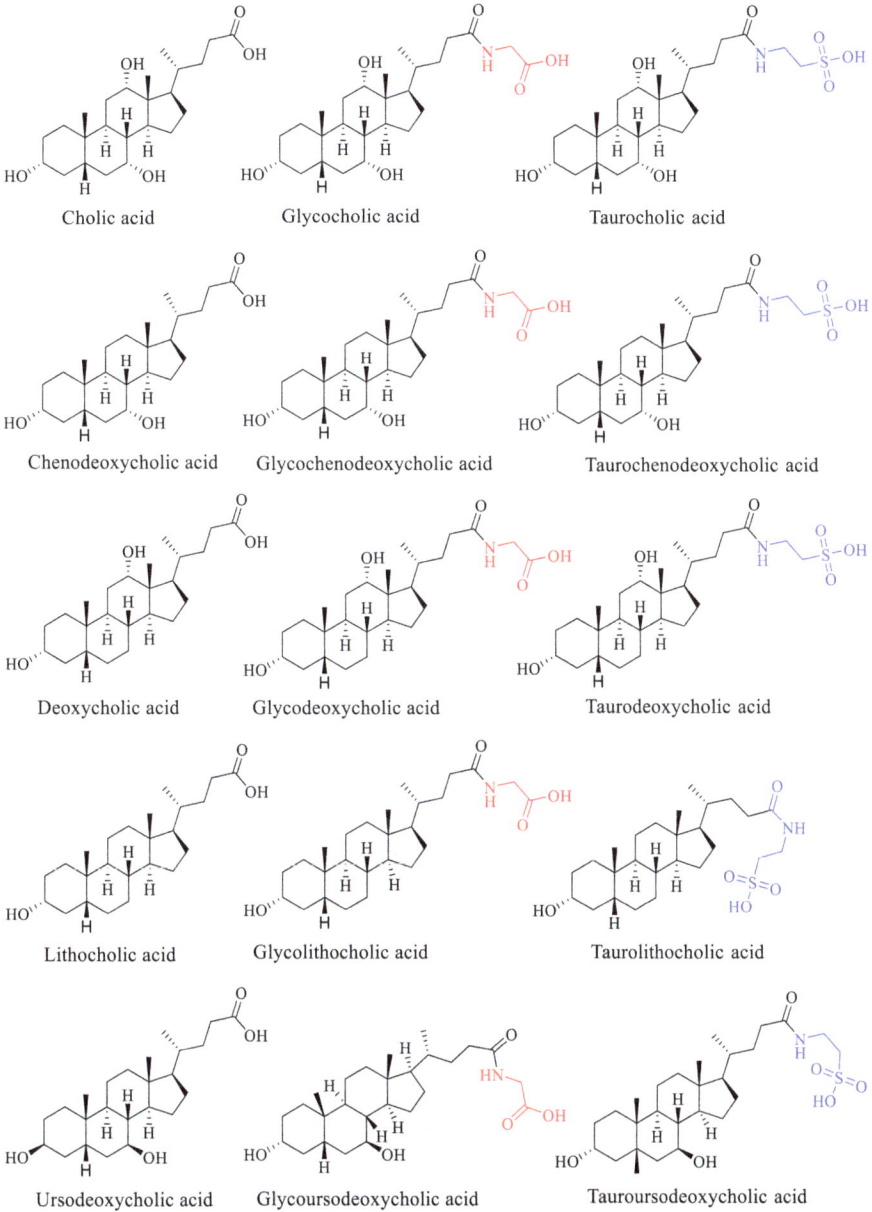

Figure 13.17 Common bile acids in humans. The glycine and taurine structures in the bile acid conjugates are shown in red and blue, respectively.

Cholic acid

Glycocholic acid

Taurocholic acid

Chenodeoxycholic acid

Glycochenodeoxycholic acid

Taurochenodeoxycholic acid

Deoxycholic acid

Glycodeoxycholic acid

Taurodeoxycholic acid

Lithocholic acid

Glycolithocholic acid

Taurolithocholic acid

Ursodeoxycholic acid

Glycoursodeoxycholic acid

Tauroursodeoxycholic acid

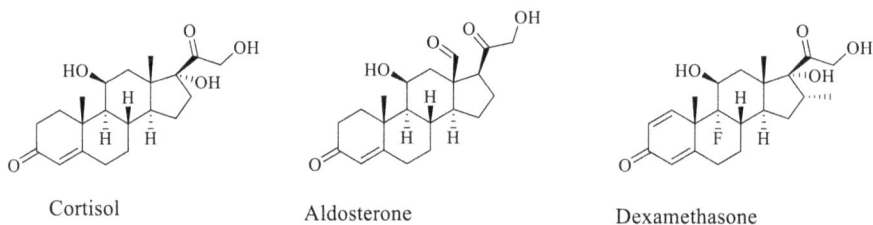

Cortisol   Aldosterone   Dexamethasone

Figure 13.18   Structures of cortisol, aldosterone, and dexamethasone.

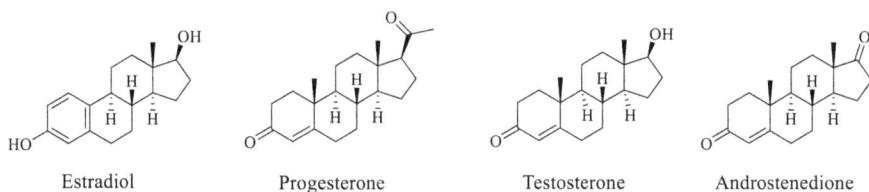

Estradiol   Progesterone   Testosterone   Androstenedione

Figure 13.19   Structures of sex hormones.

used approaches to contraception in history is the use of synthetic female sex hormones to prevent ovulation and/or conception. On the other hand, the synthetic analogues of testosterone (Figure 13.19), anabolic steroids, are used and are often abused to accelerate muscle development. They have many side effects, however, including heart-related disorders.

Triterpenoids have ecological significance and play a role in interspecies communications (for example, see Figure 13.20). Cucurbitacins (cucurbitacin B) and quassinoids (*e.g.* quassin) are highly oxygenated triterpenes with an extremely bitter taste. When they occur in plants, they deter herbivores. They also have numerous pharmacological properties. Limonin is a good example of these compounds as a citrus bitter principle and, based on this structural moiety, the limonoid azadirachtin (Figure 13.20) extracted from the neem tree (*Azadirachta indica*) is among the most potent and effectively utilised insect anti-feedant compounds in use today.

A good example of a steroidal drug is digoxin (Figure 13.21), which is used to treat heart conditions. As a class of drugs, digoxin and digitoxin belong to the cardiac glycosides and are used to increase the force of heart contraction as they inhibit the cardiac Na^+,K^+-ATPase enzyme. They are used in the treatment of atrial fibrillation, atrial flutter, and congestive heart failure. The discovery of such drugs was based on traditional medicine, digitalis, which is derived from the foxglove plant, *Digitalis purpurea*, and has been used for thousands

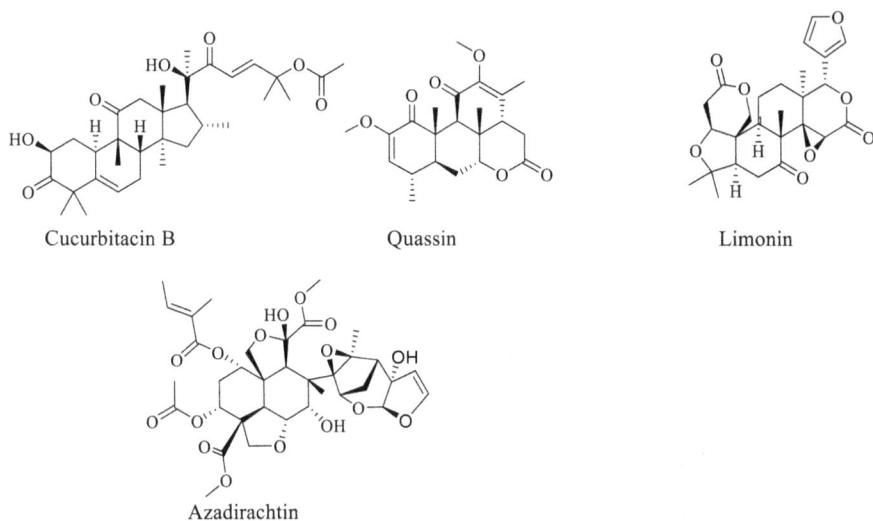

Cucurbitacin B   Quassin   Limonin

Azadirachtin

Figure 13.20 Structures of some bitter triterpenes with diverse pharmacological effects.

of years. The structure of digoxin is based on a triterpene skeleton containing three sugar units. On the other hand, diosgenin is a hydrolysis product without the sugar units (Figure 13.21) that is used in the commercial synthesis of cortisone, pregnenolone, and progesterone. There are many triterpenes in Nature with diverse pharmacological properties and their structures range from simple phytosterols to complex glycosides such as saponins. Details of these compounds are beyond the scope of this book.

13.3.1.6 Tetraterpenes

As shown in Figure 13.3, tetraterpenes are formed when two units of 20-carbon skeleton (diterpenoid) precursors join together to form 40-carbon terpenoids. The most prevalent tetraterpenes of both pharmaceutical and nutritional importance are the carotenoids. These are largely lipophilic compounds present in plants, algae, and some bacteria and fungi with their characteristic colouration of yellow, orange, and red. One of their uses is as a natural food colourant, *e.g.* carotenoids extracted from the marine alga *Dunaliella salina*. Industrial applications also include the extraction of marigold (*Tagetes patula* L.) in the clothing industry. Saffron (*Crocus sativus* L.) has been used for centuries in Asia and especially Persia (now Iran) as a food spice and colourant and for colouring clothing and fabrics. Carotenoids are

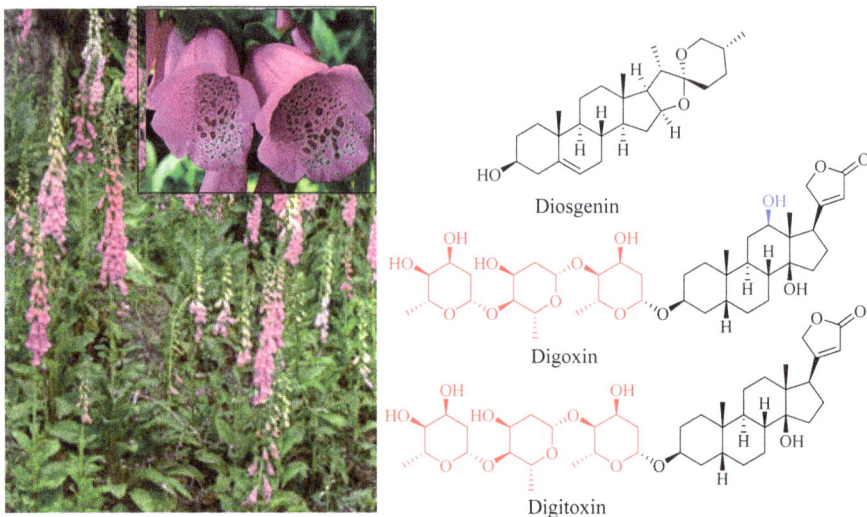

Figure 13.21 Structures of digoxin and diosgenin. Not that digoxin is a sapo-
nin, which is composed of a sugar part and a triterpene skeleton.
Also note that the presence of sugar units in the structure of
digoxin makes it water soluble, whereas diosgenin is soluble in
organic solvents such as chloroform but not water. Now largely
used as an ornamental plant, *Digitalis purpurea* (foxglove) has
been a source of the cardiac glycoside digoxin and the related
compound digitoxin. These compounds differ from each other
only in the presence of one more hydroxyl group in digoxin. Eating this plant can cause nausea, abdominal pain, vomiting, cardiac dysrhythmias, and hyperkalaemia (high level of potassium
in the blood). Foxglove image: Reproduced from https://com-
mons.wikimedia.org/wiki/File:Foxglove_-_Digitalis_purpurea.
jpg, under the terms of the CC BY-SA 4.0 license, https://cre-
ativecommons.org/licenses/by-sa/4.0/deed.en. Image Credit:
Jim Evans.

generally divided into two classes: compounds with only the hydrocarbon skeleton or no oxygen that we call carotenes (*e.g.* β-carotene,
α-carotene, lycopene, and phytoene) and those with one or more oxygen atoms in the molecule called xanthophylls (*e.g.* lutein, zeaxanthin,
astaxanthin, canthaxanthin, α- and β-cryptoxanthin, and fucoxanthin)
(Figures 13.22 and 13.23).

A characteristic feature of carotenoids is their ability to absorb light
in the visible range of the electromagnetic spectrum. This is because
of the large number of conjugated double bonds (often more than
nine) in their molecule that absorb light energy. They have a role in
photosynthesis in collaboration with chlorophyll and they also protect
biomolecules from oxidative damage – they are a natural antioxidant

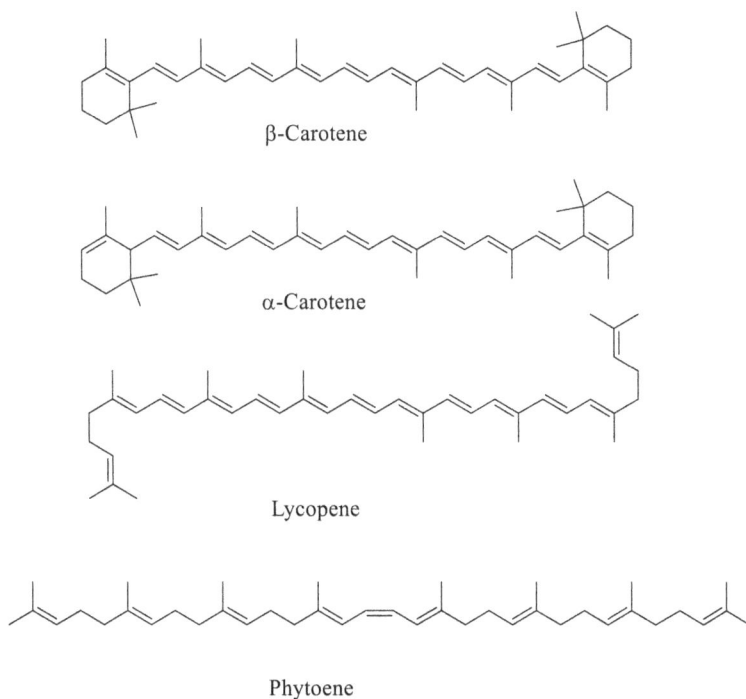

β-Carotene

α-Carotene

Lycopene

Phytoene

Figure 13.22 Structures of carotenes: β-carotene, α-carotene, lycopene, and phytoene.

and offer photoprotection. Vegetables and fruits are good sources of carotenoids; the list is long, and includes apricots, carrots, corn, guava, kale, mangoes, mustard, nectarines, tangerines, peaches, pink grapefruits, pumpkins, squash, sweet potatoes, tomatoes, and watermelons. Whereas carrots are rich in β- and α-carotene, to which their orange–yellow colour is due, lycopene contributes to the red–orange colour in tomato fruits. Lycopene is also found in watermelons and pink grapefruits. It has numerous biological effects but primarily serves as an antioxidant. The main source of carotenoids is plants but some fish, such as salmon, store them at high levels from their phytoplankton diet. Astaxanthin is the main carotenoid of salmon and is also found in other freshwater organisms and marine organisms such as crayfish and lobsters. Lutein is also common in these organisms but it should be noted that modern fish farms may add carotenoids to the diet of their fish to give them a desirable reddish colour. The global carotenoids market in 2019 was estimated to be around US$1.5 billion and it is expected to rise to US$2 billion by 2026. This market largely includes their use as feeds, foods and beverages, dietary supplements,

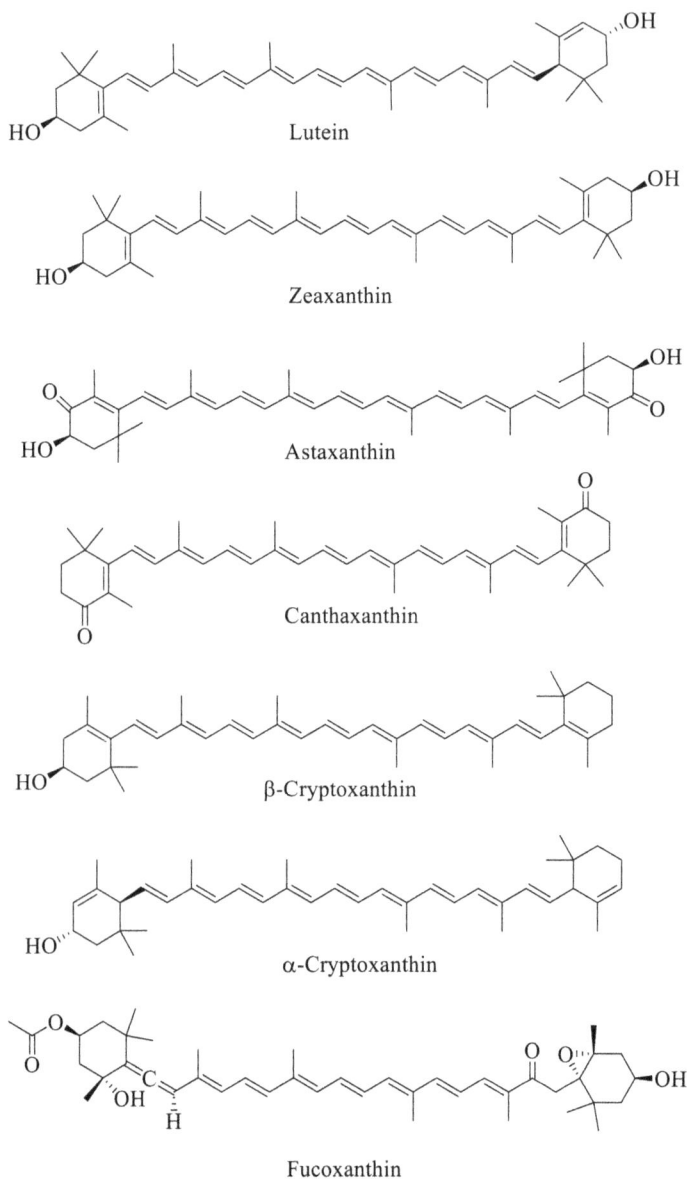

Figure 13.23 Structures of xanthophylls: lutein, zeaxanthin, astaxanthin, canthaxanthin, α- and β-cryptoxanthin, and fucoxanthin.

cosmetics, and pharmaceuticals and formulations. The most utilised carotenoids in this business are astaxanthin, β-carotene, lutein, lycopene, canthaxanthin, and zeaxanthin.

Apocarotenoids are compounds formed from the degradation or cleavage of carotenoids. They include the vitamin A retinoids, namely

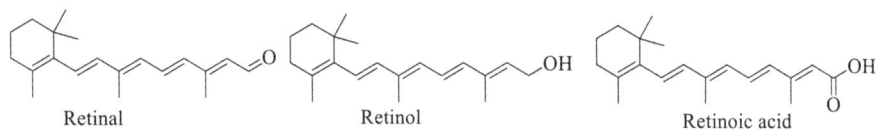

| Retinal | Retinol | Retinoic acid |

Figure 13.24 Structures of retinoids with vitamin A activity. The structures of retinal, retinol, and retinoic acid are shown.

retinal, retinoic acid, and retinol (Figure 13.24), and the plant hormone abscisic acid. Hence they are often called tetraterpenoid-derived phytohormones. These compounds are formed by both enzymatic and non-enzymatic breakdown of carotenoids in both plants and mammalian tissues. The carotenoid precursors of vitamin A are called provitamin A carotenoids, which are mainly represented by β-carotene. The formation of the photosensitive pigments that detect light in our eyes is based on the retinoid 11-*cis*-retinal. That is why vitamin A deficiency was recognised long ago as a cause of night blindness. There is also what is called the macular pigment, which comprises lutein, zeaxanthin, and *meso*-zeaxanthin at the retinal macula (central area of the retina, which is yellow pigmented). These compounds are used to optimise visual performance and have antioxidant properties.

In some organisms such as marine sponge (*Phorbas gukhulensis*), *diterpenoids undergoing dimerisation to form* tetraterpenoid compounds have been noted. Compounds named gukulenins have been shown to display cytotoxicity against cancer cells at very small doses.

13.3.2 Polyketides

Polyketides are a large group of natural products that are synthesised based on the action of enzymes called polyketide synthases. The biosynthesis process that starts from acetyl-CoA occurs in bacteria, fungi, plants, and some marine animals. Through the malonyl-CoA intermediate, acetyl-CoA is condensed to form a long-chain polyketide (Figure 13.25), following which different forms of cyclisation occur to form diverse natural products. The remarkable wonder of the natural world in this case is the polyketide synthases in these organisms that we are now manipulating through genetic engineering mostly to maximise the yield of these valuable natural products. A large number of clinically useful drugs are derived from the polyketide pathway. The most important sources of polyketide-based drugs are plants and bacteria, including the genus *Streptomyces*.

Macrolides are a group of polyketide-based compounds with a lactone-carrying macrocyclic 14–16-membered ring system. Good

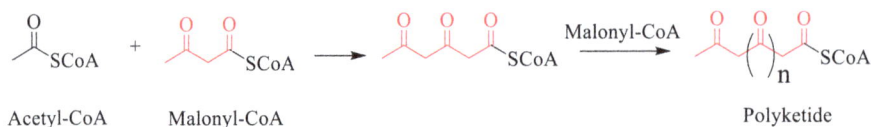

Figure 13.25 The polyketide pathway of biosynthesis. Through the malonyl-CoA intermediate, a large number of acetyl-CoA units can be condensed to form a long polyketide chain. Fatty acids are synthesised through the same process where 2-carbon skeleton (from acetyl-CoA) is added at a time. The polyketide then cyclises to form a variety of products that are unique to the living organisms that produce them.

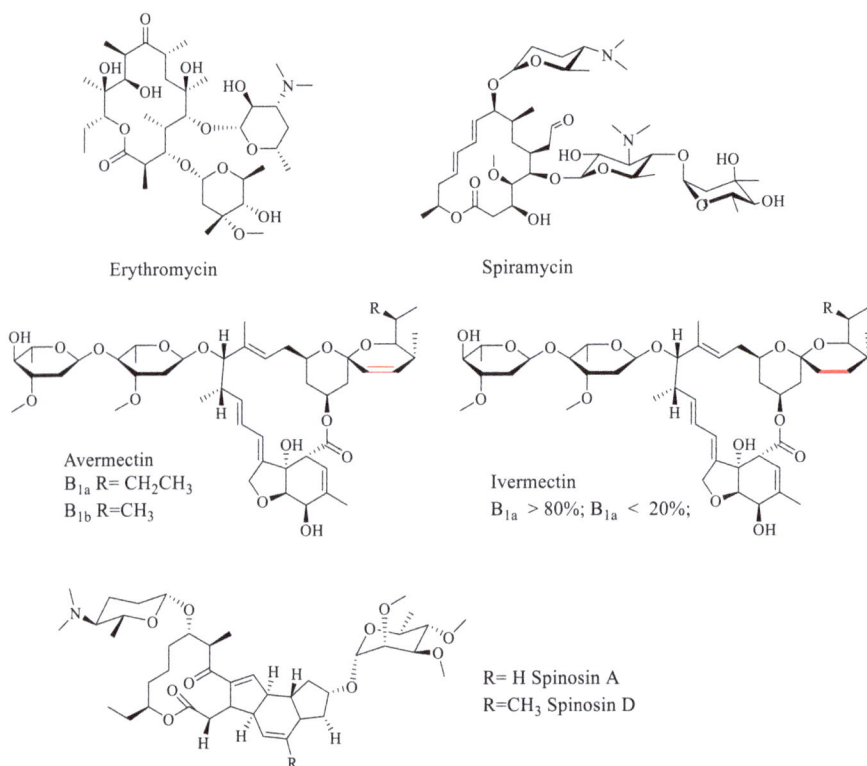

Erythromycin

Spiramycin

Avermectin
B_{1a} R= CH_2CH_3
B_{1b} R=CH_3

Ivermectin
$B_{1a} > 80\%$; $B_{1a} < 20\%$;

R= H Spinosin A
R=CH_3 Spinosin D

Figure 13.26 Structures of some macrolide derivatives of natural products isolated from microorganisms. Note the structural similarity between avermectin and ivermectin and their difference highlighted in red. The drug as a mixture of the two components, B_{1a} and B_{1b}, is also shown.

examples (see Figure 13.26) include useful antibiotics (*e.g.* erythromycin, first isolated from the bacterium *Saccharopolyspora erythraea*, and spiramycin, first isolated from *Streptomyces ambofaciens*), anthelmintics (*e.g.* avermectin and ivermectin isolated from *Streptomyces* sp.), and some insecticides such as spinosad (a mixture containing spinosyn A and D from *Saccharopolyspora spinosa*).

Other semi-synthetic derivatives of erythromycin are also worth mentioning and include clarithromycin, azithromycin, roxithromycin, telithromycin (Ketek), solithromycin, and nafithromycin (Figure 13.27). This is a good example of drug discovery where natural products can be modified to obtain drugs that are either more efficacious or have a better safety profile.

Eighteen-membered macrolactone antibiotics represented by tiacumicins have also been discovered in bacteria in recent years (Figure 13.28).

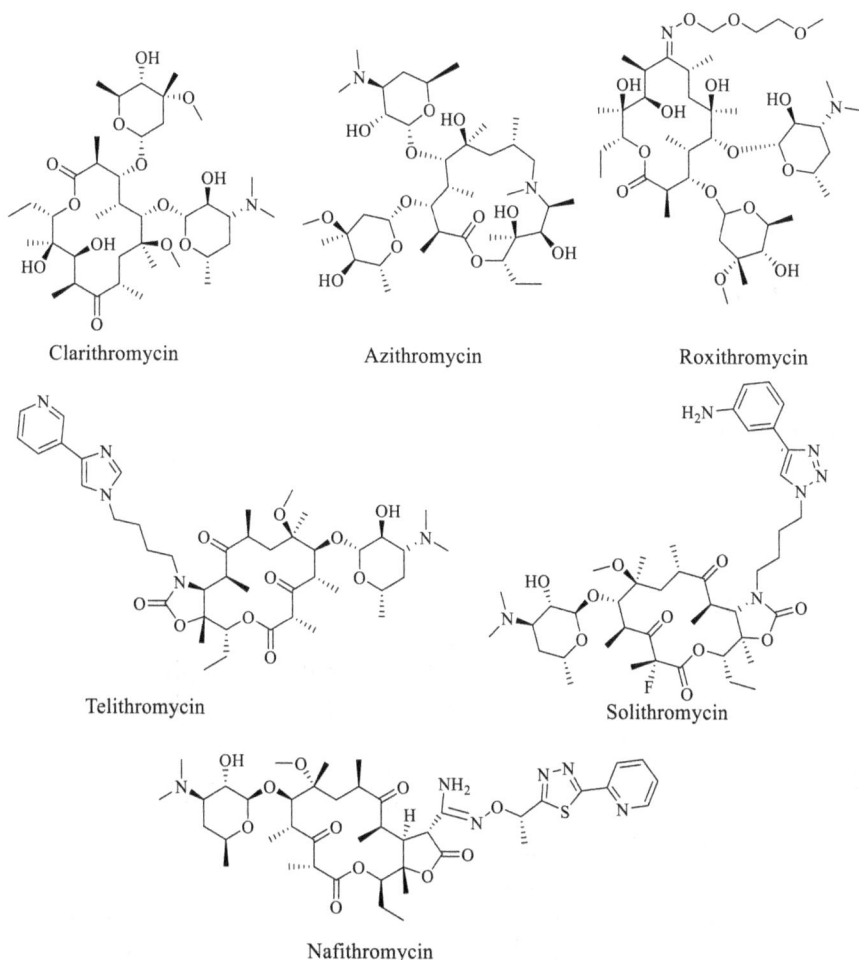

Clarithromycin

Azithromycin

Roxithromycin

Telithromycin

Solithromycin

Nafithromycin

Figure 13.27 Semi-synthetic derivatives of erythromycin.

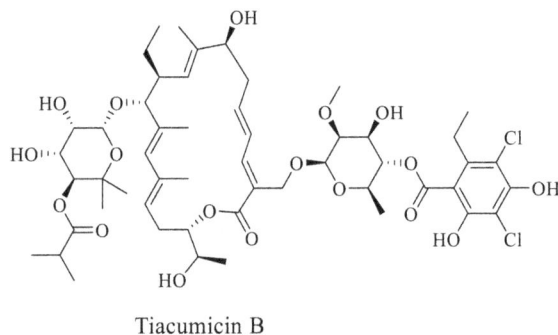

Tiacumicin B

Figure 13.28 The structure of tiacumicin B as an example of an 18-membered macrolactone.

Another group of antibiotics called ansamycins (Figure 13.29) are polyketide-based drugs originating from bacteria. Structurally, they also have a cyclic ring system with aliphatic chain bridges at two positions. This group includes the rifamycin antibiotics (first isolated from *Streptomyces mediterranei*), which are effective in the therapy of mycobacterial diseases such as tuberculosis and leprosy. There are also rifamycin derivatives such as rifampicin (or rifampin), rifabutin, rifapentine, rifalazil, and rifaximin. The ansamycins class also includes the anticancer drugs geldanamycin and macbecin.

Other useful drugs based on the polyketide skeleton include polyunsaturated organic compounds called polyenes. Common antifungal drug therapies originally isolated from *Streptomyces* species including amphotericin, nystatin, and pimaricin (or natamycin) belong to this group. The structures displayed in Figure 13.30 show the massive macrolide structure with conjugated double bonds and many functional groups together with a sugar attachment.

The polyether structural group (Figure 13.31) is represented by the antibiotic monensin (isolated from *Streptomyces cinnamonensis*), which is an ionophoric antibiotic used to treat bacterial, fungal, and parasitic infections. These antibiotics are called ionophores because they form complexes with some ions and facilitate their transport across cell membranes. Such compounds are also used as cattle feed additives to increase feed efficiency and body weight gain. Nigericin and nanchangmycin are other examples of polyethers biosynthesised through the polyketide pathway.

Tetracyclines (see Figure 13.32) are broad-spectrum antibiotics of polyketide origin. They are effective against both Gram-positive and Gram-negative bacteria and also against chlamydiae, mycoplasmas, and even protozoan parasites. The original tetracycline drugs isolated

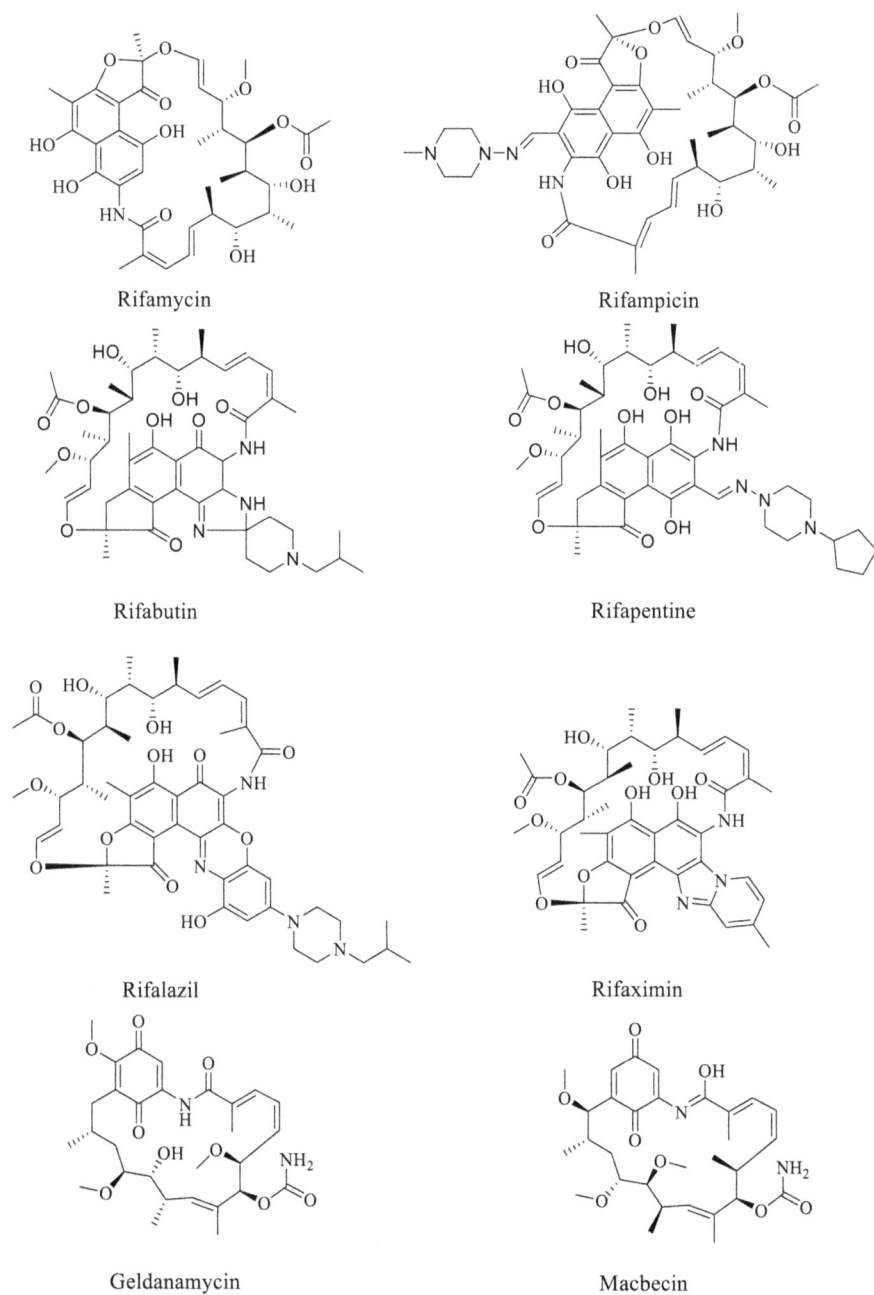

Rifamycin

Rifampicin

Rifabutin

Rifapentine

Rifalazil

Rifaximin

Geldanamycin

Macbecin

Figure 13.29 Structures of ansamycins.

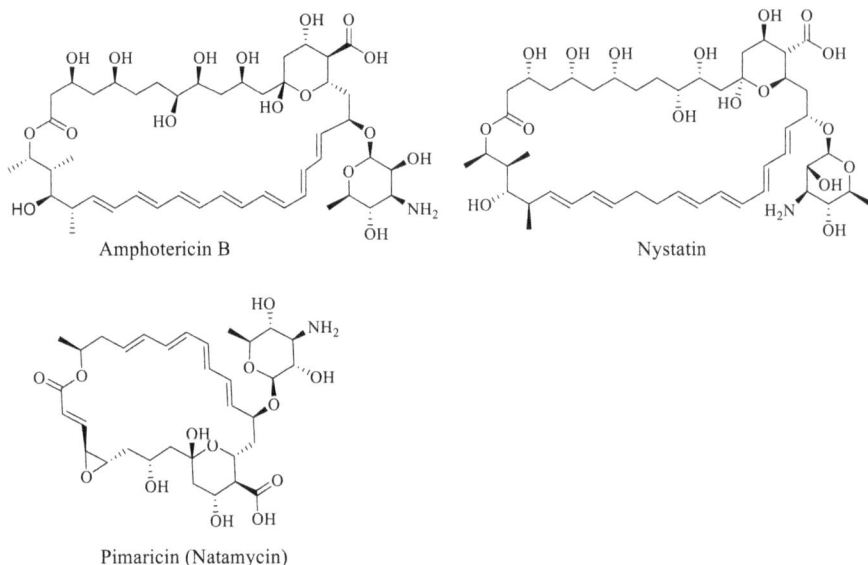

Amphotericin B

Nystatin

Pimaricin (Natamycin)

Figure 13.30 Structures of some polyenes.

from *Streptomyces* species were chlortetracycline, oxytetracycline, and tetracycline. We further have the semi-synthetic derivatives of tetracyclines, which include doxytetracycline (doxycycline), minocycline, tigecycline, omadacycline, and sarecycline. An important member of tetracyclines produced by *Streptomyces* is doxorubicin, which has been effectively used clinically to treat cancers, including breast cancer, solid tumours in children, lymphomas, and sarcomas of other types.

Organic compounds belonging to the polyketide pathway in plants are best represented by anthraquinones (Figure 13.33), which also occur in fungi and lichens. Their structures are composed of three benzene rings and a diketone moiety (quinone) called the 9,10-anthracenedione skeleton. The derivatives of anthraquinones with one less ketone functional group (anthrones) and their dimeric structures are also common in plants. Plants known for their anthraquinone composition such as *Aloe* species, rhubarb, *Rhamnus*, and *Senna* (*Cassia*) species have characteristic laxative properties. The anthraquinones in these plants mostly occur as glycosides and include physcion, chrysophanol, aloe emodin, rhein, and sennosides (Figure 13.33). As drug molecules, the *Senna* leaves and pods, sold as a laxative as Senokot, have principal active components called sennoside A and B. These compounds are dianthrone glycosides.

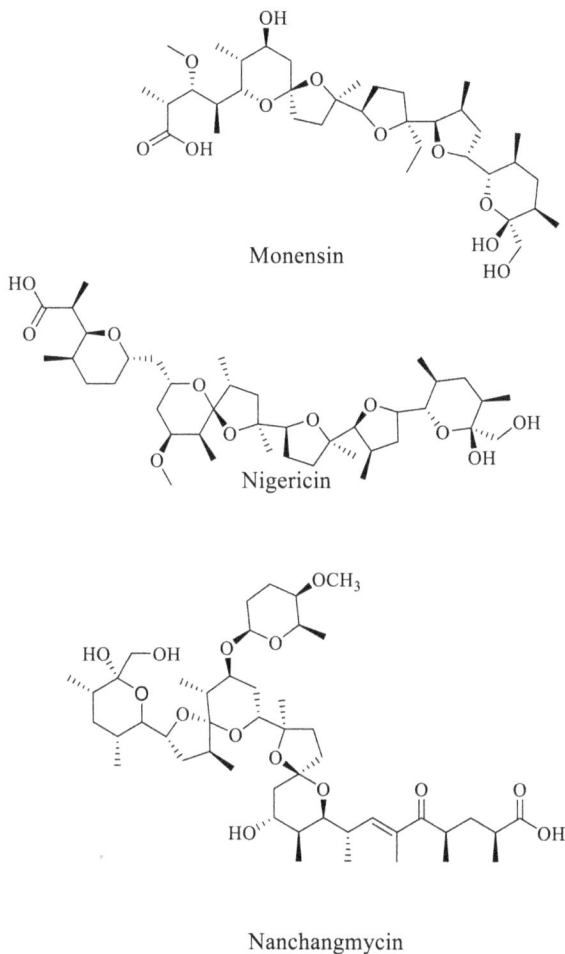

Monensin

Nigericin

Nanchangmycin

Figure 13.31 Structures of some antibiotics of the polyether class.

In *Aloe vera*, several anthraquinones occur, while the glycosides include aloin (Figure 13.33).

The dimeric anthraquinone derivative hypericin (Figure 13.34) from the medicinal plant St. Johns' wort (*Hypericum perforatum* L, Hypericaceae) has pharmacological effects, including antidepressant activity. Hypericin is also a photosensitiser and can be activated by light or UV irradiation in phototherapy. Skin phototoxicity is also common in these kinds of compounds, including fagopyrins (Figure 13.34), which are found in common buckwheat leaves.

Note that fatty acids, although not very common as drug molecules, are also synthesised in Nature through the polyketide pathway.

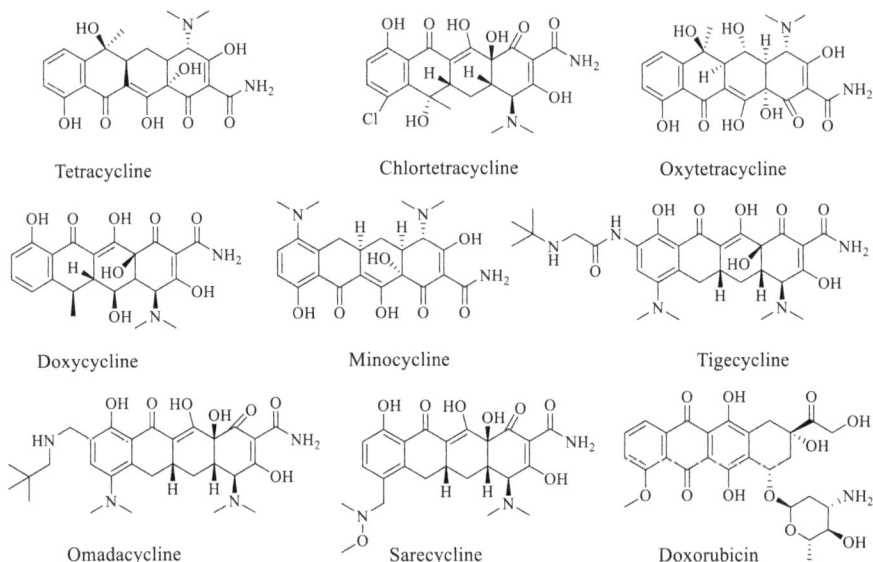

Tetracycline   Chlortetracycline   Oxytetracycline

Doxycycline   Minocycline   Tigecycline

Omadacycline   Sarecycline   Doxorubicin

Figure 13.32 Examples of natural tetracyclines and their semi-synthetic derivatives.

13.3.3 The Shikimic Acid Pathway

Many natural phenolic compounds trace their biosynthetic origin to aromatic amino acids such as phenylalanine, tyrosine, and tryptophan through an intermediate called shikimic acid. While the pathway starts from primary metabolites such as phosphoenolpyruvate and D-erythrose-4-phosphate, the aromatic amino acid precursors are also primary metabolites. Hence, strictly, the biosynthesis pathway of most of the phenolic compounds can be described as that starting from these aromatic amino acids.

13.3.3.1 Phenylpropanoids and Derivatives

One of the most diverse and abundant natural products are phenylpropanoids (with a six-carbon phenyl group joined with a three-carbon chain). They include cinnamic acid, p-coumaric acid, ferulic acid, and caffeic acid, which are also incorporated in the structures of many other natural products (Figure 13.35). For example, caffeic acid derivatives occur in Nature as caffeic acid phenethyl ester (a component of honeybee wax), rosmarinic acid (in rosemary), caffeoylquinic acid esters (*e.g.* chlorogenic acid), and salvianolic acid (a component of the Asian medicinal plant *Salvia miltiorrhiza*). These compounds display

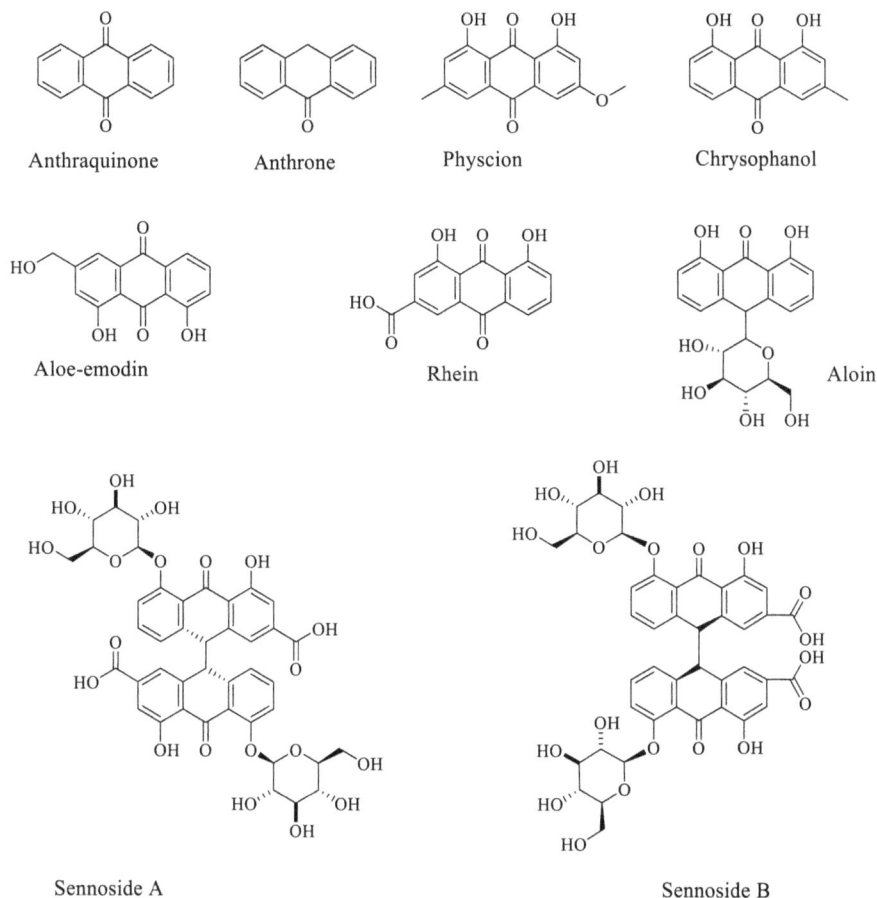

Figure 13.33 Examples of some plant anthraquinones and their derivatives.

numerous pharmacological activities including antioxidant, anti-inflammatory, and anticancer effects.

One of the by far most studied natural phenolic acids are the stilbenes (Figure 13.36), which are represented by resveratrol. They are mostly found in the Vitaceae plant family that includes the grape vine, *Vitis vinifera* L. These are compounds known for health benefits through their antioxidant, chemoprevention, and a range of other biological properties.

Coumarins are phenylpropanoid derivatives with a basic coumarin skeleton, as shown in Figure 13.37. As a class of drugs, they include classic anticoagulants such as warfarin, a synthetic drug, which is a vitamin K antagonist. Hymecromone (umbelliferone) **is choleretic whereas** armillarisin A and novobiocin (an aminocoumarin that is

St. John's wort (*Hypericum perforatum*)   Buckwheat (*Fagopyrum esculentum*)

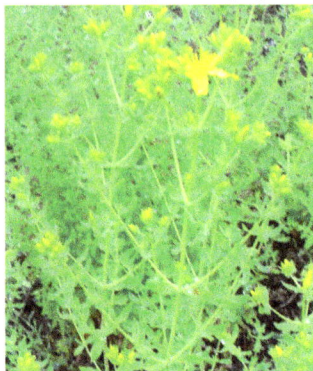

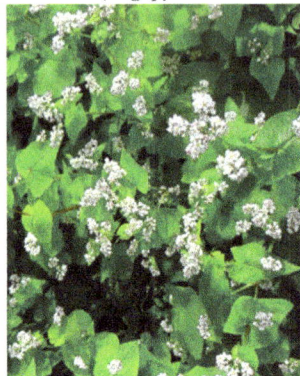

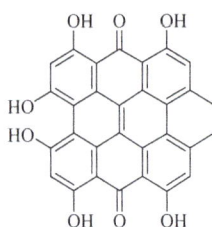

Hypericin

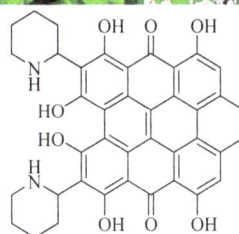

Fagopyrin

Figure 13.34 Structures of hypericin and fagopyrin. The images of the plants, which are the source of the indicated compounds, were taken in our medicinal gardens.

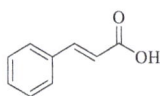

Cinnamic acid

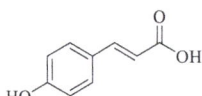

p-Coumaric acid

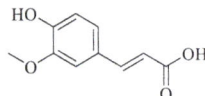

Ferulic acid

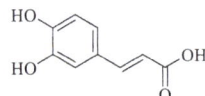

Caffeic acid

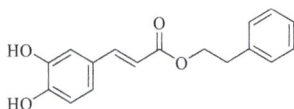

Caffeic acid phenethyl ester

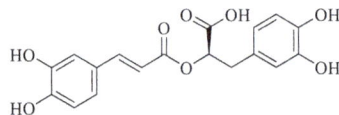

Rosmarinic acid

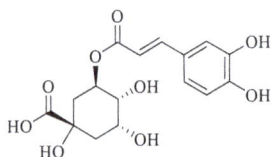

Chlorogenic acid

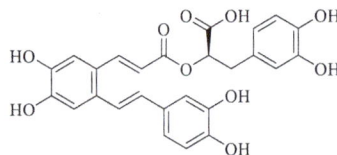

Salvaianolic acid A

Figure 13.35 Examples of phenylpropanoids and their derivatives.

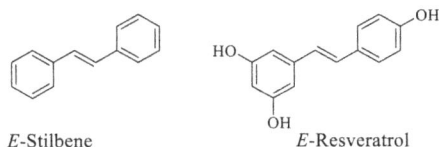

E-Stilbene   *E*-Resveratrol

Figure 13.36 Structures of stilbene and resveratrol.

produced by the actinomycete *Streptomyces niveus*) are antibiotics. Many synthetic coumarin-based drugs are also in use today to treat human diseases. For example, ensaculin is an NMDA (*N*-methyl-D-aspartate) receptor antagonist and a 5HT1A receptor agonist and is used to treat dementia. Coumarins are also known for their toxicity. In this regard, carcinogenicity and hepatotoxicity are subjects extensively studied in the field.

The linking of two phenylpropanoid units forms lignans, which are very important as medicines, classically represented by podophyllotoxin as an anticancer compound (Figure 13.38). This compound also serves as a skeleton for the synthesis of several synthetic anticancer agents (*e.g.* etoposide and teniposide) in clinical use today. Further polymerisation of phenylpropanoids could lead to structural components of plants, *i.e.* lignins, that form the rigid structure of cell walls in woody vascular plants. Many plant lignans (see Figure 13.38) found in cereals such as flaxseeds and foods (*e.g.* pinoresinol, lariciresinol, secoisolariciresinol, syringaresinol, and sesamin) are metabolised by intestinal bacteria to form mammalian lignans (*e.g.* enterodiol and enterolactone). Many of these compounds are also called phytoestrogens since they activate oestrogen receptors.

Other derivatives of phenylpropanoids include simple phenolic acid or C_6–C_1 (aromatic ring with one carbon addition mostly as carboxylic acid) compounds that are represented by gallic acid, *p*-hydroxybenzoic acid, vanillic acid, and sinapic acid (Figure 13.39). These compounds, particularly gallic acid, are also incorporated in various structures. The dimeric structure ellagic acid can polymerise to form tannins (*e.g.* tannic acid). A classic example is phenolic acids incorporated into glucose (or other sugars, see Figure 13.39) as ester derivatives to give what are called hydrolysable tannins (*e.g.* gallotannins and ellagitannins). 1,2,3,4,6-Pentagalloylglucose (a gallotannin) and punicalagin (an ellagitannin) are antioxidants and pharmacologically active compounds isolated from numerous medicinal plants.

In various chapters of this book, the structure and pharmacological effects of aspirin are highlighted. Indeed, its discovery from traditional medicinal uses of plants to chemical synthesis is a success

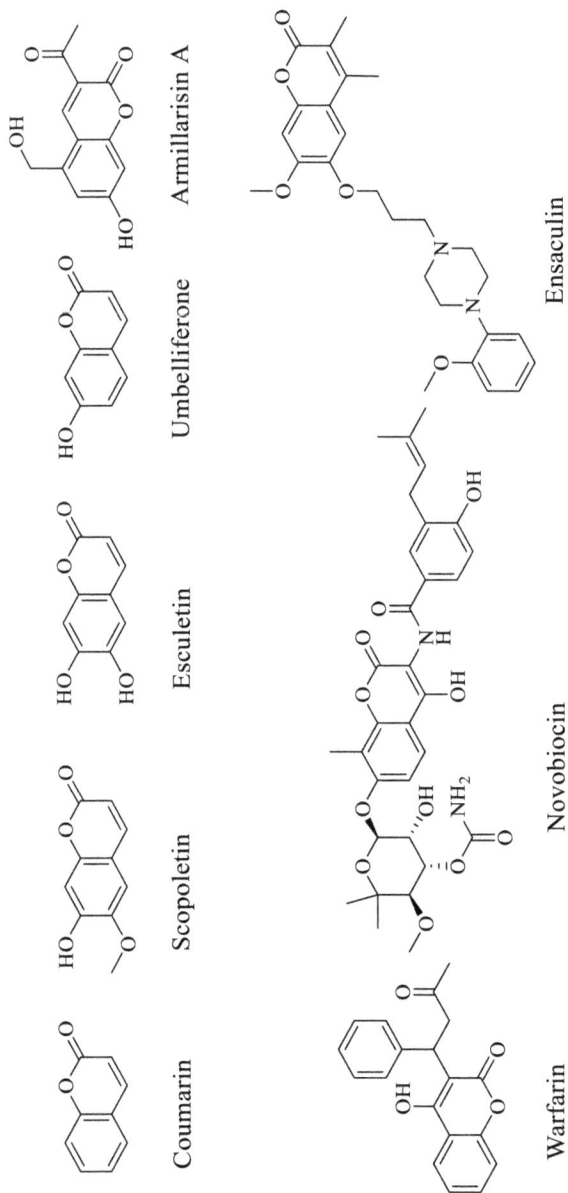

Figure 13.37 Structures of some coumarins.

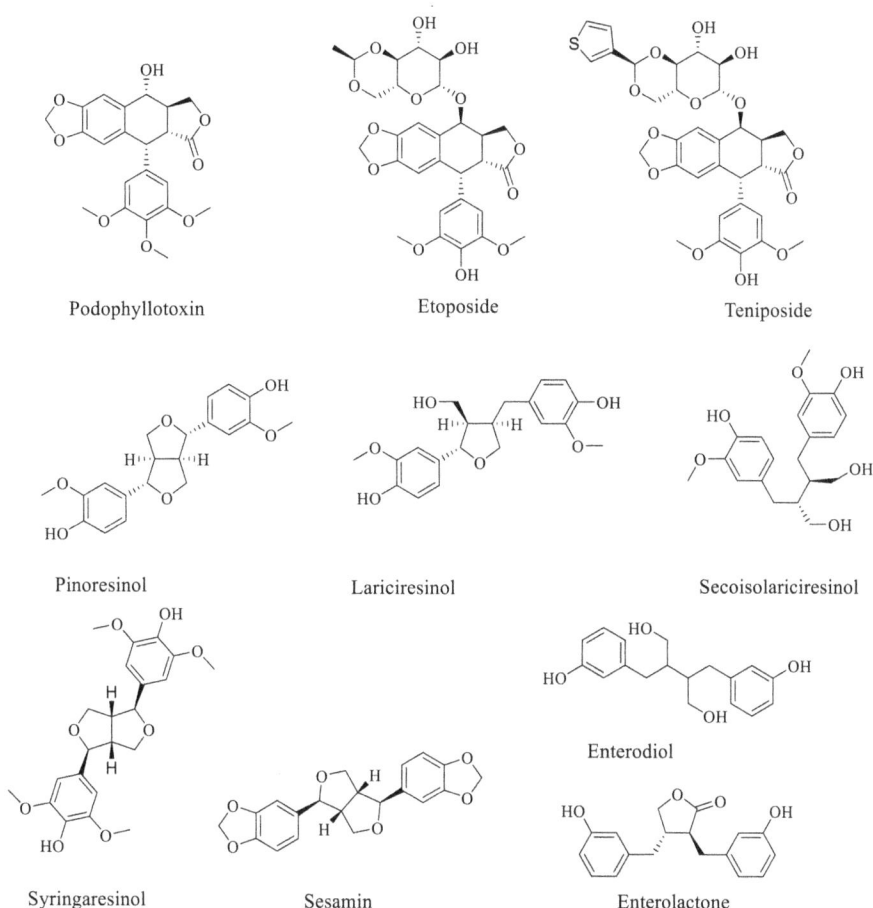

Figure 13.38 Examples of some lignans. Podophyllotoxin was originally isolated from the roots and rhizomes of medicinal plants, *Podo-
phyllum* species. It is still used today for conditions including
the treatment of genital warts. Inspired by podophyllotoxin,
etoposide and teniposide are synthetic anticancer derivatives
that are extensively used to treat cancers such as testicular,
breast, pancreatic, lung, stomach, and ovarian cancers. In our
laboratories, we have isolated from plants several derivatives
of podophyllotoxin with potent anticancer activities *in vitro*.
The structures of other lignans are also shown.

story of medicine used for over two millennia. The use of willow bark
by ancient civilisations (from the Greeks to ancient Egyptians) as far
back as 1500 BCE has been well described in the literature. It was in
1828 that a crystalline compound was extracted from the plant as a
bitter principle and named salicin (Figure 13.39). Based on the study
of the anti-inflammatory effect of this compound, further research on

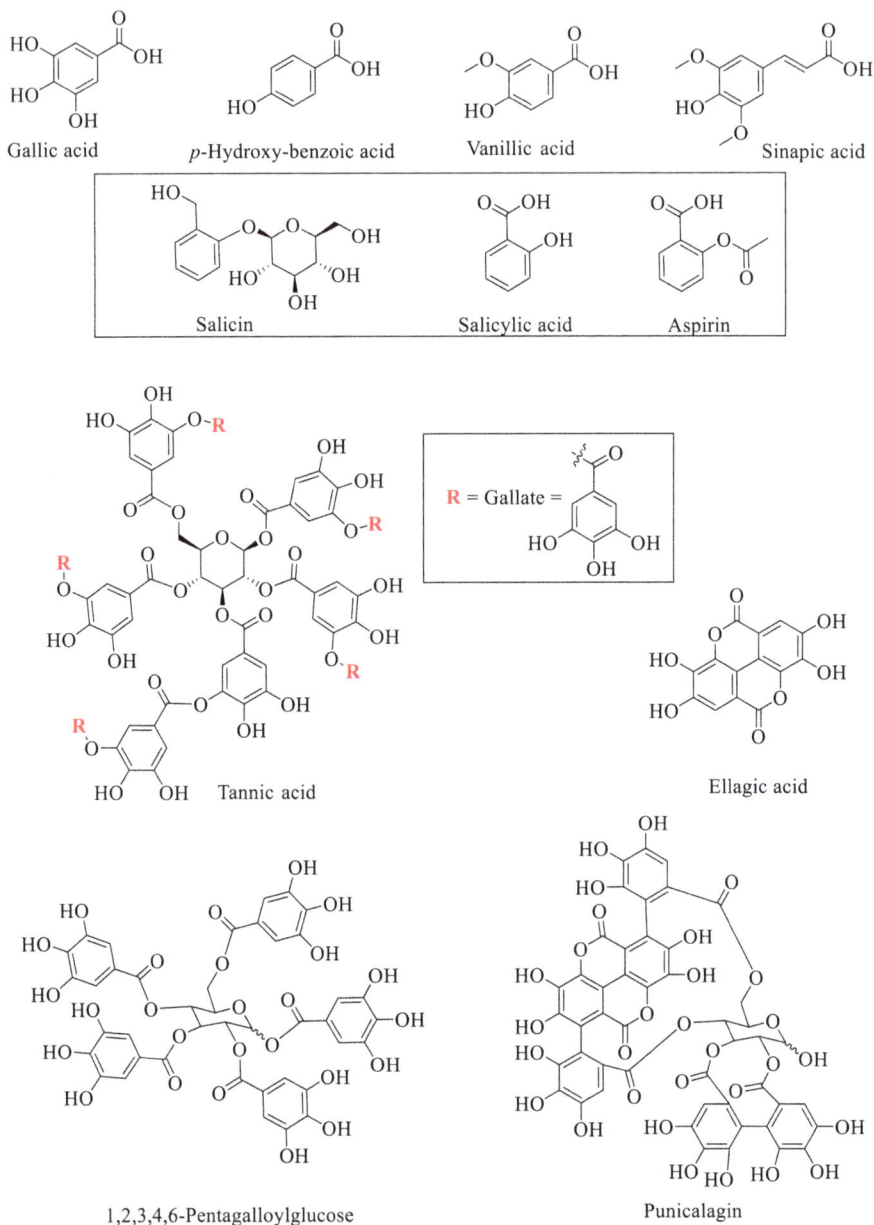

Gallic acid   *p*-Hydroxy-benzoic acid   Vanillic acid   Sinapic acid

Salicin   Salicylic acid   Aspirin

R = Gallate =

Tannic acid   Ellagic acid

1,2,3,4,6-Pentagalloylglucose   Punicalagin

Figure 13.39 Structures of some common phenolic acids and derivatives. Gallic acid and related phenolic compounds are found in many fruits and vegetables either on their own or incorporated into other structural groups. They also condense to form polymers such as tannins. Aspirin is a good example of a small-molecule drug, and its discovery was based on a study of a willow tree that led to the identification of salicin and acetylsalicylic acid.

salicylic acid, which is also a common natural product, led to the synthesis of aspirin (Figure 13.39) at Bayer in 1897. Aspirin, as a simple acetylation product of salicylic acid, has less irritant properties than salicylic acid, and is still in use today as an over-the-counter drug.

13.3.3.2 Flavonoids

Flavonoids are among the most ubiquitous natural products, with diverse pharmacological activities. Being phenolics, they also display potent antioxidant properties to which the health benefit effects of many fruits and vegetables are attributed. Biosynthetically, they are formed from a mixed pathway: shikimic acid (source of phenylpropanoids) and acetate–polyketide [source of aromatic C_6 (aromatic unit)], leading to their 15-carbon skeleton. Their basic structure with the classic three-ring system is shown in Figure 13.40.

Depending on the presence or absence of the C-4 ketone group, the double bond in the C-ring, position of attachment of the B-ring, *etc.*, flavonoids can be categorised into several sub-classes. Some good examples of these structural groups are presented in Figure 13.41. More diversity of flavonoids comes through glycosylation (addition of sugars) at various positions, either directly attached to the carbon or through an oxygen bridge and other groups. Terpenoids, phenylpropanoids, and gallate derivatives are also common structural groups added to flavonoids. That is why several thousand different flavonoid structures have been isolated from Nature.

Contributing to the diverse colouring in plants (*e.g.* flowers and fruits) and biological effects, flavonoids play a vital role in plant ecology and survival. They protect plants from ultraviolet (UV) radiation, pests, and microbial infections. They also have therapeutic implications that cannot be included here owing to their great diversity.

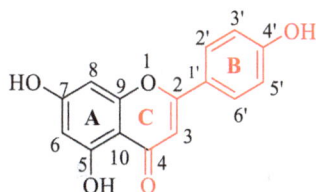

Figure 13.40 The flavonoid skeleton. Ring A originates from the acetate–polyketide pathway whereas rings B and C are phenylpropanoid skeletons originating from the shikimic acid pathway. Many structural groups based on variations of ring formation, number, and position of hydroxyl groups, sugars, and other groups added at various sites, *etc.*, are known.

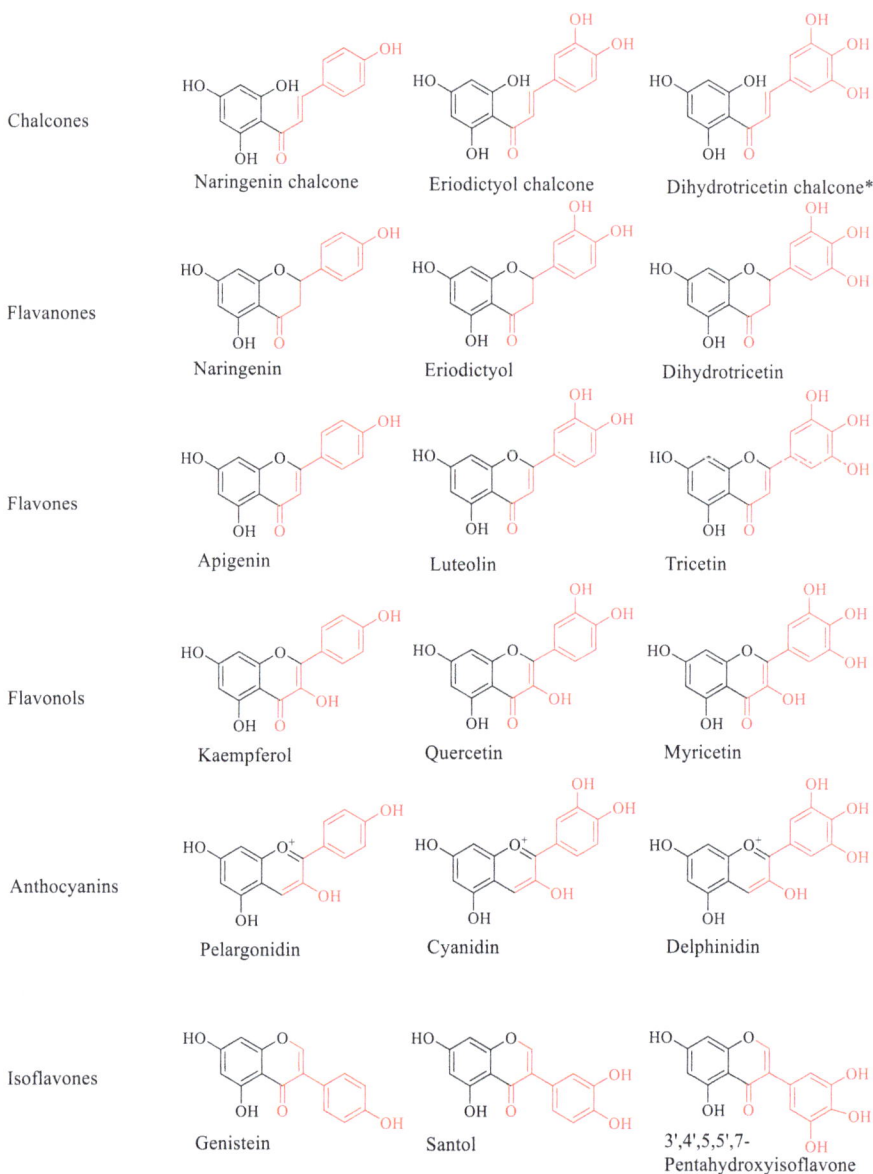

Figure 13.41   Major structural classes of flavonoids. *Known in the literature by many other names (*e.g.*, 2',3,4,4',5,6'-hexahydroxychalcone).

The potent antioxidant effect of flavonoids is mostly linked to their diverse biological effects, although they have also been shown to display specific/selective pharmacological effects. From antimicrobial effects, including antiviral properties, to complex diseases such as diabetes and neurological disorders (*e.g.* Alzheimer's disease), flavonoids are known to display pharmacological effects *in vitro*, *in vivo* (in

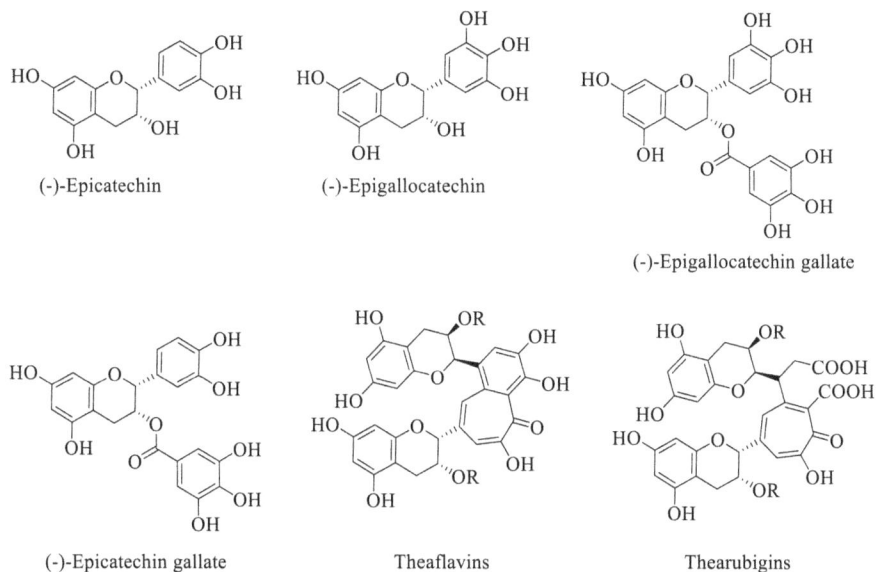

(-)-Epicatechin

(-)-Epigallocatechin

(-)-Epigallocatechin gallate

(-)-Epicatechin gallate

Theaflavins

Thearubigins

Figure 13.42 Major flavonoids of tea. Flavonoids in tea either exist as derivatives of (−)-epicatechin including (−)-epicatechin gallate, (−)-epigallocatechin, and (−)-epigallocatechin-3-gallate, or are polymerised to form complex structures such as theaflavins and thearubigins. These structures are very complex, and the indicated R groups represent either gallate or other structures.

animals), and under clinical (in humans) conditions. As dietary components, their presence in the most conspicuous fruits due to their colouration, such as blueberries, and beverages including tea contributes to the claimed health benefits. In the case of tea, the structures of the flavonoid skeleton (−)-epicatechin incorporating gallate and other derivatives are shown in Figure 13.42.

13.3.4 Alkaloids

13.3.4.1 Classification Based on Amino Acid Origin

By far the most biologically active group of organic compounds is the alkaloids, which are nitrogenous compounds. Most of the clinically useful drugs belong to this group. Biosynthetically they are formed, with a few exceptions, from amino acids. Some that can be mentioned include morphine, codeine, coniine, quinine, scopolamine, hyoscyamine, atropine, caffeine, sanguinarine, and berberine. There are also several toxins such as strychnine. One may group alkaloids based on their biosynthetic origins. For example, ornithine can give

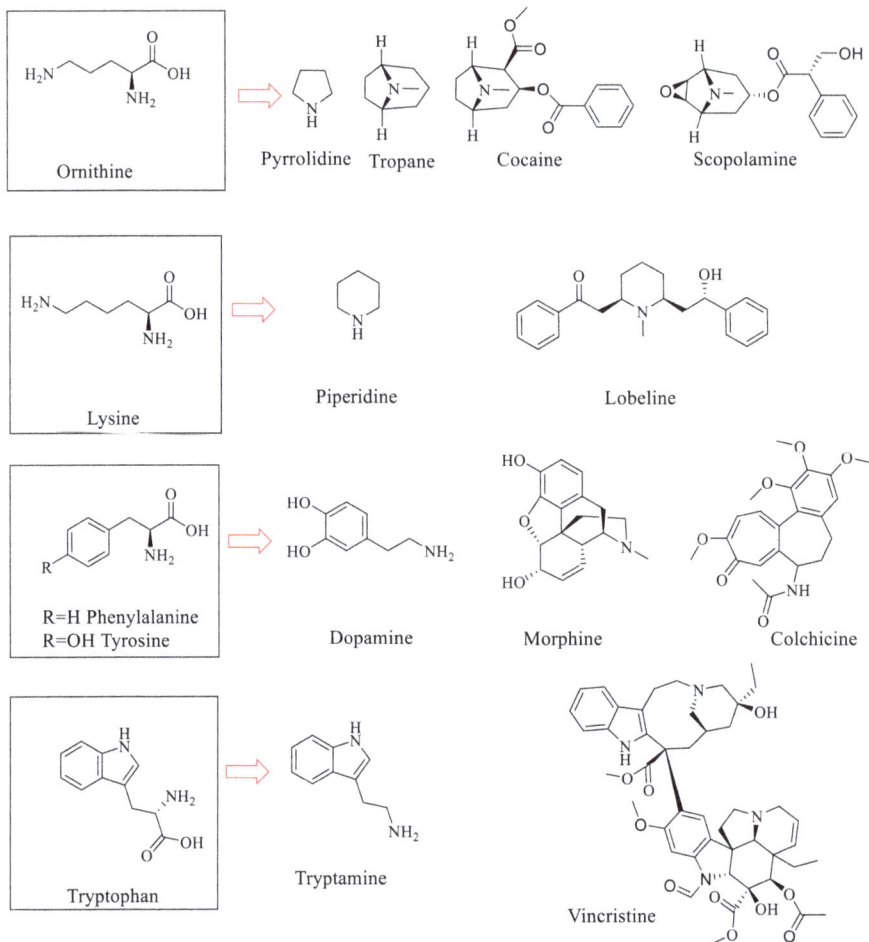

Figure 13.43 Examples of the biosynthesis of alkaloids from amino acids.

rise to a structural class called pyrrolidine, pyrrolizidine, and tropane alkaloids; lysine gives rise to piperidine, pyridine, and quinolizidine alkaloids; phenylalanine and tyrosine yield isoquinoline alkaloids; and tryptophan forms indole alkaloids. Some of these examples are shown in Figure 13.43.

13.3.4.2 Classification of Alkaloids Based on the Structural Skeleton

Instead of their amino acid origin, many alkaloids are also named based on their immediate structural precursors. For example, those originating from ornithine and based on the pyrrolidine precursor are called pyrrolidine alkaloids. Atropine, cocaine, and scopolamine are based on a tropane skeleton (8-azabicyclo[3.2.1]octane) and are therefore called tropane alkaloids. On a similar basis, we also have pyrrolidine, piperidine (*e.g.* coniine, lobeline, and cynapine), quinolizidine (*e.g.* lupinine, spareine, lupanine, matrine, and ormosanine), indolizidine (*e.g.* castanospermine), isoquinoline (*e.g.* emetine, codeine, morphine, thebaine, imerubrine, lycorine, and protopine), pyridine (nicotine, nornicotine, anabasine, and actinidine), acridine (*e.g.* acronicine), quinoline (quinine, quinidine, and cinchonine), indole (*e.g.* ajmalicine, ergotamine, strychnine, reserpine, vincamine, vinblastine, vincristine, and vindesine), imidazole (*e.g.* histamine and pilocarpine), purine (*e.g.* aminophylline, caffeine, theobromine, and theophylline), phenethylamine (*e.g.* cathinone, tyramine, ephedrine, pseudoephedrine, mescaline, catecholamine neurotransmitters such as noradrenaline, dopamine, and the hormone adrenaline), and benzylamine (*e.g.* capsaicin, dihydrocapsaicin, and nordihydrocapsaicin) alkaloids, among others (see Figure 13.44). Other structural classes such as steroids and diterpenes can also incorporate nitrogen later after their biosynthesis to become steroidal (*e.g.* solanidine) and

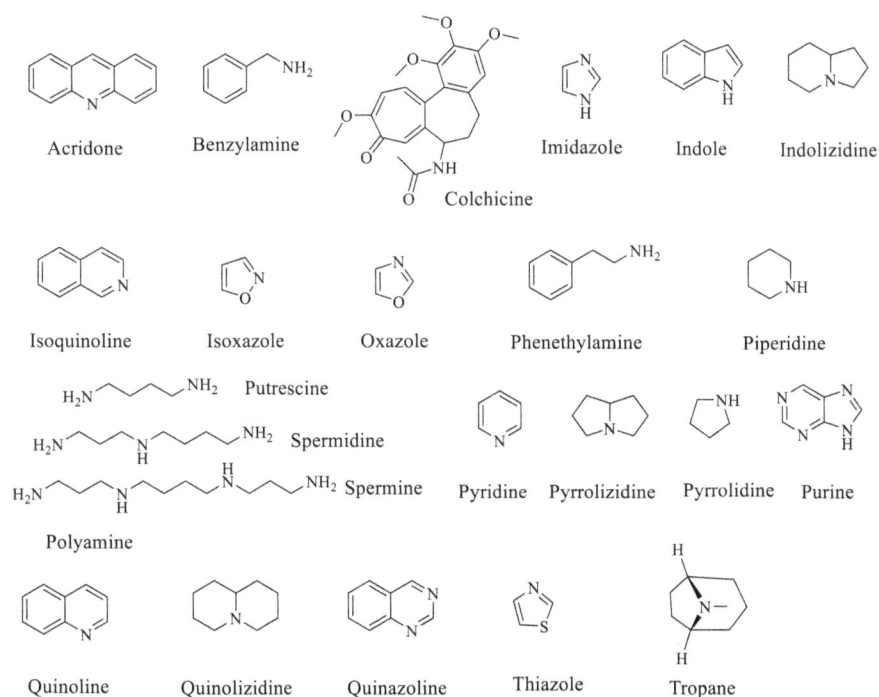

Figure 13.44 Classification of alkaloids based on their structural skeleton.

diterpenoid (*e.g.* aconitine and delphinine) alkaloids, respectively. Alkaloids may also occur in acyclic structures such as putrescine, spermidine, and spermine (Figure 13.44), all of which are derived from ornithine and are present in the human body in good concentrations. Pyrrolizidine alkaloids (*e.g.* senecionine, heliotrine, and clivorine) are known for their toxicity, and contamination of food and medicine with these compounds needs to be monitored.

13.3.4.3 Some Examples of Natural Alkaloids and Their Derivatives as Drugs

13.3.4.3.1 Coffee and Tea – Caffeine; and Tobacco – Nicotine

Caffeine (improves concentration and stimulates memory) and nicotine (improves memory and concentration) are good examples of alkaloids in legal use today as stimulants (see Figure 13.45). Coffee and tea are by far the most consumed beverages in the world and their stimulant effect is due to caffeine, which has numerous pharmacological effects but primarily acts as a CNS stimulant. Among the well-established mechanisms involving caffeine is the blocking of adenosine receptors that are known to slow CNS activity, *i.e.* caffeine reverses the drowsiness or sleepy feeling activity induced by adenosine in the brain. As an alkaloid, caffeine is often called a *pseudoalkaloid* because it does not originate from an amino acid. Instead, it originates from the purine base as with other alkaloids such as theobromine and theophylline (Figure 13.45), which have diverse pharmacological effects such as bronchodilation, vasodilation, and muscle relaxation. In addition to coffee and tea, caffeine, theobromine, and theophylline are also found in several other beverages such as cocoa and cola drinks.

Nicotine is largely consumed as cigarettes and cigars and is a stimulant, inducing a pharmacological effect by stimulating nicotinic acetylcholine receptors. As the name implies, the receptors are named as such because of the specific activity of nicotine to these receptors located at the neuronal junction between two neurons (ganglion) and the neuromuscular junction of the skeletal muscles. Nicotine is highly addictive and is used clinically for treating cigarette smokers to relieve nicotine dependence.

The nicotine molecule has one chiral centre and hence exists in *R* and *S* enantiomeric forms (Figure 13.46). However, only the (*S*)-(−)-nicotine enantiomer occurs naturally in tobacco, although the smoking condition appears to convert some of the natural (*S*)-(−)-nicotine into (*R*)-(+)-nicotine. Highlighting the significance of chirality in biological activity once again, the *S* isomer of nicotine is significantly more potent than the *R* isomer.

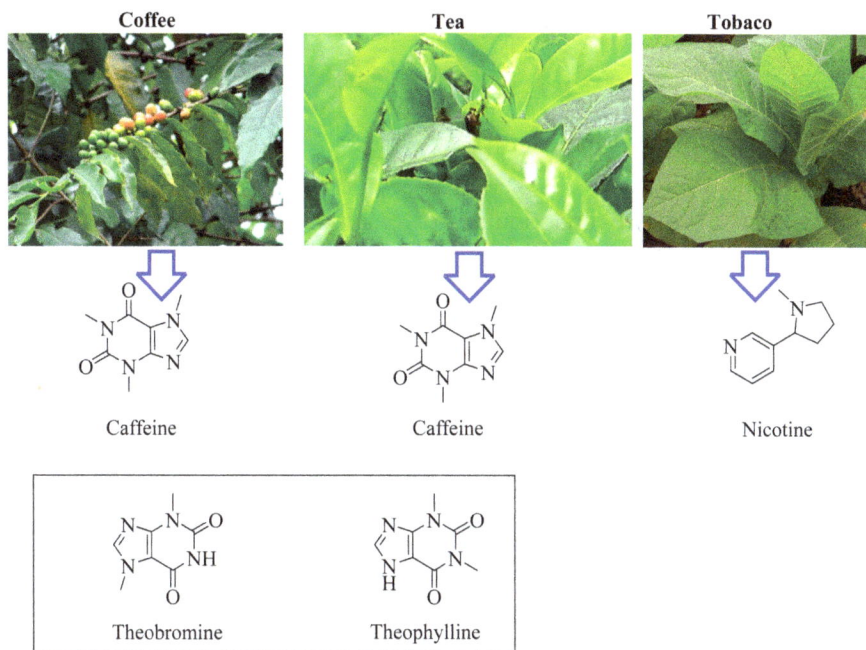

Figure 13.45 Structures of caffeine and nicotine. Also present in coffee and tea are theobromine and theophylline, which are also pseudoalkaloids. Coffee plant image: Reproduced from https://en.wikipedia.org/wiki/Coffea_arabica#/media/File:Starr_070308-5472_Coffea_arabica.jpg, under the terms of the CC BY 3.0 license, https://creativecommons.org/licenses/by/3.0/deed.en. Image Credit: Forest & Kim Starr. Tea plant image: Reproduced from https://mrj.wikipedia.org/wiki/%D0%A4%D0%B0%D0%B9%D0%B-B:%C3%87ay-1.jpg, image in the public domain. Tobacco plant image: Reproduced from https://commons.wikimedia.org/wiki/File:Patch_of_Tobacco_(Nicotiana_tabacum_)_in_a_field_in_Intercourse,_Pennsylvania.jpg, under the terms of the CC BY-SA 4.0 license, https://creativecommons.org/licenses/by-sa/4.0/deed.en. Image Credit: ©2006 Derek Ramsey (Ram-Man).

13.3.4.3.2 Chondrodendron tomentosum – Curare – Arrow Poison

(+)-Tubocurarine (D-tubocurarine), (−)-curine [(−)-bebeerine], and (+)-isochondrodendrine [(+)-isobebeerine] (Figure 13.47) are components of the curare poison, which has been used by indigenous people in Central and South America as an arrow poison. Represented by (+)-tubocurarine as the main component of curare, these are compounds that cause muscle paralysis by blocking the nicotinic acetylcholine receptors located at the neuromuscular junction of skeletal muscles. From simple observation to laboratory experiments, these alkaloids have transformed our knowledge and therapeutics in the field of muscle relaxants.

R-(+)-Nicotine   S-(-)-Nicotine

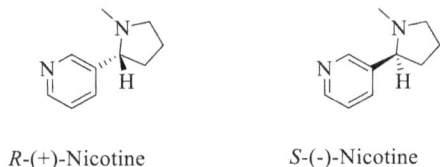

Figure 13.46 The two enantiomers of nicotine. The tobacco plant contains the S-(–)-nicotine form but some degree of change to R-(+)-nicotine occurs during smoking.

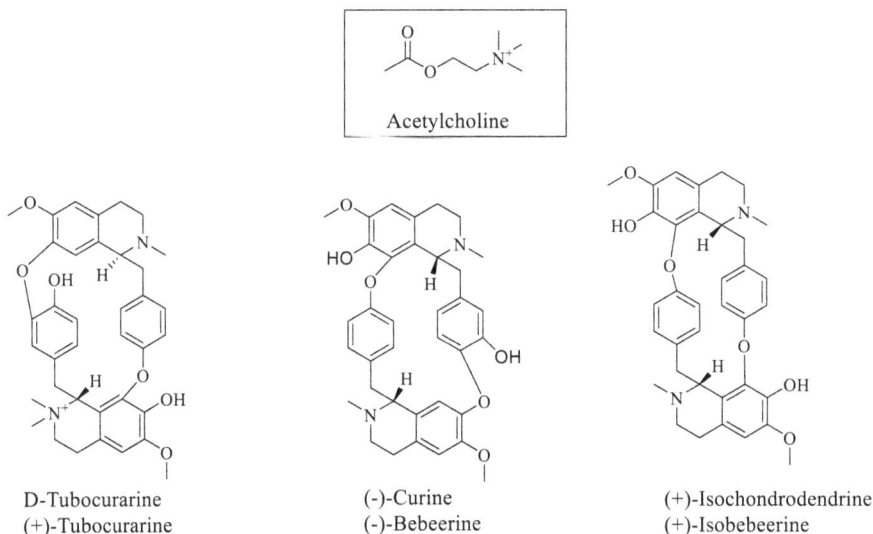

Acetylcholine

| D-Tubocurarine | (-)-Curine | (+)-Isochondrodendrine |
| (+)-Tubocurarine | (-)-Bebeerine | (+)-Isobebeerine |

Figure 13.47 Alkaloidal components of curare. These are compounds that bind to acetylcholine receptors and inhibit neurotransmission in skeletal muscles, resulting in muscle paralysis. The poison dart or arrow coated with curare allows these compounds to enter the bloodstream of hunted animals, leading to muscle paralysis. Because these compounds are charged, they are not absorbed from the gut, *i.e.* eating the poisoned animal does not harm the hunters.

Based on studies of the chemistry and pharmacology of (+)-tubocurarine, several synthetic muscle relaxants in clinical use today have been developed. Some examples of (+)-tubocurarine-inspired drugs include decamethonium, suxamethonium, atracurium, cisatracurium, rocuronium, pancuronium, vecuronium, and mivacurium (Figure 13.48).

These muscle relaxant compounds, being positively charged, are prepared in a salt form (*e.g.* atracurium or cisatracurium besylate, rocuronium or vecuronium bromide, pancuronium dibromide, suxamethonium chloride, decamethonium bromide, *etc.*). The compounds are synthesised based on the distance between the two nitrogen

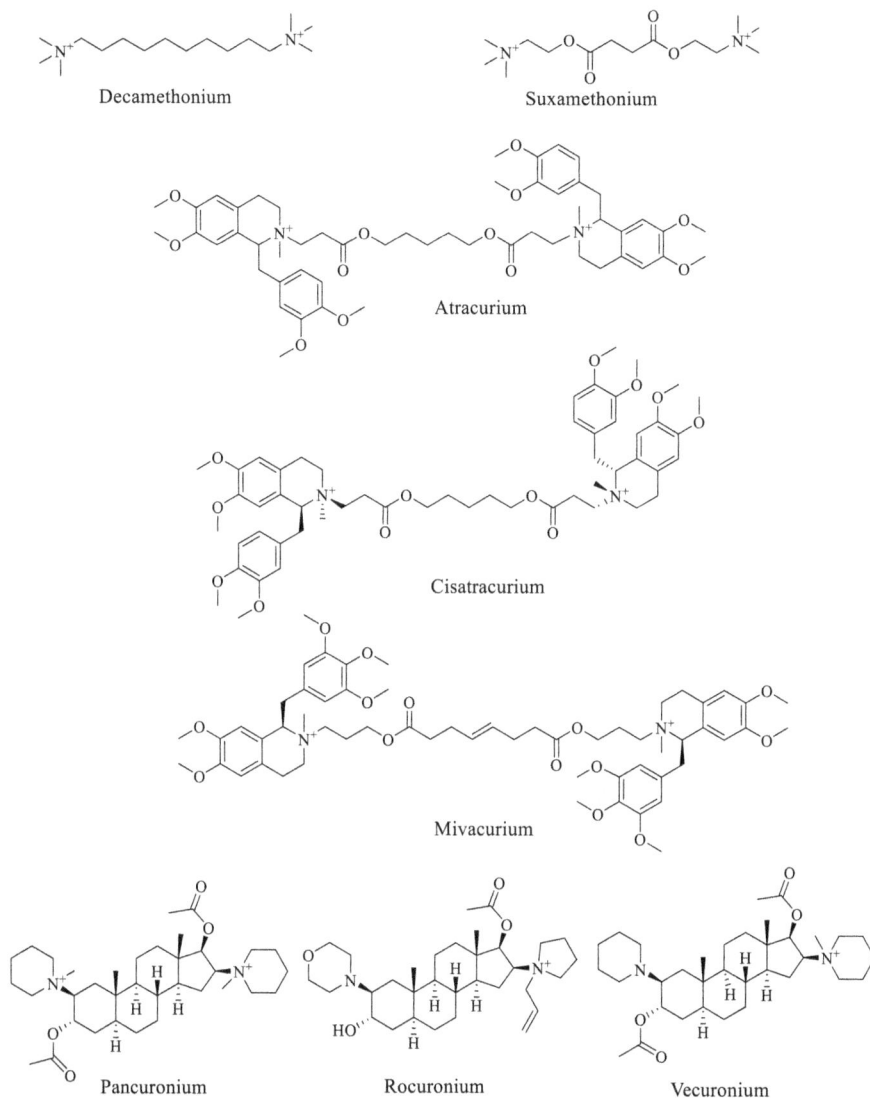

Figure 13.48 Structures of clinically useful muscle relaxants obtained by (+)-tubocurarine-inspired synthesis. Natural product-inspired drug discovery starts by observing the structure of the active compounds. In (+)-tubocurarine, the two nitrogen atoms, which are charged, are separated from each other by a distance of about 10 carbon bonds. Decamethonium and suxamethonium are results of this observation whereas others are based on the same principle but are derived from other skeletons such as steroidal skeletons (pancuronium, rocuronium, and vecuronium).

atoms in the tubocurarine skeleton, which play a role in binding to acetylcholine receptors (nicotinic acetylcholine receptors) at the neuromuscular junction of skeletal muscles.

13.3.4.3.3 *Papaver somniferum* – Opium Poppy

Alkaloids are the main components responsible for the biological activity of opium. Morphine is the major alkaloidal component, which is still in clinical use today as an analgesic, and others include the antitussive (cough relief) and analgesic drug codeine, the morphine antagonist thebaine, and papaverine (Figure 13.49), which is a vasodilator used to treat gastrointestinal disorders. Morphine, as an agonist, acts by binding to its opioid receptors (called MOP) subtypes. These receptors are classified as the mu (μ), delta (δ), and kappa (κ) opioids, representing MOP, DOP, and KOP, respectively. Morphine mainly targets the MOP subtypes and has little effect on other opioid receptor types (DOP and KOP).

In the analgesia field, semi-synthetic opioid agonists of morphine derivatives are used clinically and include hydrocodone (Vincodin) and oxycodone (OxyContin) (Figure 13.50). These drugs have a prolonged effect in the treatment of pain but are highly addictive. Morphine-inspired synthesis (synthetic opioids) also led to clinically useful drugs in analgesia and pain relief. They include dextropropoxyphene, tramadol, meperidine (Demerol), and methadone (Figure 13.50). In addition to being a MOP receptor agonist, methadone possesses other pharmacological effects (*e.g.* as an *N*-methyl-D-aspartate receptor antagonist) and its analgesic effect lacks the side effect of morphine of inducing euphoria.

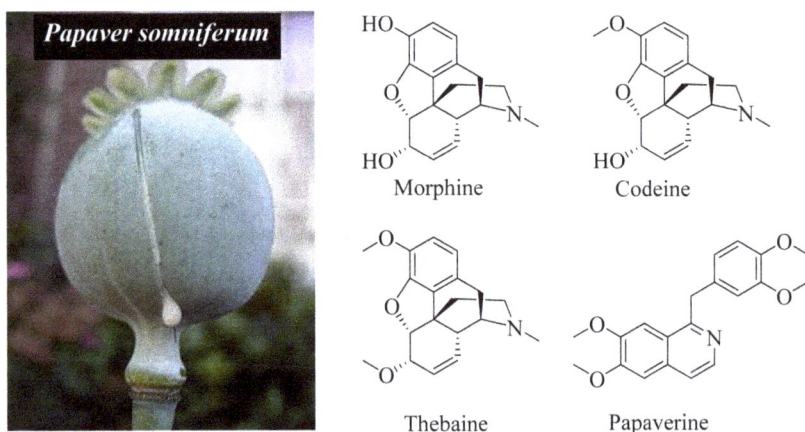

Figure 13.49 Structures of opium alkaloids. Beyond being a garden or ornamental plant, the opium poppy (*Papaver somniferum*) has thousands of years of history as a medicine. The principal components shown are still in clinical use today. Poppy image: Image Credit KGM007, image in the public domain.

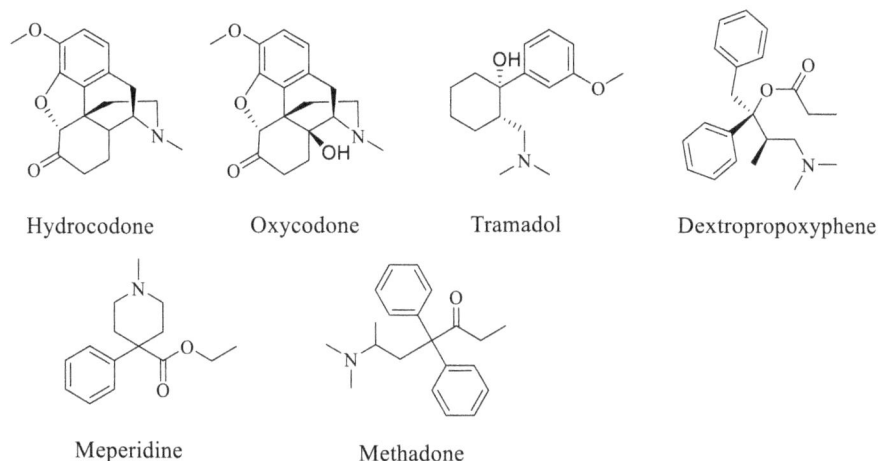

| Hydrocodone | Oxycodone | Tramadol | Dextropropoxyphene |

| Meperidine | Methadone |

Figure 13.50 Examples of semi-synthetic derivatives of morphine and morphine-inspired synthetic analogues. Dextropropoxyphene, tramadol, meperidine, and methadone are synthetic opioids, and hydrocodone and oxycodone are semi-synthetic derivatives of morphine.

Opium – Key Facts

- Opium – among the oldest recorded medical prescriptions – before 2000 BCE.
- Opium contains around 24 alkaloids, including morphine, codeine, and papaverine.
- Morphine was first extracted from opium in a pure form in the early nineteenth century.
- Codeine was first isolated in 1830 and has been used mainly as a cough remedy.
- Opium still serves as a raw material to produce numerous drugs:

  o Legal drugs such as morphine, codeine, hydromorphone, oxycodone, and hydrocodone.
  o Illegal drugs such as heroin.

- Heroin, as the first semi-synthetic opioid, was synthesised in 1874 – apparently to resolve the addiction issue of morphine.
- From 1898 to 1910, heroin was marketed with a claim of being a non-addictive morphine substitute and cough medicine for children.
- Commercially produced in the mid-nineteenth century, morphine has been used as an alternative to opium and to tackle opium addiction.

13.3.4.3.4 *Catharanthus roseus – Vinca Alkaloids*

Other classic examples of drugs obtained from natural sources are represented by vinblastine and vincristine, which are alkaloids isolated from *Catharanthus roseus* (Figure 13.51). They are anticancer agents with clinical application in the treatment of leukaemia, Hodgkin's lymphoma, lung cancer, and breast cancer. Since their

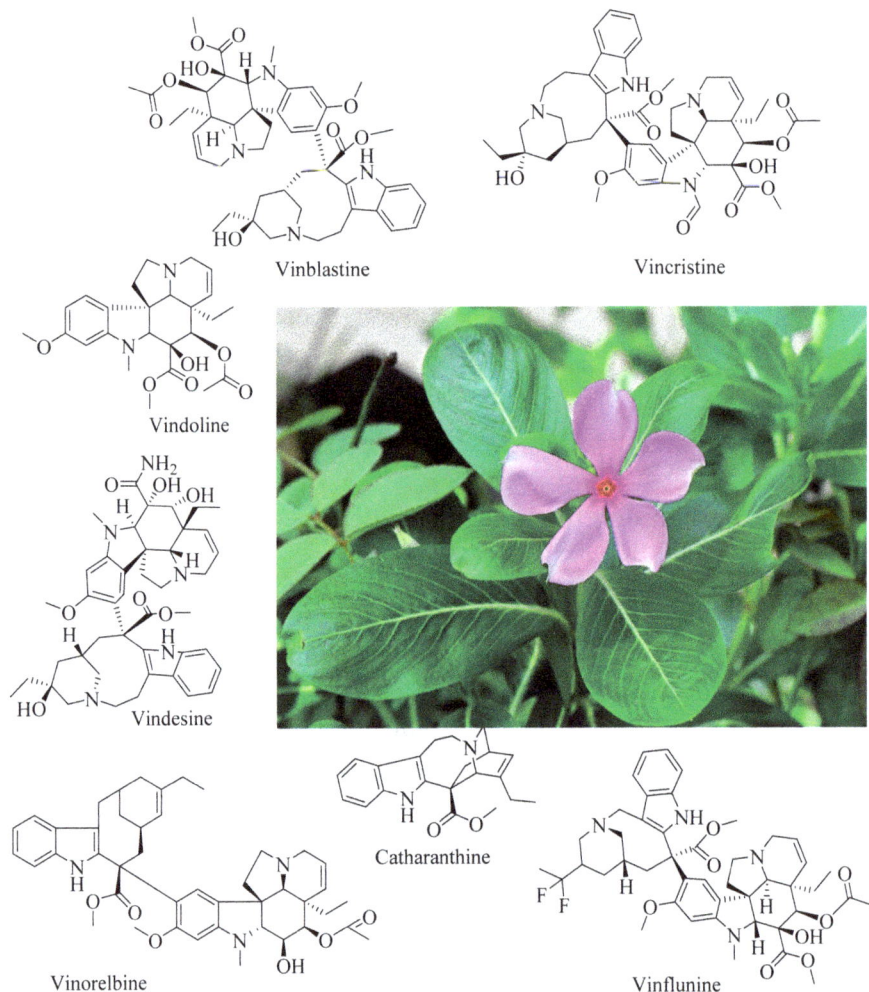

Figure 13.51 Structures of *Vinca* alkaloids and semi-synthetic derivatives. Image of *Catharanthus roseus*: Reproduced from https://commons.wikimedia.org/wiki/File:Catharanthus_roseus24_08_2012_(1).JPG, under the terms of the CC BY-SA 3.0 license, https://creativecommons.org/licenses/by-sa/3.0/deed.en. Image Credit: Joydeep.

approval in the early 1960s, research on these compounds has intensified, especially given their extremely low yield from natural sources and as an attempt to make semi-synthetic derivatives. The study of the relatively better yield of vinblastine led to the clinically useful anticancer semi-synthetic derivative vindesine, which is effective in treating melanoma and acute lymphoblastic leukaemia. Alkaloids with lower efficacy but abundantly found in plants (*e.g.* catharanthine and vindoline) have also been used to synthesise anticancer agents. Vinorelbine and vinflunine (Figure 13.51) are good examples of such research exercises.

13.3.4.3.5 *Erythroxylum coca*: Natural Tropane Alkaloids and Synthetic Analogues

Representing the tropane class of alkaloids, *cocaine* isolated from *Erythroxylum coca* has numerous pharmacological properties. Despite its narcotic and euphoriant effects, cocaine has clinical uses, including in topical and local anaesthesia. Interestingly, cocaine-inspired synthesis led to the identification of procaine as a common local anaesthetic without a narcotic side effect. Cocaine also contributed to the development of some clinically useful semi-synthetic derivatives. These include (see Figure 13.52) N-butylscopolamine, which is an antimuscarinic anticholinergic agent used against intestinal spasms, ipratropium as an anticholinergic used to dilate airways in the lung to treat bronchitis and asthma, tiotropium bromide as a long-acting bronchodilator used to treat chronic obstructive pulmonary disease and asthma, and homatropine as a muscarinic acetylcholine receptor antagonist (anticholinergic) used in heart and eye disorders (used in eye drops to treat cycloplegia, which is paralysis of the ciliary muscle of the eye, and as a mydriatic).

13.3.4.3.6 Other Examples of Tropane Alkaloids

A further example of tropane alkaloids (see Figure 13.53) of natural origin is atropine, which is a classic acetylcholine antagonist acting at muscarinic receptors. It reverses the effects of nerve agents and pesticide poisonings. By reversing the effect of acetylcholine or parasympathetic nervous system activation, atropine has application in surgery to decrease saliva production. Commonly known as belladonna or deadly nightshade, the source plant of atropine is *Atropa belladonna*, which has a long history of medicinal and poisonous properties. This plant is a member of the Solanaceae family, which is known for alkaloidal constituents. Another compound that

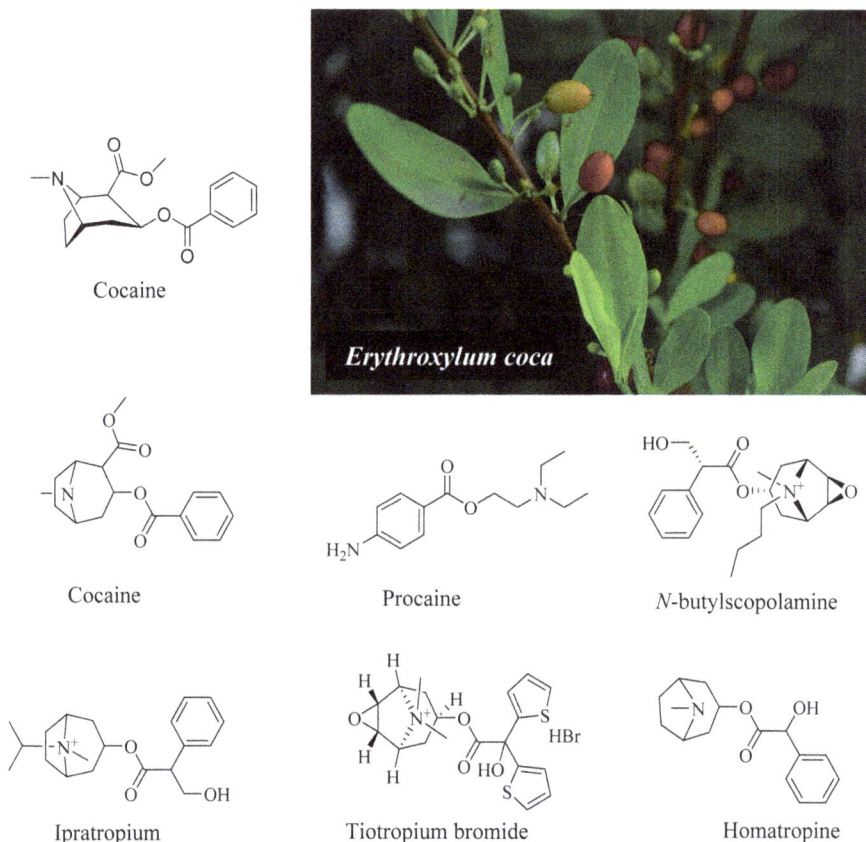

Figure 13.52 Structures of cocaine and its synthetic and semi-synthetic derivatives. Note the two forms of structural presentation of cocaine for the bicyclic tropane *ring* skeleton. *Erythroxylum coca* or coca is the common source of cocaine as a drug of abuse in the street. Coca plant image: Reproduced from https://commons.wikimedia.org/wiki/File:Coca_(Erythroxylum_coca)_en_Meta_(Colombia)_1.jpg, under the terms of the CC BY 4.0 license, https://creativecommons.org/licenses/by/4.0/deed.en. Image Credit: Danna Guevara.

can be isolated from this plant is scopolamine (hyoscine), which is also found in other members of the Solanaceae family such as *Hyoscyamus niger*. Scopolamine, as a muscarinic receptor antagonist, is used to control motion sickness or prevent nausea and vomiting induced by motion. Several species of *Datura* (*e.g. D. stramonium*) also contain tropane alkaloids, including atropine, hyoscyamine, and scopolamine.

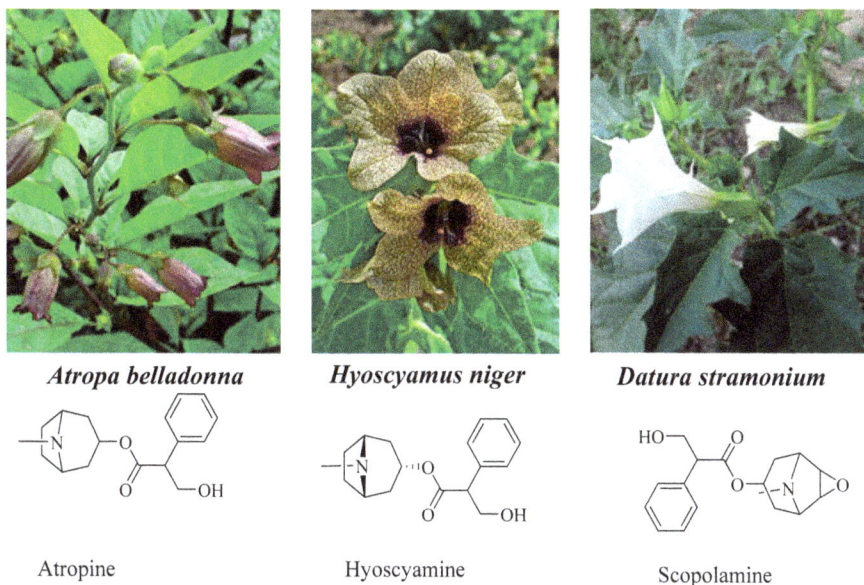

Atropa belladonna   **Hyoscyamus niger**   **Datura stramonium**

Atropine   Hyoscyamine   Scopolamine

Figure 13.53 Structures of tropane alkaloids: atropine, hyoscyamine, and scopolamine. Note that atropine is a mixture of stereoisomers, one of which is hyoscyamine as the (*R*)-(+)-*hyoscyamine* isomer, which about twice as *potent* as atropine (racemic mixture). *Atropa belladonna*: Reproduced from https://commons.wikimedia.org/wiki/File:Atropa_belladonna_001.JPG, under the terms of the CC BY-SA 3.0 license, https://creativecommons.org/licenses/by-sa/3.0/deed.en. Image Credit: H. Zell. *Hyoscyamus niger*: Reproduced from https://commons.wiki-media.org/wiki/File:Hyoscyamus_niger_0002.JPG, under the terms of the CC BY-SA 3.0 license, https://creativecommons.org/licenses/by-sa/3.0/deed.en. Image Credit: H. Zell. *Datura stramonium*: Reproduced from https://commons.wikimedia.org/wiki/File:DATURA_STRAMONIUM_-_GUIXERS_-_IB-615.JPG, under the terms of the CC BY-SA 3.0 license, https://creativecommons.org/licenses/by-sa/3.0/deed.en. Image Credit: Isidre Blanc.

13.3.4.3.7 *Cinchona* Species (Cinchona Bark) – The Discovery of Chloroquine and Hydroxychloroquine

The principal components of *Cinchona* alkaloids include cinchonine, cinchonidine, quinine, quinidine, and two stereoisomers, dihydro-quinine and dihydroquinidine (Figure 13.54). The isolation of quinine led to the discovery of the synthetic compound chloroquine as one of the most successful therapeutic agents for human diseases. Two common sources in the production of quinine are *Cinchona pubescens* [also known as Red Cinchona and Quina (Quechua)] and *Cinchona officinalis.*

Cinchona Bark and Quinine – Key Facts

- The potential of cinchona bark for the treatment of malaria was identified in the early 1630s – it used to be known as 'Jesuits' 'bark', 'cardinal's bark', or 'sacred bark'.
- Quinine was extracted from the bark, and isolated in 1820 to replace the bark as a treatment for malaria.
- Other alkaloids of the bark such as quinidine, cinchonine, and cinchonidine are also effective against malaria.
- Quinine was preferred because it was found to be abundant in Javan cinchona bark as compared with the original South American source.
- Quinine was used until the 1940s, when it was replaced with chloroquine.
- Hydroxychloroquine is a less toxic analogue of chloroquine and has been extensively used in malaria treatment.
- Chloroquine and hydroxychloroquine were thought to have efficacy against the virus (SARS-CoV-2) that causes COVID-19, although clinical trials did not prove this claim.
- Purified quinine and/or cinchona bark is still used to flavour tonic water, many bitter lemon cocktails, and other beverages.

13.3.4.3.8 Poison Hemlock (*Conium maculatum*) – Piperidine Alkaloids

Native to Europe, poison hemlock of the family Umbelliferae has been known as a poisonous or toxic plant due to its piperidine alkaloids. The alkaloids are represented by coniine and γ-coniceine, the latter being more toxic. The list of alkaloids in the flowers and fruits of this plant is long, however, and includes coniine, N-methylconiine, conhydrine, pseudoconhydrine, and γ-coniceine (Figure 13.55). Neurotoxicity (neuromuscular blockade, especially in skeletal muscles such as respiratory muscles) is the main pharmacological effect of these alkaloids, although some are teratogenic. According to legend, hemlock was used to kill condemned prisoners in ancient Greece and the death of Socrates (Figure 13.55) was known to be attributed to drinking a potion of this plant.

13.3.4.3.9 Ergot Alkaloids – Indole Alkaloids

The disease called ergotism is caused by the parasitic ergot fungus *Claviceps purpurea*, which infects rye and other grains. Eating contaminated grains causes the classic symptoms of ergotism such as

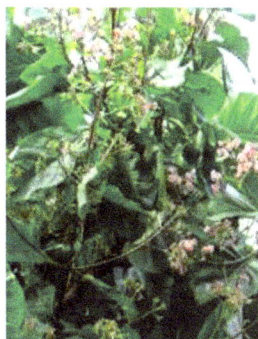 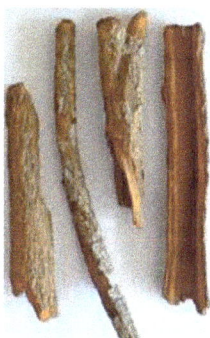 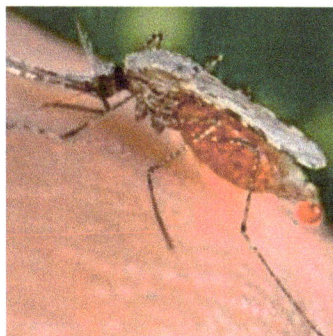

Cinchona pubescens   **Cinchona bark**   *Anopheles mosquito* **feeding**

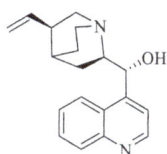 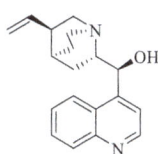 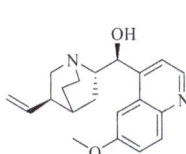 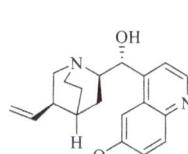

Cinchonine   Cinchonidine   Quinine   Quinidine

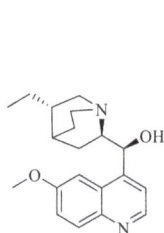 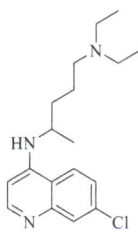 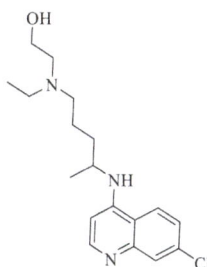

Dihydroquinine   Chloroquine   Hydroxychloroquine

Figure 13.54 Structures of *Cinchona* alkaloids and quinine-inspired synthetic antimalarial agents (chloroquine and hydroxychloroquine). The malaria parasite of various *Plasmodium* species is transmitted through mosquito bites. The earliest therapy was cinchona bark from which the antimalarial compounds were isolated, and further research on these compounds led to the discovery of chloroquine and hydroxychloroquine. *Cinchona pubescens*: Reproduced from https://commons.wikimedia.org/wiki/File:RUBIACEAE_Cinchona_pubescens.jpg, under the terms of the CC BY-SA 3.0 license, https://creativecommons.org/licenses/by-sa/3.0/deed.en. Image Credit: Klockrike. Cinchona bark: Reproduced from https://commons.wikimedia.org/wiki/File:Cinchona_officinalis_001.JPG, under the terms of the CC BY-SA 3.0 license, https://creativecommons.org/licenses/by-sa/3.0/deed.en. Image Credit: H. Zell. *Anopheles* mosquito feeding. Image Credit: Jim Gathany, image in the public domain.

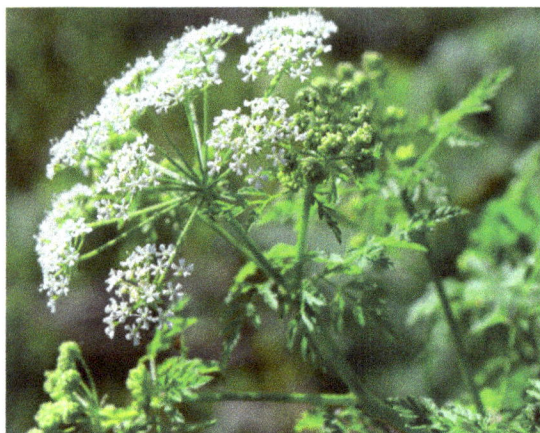

Poison hemlock   Socrates

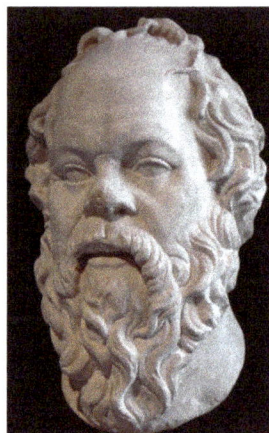

Coniine   γ-Coniceine   Conhydrine   *N*-Methyl coniceine   Pseudoconhydrine

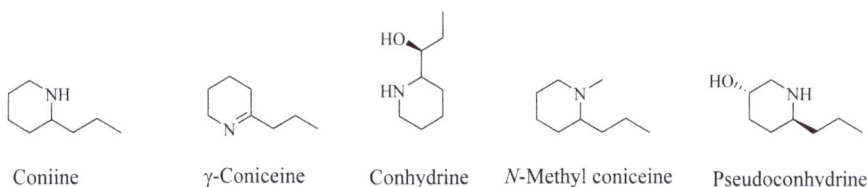

Figure 13.55 Alkaloids of poison hemlock. The plant *Conium maculatum* is known for its toxicity due to the presence of piperidine alkaloids, the structures of the main components of which are shown. In ancient Greece, condemned prisoners were killed by potions of hemlock. The legendary Socrates, condemned for corrupting the minds of the young men in Athens in 399 BCE, was said to have chosen hemlock tea to carry out his death sentence. Poison hemlock image: Reproduced from https://en.wikipedia.org/wiki/Conium_maculatum#/media/File:Poison_Hemlock.jpg, under the terms of the CC BY-SA 4.0 license, https://creativecommons.org/licenses/by-sa/4.0/. Image Credit: Djtanng. Socrates: Reproduced from https://commons.wikimedia.org/wiki/File:Socrate_du_Louvre.jpg, under the terms of the CC BY-SA 2.5 license, https://creativecommons.org/licenses/by-sa/2.5/deed.en. Image Credit: Sting.

nausea, vomiting, headache, and psychosis, among others. The ergot alkaloids responsible for this disease are grouped into three types: clavines, lysergic acid amides (ergoamides), and peptides (ergopeptines or d-lysergic acid peptide derivatives) (Figure 13.56). One of the ergot alkaloids of therapeutic value is ergotamine, which is a potent vasoconstrictor. Ergot alkaloids have also been used in the development of lysergic acid diethylamide (LSD), which is hallucinogenic and used in the treatment of schizophrenia. In addition to *Claviceps*, several alkaloids belonging to the group have also been isolated from the fungus genera *Aspergillus*, *Rhizopus*, and *Penicillium*.

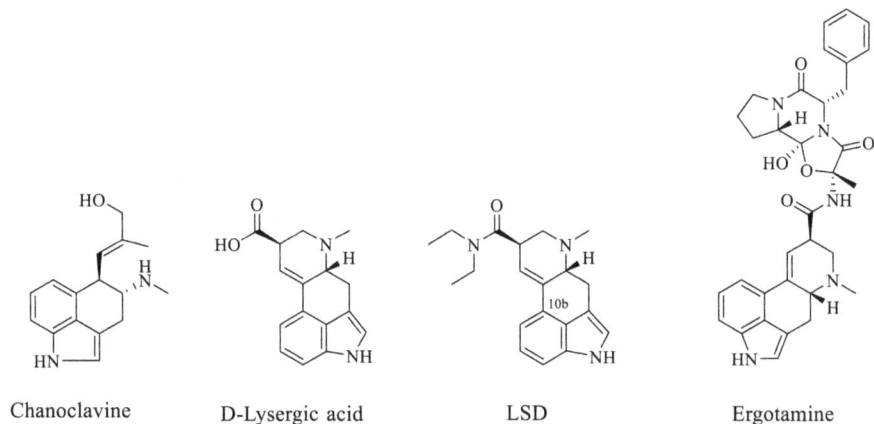

| Chanoclavine | D-Lysergic acid | LSD | Ergotamine |

Figure 13.56 Structures of some ergot alkaloids and LSD.

Ergot Alkaloids – Key Facts

- Over 80 ergot alkaloids, including lysergic acid, are produced by the parasitic fungus *Claviceps purpurea* and others.
- They increase uterine motility/contraction, and also have several cardiovascular and neuronal effects. They reduce prolactin secretion.
- Historically, they are known to poison and cause death in humans (ergotism) due to contaminated flour (*e.g.* rye flour).
- They have medicinal applications – migraine headaches, Parkinson's disease, stimulation of uterine contractions in childbirth.

13.3.4.3.10 Natural Hallucinogenic Alkaloids and Related Compounds

Readers should bear in mind that alkaloids with numerous biological properties both as medicines and toxins have been isolated from micro and macro fungi, animals including toads, fish, insects, millipedes, and several marine organisms.

Classic examples of alkaloids from mushrooms as hallucinogenic compounds have been identified from various genera, including *Psilocybe* and *Panaeolus* species. Psilocybin and psilocin (Figure 13.57) are good examples that were obtained from the sacred mushroom of Mexico, teonanácatl, and also many others. Hallucinogenic mushrooms are also called magic mushrooms, and are also sources of common substance abuse. *Psilocybe semilanceata* with a wide distribution throughout the world is a source of psilocybin. Several other

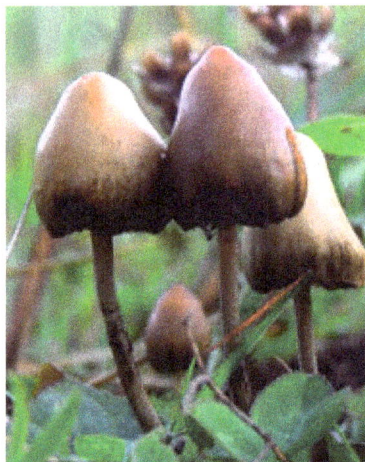
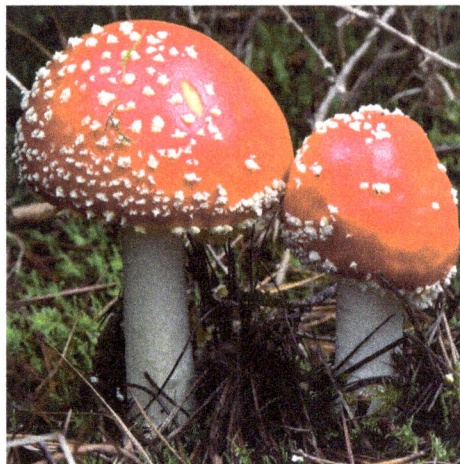

Psilocybe semilanceata   *Amanita muscaria*

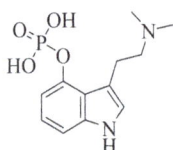
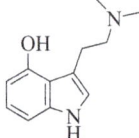
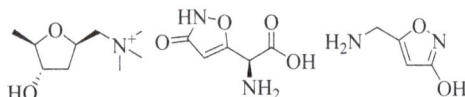
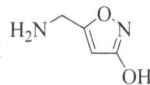

Psilocybin   Psilocin   Muscarine   Ibotenic acid   Muscimol

Figure 13.57 Examples of drugs from mushroom sources. Psilocin is the most common hallucinogenic compound, isolated from magic mushrooms (mostly known in the USA as liberty cap) such as *Psilocybe semilanceata*. These fungi have been used since prehistoric times and their symptoms, which mostly appear within an hour, include euphoria, hallucinations, altered sense of time and space, and depersonalisation. These symptoms are said to be similar to those with LSD, although they have a shorter duration of action. Muscarine has been isolated from various mushrooms and its identification from *Amanita muscaria* helped in understanding the pharmacology of acetylcholine receptors. The most toxic and hallucinogenic compounds of the fungus are also shown. *Psilocybe semilanceata*: Reproduced from https://en.wikipedia.org/wiki/File:Psilocybe_semilanceata_6514.jpg, under the terms of the CC BY-SA 3.0 license, https://creativecommons.org/licenses/by-sa/3.0/deed.en. Image Credit: Arp. *Amanita muscaria*: Reproduced from https://en.wikipedia.org/wiki/Amanita_muscaria#/media/File:Amanita_muscaria_Marriott_Falls_1.jpg, under the terms of the CC BY-SA 3.0 license, https://creativecommons.org/licenses/by-sa/3.0/deed.en. Image Credit: J. J. Harrison.

mushroom genera known to be good sources of psilocybin include *Copelandia*, *Gymnopilus*, *Inocybe*, *Panaeolus*, *Pholiotina*, and *Pluteus*. Their pharmacology is well established: for example, psilocin is a serotonin or 5-HT receptor (5-HT$_{1A}$, 5-HT$_{2A}$, and 5-HT$_{2C}$ receptor subtypes) agonist. Psilocybin is dephosphorylated in the body to yield its active metabolite, psilocin. Another good example of a mushroom-derived drug is muscarine (Figure 13.57), which was originally isolated from *Amanita muscaria*. The classification of acetylcholine (neurotransmitter) receptors into nicotinic and muscarinic types was originally based on the selective effect of nicotine and muscarine as agonists to these receptors, respectively. Hence muscarine mimics acetylcholine and, through action on muscarinic receptors, which are located on smooth muscle cells, it slows the heart and increases the activity of the gastrointestinal system. The most poisonous compounds of this mushroom are, however, ibotenic acid and its decarboxylation product, muscimol (Figure 13.57), which are structural analogues of two CNS neurotransmitters: glutamic acid (excitatory) and γ-aminobutyric acid (GABA) (inhibitory). Ingestion of the mushroom induces an initial excitatory effect (elation, giddiness, hyperactivity, and muscle tremors) followed by inhibitory (tiredness and deep sleep) phases of pharmacological effects.

Hallucinogenic alkaloids are also common in plants and a good example is the peyote cactus (*Lophophora williamsii*). The main bioactive compound is mescaline (Figure 13.58) – although it is not as potent as psilocybin, its hallucinogenic effect has been well documented. The buds and leaves of the khat (*Catha edulis*) are chewed in many countries for stimulant and euphoric effects. The two alkaloidal compounds present, cathinone and cathine (Figure 13.58), have pharmacological activities similar to those of amphetamine.

13.3.4.4 Miscellaneous Alkaloids

In terms of structural classes, there are also numerous miscellaneous alkaloids or nitrogen-containing biologically active compounds in Nature. For example, glucosinolates and isothiocyanates are biologically active compounds that plants use as a defence against pathogens and herbivores. These compounds also display numerous pharmacological activities. Glucomoringin and moringin are good examples, isolated from *Moringa* species such as *Moringa stenopetala* and *Moringa oleifera*. Upon damage to the plant tissues, the enzyme myrosinase digests the glucoseinolate (glucomoringin) to release the bioactive compound moringin (Figure 13.59).

In some plants, terpenoids such as diterpenes and steroids incorporating nitrogen atom(s) are commonly found. Good examples are the plant families Solanaceae (potato and tomato families), Buxaceae, Apocynaceae, and Liliaceae, which are sources of several biologically active steroidal alkaloids and their semi-synthetic derivatives.

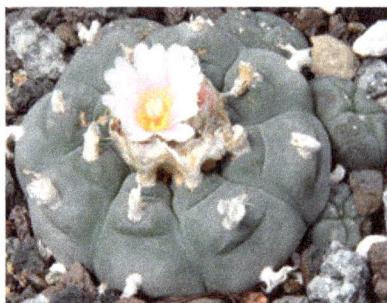

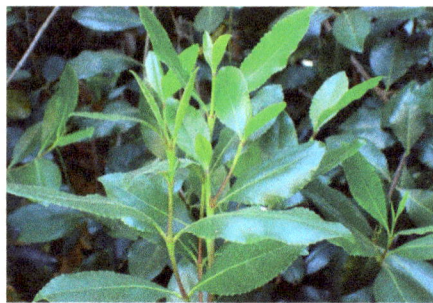

Lophophora williamsii

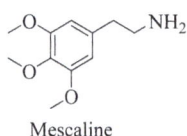

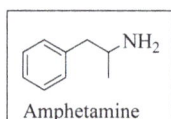

Mescaline

Amphetamine

Catha edulis

Cathinone   Cathine

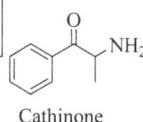

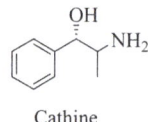

Figure 13.58 Structures of mescaline from the peyote cactus (*Lophophora williamsii*) and cathinone and cathine from khat (*Catha edulis*). Note the similarity of the khat alkaloids to amphetamine, and they also have a chiral centre like amphetamine (see Chapter 6). *Lophophora williamsii*: Reproduced from https://en.wikipedia.org/wiki/File:Lophophora_williamsii_pm.jpg, under the terms of the CC BY 3.0 license, https://creativecommons.org/licenses/by/3.0/deed.en. Image Credit: Peter A. Mansfeld. *Catha edulis*: Reproduced from https://commons.wikimedia.org/wiki/File:Catha_edulis_kz01.jpg, under the terms of the CC BY-SA 4.0 license, https://creativecommons.org/licenses/by-sa/4.0/deed.en. Image Credit: Krzysztof Ziarnek, Kenraiz.

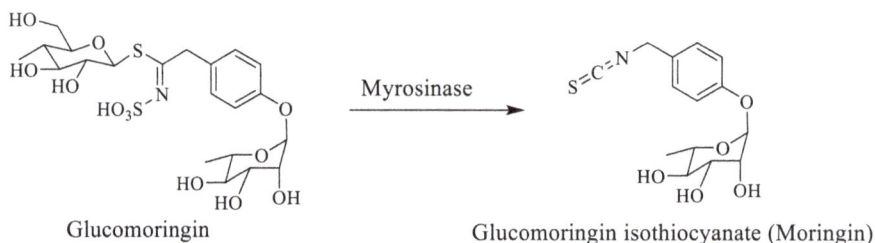

Glucomoringin   Glucomoringin isothiocyanate (Moringin)

Myrosinase

Figure 13.59 *Alkaloids from* Moringa species. Glucosinolates are a large group of plant secondary metabolites mainly produced as defensive chemicals but they also have nutritional and medicinal values. When cleaved by myrosinase enzymes in the plant, which is released during tissue damage, a range of bioactive compounds, including isothiocyanates, are released.

Prototype bioactive compounds include α-chaconine, α-solanine, sola-nidine and solasodine (from *Solanum tuberosum*), *tomatidine* (*from* unripe tomatoes), *and* veratramine and jervine (from *Veratrum* species) (Figure 13.60). Several compounds of this nature have also been iso-lated from marine sources (*e.g.* sponge) and amphibians such as toads (see Section 13.5). Note that these compounds also exist in Nature both in glycosylated form (with sugars attached in the same way as in sapo-nins), hence called glycoalkaloids, and in aglycone form (without sug-ars) (Figure 13.60). Owing to their known toxicity, commercial potato breeds with low concentrations of these compounds are selected. The pharmacological activities of these compounds, including anticancer effects, have been extensively studied in recent years. Nitrogen atoms

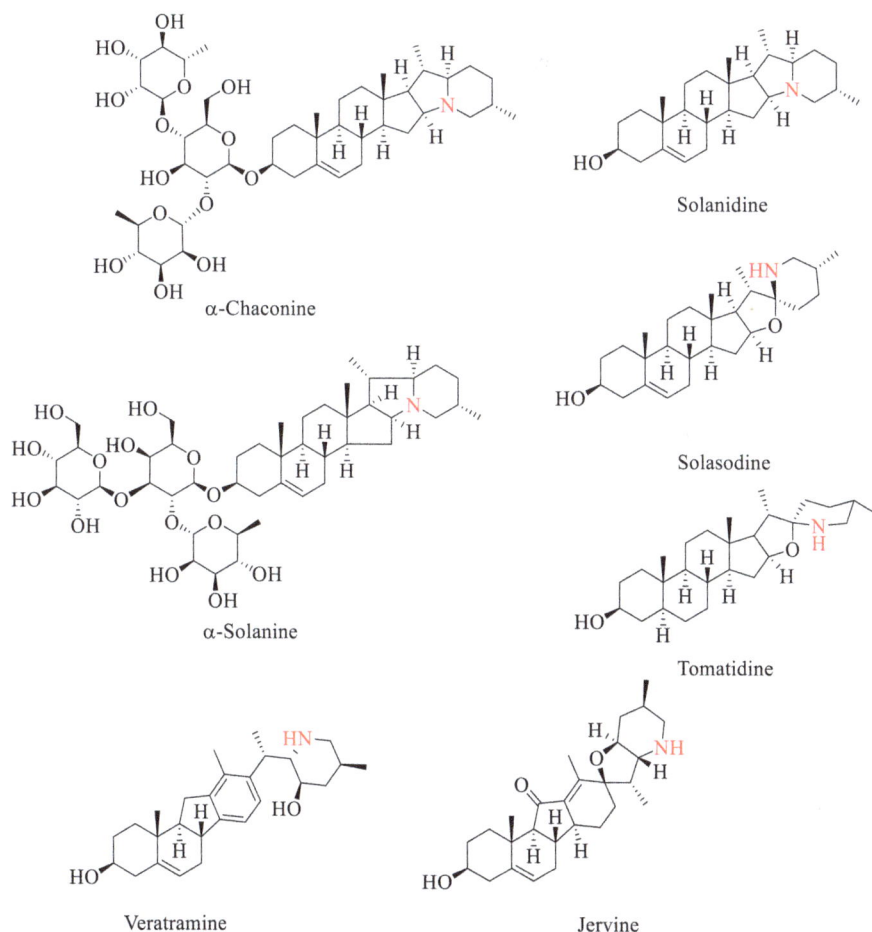

Figure 13.60 Structures of representative steroidal alkaloids.

can also be incorporated in other terpenoid classes such as sesqui-terpenes. As shown for the synthetic muscle relaxants (Figure 13.48) obtained through inspiration by the natural alkaloid D-tubocurarine, steroids can also be chemically modified to incorporate nitrogen.

13.3.4.5 Other Compounds from Mixed Biosynthesis Pathways – Cannabinoids

Many natural products are derived from mixed biosynthesis pathways. For example, we have seen flavonoids (Section 13.3.3.2) as products from both the acetate–polyketide pathway and the shikimic acid pathway. Another good example of a mixed pathway is cannabinoids, which have their biosynthetic origin in the terpenes and the polyketide pathway. In a classic example of this pathway (Figure 13.61), geranyl pyrophosphate (a precursor of monoterpenes) combines with olivetolic acid to yield can-nabigerolic acid, the immediate precursor of cannabinoids or phytocan-nabinoids (see Figure 13.61) that we find in *Cannabis sativa*. The types of compounds obtained through this pathway are cannabidiolic acid (CBDA), Δ^9-tetrahydrocannabinolic acid (Δ^9-THCA), cannabigerolic acid (CBGA), cannabidiol (CBD), Δ^9-tetrahydrocannabinol (Δ^9-THC), cannabi-nol (CBN), Δ^9-tetrahydrocannabivarin (Δ^9-THCV), cannabidivarin (CBDV), cannabigerol (CBG), and cannabichromene (CBC). Of these, CBDV is a non-psychoactive cannabinoid. Readers should note that cannabinoids in the form of the illicit drug cannabis have a long history of use as med-icines and drugs of abuse. Apart from their addictive effect, they have a profound effect on brain function and affect memory and mood. Their effect is mediated through receptors (cannabinoid receptors), which respond to our own internal cannabinoids (called endocannabinoids). Δ^9-THC is the main constituent of cannabis and has a potent analgesic effect along with relaxation, dysphoria, tolerance, and, of course, depen-dence. There are also several synthetic cannabinoids, some of which are substances of abuse. Some of them are by orders of magnitude more potent than the natural analogues. Research is also ongoing to synthe-sise compounds that retain the beneficial effect of cannabinoids without inducing addictive behaviour.

13.4 Microbial Toxins

13.4.1 Mycotoxins

The word 'mycotoxin' is derived from the Greek word '*mycos*', meaning fungus, and the Latin word '*toxicum*', meaning poison. Certain fila-mentous fungi such as moulds produce toxins that we call mycotoxins.

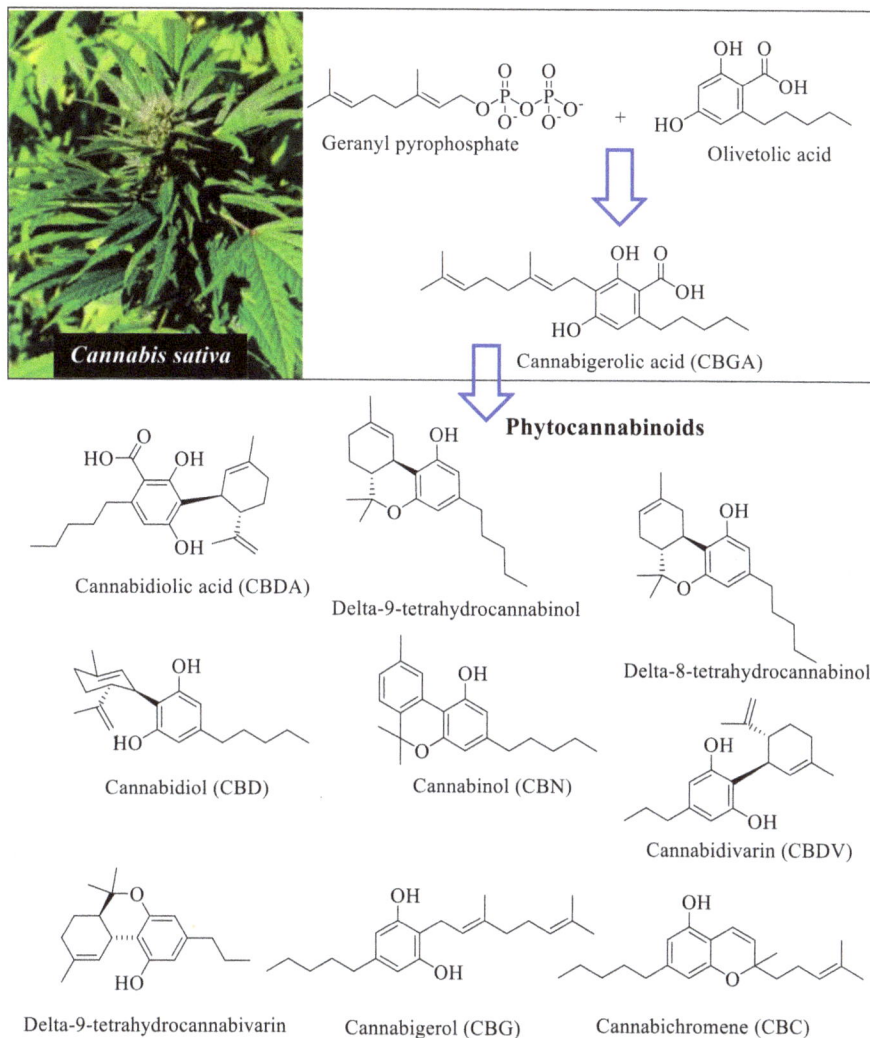

Figure 13.61 Biosynthesis of phytocannabinoids in cannabis (*Cannabis sativa*). *Cannabis sativa*: Reproduced from https://commons.wikimedia.org/wiki/File:Cannabis_sativa_2.jpg, under the terms of the CC BY-SA 4.0 license, https://creativecommons.org/licenses/by-sa/4.0/deed.en. Image Credit: Thayne Tuason.

Since some of these fungi are parasitic to crops, they are ingested by humans in contaminated food. Hundreds of these toxins are known and may be grouped into several classes.

13.4.1.1 Aflatoxins

Produced by the moulds *Aspergillus flavus* and *Aspergillus parasiticus*, aflatoxins are potent hepatotoxic, genotoxic, and carcinogenic agents. There

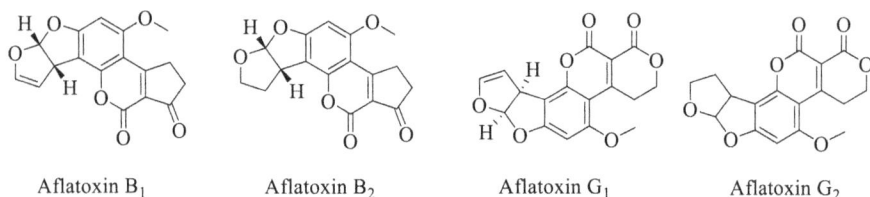

Aflatoxin B$_1$ Aflatoxin B$_2$ Aflatoxin G$_1$ Aflatoxin G$_2$

Figure 13.62 Structures of common aflatoxins.

are four major aflatoxins, named aflatoxin B$_1$, B$_2$, G$_1$, and G$_2$ (Figure 13.62). Of these, the B$_1$ form is the most toxic and is the second most carcinogenic compound known after the synthetic polychlorinated biphenyl groups. Since *Aflatoxin flavus* thrives well in a warm, humid climate, food contamination by aflatoxins is common in tropical countries.

13.4.1.2 Trichothecenes

Based on the sesquiterpenoid class of terpenoids, trichothecenes are a group of toxic compounds produced by many *Fusarium* species, *Baccharis megapotamica*, *Myrothecium roridum*, *Myrothecium verrucaria*, *and Stachybotrys atra.* These compounds are divided into subgroups A–D, but types A and B are the most common (Figure 13.63). Type A is represented by neosolaniol, HT-2 toxin, T-2 toxin, T-2 triol, T-2 tetraol, and diacetoxyscirpenol (DAS). Type B trichothecenes are represented by deoxynivalenol (DON), 3-acetyl-DON, 15-acetyl-DON, nivalenol, and fusarenon X. The *Fusarium* species appear to be the most important and are sources of over 150 toxins of this kind.

13.4.1.3 Fumonisins

Mostly affecting corn and corn-based foods, these toxins are produced by *Fusarium* moulds. The most common is fumonisin B$_1$ (FB$_1$) (Figure 13.64) [the B$_2$ (FB$_2$) and B$_3$ (FB$_3$) forms are also common] and they are implicated in oesophageal cancer.

13.4.1.4 Zearalenones

Represented by zearalenone (known as F-2 toxin), these are non-steroidal oestrogenic mycotoxins (Figure 13.65) produced by *Fusarium* species (*e.g. F. graminearum*). Zearalenone has an oestrogenic effect, which means that it stimulates oestrogenic receptors in the same way as oestrogen (oestradiol) does to induce an oestrogenic response. The compound also induces hepatotoxicity and immunotoxicity.

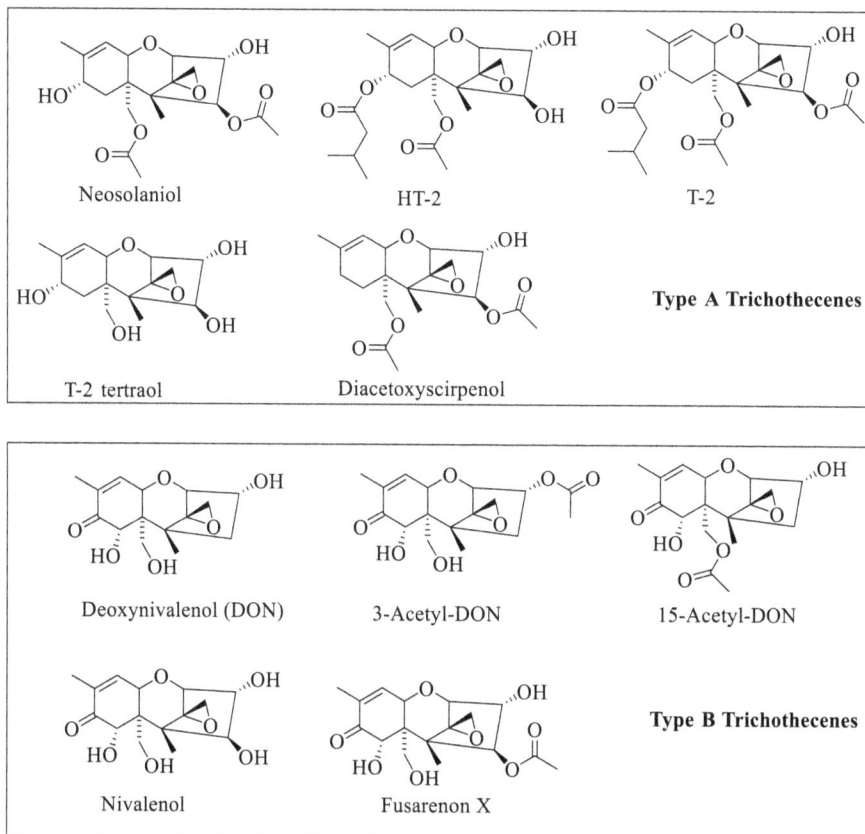

Figure 13.63 Structures of trichothecene mycotoxins.

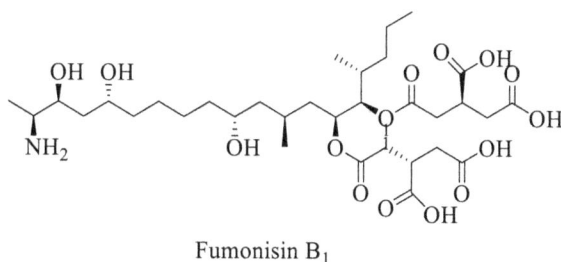

Fumonisin B_1

Figure 13.64 Structure of fumonisin B_1.

13.4.1.5 Ochratoxins

Represented by ochratoxin A (Figure 13.65) (ochratoxin B, C, and D also occur) as the most abundant and most toxic member, they are produced by fungi such as *Aspergillus ochraceus*, and *Penicillium* species. Cereals and grain products are the main sources of contamination.

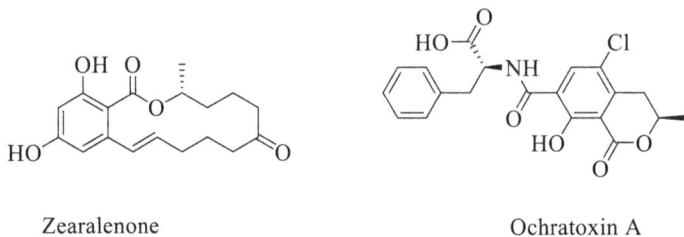

Zearalenone   Ochratoxin A

Figure 13.65   Structures of zearalenone and ochratoxin A.

13.4.1.6   Ergot Alkaloids

These are discussed in Section 13.3.4.3.9.

13.4.2   Bacterial Toxins

Various pathogenic bacteria have evolved to produce toxins as virulence factors to help them colonise their host. Some toxins are located inside bacteria and are actively excreted by the live bacteria. These are called *exotoxins* and include neurotoxins (affecting the nervous system), enterotoxins (affecting intestinal mucosa), and cytotoxins (affecting all tissues). Exotoxins of a protein nature from *Botulinum*, *Clostridium*, and *Diphtheria* poisons may also act like enzymes to function as ADP-ribosylating proteins, or as phospholipase, adenylate cyclase, metalloprotease, deamidase, protease, and deoxyribonuclease. On the other hand, some toxins are called *endotoxins* as they are firmly attached either in the cell wall or inside the bacteria and are discharged into host tissues upon bacterial cell death. Bacterial toxins affect host organisms in the following ways:

Cell membrane damage: In many cases, bacterial exotoxins destroy cells and tissues as a whole or act in specific areas of cells to make pores. They use enzymes for such hydrolysis and disrupt lipid bilayers. Pore-forming toxins include cytotoxic proteins such as α-toxins from *Staphylococcus aureus* and *Clostridium perfringens*. When bound to the cell membrane, they make channels or pores that allow the free movement of materials in and out of the cells (cell swelling), leading to cell death. *Staphylococcus aureus* α-toxin is a good example.

Protein synthesis inhibition: Bacterial toxins mostly interfere with ribosomal RNA by targeting ADP-ribosylating elongation factor 2. In terms of our organic chemistry topic, ADP-ribosylation by bacterial ADP-ribosylating exotoxins is a covalent modification reaction in which the nicotinamide adenine dinucleotide donor (NAD^+) molecule transfers the ADP-ribose moiety to an amino acid (*e.g.* Arg, Asn, Thr,

Cys, or Gln) substrate acceptor in a protein. The reaction liberates nicotinamide (Figure 13.66). This results in post-translational modification of proteins and the cholera and heat-labile enterotoxin particularly target GTP-binding proteins through this mechanism.

Activation of second messenger pathways: Toxins can affect the signal transduction pathways of cells. In some cases, the toxins act like phospholipase A_2 or other enzymes involved in cell signalling. One of the most important cell-signalling second messengers is cyclic adenosine monophosphate (cAMP), the activity of which has been shown to be increased by protein exotoxins of cholera toxin from *Vibrio cholerae*, heat-labile enterotoxins of *Escherichia coli*, and pertussis toxin of *Bordetella pertussis*. The toxins do this either by modifying the function of key enzymes or through acting in the same way as the host enzymes (*e.g.* adenylate cyclase that produces cAMP).

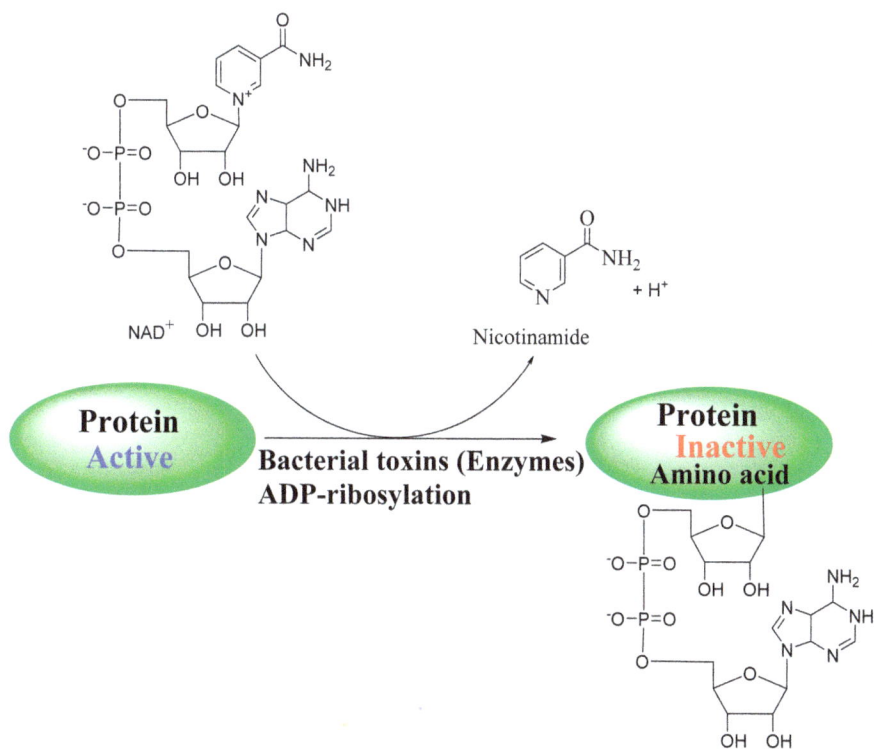

Figure 13.66 Typical reaction catalysed by ADP-ribosylating exotoxins. The toxins act like enzymes and add ADP-ribose from the NAD⁺ to amino acid acceptors of host target proteins. The reaction is an example of covalent bond formation between drugs and their targets (see Chapter 12).

Inhibition of release of neurotransmitters: *Clostridium botulinum* (botulinum neurotoxin) and *Clostridium tetani* (tetanus neurotoxin) are good examples. In the case of botulinum neurotoxins, they act like metalloproteases through which they block synaptic transmission by preventing the release of acetylcholine at the motor neurones. Through enzymatic action, the toxin degrades specific proteins (SNARE proteins) that are required for the neurotransmitter vesicle fusion with the nerve terminal cell membrane to release acetylcholine. This results in muscle paralysis. In the case of tetanus neurotoxin, its mode of action is similar to that of botulinum toxin but it affects specific neurons called inhibitory neurons in the CNS (instead of the peripheral nervous system). Inhibiting the 'inhibitory neurones' means that the motor activity is increased, leading to muscle contraction. This also ends up in muscle paralysis. The ability of tetanus neurotoxins to be transported to the CNS through motor neurons is an interesting therapeutic mechanism of drug delivery from the peripheral nervous system to the CNS.

Activation of host immune response: Toxins may trigger immune cells such as T cells and these include endotoxins that cause shock. Endotoxins are composed of lipopolysaccharides that are found in the cell walls of mostly Gram-negative bacteria. They induce inflammation and death by multiple organ failure. Lipid A (Figure 13.67), the active moiety of lipopolysaccharides or endotoxins, is composed of two glucose amine sugars with fatty acids attached. It also has two phosphate

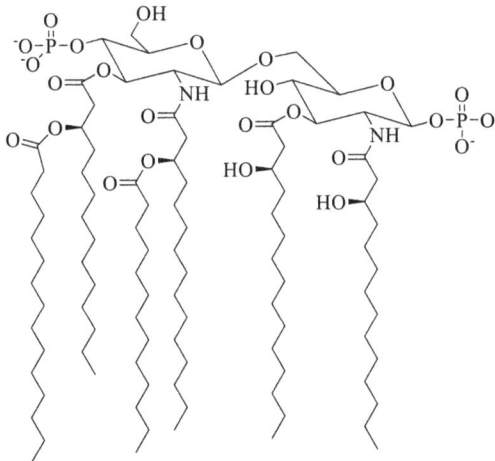

Figure 13.67   Structure of lipid A, the active component of bacterial endotoxin. Bacterial endotoxin is a lipopolysaccharide with the active component regarded as lipid A.

groups, hence it is a phosphoglycolipid. Drugs that bind with lipid A both through ionic interactions *via* the phosphate groups and lipid–lipid interactions *via* the fatty acid units can firmly bind to lipopoly-saccharides and detoxify them. Polymyxin B is an antibiotic that does this job, and it is also used to purify blood in patients with sepsis. Melittin from bee venom also does this, but it is too toxic to be used as a drug to tackle bacterial endotoxins.

Note that bacterial toxins are not always bad – they can be used effectively in therapeutics and research. Their specific binding with certain biological targets in the cells makes them valuable as markers in cell biology studies. For example, cholera toxin B binds specifically to gangliosides (sialic acid-containing glycosphingolipids) within the cell membrane. They are also used to deliver large proteins into the cytosolic compartment of target cells, and these can include nucleic acids, liposomes, and drug nanoparticles. Botulinum toxin is used to treat dystonia, disorders, and muscular atrophy.

13.5 Drugs from Animal Sources

The production of human insulin in use today for the treatment of diabetes is a success story of recombinant DNA technology or genetic engineering. As with the history of its usage in earlier days, insulin is still extracted from the pancreas of cattle and pigs and sold as pharmaceutical products. A similar story of hormonal insufficiency is hypothyroidism, which has been treated by using sheep thyroid or thyroxine, or similarly from pigs and cows for therapies such as hypertension. In both cases of insulin and thyroid hormone replacement therapy, the hormones are extracted and carefully purified to isolate the active hormone ingredients. The extraction of gonadotropin hormone from animal pituitary glands has also been exploited for the treatment of infertility in humans. All these approaches were successful because the chemical structures and activity of the hormones in animals are very similar to those in humans. Experimental studies in the laboratory extensively use animal enzymes such as lipases and proteases of the digestive enzymes, or blood cells of all kinds, *etc.* Animal products are also used in vaccine production.

The list of drugs sourced from pigs is impressive. They include anti-coagulants such as clexane, fragmin, heparin sodium, and heparinised saline. Porcine gelatins are used in vaccine production. Bovine products also include immune supplements, digestive supplements, immunoactive proteins, and others in vaccine production. Bovine serum albumin, which is used extensively in tissue and cell culture studies, is also used in biotechnology and vaccine products. Other animal sources extensively used in medicine include Chinese hamster ovary (CHO) cells, mice in numerous antibody-based therapies, horses in medicines, primarily antivenom therapeutics, chicken eggs in vaccine production, *etc.*

Of both nutritional and medicinal interest, the cod liver is used as a source of valuable vitamins such as vitamins A and D. Cod liver oil, often formulated and encapsulated, is also widely available to the public as a food supplement.

Several toxins of animal origin have been exploited in scientific studies, particularly pharmacology and pharmaceutical/clinical developments. Some of these have already been developed as drugs and are described in Table 13.2.

Table 13.2 Examples of animal protein toxins and drugs.

Source of venom	Description
Black widow spider	The bite of a *black widow spider* (*Latrodectus* species such as *Latrodectus mactans*) *has* neurotoxic venom called α-latrotoxin. The protein in this venom initiates the exocytosis of the neurotransmitter in the absence of nerve impulse or neurotransmitter release such as acetylcholine. The vesicles carrying acetylcholine are, however, not recovered after fusion with the cell membrane, hence the venom irreversibly inhibits vesicle recycling.
Scorpion	Scorpion venom, which is used effectively to immobilise prey, has neurotoxins. The venom also contains mucopolysaccharides, enzymes (hyaluronidase, phospholipase, and acetylcholinesterase), serotonin, histamine, protease inhibitors, and histamine releasers. The venom induces the release of serotonin that causes the pain immediately after envenomation.
	One of the most studied scorpions is *Leiurus quinquestriatus*, which inhabits North Africa and the Middle East. A 36-amino acid peptide found in the venom called chlorotoxin has been developed for the treatment and diagnosis of brain tumours (glioma) since it selectively blocks small-conductance chloride channels. It also has other pharmacological effects that are being studied.
Many-banded krait (*Bungarus multicinctus*)	The snake venom contains α-bungarotoxin, which is an example of α-neurotoxins. The toxin binds to nicotinic acetylcholine receptors located at the neuromuscular junction, resulting in skeletal muscle paralysis. Death can occur mostly from paralysis of the respiratory muscle, the diaphragm. In addition to the α-bungarotoxins, the venom contains β-bungarotoxins, which bind to the nerve terminus to inhibit the release of acetylcholine.

Table 13.2 (continued)

Source of venom	Description
Eastern green mamba snake	The venom of the eastern green mamba snake (*Dendroaspis angusticeps*, *D. polylepis*, *D. viridis*, and *D. jamesoni*) has neurotoxic components, including those acting at the post-synaptic acetylcholine receptors, called α-neurotoxins, dendrotoxins, and muscarinic toxins.
Brazilian lancehead snake (*Bothrops moojeni*)	*Batroxobin* is a purified venom used to break down fibrinogen in infarctions in the brain and myocardial (angina) and other cases such as surgery. An autologous fibrin sealant preparation from this venom source is also available in surgical operations.
Jararaca pit viper snake (*Bothrops jararaca*)	The Brazilian arrowhead viper (*B. jararaca*) with peptide inhibitors is a source of antihypertensive agents. Now obtained by synthesis, *captopril* is a well-known antihypertensive agent that acts through inhibition of the angiotensin-converting enzyme. Another product of this snake venom that is obtained by synthesis is *enalapril*, which is used for the same purposes as captopril.
Common lancehead snake (*Bothrops atrox*)	Common in both North and South America, this snake has a source of venom that was developed into *batroxobin*, which is used clinically to treat sudden deafness, acute cerebral infections, and angina pectoris. It is known to break down fibrinogen Aα chains. A platelet gel preparation (PLATELEX-ACT) for topical applications has also been developed.
Chinese cobra (*Naja naja atra*)	The purified venom (*cobratide*) that is known to block nicotinic acetylcholine receptors is used clinically to treat chronic arthralgia and neuropathic headache.
Pygmy rattlesnake (*Sistrurus miliarius*)	Common in the southern USA, this pit viper snake is a source of anticoagulant agent. Now obtained through synthesis, a product called *eptifibatide* is used in the therapy of coronary diseases for its effect as an anticoagulant. It works by inhibiting the binding of GPIIb/IIIa to ligands such as fibrinogen, von Willebrand factor, and others.
Saw-scaled viper snake (*Echis carinatus*)	Common in the dry regions of Africa and Asia, this snake is a source of venom that is useful as an anticoagulant agent. Now obtained by synthesis, *tirofiban* is useful in the treatment of coronary disease due to its anticoagulant effect. It inhibits the binding of fibrinogen with GPIIb/IIIa.
Honeybee (*Apis mellifera*)	The whole venom is used clinically to treat inflammatory diseases, particularly pain associated with osteoarthritis and multiple sclerosis. The principal toxic component in the honeybee venom (*Apis mellifera*) is *melittin*. Composed of 26 amino acid residues, it has been shown to have numerous pharmacological properties that are under active research.
European medicinal leech (*Hirudo medicinalis*)	In leech therapy, a few leeches are used to drain blood during surgery. Leeches have chemicals that inhibit platelet aggregation, hence inhibiting blood coagulation. The synthetic product *bivalirudin* is used as an anticoagulant in coronary disease for its antithrombin effect. Another synthetic (recombinant) product, *desirudin*, acts as an antithrombin agent to prevent venous thrombosis. Other medicinal leaches include *H. verbana*, *H. troctina*, and *H. orientalis*.

(*continued*)

Table 13.2   (continued)

Source of venom	Description
Cone snails	These venomous snails mostly produce small peptides 10–30 amino acids in length. They occur in large numbers and their diverse effects include blockade of ion channels (Na^+, K^+, and Ca^{2+} channels) or receptors, including the nicotinic acetyl-choline receptor. Derived from the cone snail *Conus magus*, *ziconotide* is an analgesic agent used clinically to treat chronic pain. It is a calcium channel antagonist.
Sun anemone (*Sticho-dactyla helianthus*)	This is a common sea anemone in the Caribbean islands. A small basic peptide with 35 amino acid residues called *sticho-dactyla* toxin has been shown to block potassium channels, with therapeutic implications for inflammatory and autoimmune diseases.
Northern short-tailed shrew (*Blarina brevicauda*)	Inhabiting the north-eastern region of North America, the potent venom in its saliva with a kallikrein-like protease effect is used to paralyse and subdue its prey. A 54-amino acid peptide from this venom called *soricidin* is an inhibitor of ion channels (*e.g.* sodium channel and TRPV6 calcium channel). Since the TRPV6 calcium channel is highly expressed in epithelial cell cancers, *soricidin* is being developed for cancer therapy, including breast, ovarian, and prostate cancers.
Gila monster lizard (*Heloderma suspectum*)	Proteins and peptides from the venomous saliva of this reptile were pioneered as drugs for diabetes. *Exenatide*, which is now synthesised with other variants, is in clinical use for type-2 diabetes. It is a glucagon-like peptide-1 receptor agonist. Other synthetic peptides inspired from this research include *lixisenatide*.

Note that animals also use low molecular weight compounds (non-protein compounds) as toxins. Many amphibians such as *Bufo* toads and *Phyllobates* species have skin secretions that are toxins containing alkaloids (see Figure 13.68). Among the toxins of amphibians are batrachotoxins (they keep voltage-gated sodium channels open) from *Phyllobates* species that have traditional application in Colombia in poison darts (from Colombian poison dart frogs) for hunting. Batrachotoxins (*e.g.* batrachotoxin) are useful in pharmacology research but are too toxic for clinical use. Chemically, they are steroidal alkaloid neurotoxins. Other toxins produced by these amphibians include pumiliotoxins (*e.g.* pumiliotoxins A and B) and histrionicotoxins. An example of histrionicotoxins is histrionicotoxin (others include isodihydrohistrionicotoxin and allodihydrohistrionicotoxin), which was also identified from *Dendrobates histrionicus* from western Colombia. The *Bufo* toads are known to produce a cardiac glycoside toxin called bufotoxin. They also make tryptamine (hallucinogenic) and bufotenine. Some toxins are also acquired from their diet.

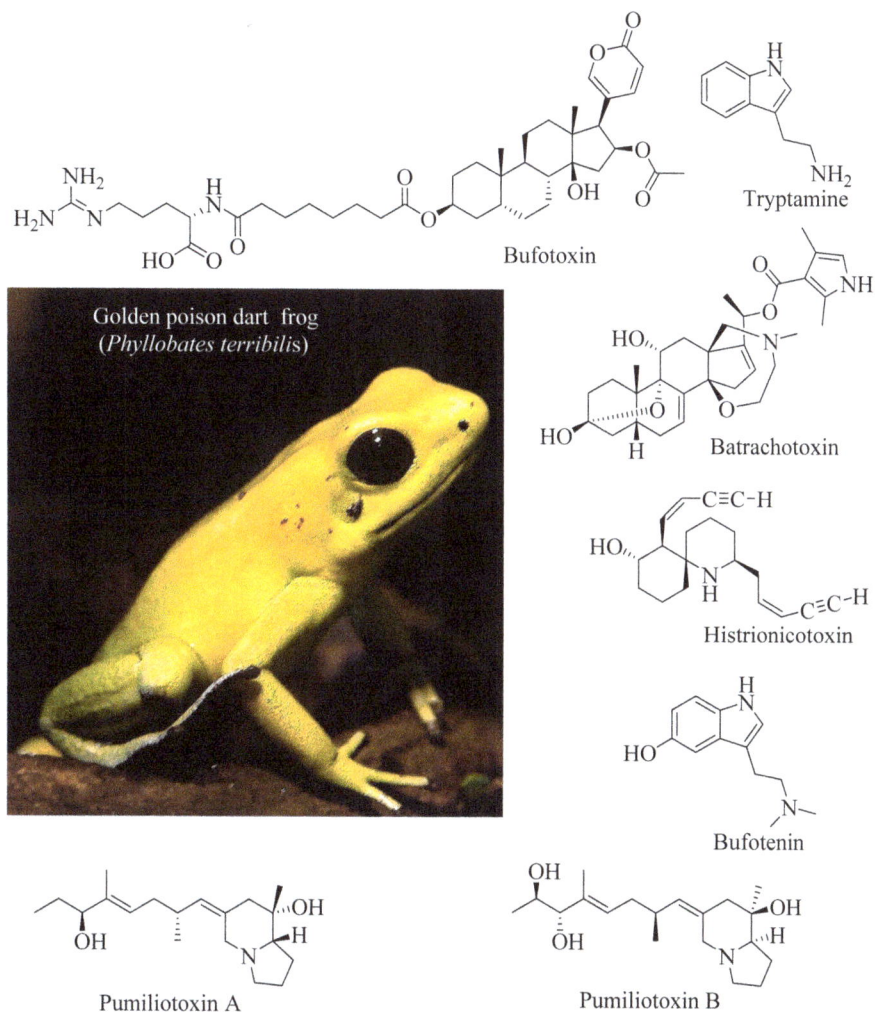

Bufotoxin

Tryptamine

Golden poison dart frog
(*Phyllobates terribilis*)

Batrachotoxin

Histrionicotoxin

Bufotenin

Pumiliotoxin A

Pumiliotoxin B

Figure 13.68 Structures of some alkaloid-based toxins isolated from the skins of amphibians. These alkaloids have unique structures with several functional groups. Note that batrachotoxin and bufotoxin are based on steroidal lactones just like cardiac glycosides discussed in Section 13.3.1.5. The compounds from the skin secretions of frogs such as the golden poison frog (*Phyllobates terribilis*) are used on poison darts in Colombia. *Phyllobates terribilis*: Reproduced from https://commons.wikimedia.org/wiki/File:Schrecklicherpfeilgiftfrosch-01.jpg, under the terms of the CC BY-SA 2.0 DE license, https://creativecommons.org/licenses/by-sa/2.0/de/deed.en. Image Credit: Wilfried Berns.

Of the poisonous fishes, the puffers in the family Tetraodontidae are sources of one of the most potent neurotoxins, tetrodotoxin (see Section 12.3.1). Like other sea animals (*e.g.* porcupinefish and blue-ringed octopus), the puffers acquire this toxin from bacteria such as *Vibrio alginolyticus* and *Pseudomonas tetraodonis*, which have a symbiotic relationship with the fish. The toxin blocks sodium ion channels located on neurones, thereby causing paralysis. Nausea, vomiting, and respiratory failure are classic symptoms of tetrodotoxin poisoning but a small dose may simply be felt as a tingling sensation in the fingers and toes.

13.6 Mineral Sources

Minerals of normal body composition can be applied as medicines where there is a medical issue associated with their deficiency. The common deficiencies such as iron in anaemia and iodine in hypothyroidism are good examples. Other minerals including zinc and salts such as gold salts (for rheumatoid arthritis) and mercury salts (for syphilis) have been used in therapy. The therapeutic potential of other minerals including fluorine, borax, and selenium is also known. Numerous petroleum-based products have also been used in diagnosis and pharmaceutical preparations of drugs.

13.7 Semi-synthetic and Synthetic Sources

Once a biologically active compound has been isolated from natural sources and proven to be efficacious, other alternative means of sourcing the compound need to be investigated. In many cases, altering the structure of the compound or minor modification may lead to significant improvements in its efficacy. While sourcing drugs from natural sources has its own challenges, it may be even more difficult when the yield of the compound from natural sources is very low. For example, the anticancer agent taxol (paclitaxel) was originally developed by extracting it from the bark of the Pacific yew tree, *Taxus brevifolia*. Unfortunately, the yield of this compound was in the order of 0.004–0.01%. To obtain 1 kg of taxol, several hundred thousand kilograms of yew tree bark were required. This was not economically viable or sustainable as it would lead to the extinction of the plant. One alternative was to extract the precursor of taxol, 10-deacetylbaccatin III, from the common garden yew plant relative *Taxus baccata* and convert it to taxol by chemical reactions.

Semi-synthetic versions of taxol such as docetaxel and cabazitaxel are now commercially available. Numerous antibiotics, some of which have already been described in previous chapters, are modified to yield semi-synthetic drugs. Whereas penicillin G is a natural product, ampicillin, amoxicillin, and methicillin are semi-synthetic antibiotics. In the area of narcotics, morphine and codeine are natural products whereas heroin is a semi-synthetic drug. In fact, several other derivatives of opium alkaloids with a morphine-like effect have been developed and include benzylmorphine (peronine), ethylmorphine (dionine), diacetylmorphine (heroin), dihydrodesoxymorphine-D (desomorphine), ethyldihydromorphinone, methyldihydromorphinone (metopon), monoacetylmorphine, α-, β-, and γ-isomorphine, tetrahydroxydesoxymorphine, dihydromorphinone (dilaudid), allopseudocodeine, heterocodeine, isocodeine, pseudocodeine, dihydrocodeinone (dicodid), dihydrohydroxycodeinone (eucodal), and morpholinylethylmorphine (pholcodin).

In the above examples, we have seen that semi-synthetic drugs are hybrids between natural and synthetic compounds. They are neither completely natural, nor are they completely synthetic. On the other hand, drugs can be made from starting materials that are not found in Nature and hence are called synthetic. These are built in the laboratory from smaller blocks and hence are anthropogenic. The list of synthetic drugs is far too long to include here. The anticancer drugs methotrexate (MTX) and sorafenib (Nexavar) are good examples. In drug abuse areas, there are synthetic drugs such as bath salts, synthetic cathinone (Flakka), 3,4-methylenedioxymethamphetamine (MDMA, Molly, or Ecstasy), synthetic cannabinoids (K2 or Spice), synthetic alternative to LSD (Smiles), and crystal meth.

Undoubtedly, Nature has provided the bulk of resources to treat human diseases and as such earlier chemistry studies were largely designed to quench the thirst of scientists' fascination in the natural world, be it in medicine or organic chemistry. Since then, organic synthesis has evolved through combinatorial organic synthesis to obtain large numbers of small molecules in a short period of time and at low cost. While the development of a library of small molecules was the focus of many pharmaceutical companies in the late twentieth century, advances in science have now transformed the dream of obtaining millions of new chemical entities in just a few months into reality. For those readers who pursue this line of study, the thousands of new chemical entities entering the scientific literature each year could be an inspiration to study their potential as drug molecules.

13.8   Recombinant DNA Technology

One may take a small piece of DNA from one organism and combine it with another strand of DNA from the same or another organism. The resulting DNA is called recombinant DNA (rDNA) or a 'chimera'. Recombinant DNA technology has been extensively exploited to develop vaccines by targeting a specific antigen instead of the whole pathogenic organism. By using this technology, human proteins such as hormones (*e.g.* insulin) can be made in microorganisms. The future of gene therapy is also based on treating or preventing disease by using recombinant DNA technology to replace defective genes. Antibodies and various other protein-based drugs are produced through this technology. Pharmaceutical products obtained through rDNA technology are divided into the following three groups:

- Human protein replacement – *e.g.* insulin and human growth hormone when they are deficient.
- Therapeutic agents – insulin and growth hormones can also be included in this group, but we also have interferon (IF, such as IFα2a, IFα2b, IFβ1a, IFβ1b, IFγ1b, PEGylated IFα2a, PEGylated IFα2b, *etc.*), factor VIII, erythropoietin, *etc.*
- Vaccines – advances in DNA technology have long culminated in delivering genetically engineered DNA to induce an immune response. Using this technology, we generate recombinant protein vaccines (whole protein or polypeptide vaccines) or rDNA vaccines. In the case of the DNA vaccines (also called third-generation vaccines), the strand of DNA or plasmid containing the DNA sequence for encoding a specific antigen(s) that elicits an immune response is introduced. Advances in vaccine development can be further explained by the approaches developed for COVID-19 vaccines, which include the following:

    ○ Using an inactive or weakly virulent virus as vaccine (*inactivated or weakened virus vaccines or whole virus vaccines*) that does not cause the disease but has the ability to stimulate the immune response. Chemicals, heat, or radiation can be used to inactivate or kill the virus. As shown for the MMR, chickenpox, and shingles vaccines, the weakened version of the virus can be used as a vaccine alternative.
    ○ Using protein or a protein fragment of the viral antigen (protein-based vaccine) that stimulates an immune response. The viral surface proteins (harmless S proteins) as harmless tools that activate the immune system can be used as vaccines.

This approach has been used successfully in the prevention of many viral diseases such as hepatitis B and acellular pertussis, which employ protein subunits. Similarly, polysaccharide vaccines are also available and include pneumococcal and the MenACWY vaccines.

o Using a safe virus (viral vector vaccines) that cannot cause disease but serves as a vehicle to introduce the virus proteins that initiate an immune response. Upon entry of the viral vector into host cells, it delivers genetic material from the COVID-19 virus that contains the instructions for making copies of the viral surface protein (S protein). This approach is often described as smuggling the instructions for making antigens from the disease-causing virus into cells to initiate protective immunity against it. The Ebola vaccine was developed using this technology and it led to the development of vector vaccines such as the AstraZeneca and Janssen COVID-19 vaccines. In the case of the AstraZeneca vaccine, a genetically modified vector of chimpanzee adenovirus ChAdOx1 was used to sneak the genetic blueprint of the COVID-19 virus surface proteins.

o Genetically engineered RNA or DNA (RNA and DNA vaccines or nucleic acid vaccines) to generate a protein that stimulates an immune response. The genetically engineered mRNA vaccine is similar to the DNA vaccine in that it carries instructions for making the viral surface proteins (S protein), which is recognised by the immune system. The Pfizer–BioNTech BNT162b2 and Moderna vaccines are good examples of COVID-19 mRNA vaccines.

13.9 Overview of Drug Discovery and Development

In earlier chapters of this book, we have seen how a drug molecule can act in a biological system through its functional groups and well-defined isomerism. In this chapter, we also looked at several examples of organic compounds and drug molecules of natural, semi-synthetic, or synthetic origin. A drug molecule may be a simple low molecular weight molecule such as that of aspirin or could be a complex metabolically or genetically engineered protein such as vaccines and protein-based drugs. Although the emphasis of this book is on the basic chemistry of drug molecules, it is important to summarise the process of drug discovery approaches and development to appreciate how an organic compound is transformed to become a drug.

When we say that the typical drug discovery and development cycle requires 12–15 years of research and multi-million dollar/pound investment, it is for good reason for the following processes.

13.9.1 Early Drug Discovery Process – Preclinical Development

You may identify the biological activity of an organic compound through basic research or a systematic drug discovery study in a pharmaceutical company. This is what we call lead identification. Ideally, we may identify a biological target that links the diseases and search for drugs that target the process. In the case of cancer, we may grow cancer cells *in vitro* and look for organic compounds that kill them, or we select a specific protein, receptor, enzyme, or sub-cellular processes as cancer targets. We thus have a validated biological target for screening compounds to detect initial activity. Pharmaceutical companies have libraries of thousands or millions of compounds to screen for biological activity.

Identified active compounds or hits go through further research in animals, tissue cultures, and other assays to identify the selectivity of the identified hits – this is what we call secondary assays for selecting an ideal drug-like candidate. This can further go through animal studies to study the pharmacological efficacy (on the disease in question) and toxicology studies. In the case of cancer, we may inoculate cancer cells in animals and study the potential of the active compounds to increase the life span of the diseased animals. In diabetes, we initiate the disease in animals and see if the sugar control is improved in these animals by the active compound. The doses are also selected, and potential adverse effects are monitored in animals. It is only after all these preclinical studies for the selected drug-candidate have been concluded that clinical trials in humans are then considered. The overall process of the drug discovery stages is shown in Figure 13.69.

Of high relevance to our topic on basic chemistry is the hit discovery process using the validated disease target. This involves the following:

High-throughput screening: If we have a large library of potentially bioactive compounds, we randomly screen them all against the validated target. This is an expensive process and can be met only by large pharmaceutical companies. In biological assays, we often do this using tissue culture or protein-based targets in multi-well plates (*e.g.* 384 wells or even more). Taxol as an anticancer compound was discovered through such a random screening approach.

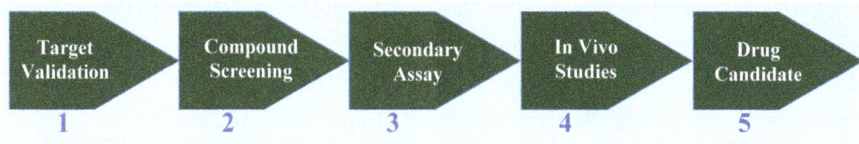

Figure 13.69 Biological screening assays in drug discovery. Experimental research on molecular, cellular, and animal studies helps in the identification of a biological target for a specific disease (1); various approaches to screening assays may be used to identify a biologically active compound that we may call a hit (2); further *in vitro* and *in vivo* studies help to validate the biologically active compound as a drug lead (3); animal studies are used to determine the pharmacological efficacy in a disease model and also to determine toxicity (4); finally, the selected drug through preclinical studies is considered for human trial studies (5).

Focused screening: If we know that a certain class of compounds show biological activity in the chosen target, then we can screen similar compounds in the validated assy. This reduces the cost of the assay and increases the chance of identifying an active compound, but you should check that the existing patent on the known compounds does not cover the closely related structure that you are working on. In the case of traditional medicines already used for a specific disease, we choose them in the screen to test their efficacy. The discovery of many drugs such as artemisinin as an antimalarial drug was based on this approach. For plants, we call this an *ethnobotanical approach of drug discovery programme*.

Fragment screening: You may have small fragments (or very small compounds) with weak activity in the identified assay but when you join them chemically you may obtain a larger structure with greater potency. This approach is now becoming common, and compounds normally discarded because of their weaker millimolar-level activity range are used to build a potent drug. This is often done by using nuclear magnetic resonance (NMR) spectroscopy as a technique and hence it is called an *NMR screen*.

Structure-aided drug design and virtual screening: Based on the crystal structure of the biological target molecule and the drug candidate, computational docking studies can be performed to predict the selectivity, potency, and ways of structural improvements. X-ray structures of a vast array of protein targets and ligands are now available along with various docking models.

Physiological or tissue-based screening: Instead of cellular or protein-based assays, we use tissue-based assays that are more relevant to the disease process or close to the *in vivo* environment.

In the lead identification and optimisation process, terminologies other than pharmacological efficacy that we encounter include absorption, distribution, metabolism, and excretion (ADME) properties in addition to physicochemical and pharmacokinetic (PK) measurements. The physicochemical properties of the drug that we have addressed in several chapters of this book are of relevance to this. The solubility of the drug in water, its lipophilicity, the form in which it is administered, and how it is transported and eliminated within the body are key parameters to be investigated.

13.9.2   Clinical Studies

The approval process for a new drug involves a new drug application to the relevant authorities, *e.g.* the Food and Drug Administration (FDA) in the USA. The initial application (*e.g.* Investigational New Drug application) is intended in essence to obtain approval to start trials on humans through three stages that we call Phase 1, Phase 2, and Phase 3 of human clinical studies. These studies are designed to prove the pharmacological efficiency and pharmacokinetic profile of the drug to be developed and to examine possible adverse effects for the various dose ranges of the drug.

- *Phase 1*: Involves 20–200 healthy subjects or patients with the disease intended to be treated with the drug.
- *Phase 2*: Several hundred patients participate in the trial to assess the efficacy of the drug in the disease to be treated and register any adverse effects or toxicities.
- *Phase 3*: Several hundred to several thousand patients participate to assess both the efficacy and adverse effects.

Once the relevant clinical trials have been completed, the second stage of the application process (new drug application) is needed for marketing approval of the drug. Hence data starting from the chemistry of the drug, its manufacturing process and preparation of the dosage forms, data on animal studies on the pharmacological efficacy and toxicology profile, human studies on the bioavailability of the drug, and complete pharmacokinetic profile and the clinical trial data must be included. The drug discovery processes are summarised in Figure 13.70.

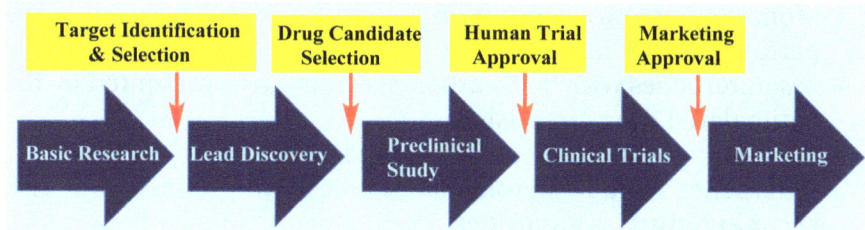

Figure 13.70 The overall process of drug discovery. Basic research on target identification takes years of research and is often based on a literature search of the relevant field. Lead discovery is a multi-year process while preclinical development and clinical trials take several years to complete. Along these lines, we have costs associated with patents and scientific studies from screening to approvals (investigational new drug application and new drug or market approvals).

13.10 Summary

In this chapter, we have learned the following:

- Natural products include crude preparations of extracts from natural sources and purified compounds.
- Plants and microorganisms are common sources of drugs, but marine organisms are beginning to be utilised.
- Primary metabolites include metabolic reaction products of proteins, carbohydrates, DNA, and lipids that are involved in the immediate survival of the species – anabolic and catabolic reactions.
- Secondary metabolites are what we call the terpenoids, alkaloids, *etc.* – used in defence against pathogenic organisms or for the long-term survival of the organism.
- Several million chemical compounds in Nature are synthesised through a handful of biosynthetic pathways.
- Terpenoids are made from five-carbon isoprene units and divided based on the number of these units in the skeleton: monoterpenes, diterpenes, triterpenes, *etc.*
- Terpenoids are mainly products of the malonic acid pathway.
- The smallest terpenoids are hemiterpenes but in Nature monoterpenes are the common smaller units.
- The diversity in terpenoids comes from the loss of the phosphate group in the precursor molecule that leads to cyclisation in different formats and reactions such as addition, reduction, oxidation, hydroxylation, glycosylation, *etc.*

- Monoterpenes are common in essential oils and are used in the perfumery/fragrance industry.
- Sesquiterpenes with a 15-carbon skeleton are represented by the antimalarial drug artemisinin.
- The best known diterpene is the anticancer drug taxol.
- Triterpenes include steroids and cholesterol products and also occur in Nature as glycosides.
- Tetraterpenes are represented by carotenoids such as β-carotene.
- The polyketide pathway in microorganisms is a common source of drugs such as erythromycin, rifamycin, amphotericin, tetracycline, *etc.* Several semi-synthetic and synthetic analogues are available.
- The polyketide pathways in plants are represented by the laxative compounds of Senokot.
- The shikimic acid pathway is a major source of phenolic compounds – this is *via* aromatic amino acids such as tyrosine and phenylalanine.
- Compounds of mixed biosynthetic origin include flavonoids (acetate plus shikimate), cocaine (amino acid and polyketide) and cannabinoids (acetate/polyketide pathway and the shikimic acid pathway).
- Many drug molecules belong to the alkaloid class – mostly originating from amino acids.
- Alkaloids are classified based on their structural skeleton or biosynthetic origin – which amino acid they originated from.
- Examples of plant-based alkaloids as drugs include caffeine and nicotine as stimulants, muscle relaxants of the curare compounds, opium alkaloids such as morphine and codeine, anticancer compounds of the *Vinca* alkaloids, cocaine and atropine of the tropane alkaloids class, atropine and related compounds, antimalarial *Cinchona* compounds, and piperidine alkaloids of the poison hemlock.
- Of the microorganisms, ergot alkaloids and protein toxins are common and mushrooms are sources of diverse pharmaceutical agents and hallucinogenic compounds. Microbial toxins include mycotoxins and bacterial toxins and are clinically important.
- Drugs from animal sources include hormones and toxins.
- In addition to synthetic and semi-synthetic routes, recombinant DNA technology offers the generation of novel vaccines and drugs.
- Drug discovery is a long and rather expensive process. Several years are required to test drugs and develop them through a series of clinical trials. Guaranteeing the quality, efficacy, and safety of drugs is paramount to regulatory authorities as with the scientific community.

13.11 Problems

Questions 1–6: Hemiterpenes are derivatives of isoprene. Name the structures shown in Figure 13.71.

1. _____.
2. _____.
3. _____.
4. _____.
5. _____.
6. _____.

Questions 7–10. In Figure 13.72, identify the following:

7. Which compounds are monoterpenes?
8. Which compounds are sesquiterpenes?
9. Which compound represents phenolic (derived from shikimic acid) compounds?
10. Which compound is an alkaloid?

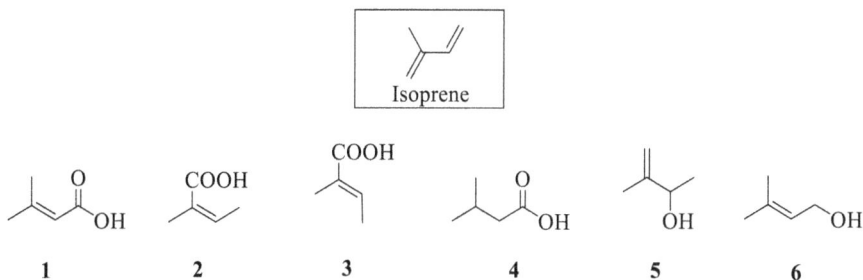

Figure 13.71 Questions 1–6.

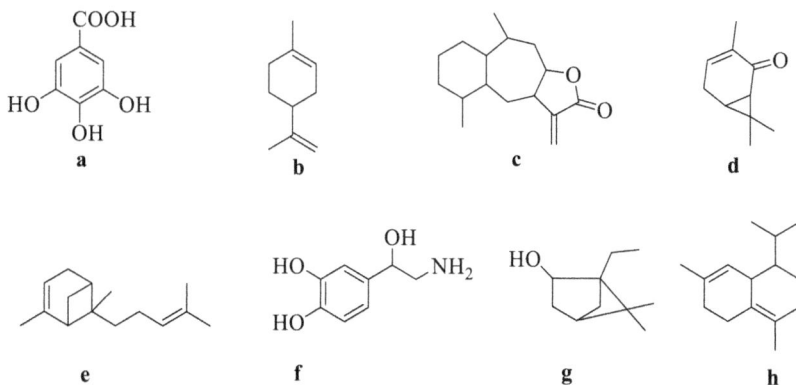

Figure 13.72 Questions 7–10 are based on structures **a–h**.

Questions 11–13. Name two important biologically active compounds in each of the following classes:

11. Sesquiterpenes.
12. Diterpenes.
13. Triterpenes.

Questions 14–19 are related to carotenoids:

14. From the biosynthesis point of view, how do we classify carotenoids?
15. Looking into the structures of α- and β-carotene (Figure 13.22), which structural group do they represent?
16. Give two examples of oxygenated carotenoids (called xanthophylls).
17. What do you think about the solubility of carotenoids?
18. What is the structural difference between lutein and zeaxanthin?
19. What is the pharmacological significance of carotenoids?

Questions 20–27 are based on Figure 13.73, which shows semi-synthetic derivatives (**a–d**) of a compound:

20. What is the reaction called in the synthesis of compound **a**?
21. What happens to the polarity of the compound by making derivative **a**?
22. What is the reaction called in the synthesis of compound **b**?

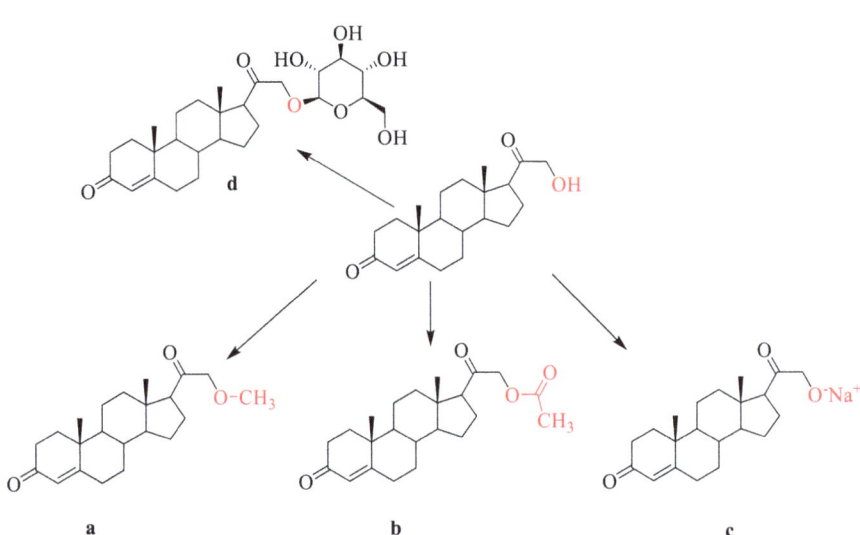

Figure 13.73 Questions 20–27.

23. What happens to the polarity of the compound by making derivative **b**?
24. What reaction do you undertake to make compound **c**?
25. What happens to the polarity of the compound by making derivative **c**?
26. What is the reaction called in the synthesis of compound **d**?
27. What happens to the polarity and solubility of the compound by making derivative **d**?
28. Heroin is a semi-synthetic product of morphine which was developed with the aim of abolishing the addictive effect of morphine. It is an acetylated product of morphine (Figure 13.49). Show this acetylation reaction and the product.

Questions 29–32: Hydrocortisone, prednisone, and dexamethasone are synthetic glucocorticoids (analogues of an adrenal steroid such as cortisone) with anti-inflammatory and immunosuppressant properties. Hydrocortisone is a short-acting drug whereas prednisone is 4–5 times more potent than hydrocortisone and has an intermediate duration of action of around 12 h. On the other hand, dexamethasone is over 25 times more potent than hydrocortisone and has a long duration of action of up to 24 h. Based on the structures shown in Figure 13.74, identify the structural groups to which these differences can be attributed:

29. In what way does hydrocortisone differ from cortisone?
30. In what way does prednisone differ from hydrocortisone?
31. In what way does dexamethasone differ from prednisone?
32. On what basis do you think they differ in their potency and duration of action?
33. Using taxol (also called paclitaxel) as an example, research how drug development is a long and expensive process.
34. Protein-based drugs have several advantages (*e.g.* higher potency and selectivity) in therapeutic applications compared with small-molecule organic drugs. What would be their limitations?
35. What are pseudoalkaloids? Give an example.

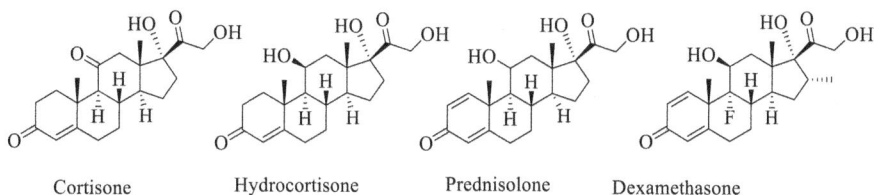

Cortisone   Hydrocortisone   Prednisolone   Dexamethasone

Figure 13.74 Questions 29–32 are based on structures of four steroids: cortisone, hydrocortisone, prednisone and dexamethasone.

36. Alkaloids belong to which functional group?
37. What range of pH values (less than or greater than 7) do you expect for alkaloids?
38. What are the two most common functional groups in aflatoxins?
39. Cannabinoids are largely lipophilic or non-polar and hence not water soluble. If you have to make a drug preparation without altering their structure (*e.g.* by salt formation), what approach do you take?
40. Vitamin E represents a group of fat-soluble compounds such as tocopherols and tocotrienols. They have alpha, beta, gamma, and delta variants. Research their biosynthesis and identify their structural variations.

13.12 Solutions to Problems

1. 3-Methylbut-2-enoic acid.
2. (*Z*)-2-Methylbut-2-enoic acid.
3. (*E*)-2-Methylbut-2-enoic acid.
4. 3-Methylbutanoic acid.
5. 3-Methylbut-3-en-2-ol.
6. 3-Methylbut-2-en-1-ol.
7. **b**, **d**, and **g**.
8. **c**, **e**, and **h**.
9. **a** and **f**.
10. **f**.
11. Sesquiterpenes – artemisinin and parthenolide.
12. Diterpenes – taxol and ginkgolides.
13. Triterpenes, choices from steroids, digitoxin, *etc.*
14. Tetraterpenes.
15. Alkenes or cycloalkenes.
16. See Figure 13.23.
17. Insoluble in water or soluble in organic solvents.
18. See Figure 13.23 – position of the double bond and stereochemistry of the hydroxyl group. Note the three chiral centres in lutein *versus* two in zeaxanthin.
19. Antioxidant, provitamin A, *etc.*
20. Methylation.
21. Became non-polar – hydrogen bonding removed.
22. Acetylation.
23. Became non-polar – hydrogen bonding removed.

24. Alcohols react with active metals such as sodium to form a sodium salt.
25. A salt is water soluble.
26. Glycosylation – addition of sugar.
27. Become more water soluble – more polar.
28. See Figure 13.75.
29. Ketone *versus* alcohol functional group.
30. Extra double bond in prednisone.
31. Fluorine incorporated in the ring system and another minor difference is the extra methyl group in dexamethasone.
32. Differences in receptor binding potency and pharmacokinetic profile such as metabolism differences.
33. See the following:

   ○ The development of this drug took around 30 years.
   ○ The crude extract of the bark of the Pacific yew, *Taxus brevifolia*, was shown to have an anticancer effect in the 1960s.
   ○ The active component was isolated in 1969 and its chemical structure was determined in 1971.
   ○ It was selected for clinical trial in 1977 and a Phase 1 trial started in 1983.
   ○ First approval as an anticancer agent came in 1992.
   ○ The entire process was a result of hard work and large amounts of money poured into the development.
   ○ The benefit for the developers – by 2000 taxol had annual sales of about US$2.1 billion per year.

34. Short circulating half-life, lack of membrane permeability, and poor oral bioavailability, potential immunogenicity, and conformational instability during storage and transportation.
35. Alkaloids that are not derived from amino acids are called pseudoalkaloids. Caffeine, theobromine, and theophylline are

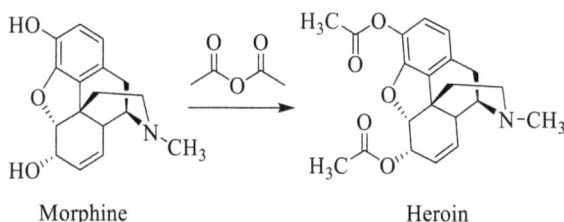

Morphine   Heroin

Figure 13.75 Answer to question 28. A simple acetylation reaction by reagents such as acetic anhydride can give diacetylmorphine or heroin.

examples of pseudoalkaloids. Some steroids or terpenoids incorporate nitrogen atoms into their structure at a later stage of their biosynthesis and are also called pseudoalkaloids.

36. Amine.
37. Basic or amine means a pH greater than 7.
38. See Figure 13.61 – ether (mostly aromatic ethers) and ketone.
39. The best way is formulation to make them compatible with aqueous media. Micro- or nano-emulsions of cannabinoids are now available for water solubility.
40. This is your project as extra reading material. Tocopherols and tocotrienols differ from each other in the number of double bonds – trien referring to three extra double bonds in tocotrienols. In both cases '-ol' refers to the alcohol or phenol structural moiety, in this case they have phenol. The alpha, beta, gamma, and delta variants are based on the position and substitution pattern of the methyl groups in the phenol ring. You should note that a terpenoid (isoprene) skeleton is in the molecule and also a phenolic moiety, suggesting a mixed biosynthesis route. You can also research on how they do their job as antioxidants – oxidation–reduction reactions.

References

1. S. Habtemariam, *Int. J. Mol. Sci.*, 2017, **19**(1), 4.
2. S. Habtemariam, *Molecules*, 2018, **23**(1), 117.

Subject Index